T0329699

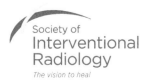

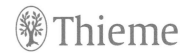

Digestive Disease Interventions

Baljendra S. Kapoor, MD, FSIR, FCIRSE
Associate Professor of Radiology
Cleveland Clinic Foundation
Cleveland, Ohio

Jonathan M. Lorenz, MD, FSIR
Professor of Radiology
Section of Interventional Radiology
The University of Chicago
Chicago, Illinois

640 illustrations

Thieme
New York • Stuttgart • Delhi • Rio de Janeiro

Executive Editor: William Lamsback
Managing Editor: J. Owen Zurhellen IV
Director, Editorial Services: Mary Jo Casey
Production Editor: Naamah Schwartz
International Production Director: Andreas Schabert
Editorial Director: Sue Hodgson
International Marketing Director: Fiona Henderson
International Sales Director: Louisa Turrell
Director of Institutional Sales: Adam Bernacki
Senior Vice President and Chief Operating Officer: Sarah Vanderbilt
President: Brian D. Scanlan

Library of Congress Cataloging-in-Publication Data

Names: Kapoor, Baljendra S., editor. | Lorenz, Jonathan, editor.
Title: Digestive disease interventions / [edited by] Baljendra S. Kapoor, Jonathan M. Lorenz.
Description: First edition. | New York : Thieme, [2018] | Includes bibliographical references and index.
Identifiers: LCCN 2017057088| ISBN 9781626233744 (hardcover : alk. paper) | ISBN 9781626233751 (ebook)
Subjects: | MESH: Digestive System Diseases–radiotherapy | Radiology, Interventional–methods
Classification: LCC RC806 | NLM WI 140 | DDC 616.3/0642–dc23
LC record available at https://lccn.loc.gov/2017057088

Thieme Publishers New York
333 Seventh Avenue, New York, NY 10001 USA
+1 800 782 3488, customerservice@thieme.com

Thieme Publishers Stuttgart
Rüdigerstrasse 14, 70469 Stuttgart, Germany
+49 [0]711 8931 421, customerservice@thieme.de

Thieme Publishers Delhi
A-12, Second Floor, Sector-2, Noida-201301
Uttar Pradesh, India
+91 120 45 566 00, customerservice@thieme.in

Thieme Publishers Rio de Janeiro, Thieme Publicações Ltda.
Edifício Rodolpho de Paoli, 25º andar
Av. Nilo Peçanha, 50   Sala 2508
Rio de Janeiro 20020-906 Brasil
+55 21 3172-2297 / +55 21 3172-1896

Cover design: Thieme Publishing Group
Typesetting by Thomson Digital, India

Printed in The United States of America by
King Printing Company, Inc.   5 4 3 2 1

ISBN 978-1-62623-374-4

Also available as an e-book:
eISBN 978-1-62623-375-1

Important note: Medicine is an ever-changing science undergoing continual development. Research and clinical experience are continually expanding our knowledge, in particular our knowledge of proper treatment and drug therapy. Insofar as this book mentions any dosage or application, readers may rest assured that the authors, editors, and publishers have made every effort to ensure that such references are in accordance with **the state of knowledge at the time of production of the book**.

Nevertheless, this does not involve, imply, or express any guarantee or responsibility on the part of the publishers in respect to any dosage instructions and forms of applications stated in the book. **Every user is requested to examine carefully** the manufacturers' leaflets accompanying each drug and to check, if necessary in consultation with a physician or specialist, whether the dosage schedules mentioned therein or the contraindications stated by the manufacturers differ from the statements made in the present book. Such examination is particularly important with drugs that are either rarely used or have been newly released on the market. Every dosage schedule or every form of application used is entirely at the user's own risk and responsibility. The authors and publishers request every user to report to the publishers any discrepancies or inaccuracies noticed. If errors in this work are found after publication, errata will be posted at www.thieme.com on the product description page.

Some of the product names, patents, and registered designs referred to in this book are in fact registered trademarks or proprietary names even though specific reference to this fact is not always made in the text. Therefore, the appearance of a name without designation as proprietary is not to be construed as a representation by the publisher that it is in the public domain.

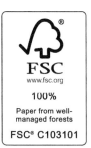

FSC
www.fsc.org
100%
Paper from well-managed forests
FSC® C103101

Dedicated to my teacher, David Hunter, MD, Professor Emeritus at the University of Minnesota, for constantly inspiring me, and to my wife Simar and my son Vij, for their enormous patience, love, and support during this project.

– BSK

Dedicated to my wife, Cynthia, and my kids, Anna and Matthew, life's greatest gifts. And to my co-editor, Baljendra S. Kapoor, who created the annual meeting of Digestive Disease Interventions as well as this textbook and continues to inspire his family of colleagues across the country with his selfless friendship, guidance and leadership.

– JML

Contents

Preface

Inspiration for this book originated from the expertise and enthusiasm we have witnessed by colleagues and participants of the annual Digestive Diseases Interventions meeting, organized by the American Society of Digestive Disease Interventions and endorsed by the Society of Interventional Radiology. This unique meeting travels the country and brings together an internationally renowned, multidisciplinary group of experts in the management of gastrointestinal disorders. This annual exchange of knowledge and technical expertise between interventional radiologists and their multidisciplinary colleagues has been a remarkable example of friendship and cooperation with the common goal of improving the care of our patients with gastrointestinal disorders. We are forever indebted to those experts for the generous time and effort they have contributed to these pages.

As our understanding of gastrointestinal disorders advances, so too does the evolution of cutting-edge, minimally invasive therapies that minimize morbidity, maximize patient comfort and improve clinical outcomes over prior options. Interventional radiology has evolved from a procedure-based subspecialty of radiology to a patient-based, clinical specialty that works in concert with experts in internal medicine, gastroenterology, oncology and surgery to perform direct, state-of-the-art clinical management. As a result, interventional radiologists are integral to the management of patients with a wide range of gastrointestinal disorders and often provide the critical or sole therapeutic option. This textbook is a comprehensive compilation of 30 chapters that review the multidisciplinary management of gastrointestinal disorders with an emphasis on management options offered by interventional radiologists. As such, the target audience is primarily practitioners, fellows and residents in the field of interventional radiology, but these pages are a valuable resource for our friends and colleagues in medical and surgical subspecialties that manage gastrointestinal disorders.

Baljendra S. Kapoor, MD, FSIR, FCIRSE
Jonathan M. Lorenz, MD, FSIR

Acknowledgments

We owe a debt of gratitude to Megan Griffiths, editorial assistant, Imaging Institute of the Cleveland Clinic. Without her technical and editorial expertise, this book would not exist. We would also like to thank William Lamsback and J. Owen Zurhellen at Thieme Publishers for their expertise, encouragement, and support.

Contributors

Rachel Abou Mrad, MD
Advocate Christ Medical Center
Oak Lawn, Illinois

Olaguoke (Goke) Akinwande, MD
Assistant Professor of Radiology
Division of Interventional Radiology
Mallinckrodt Institute of Radiology
Washington University School of Medicine
Saint Louis, Missouri

Ashley Altman, MD
The University of Chicago
Chicago, Illinois

Ronald S. Arellano, MD, FACR, FSIR
Associate Professor of Radiology
Division of Interventional Radiology
Massachusetts General Hospital
Harvard Medical School
Boston, Massachusetts

Federico N. Aucejo, MD
Associate Professor of Surgery
Director, Liver Cancer Program
Surgical Director, Liver Tumor Clinic
Co-Director, Liver Tumor Center of Excellence
Cleveland Clinic Lerner School of Medicine
Digestive Disease and Surgery Institute
Cleveland Clinic Foundation
Cleveland, Ohio

Christopher R. Bailey, MD
Radiology Resident
Russell H. Morgan Department of Radiology and
  Radiological Science
The Johns Hopkins Hospital
Baltimore, Maryland

David H. Ballard, MD
Mallinckrodt Institute of Radiology
Washington University School of Medicine
St. Louis, Missouri

Richard A. Baum, MD, MPA, MBA
Associate professor of Radiology
Section of Interventional Radiology
Brigham and Women's Hospital/Harvard Medical School
Boston, Massachusetts

Stanley Baum, MD, FSIR
Eugene P. Pendergrass Emeritus Professor of Radiology
Emeritus Chairman, Department of Radiology
University of Pennsylvania Perelman School of Medicine
Philadelphia, Pennsylvania

Kristi Bogan Oatis, MD, DABR
Assistant Professor
University of Texas Southwestern Medical Center
Children's Health Dallas
Dallas, Texas

Murthy R. Chamarthy, MD
Assistant Professor of Radiology
Division of Vascular and Interventional Radiology
University of Texas Southwestern Medical Center
Dallas, Texas

Christopher P. Coppa, MD
Assistant Professor of Radiology
Section of Abdominal Imaging
Cleveland Clinic Foundation
Cleveland, Ohio

Horacio R. V. D'Agostino, MD, FACR, FSIR
Professor of Radiology, Surgery, and Anesthesiology
Chairman, Department of Radiology
LSU Health Sciences Center Shreveport
Louisiana State University
Shreveport, Louisiana

Jon C. Davidson, MD
Assistant Professor
Fellowship Director
Department of Interventional Radiology
University Hospitals Cleveland Medical Center
Cleveland, Ohio

Miguel A. De Gregorio, MD, PhD, EBIR, FCIRSE, FSIR
Full Professor and Chairman of Interventional Radiology
Catedrático de Universidad Zaragoza
Hospita Clinico Universitario Zaragoza
IP (GITMI) Minimally Invasive Techniques Research Group
Government of Aragon
Zaragoza, Spain

Anthony M. Esparaz, MD
Chief Resident
Department of Radiology
Beth Israel Deaconess Medical Center
Harvard Medical School
Boston, Massachusetts

Nicholas Fidelman, MD
Associate Professor
Radiology and Biomedical Imaging
University of California San Francisco
San Francisco, California

Elliot K. Fishman, MD
Professor of Radiology, Surgery, Oncology, and Urology
Director, Diagnostic Imaging and Body CT
The Johns Hopkins Hospital
Baltimore, Maryland

Brian Funaki, MD, FSIR, FAHA, FCIRSE
Professor and Chief, Vascular and Interventional Radiology
University of Chicago Medicine
Chicago, Illinois

Terence P. F. Gade, MD, PhD
Assistant Professor of Radiology and Cancer Biology
Division of Interventional Radiology
University of Pennsylvania Perelman School of Medicine
Philadelphia, Pennsylvania

Suvranu "Shoey" Ganguli, MD, FSIR
Co-Director, Center for Image Guided Cancer Therapy
Associate Chief, Interventional Radiology
Massachusetts General Hospital
Assistant Professor of Radiology
Harvard Medical School
Boston, Massachusetts

Daniel B. Gans, MD
University of Virginia
Charlottesville, Virginia

Elizabeth Anne Hevert, MD
University of Miami
Miami, Florida

Kelvin Hong, MD
Associate Professor of Radiology
Division of Interventional Radiology
Johns Hopkins University
Baltimore, Maryland

Guy E. Johnson, MD, PharmD
Assistant Professor of Radiology
Section of Interventional Radiology
University of Washington
Seattle, Washington

Paul A. Jordan, MD, FRCPC, FACG
Chief of Section, Gastroenterology
Louisiana State University Health
Shreveport, Louisiana

Shellie C. Josephs, MD, FSIR
Associate Professor of Radiology
Section of Pediatric Interventional Radiology
The University of Texas Southwestern Medical Center
Dallas, Texas

Sanjeeva P. Kalva, MD, FSIR
Associate Professor of Radiology
Chief, Interventional Radiology Division
University of Texas Southwestern Medical Center
Dallas, Texas

Lisa Kang, MD
Assistant Professor of Radiology
Section of Pediatric Interventional Radiology
University of Texas Southwestern/Children's Health
Dallas, Texas

Baljendra S. Kapoor, MD, FSIR, FCIRSE
Associate Professor of Radiology
Cleveland Clinic Foundation
Cleveland, Ohio

Charles Y. Kim, MD, FSIR
Division Chief, Interventional Radiology
Associate Professor of Radiology
Duke University Medical Center
Durham, North Carolina

Hyun S. Kim, MD, FSIR
Professor of Radiology and Medicine (Medical Oncology)
Yale Cancer Center
Yale School of Medicine
New Haven, Connecticut

Stephen R. Lee, MD
Radiology Partners–Singleton
Houston, Texas

Robert J. Lewandowski, MD, FSIR
Professor of Radiology, Medicine, and Surgery
Director of Interventional Oncology
Northwestern University Feinberg School of Medicine
Chicago, Illinois

David Li, MD, PhD
Assistant Professor, Interventional Radiology
Department of Radiology
Weill Cornell Medical Center
New York, New York

R. Peter Lokken, MD, MPH
Assistant Professor of Radiology
Section of Interventional Radiology
University of Illinois Health
Chicago, Illinois

Jonathan M. Lorenz, MD, FSIR
Professor of Radiology
Section of Interventional Radiology
The University of Chicago
Chicago, Illinois

David C. Madoff, MD, FSIR, FACR
Professor of Radiology
Vice Chairman for Academic Affairs
Department of Radiology
Division of Interventional Radiology
Weill Cornell Medicine
New York, New York

Antonio Mainar, MD
Hospital Clinico Universitaro Zaragoza Lozano Blesa
Zaragoza, Spain

Kenneth Manas, MD
Louisiana State University Health
Shreveport, Louisiana

Aladin T. Mariano, MD
Clinical Fellow
Section of Body Imaging
Stanford University Medical Center
Stanford, California

Louis G. Martin, MD, FSIR, FACR
Professor of Radiology
Vascular and Interventional Radiology Section
Emory University School of Medicine
Atlanta, Georgia

K. V. Narayanan Menon, MD, FRCP, FAASLD
Medical Director of Liver Transplantation
Gastroenterology and Hepatology
Cleveland Clinic
Cleveland, Ohio

Christopher A. Molvar, MD
Associate Professor of Radiology
Section of Vascular and Interventional Radiology
Loyola University Medical Center
Maywood, Illinois

Eric J. Monroe, MD
Assistant Professor of Radiology
Section of Interventional Radiology
University of Washington
Seattle, Washington

Eunice Moon, MD
Staff Physician
Department of Vascular and Interventional Radiology
Cleveland Clinic Foundation
Cleveland, Ohio

Peter R. Mueller, MD
Division Head, Interventional Radiology
Massachusetts General Hospital
Professor of Radiology
Harvard Medical School

Arvind R. Murali, MD
Assistant Professor, Internal Medicine
Division of Gastroenterology and Hepatology
University of Iowa
Iowa City, Iowa

Gregory J. Nadolski, MD
Assistant Professor of Radiology
Division of Interventional Radiology
University of Pennsylvania Perelman School of Medicine
Philadelphia, Pennsylvania

Govindarajan Narayanan, MD
Chairman and Professor
Department of Interventional Radiology
University of Miami Miller School of Medicine
Miami, Florida

Robert O'Shea, MD, MSCE
Staff
Department of Gastroenterology and Hepatology
Cleveland Clinic
Cleveland, Ohio

Siddharth A. Padia, MD
Associate Professor of Interventional Radiology
David Geffen School of Medicine
University of California Los Angeles
Los Angeles, California

Indravadan J. Patel, MD
Assistant Professor
Case Western Reserve University School of Medicine
Section Chief, Interventional Radiology
University Hospitals Health System
Cleveland, Ohio

Mikin V. Patel, MD, MBA
Department of Radiology
University of Chicago Medical Center
Chicago, Illinois

Rex M. Pillai, MD
Professor of Radiology
Interventional Radiology
University of California, Davis
Sacramento, California

Siva P. Raman, MD
Bay Imaging Consultants
Walnut Creek, California

Charles E. Ray Jr., MD, PhD
Professor of Radiology
Acting Dean
University of Illinois College of Medicine
Chicago, Illinois

Mark J. Sands, MD, MBA, FACR
Vice Chairman of Clinical Operations and Quality
Section Head, Interventional Radiology
Imaging Institute
Cleveland Clinic Foundation
Cleveland, Ohio

David S. Shin, MD
Assistant Professor
Department of Radiology
University of Washington
Seattle, Washington

Ashraf Thabet, MD
Associate Chief
Division of Interventional Radiology
Massachusetts General Hospital
Boston, Massachusetts

Raul N. Uppot, MD
Assistant Professor of Radiology
Division of Interventional Radiology
Massachusetts General Hospital
Harvard Medical School
Boston, Massachusetts

Karim Valji, MD
Professor of Radiology
Chief of Interventional Radiology
University of Washington
Seattle, Washington

Shree Ramanan Venkat, MD
Assistant Professor of Clinical Interventional Radiology
University of Miami Miller School of Medicine
Miami, Florida

1 Intraprocedural Imaging and Navigational Tools in Digestive Disease Interventions

Stephen R. Lee, Raul N. Uppot, and Suvranu "Shoey" Ganguli

1.1 Introduction

Since its birth in 1964, the specialty of interventional radiology has relied on a variety of advanced imaging techniques to successfully perform minimally invasive procedures. Many of the advances and successes garnered by the specialty would not be possible without technological advancements, which have assisted interventional radiologists in detecting and visualizing pathology. Furthermore, the ability to perform a procedure in the least invasive fashion is predicated on the interventionalist's ability to track interventional tools accurately. In this chapter, we discuss recent advances in intraprocedural imaging and navigational tools in practice. These advances include cone-beam computed tomography (CBCT), one of the newer imaging technologies which gives the interventionalist the ability to take advantage of spatial information provided by conventional CT in a standard fluoroscopy suite. Current navigational tools in development and practice, including trajectory guidance, image fusion, and body global positioning systems, will also be discussed.

1.2 Cone-Beam CT

1.2.1 Background

With increasing complexity of current vascular interventions, interventionalists not only rely on vascular anatomy, but also require information about the surrounding soft tissues. CBCT allows for visualization of structures in a standard two-dimensional (2D) planar view and also gives the operator the ability to acquire cross-sectional CT-like images intraprocedurally in a relatively seamless fashion.

Although CBCT has only been implemented into clinical practice within the past decade, its development began in the 1980s. Feldkamp and colleagues were among the first to describe an algorithm to integrate 2D projectional image sets to create a 3D dataset. The method they described was based on a convolution back-projection formula, which was computationally less intensive and faster than iterative methods proposed earlier.[1] However, in spite of this early computational advance, early implementations of CBCT suffered from poor spatial and contrast resolution due to the limitations of image-intensifier systems and charge-coupled devices.

It was in the early 2000s that the clinical utility of CBCT again began to be investigated. With the development of flat panel detectors (FPDs), several advantages of this new technology could be translated to CBCT. FPDs were markedly more compact than image-intensifier systems. Because CBCT relies on acquisition of a series of X-ray projection images about a center of rotation covering at least a 200-degree angular range, having a smaller and lighter detector provided a mechanical advantage over image intensifier–based systems.

The larger area of the FPDs also translated into a larger volume that could be imaged. Modern detectors typically cover an area of 19×25 cm to 30×40 cm, which translates to a reconstructed volume of $25 \times 25 \times 19$ cm to $30 \times 30 \times 40$ cm.

Finally, imaging performance attributes of FPDs seemed well suited for CBCT. Unlike image-intensifier systems, FPDs were not affected by geometric distortion and veiling glare, the effects of which would be exaggerated upon integration of 2D planar images into a 3D dataset. Because CBCT relies on reconstruction of linear attenuation coefficients in a similar fashion to CT, the excellent CT number linearity of FPDs provided accurate density measurements on the reconstructed datasets. The high detective quantum efficiency, high frame rate, and dynamic range also contributed to improved image quality over previous systems.[2]

1.2.2 Equipment, Technical Factors, and Radiation Dose

There are three CBCT systems commercially available in the United States: DynaCT (Siemens Medical Solutions, Forchheim, Germany), XperCT (Phillips Medical Systems, Eindhoven, the Netherlands), and Innova CT (GE Healthcare, Waukesha, WI). All three systems have the ability to obtain varying numbers of projections, typically between 200 and 600, within 5 to 20 seconds at varying tube currents, depending on the protocol used. A typical abdominal imaging protocol consists of around 300 projections, 5- to 10-ms pulses per projection at 120 kVp over a 200-degree arc. It is important to note that imaging speed is ultimately limited by intrinsic physical properties of the CsI scintillator, which suffers from some degree of lag.[3] This sets the lower limit of imaging time at around 3 seconds. In any case, shorter imaging times are likely not desirable for most applications as current speeds are within normal thresholds for patient breath-holds. Furthermore, the faster C-arm rotational speeds required for faster imaging increase the potential for mechanical patient injury.

Although initially a major limitation in clinical use, the time required for volumetric reconstruction and postprocessing has fallen dramatically over the past few years. Current systems are capable of delivering full-resolution images in less than 15 seconds after acquisition. In most modern clinical implementations of CBCT systems, images are reviewed on a separate 3D workstation in the control room, but increasingly, vendors are engineering systems for in-room manipulation of images with a sterile input device or touch screen. Because a 3D dataset is generated, standard axial, sagittal, and coronal reformations are possible, as well as 3D renderings. Most recently, additional postprocessing algorithms integrated into clinical practice offer the ability to correct for photon starvation or metallic artifacts.

In spite of the continuing advances in CBCT technology, which decrease image acquisition time, one of the remaining

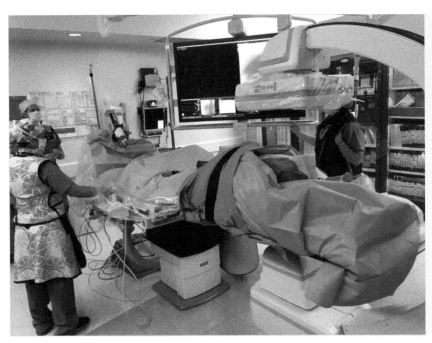

Fig. 1.1 All obstructing lines and equipment must be secured prior to acquisition of CBCT. This transition typically takes 5 to 10 minutes depending on the familiarity of the interventional radiology team with CBCT.

factors precluding its seamless integration into clinical workflow is the setup time required to transition from 2D projectional imaging to 3D cross-sectional acquisition.[4] In our own clinical practice, this transition typically takes at least 5 to 10 minutes, depending on the familiarity of the operator, technologist, and nursing staff with CBCT (▶ Fig. 1.1). During this time, any obstructing equipment—lead shields, intravenous lines, arm boards, anesthesia equipment—must be cleared from the path of the C-arm. For larger patients, their arms may need to be repositioned above their heads to decrease their overall transverse dimension to allow passage of the C-arm; this also notably improves image quality with decreased beam hardening artifacts through the abdomen. Patients must also be positioned to ensure that the area of interest is included in the acquired image set. Lateral and anteroposterior projections are used to ensure the targeted areas are included in both the transverse and craniocaudal dimensions. A final test rotation of the C-arm must also be performed to ensure that no obstructions are present in the path of the C-arm.

1.2.3 Applications of Cone-Beam CT and Navigation

Vascular Intervention

Hepatic Arterial Intervention

One of the most common uses of CBCT in vascular body interventions today is in the setting of hepatic arterial interventions performed for hepatocellular carcinoma (HCC) and metastases. CBCT assists interventionalists in overcoming two of the potential challenges in hepatic arterial interventions: lesion visibility and lesion targeting.

Treatment algorithms of HCC and metastases rely on cross-sectional imaging (CT or magnetic resonance imaging [MRI]) to identify and characterize potential lesions. The ability of interventionalists to treat lesions of concern is predicated on lesion

visibility intraprocedurally. With only digital subtraction angiography (DSA) imaging, interventionalists must heavily rely on the arterial phase of image acquisition to both identify the lesions of concern and determine the best approach to treatment with regard to the degree of vessel subselection and appropriate catheter/wire selection. CBCT affords the operator the ability to acquire cross-sectional images such that direct comparison to preprocedure imaging is possible (▶ Fig. 1.2).

As shown by Miyayama and colleagues, sensitivity for detection of small HCCs during chemoembolization is equivalent to contrast-enhanced MRI when dual-phase (hepatic arterial and arterioportal phases) CBCT is employed.[5] In their series of 68 tumors, nonselective DSA also failed to detect 19 tumors seen on preprocedure CT or MRI. Eight of the 68 tumors treated were also not seen on preprocedure imaging, apparent only on intraprocedural CBCT. The added value of dual-phase imaging appears to be an important future direction (▶ Fig. 1.3). In an earlier study of 82 tumors, Loffroy and colleagues showed the utility of dual-phase CBCT. Sensitivities of arterial and venous phases alone for detection of HCC were 71.9 and 86.6%, respectively. Overall sensitivity when both arterial and venous phases were evaluated improved to 93.9%. Notably, of 23 tumors that were not identified on arterial phase, 17 were detected on venous phase.[6] See ▶ Table 1.1 for a standard CBCT dual-phase imaging protocol.

A second challenge frequently encountered by interventionalists during hepatic arterial interventions is difficulty in confidently defining the arterial anatomy in regard to both the tumor-feeding branches and nearby nontarget extrahepatic arteries. Recognition of variant arterial anatomy supplying the small bowel, stomach, diaphragm, and skin is requisite for safely performing hepatic arterial chemoembolization and radioembolization. Failure to recognize these variants can result in nontarget embolization to these structures.[7] CBCT is a useful tool to identify vessels not initially apparent on DSA. CBCT also allows the operator to clearly identify the origins and supplies of indeterminate vascular structures, obviating the need for multiple

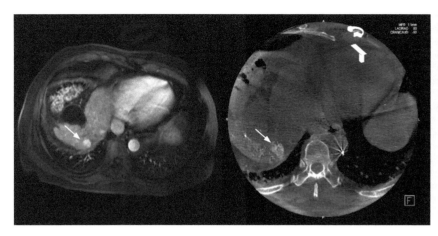

Fig. 1.2 Contrast-enhanced MRI shows an enhancing HCC in segment 7 of the liver (*white arrow*). Intraprocedural CBCT obtained after selection of the presumed feeding vessel supplying the targeted HCC confirms appropriate microcatheter position to minimize nontarget embolization.

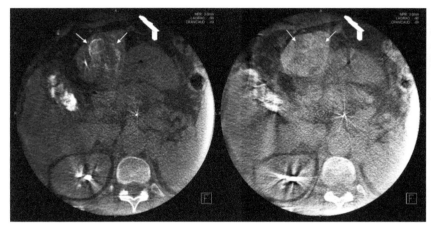

Fig. 1.3 Dual-phase CBCT performed during transcatheter arterial chemoembolization of a left hepatic lobe HCC. Arterial phase CBCT demonstrates heterogeneous enhancement of the lesion of interest (*white arrows*). Delayed phase CBCT demonstrates that the lesion of interest becomes hypodense to background liver parenchyma (*white arrows*).

vessel subselections and DSAs from various projections to confirm that intervention may be performed without risk of nontarget embolization.[4]

In addition to identifying potential nontarget vessels, CBCT has also been shown to be useful in assisting the operator in identifying the tumor-feeding branch(es) (▶ Fig. 1.4). Currently, there are two systems that can detect the tumor-feeding branch(es) and guide microcatheter positioning (Flight Plan for Liver, GE Healthcare, Chalfont St Gilles, England or EmboGuide, Philips Healthcare, Best, the Netherlands). After acquisition of a CBCT volume, 3D segmentation of the lesion of interest is performed. The system then analyzes the lesion of interest and identifies and annotates potential feeding vessels. The potential vessels are then projected as an overlay and the roadmap is registered to the live view. The roadmap will make adjustments according to C-arm angulation, table translation, and magnification changes. The clinical utility of this system has been verified. In a study of 68 tumors, 81 of 100 tumor-feeding branches could be identified using the detection software in conjunction with CBCT. When nonselective DSA was used alone, only 38 of the 100 branches could be identified. There were also 27 false-positive branches when only nonselective DSA was used.[5]

Portal Vein Intervention

Portal Vein Embolization

CBCT may be used to delineate portal venous anatomy during portal vein embolization procedures. Although portal venous variant anatomy is present in only 10 to 15% of patients, nontarget embolization of portal vein branches can affect the potential

Table 1.1 CBCT systems and specifications available in the United States

Vendor	Commercial name	External detector size and maximum FOV (cm)	Matrix size	Voxel size (mm)	Frame rate (fps)	Maximum number of projections	Gantry angular velocity (degrees/s)	Gantry angular range (degrees)
Phillips	Allura Xper FD20	42 × 50 30 × 40	2,560 × 2,048	0.35	12	310 (30 fps) 620 (60 fps)	25–55	200
GE	Innova 3D	41 × 41	512 × 512	0.4	30	600	Up to 40	222
Siemens	Syngo Dyna CT	30 × 40	1,920 × 2,480	0.3	60	Protocol dependent (maximum 1 image/degree)	Up to 60 (90 for multiaxis solution)	200 (400 for multiaxis solution)

Abbreviation: FOV, field of view.

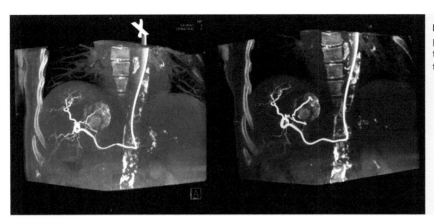

Fig. 1.4 Use of 3D maximum intensity projections assists the operator in identifying the tumor feeding branches during transradial transcatheter arterial chemoembolization.

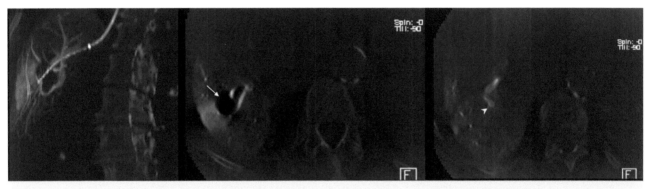

Fig. 1.5 Cone-beam CT obtained during TIPS procedure. 3D reformation of the TIPS sheath during balloon occlusion portogram. The air-filled structure in the right hepatic vein represents the Fogarty balloon catheter (*white arrowhead*). The wedged portogram shows parenchymal staining with reflux into a branch of the portal vein (*white arrow*). Adequate right portal and right hepatic branches are identified for TIPS creation.

success of future liver resection.[8] Furthermore, in the setting of anticipated extended left or right hepatectomies, CBCT allows for clear visualization of segment IV branches. Portal venous anatomy can be visualized with 30% dilute contrast injected at a rate of 3 mL/s with an imaging delay of 4 seconds for main portal vein injection and a delay of 2 seconds for left portal vein injections.[4]

Transjugular Intrahepatic Portosystemic Shunts

One of the most challenging aspects of transjugular intrahepatic portosystemic shunt (TIPS) creation is the transhepatic puncture into the portal vein. The standard approach for portal vein puncture guidance is to perform a wedged CO_2 portogram after catheterization of the right hepatic vein. The operator must rely on 2D imaging, oftentimes in more than one obliquity, to determine the location and course of the right portal vein with respect to the chosen transvenous puncture site. Multiple "blind" punctures may be required to access the portal vein, some of which may be inadvertently extracapsular or into an extrahepatic portion of the portal vein.

CBCT has the potential to provide guidance in this portion of the procedure. Wallace and colleagues described a technique in which a wedged CO_2 portogram is performed from the transjugular hepatic vein access during CBCT acquisition.[4] Two 60-mL syringes with CO_2 are connected to the balloon occlusion catheter via injection tubing and a three-way stopcock. The operator stands behind lead shields while CBCT images are acquired and manually injects the CO_2 without an imaging delay. An 8-second image acquisition protocol is used. Images

can be reviewed on a 3D workstation, giving the operator a thorough understanding of right portal vein course and position. Distance to the liver capsule from the chosen puncture site as well as the location of the extrahepatic portion of the portal vein can also be assessed (▶ Fig. 1.5).

An image overlay can be created over the live fluoroscopic image for real-time guidance. It should be noted that misregistration artifacts are more significant during TIPS procedures than other liver-directed therapies, due to distortion of hepatic position and rotation upon introduction of the TIPS cannula. This effect may be obviated by positioning the TIPS cannula alongside the balloon occlusion catheter prior to obtaining the portogram.

Use of CBCT during TIPS formation has yet to gain widespread use, likely due to challenges in patient positioning and room setup with the transjugular approach. However, this technique is a potential problem-solving tool when performing TIPS, particularly in nonroutine cases. Sze and colleagues describe a case in which a TIPS was created in a patient with distorted liver anatomy due to polycystic liver disease and recurrent ascites. CBCT assisted in guiding portal vein puncture, a feat that would have been difficult to achieve under 2D fluoroscopic guidance, as the tract length between the hepatic and portal vein branch measured greater than 9 cm.[9] Luo and colleagues[10] described CBCT's utility in evaluating the portal vein entry site and shunt course after transhepatic portal venous access was achieved. In a series of 21 patients, seven portal vein entries were identified as inappropriate based on CBCT images. In these patients, TIPS creation from an extrahepatic puncture site or a tortuous course predisposing to stent kinking was prevented.

Thermal Ablation

Although typically performed under CT or ultrasound guidance, percutaneous ablation procedures can also be performed with the use of CBCT. Navigation systems integrated into the CBCT workflow can assist operators in precise probe placement. Abi-Jaoudeh and colleagues described their experience using CBCT to treat a variety of tumors including six HCCs and five renal cell carcinomas. In their series of 29 treated lesions, all procedures except for one were successful. Image fusion was used for 16 lesions, three of which were visible only on positron emission tomography (PET) or MRI.[11]

One potential advantage of CBCT over conventional CT guidance is the lower radiation dose associated with CBCT. Braak and colleagues compared effective dose in 92 CBCT-guided procedures with that in 137 conventional CT-guided procedures. They found a significant dose savings in the CBCT group. For upper abdominal procedures, the average effective dose was 16.1 mSv versus 20.4 mSv for the CBCT and conventional CT groups, respectively. For lower abdominal procedures, the average effective dose was 13.4 mSv versus 15.4 mSv for the CBCT and conventional CT groups, respectively.[12]

One of the technical challenges of performing ablations is ensuring adequate treatment zones. Unlike ultrasound, CBCT provides the advantage of being able to monitor both the progress and adequacy of the ablation zone during and immediately after the procedure. Intraprocedural monitoring is of particular importance when ablations are performed near structures that should be spared during ablation (e.g., central biliary ducts in liver ablation, ureter in renal ablation). CBCT has also been shown to be equivalent to traditional multidetector computed tomography (MDCT) in accessing insufficient ablation margins. In a series of 43 ablation zones, Iwazawa and colleagues report no significant difference between CBCT and MDCT in detection of insufficient margins. CBCT had a sensitivity of 90.0%, specificity of 96.4%, positive predictive value of 94.7%, and negative predictive value of 93.1%, similar to MDCT.[13]

Although ablation procedures will likely continue to be performed primarily under ultrasound and CT guidance, use of CBCT has been shown to be at least equally effective and safe as these traditional cross-sectional modalities. Use of CBCT may be a good alternative for today's busy interventional practice, especially depending on the practice setup and availability of a CT interventional suite.

Biliary

Use of CBCT in complex biliary procedures has been described.[4,14] Conventional biliary procedures rely on 2D imaging in various projections to define the biliary anatomy. This is often a challenging task, especially in the postoperative patient. In our own practice, CBCT has been used to guide biliary interventions in patients who have surgically formed bilioenteric anastomoses.

Gastrointestinal Interventions

Percutaneous gastrostomy catheters are traditionally placed using fluoroscopic guidance. In most circumstances, successful and safe placement can be achieved by insufflating the stomach with air and identifying the surrounding liver and colon with ultrasound and rectal contrast prior to the procedure. However, safe placement may not always be achievable with fluoroscopic imaging, particularly in patients who have had prior gastric surgery. In these situations, CT imaging has been found to be useful to precisely guide gastric access needle placement. However, after gastric access is achieved in the CT interventional suite, interventionalists often find it difficult to work with the wire and perform the necessary dilator and catheter exchanges without live fluoroscopic imaging. CBCT offers interventionalists the ability to take advantage of the strengths of both fluoroscopic and CT imaging. Precise gastric access can be achieved with CBCT and the remainder of the procedure may be performed with standard 2D fluoroscopic imaging. Möhlenbruch and colleagues described their experience with CBCT for placing gastrostomy tubes in 18 patients. They achieved technical success in all patients with no major complications.[15]

Biopsy

Biopsies can be performed using CBCT. A major advantage of CBCT over conventional CT is the ease with which double-angulation of the needle can be performed. Although the gantry can be angled in conventional CT-guided procedures to allow the needle to remain in-plane with the images acquired, the degree of angulation is frequently limited by the size of the gantry opening as well as the size of the patient. Angulation up to 50 degrees is possible with CBCT because of C-arm geometry, allowing the operator to perform double-angulation approaches with relative ease.[16]

Use of CBCT to guide percutaneous biopsy has been shown to be safe and effective. In a series of 41 patients, Braak and colleagues used CBCT-guided biopsy of renal masses. Only two nondiagnostic biopsy specimens were obtained, with the remainder of the biopsies matching the pathology obtained after surgical resection.[16] No major complications were reported in this series of patients.

The effective radiation doses between CBCT-guided and conventional CT-guided biopsies have also been compared. Using adult and pediatric phantoms, Ben-Shlomo and colleagues showed that use of conventional CT in biopsy procedures resulted in significantly higher effective doses. The average effective adult dose for the CBCT-guided procedures was 1.63 mSv versus 8.22 mSv for conventional CT-guided procedures. The average effective pediatric dose for the CBCT-guided procedures was 0.36 mSv versus 2.13 mSv for conventional CT-guided procedures.[17]

1.3 Navigational Tools

Navigational guidance tools integrate novel technologies into traditional imaging modality setups to help interventional radiologists perform image-guided procedures with greater efficiency, safety, and confidence. These tools broadly fall into three categories: trajectory guidance, image fusion, and body global positioning systems.

1.3.1 Trajectory Guidance

Trajectory guidance tools assist interventional radiologists in determining the correct skin entrance site, angle, and depth to

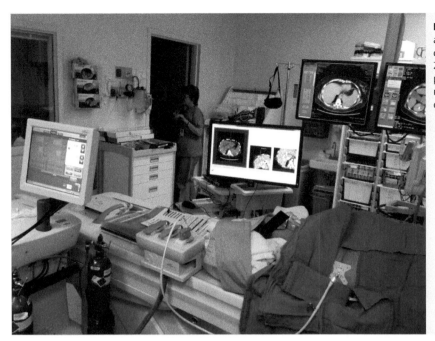

Fig. 1.6 Optical navigation used in a liver ablation. The ActiViews CT navigation system disposable camera mounts to any 11- to 20-gauge needle. Using a fiducial placed on the patient's screen, the system gives 3D information regarding needle trajectory and depth, projected on to the patient's planning CT.

a target during an image-guided procedure performed with a needle. Modern trajectory guidance tools include laser navigational systems, optical tracking systems, and CBCT-assisted navigation.

Laser Navigation Systems

Laser navigation systems (LNS) are used in conjunction with CT scanners to assist interventional radiologists in determining the appropriate skin entrance site and angle of entry during CT-guided procedures, most commonly biopsies or drainage procedures. The LNS amedo-LNSTM (amedo STS GmbH, Bochum, Germany) is one such system that can be installed in a CT interventional suite. The system consists of a laser mounted onto a mobile 220-degree rail positioned parallel to the CT gantry. After acquisition of a planning CT, the Digital Imaging and Communications in Medicine (DICOM) dataset is sent to a steering unit for intervention planning. The appropriate entry site and angle are determined and the information is transferred to the laser unit, which projects a laser beam on to the patient's skin surface. Angular information is conveyed to the operator because the laser pinpoint must be maintained on the hub of the needle for the trajectory to be correct.

This system has been compared to traditional methods in biopsy and drainage procedures. Gruber-Rouh and colleagues found that when compared to conventional techniques, use of LNS results in lower patient dose and shorter procedure time. In their study of 58 patients, mean procedure time for the LNS group versus the control group was 20.25 minutes versus 28 minutes. Mean dose length product in the LNS group versus the control group was 42.3 mGy-cm versus 59.7 mGy-cm.[18]

Optical Tracking Systems

Optical tracking systems use a camera to aid trajectory guidance. Three components are necessary for this system: (1) a fiducial placed on the patient's skin, typically with radio-opaque reference markers that can be visualized in the CT dataset,

(2) a single-use miniature camera attached to the biopsy needle, and (3) a computer workstation with tracking software. After planning images are acquired, the fiducial patch with adhesive is placed on the selected entry point on the patient's skin. A CT scan is then performed, and the images are sent to the computer workstation. This allows the acquired dataset to be referenced to the live view acquired by the miniature camera using reference markers on the fiducial patch (▶ Fig. 1.6). The tracking software then superimposes a simulated needle position on the acquired CT images, allowing the operator to align the needle to the correct trajectory.

Schubert and colleagues reported their use of an optical tracking system in 16 CT-guided procedures, 14 of which were performed successfully. Two technical failures during biopsy procedures resulted from pain-related patient movement and hypermobility of subcutaneous tissues, resulting in misregistration between the fiducial patch applied to the skin and the 3D dataset. When compared to the control group of nonnavigated procedures, the study group had a significantly longer procedure time (72.4 vs. 46.8 minutes). However, the authors noted that the optical tracking system was used only for more difficult procedures and a significantly higher proportion of cases were performed with an out-of-plane approach.[19]

1.3.2 Image Fusion

Image fusion is a process by which images from different modalities are co-registered to create an imaging overlay. This technique has allowed more information to be displayed on a single image than with a traditional single modality. One of its more common applications in diagnostic imaging today is PET/CT. By creating fusion images of both CT and PET datasets, the detailed anatomic information provided by CT can be combined with the functional information provided by PET to provide diagnostic information beyond that which either could provide alone.

In recent years, image fusion has also been applied to procedural navigation. Fusion in navigation allows an interventionalist

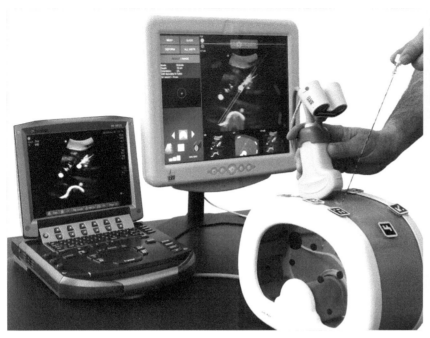

Fig. 1.7 Clear Guide Medical SCENERGY system allows the operator to fuse a CT dataset with real-time ultrasound imaging. The system uses an optical tracking device mounted to an ultrasound probe for needle tracking. Fiducial stickers are placed on the patient's skin, providing positional information, which also gives the user feedback regarding soft-tissue compression.

to target a lesion or area of interest with great accuracy during a procedure using a previously acquired dataset (▶ Fig. 1.7). It allows the operator to take advantage of both the high spatial and contrast resolution of a previously acquired CT or MRI with the high temporal resolution of the chosen intraprocedural guidance modality, typically intraprocedural ultrasound and/or an electromagnetic navigation (EMN) system.[20]

1.3.3 Image Fusion and EM Navigation Systems

EMN is commonly referred to as "body GPS" or "medical GPS" because it allows a device to be precisely tracked in relation to a patient's anatomy. It relies on Faraday's law of electromagnetic induction whereby a current is induced within a coil in a generated magnetic field. Medical EMN systems are comprised of a magnetic field generator and field sensors, both on the patient and within the interventional device. Feedback from the field sensors is provided to a processing computer by way of currents generated within the sensors in the magnetic field.[21]

EMN can be used in ultrasound- and CT-guided procedures. The EM generator should be positioned near the targeted anatomy to allow detection of field sensors also positioned near the area of interest. A radiopaque marker CT grid is placed on the patient and a procedural CT is acquired. The obtained image set is registered to a virtual 3D space created by the field sensors on the patient and in the interventional device. The procedure is then planned by marking the target within the EMN system. Visual feedback, including angle of approach and depth within the patient, is provided to the operator via the tracking device and the EMN system. A variety of methods may be used to advance the interventional device to the targeted region. If the interventional device does not have a tracking field sensor, a tracking needle can first be advanced to the region of interest. The chosen interventional device can then be advanced in tandem parallel to the tracking needle. Coaxial techniques are

also possible if a tracking inner stylet is used. The coaxial system can be advanced to the targeted region, and after confirmation of position, the tracking stylet can be removed and the biopsy or ablation device can be inserted into the cannula.

Venkatesan and colleagues demonstrated the value of EM navigation systems for targeting challenging lesions for biopsy. Previously acquired PET/CT data were co-registered with procedural CT and tracked with real-time ultrasound. In their series of 36 targeted lesions, 31 diagnostic specimens were obtained.[22] The combination of image fusion and EMN system allowed for safe and effective targeting of fluorodeoxyglucose (FDG)-avid lesions not apparent on CT or ultrasound.

1.4 Conclusion

Advances in intraprocedural imaging modalities and navigational devices are paramount to interventional radiology's continued growth and success. These technologies allow the interventionalist to visualize and navigate to pathology with greater safety, speed, and confidence. CBCT and navigational tools are excellent adjunctive technologies which allow interventionalists to perform complex abdominal interventions.

References

[1] Feldkamp LA, Davis LC, Kress JW. Practical cone-beam algorithm. J Opt Soc Am A Opt Image Sci Vis. 1984; 1(6):612–619

[2] Ning R, Chen B, Yu R, Conover D, Tang X, Ning Y. Flat panel detector-based cone-beam volume CT angiography imaging: system evaluation. IEEE Trans Med Imaging. 2000; 19(9):949–963

[3] Orth RC, Wallace MJ, Kuo MD, Technology Assessment Committee of the Society of Interventional Radiology. C-arm cone-beam CT: general principles and technical considerations for use in interventional radiology. J Vasc Interv Radiol. 2008; 19(6):814–820

[4] Wallace MJ, Kuo MD, Glaiberman C, Binkert CA, Orth RC, Soulez G, Technology Assessment Committee of the Society of Interventional Radiology. Three-dimensional C-arm cone-beam CT: applications in the interventional suite. J Vasc Interv Radiol. 2008; 19(6):799–813

[5] Miyayama S, Yamashiro M, Hashimoto M, et al. Identification of small hepatocellular carcinoma and tumor-feeding branches with cone-beam CT guidance technology during transcatheter arterial chemoembolization. J Vasc Interv Radiol. 2013; 24(4):501–508

[6] Loffroy R, Lin M, Rao P, et al. Comparing the detectability of hepatocellular carcinoma by C-arm dual-phase cone-beam computed tomography during hepatic arteriography with conventional contrast-enhanced magnetic resonance imaging. Cardiovasc Intervent Radiol. 2012; 35(1):97–104

[7] Liu DM, Salem R, Bui JT, et al. Angiographic considerations in patients undergoing liver-directed therapy. J Vasc Interv Radiol. 2005; 16(7):911–935

[8] Madoff DC, Hicks ME, Vauthey J-N, et al. Transhepatic portal vein embolization: anatomy, indications, and technical considerations. Radiographics. 2002; 22(5):1063–1076

[9] Sze DY, Strobel N, Fahrig R, Moore T, Busque S, Frisoli JK. Transjugular intrahepatic portosystemic shunt creation in a polycystic liver facilitated by hybrid cross-sectional/angiographic imaging. J Vasc Interv Radiol. 2006; 17 (4):711–715

[10] Luo X, Ye L, Zhou X, et al. C-arm cone-beam volume CT in transjugular intrahepatic portosystemic shunt: initial clinial experience. Cardiovasc Intervent Radiol. 2015; 38(6):1627–1631

[11] Abi-Jaoudeh N, Venkatesan AM, Van der Sterren W, Radaelli A, Carelsen B, Wood BJ. Clinical experience with cone-beam CT navigation for tumor ablation. J Vasc Interv Radiol. 2015; 26(2):214–219

[12] Braak SJ, van Strijen MJL, van Es HW, Nievelstein RA, van Heesewijk JP. Effective dose during needle interventions: cone-beam CT guidance compared with conventional CT guidance. J Vasc Interv Radiol. 2011; 22(4): 455–461

[13] Iwazawa J, Ohue S, Hashimoto N, Mitani T. Ablation margin assessment of liver tumors with intravenous contrast-enhanced C-arm computed tomography. World J Radiol. 2012; 4(3):109–114

[14] Kapoor BS, Esparaz A, Levitin A, McLennan G, Moon E, Sands M. Nonvascular and portal vein applications of cone-beam computed tomography: current status. Tech Vasc Interv Radiol. 2013; 16(3):150–160

[15] Möhlenbruch M, Nelles M, Thomas D, et al. Cone-beam computed tomography-guided percutaneous radiologic gastrostomy. Cardiovasc Intervent Radiol. 2010; 33(2):315–320

[16] Braak SJ, van Melick HHE, Onaca MG, van Heesewijk JPM, van Strijen MJL. 3D cone-beam CT guidance, a novel technique in renal biopsy-results in 41 patients with suspected renal masses. Eur Radiol. 2012; 22 (11):2547–2552

[17] Ben-Shlomo A, Cohen D, Bruckheimer E, et al. Comparing effective doses during image-guided core needle biopsies with computed tomography versus C-arm cone beam CT using adult and pediatric phantoms. Cardiovasc Intervent Radiol. 2015; 39(5):732–739

[18] Gruber-Rouh T, Schulz B, Eichler K, Naguib NNN, Vogl TJ, Zangos S. Radiation dose and quickness of needle CT-interventions using a laser navigation system (LNS) compared with conventional method. Eur J Radiol. 2015; 84 (10):1976–1980

[19] Schubert T, Jacob AL, Pansini M, Liu D, Gutzeit A, Kos S. CT-guided interventions using a free-hand, optical tracking system: initial clinical experience. Cardiovasc Intervent Radiol. 2013; 36(4):1055–1062

[20] Abi-Jaoudeh N, Kobeiter H, Xu S, Wood BJ. Image fusion during vascular and nonvascular image-guided procedures. Tech Vasc Interv Radiol. 2013; 16(3): 168–176

[21] Ward TJ, Goldman RE, Weintraub JL. Electromagnetic navigation with multimodality image fusion for image-guided percutaneous interventions. Tech Vasc Interv Radiol. 2013; 16(3):177–181

[22] Venkatesan AM, Kadoury S, Abi-Jaoudeh N, et al. Real-time FDG PET guidance during biopsies and radiofrequency ablation using multimodality fusion with electromagnetic navigation. Radiology. 2011; 260(3):848–856

2 Imaging of Gastrointestinal Hemorrhage and Acute Mesenteric Ischemia

Siva P. Raman and Elliot K. Fishman

2.1 Introduction

Multidetector computed tomography (MDCT) now serves as the first-line imaging modality in the emergency department for the diagnosis and risk stratification of a variety of bowel and mesenteric abnormalities. The rapidly increasing use of MDCT in the emergency setting and its increasing diagnostic efficacy have been driven by a variety of technological improvements over the last several generations of scanners, including equipment with better spatial and temporal resolution and the development of increasingly sophisticated study acquisition protocols. In particular, improvements in the temporal resolution of scanners have allowed the consistent, reproducible acquisition of images at peak arterial enhancement, greatly facilitating the evaluation of a variety of vascular disorders of the bowel and mesentery. MDCT images can now be acquired with beautiful delineation of the central mesenteric arterial vasculature (including small branch vessels), and these images can also be used to accurately gauge subtle sites of bleeding or abnormal bowel wall enhancement.

This chapter will discuss the role of MDCT in two of the most clinically important of these vascular disorders, namely acute gastrointestinal (GI) hemorrhage and acute mesenteric ischemia, with a focus on appropriate scan protocols, imaging diagnosis, and diagnostic pitfalls.

2.2 CT Protocol Design

When bowel pathology is suspected prospectively (such as in cases of bowel ischemia or acute GI bleeding), it is imperative that positive oral contrast (i.e., contrast agents with Hounsfield attenuation values > 50) not be used, as dense contrast within the bowel lumen not only will obscure sites of active bleeding or contrast extravasation but also will prevent accurate assessment of the bowel wall (in terms of either enhancement or thickness) as a result of beam hardening or streak artifact. In addition, in our particular practice, where a great deal of emphasis is placed on the creation of 3D reconstructions to aid in diagnosis, we are very cognizant that positive oral contrast material may also interfere with standard reconstruction algorithms. Instead, the patient should be scanned without the use of an enteric contrast agent; alternatively, a neutral agent (i.e., contrast agents with densities close to that of simple fluid) such as VoLumen or water should be used to achieve bowel distension without compromising optimal evaluation of bowel wall thickness and enhancement. Given the acuity of presentation of both of the disorders discussed in this chapter (GI hemorrhage and ischemia), it is not at all uncommon in our institution to scan patients in the emergency setting without using any oral contrast agent so as to not unduly delay the patient's diagnosis and treatment.[1,2]

Patients with suspected GI hemorrhage or mesenteric ischemia should be scanned using a dual-phase protocol, with the acquisition of both arterial and venous phase images after the brisk (4–5 mL/s) injection of a nonionic intravenous contrast agent (100–120 mL contrast volume). Arterial phase images are most often acquired using a bolus trigger technique (usually at approximately 30–40 s) during inspiration, whereas venous phase images are acquired using a fixed delay of approximately 50 to 60 seconds during inspiration. Images are routinely acquired using thin collimation (0.625–0.75 mm), with standard reconstruction of images into 3- to 5-mm slices for axial image review; isotropic 0.5- to 0.75-mm images are sent to an independent workstation for generation of 3D reconstructions. Commonly used 3D reconstruction techniques for the analysis of bowel and mesenteric pathology include maximum intensity projection (MIP) images, which highlight the brightest voxels in a dataset and are particularly useful for evaluation of the mesenteric vasculature, and volume-rendered images, which are 3D images created by assigning a specific color and transparency to each voxel in a dataset and are useful for providing comprehensive evaluation of the bowel.[1,2] Additionally, coronal and sagittal multiplanar reformations, which are critical for evaluation of the mesenteric vessel origins and for providing an overview of the entirety of the bowel, are automatically generated at the scanner for routine radiologist review.[1,2,3]

Dual-phase technique is critical in cases of suspected GI hemorrhage, as having two phases allows maximum sensitivity for detecting sites of active contrast extravasation (i.e., bleeding) and differentiating between sites of active bleeding and intrinsically high-density material in the bowel (e.g., medications, old barium). Intrinsically high-density material should appear identical on the two phases, whereas a true bleed should change in both size and shape.[1,2] Some practices also incorporate a third noncontrast phase (with images acquired before the administration of intravenous contrast) to better differentiate between true sites of bleeding and intrinsically high-density material, although, in theory, this distinction should be possible using a biphasic acquisition. The use of dual-energy CT for GI bleeding cases also allows for the creation of virtual noncontrast images that can aid in the interpretation of these studies without the need for a separate noncontrast acquisition.[4,5]

Dual-phase technique is also necessary in cases of mesenteric ischemia, as the two phases allow a comprehensive evaluation of the arterial and venous mesenteric vasculature for patency and offer increased sensitivity for subtle changes in bowel wall enhancement (which may be more apparent on one of the two contrast phases).[1,2]

2.3 Acute Lower GI Bleeding

Lower GI bleeding, defined as bleeding distal to the ligament of Treitz, is a very common problem in the emergency setting, accounting for up to 3% of all inpatient admissions. Although the vast majority of bleeding episodes are self-limited, rebleeding occurs in a sizable percentage of patients (up to 20%), with patients at higher risk of morbidity and mortality in the setting of rebleeding.[6]

There is no perfect radiologic modality for the evaluation of acute GI bleeding, and there has been little consensus in the literature as to the best initial option. Technetium-99m-tagged red blood cell (RBC) scans are considered quite sensitive for detecting sites of bleeding, with the ability to detect bleeding rates as low as 0.1 mL/min, and offer the advantage of potentially detecting intermittent bleeding because of their prolonged acquisition times. However, this modality suffers from poor spatial resolution and a frequent inability to accurately localize the site of bleeding, raising questions regarding its true utility in terms of guiding angiographic treatment. Moreover, tagged RBC scans do not provide information about the etiology of bleeding (e.g., diverticular disease, ischemia), also limiting its use in terms of guiding treatment.[1,2] Angiography is quite effective as a treatment modality but is relatively insensitive for the detection of bleeding, only detecting rates of bleeding of approximately 1 mL/min and higher. Moreover, angiography is insensitive to intermittent bleeds and is ineffective in identifying subtle bleeds because of its relatively limited contrast resolution. Traditionally, colonoscopy has been considered the first-line modality for the evaluation of acute GI bleeding in the emergency setting. However, colonoscopy can be technically challenging in the acute setting because of a lack of adequate bowel preparation; moreover, this procedure does not provide evaluation of the small bowel for bleeding sites.[2,6]

Overall, MDCT has been shown to be quite sensitive for detecting sites of active bleeding, is able to detect rates of bleeding as low as 0.35 mL/min, and has the additional advantage of being able to provide information about the cause of bleeding (e.g., Crohn's disease, diverticular disease, bowel ischemia). MDCT can also be used to evaluate the entirety of the bowel (both small and large bowel), unlike colonoscopy.[1,2,6] In addition, research has suggested that MDCT may be valuable for triage in the emergency department, as patients with a negative CT scan are unlikely to have subsequent episodes of rebleeding. CT may also be valuable when performed before colonoscopy to better delineate the likely site of bleeding, thus helping to guide angiographic or colonoscopy-based treatment.[7] Overall, given the rapidity of scan acquisitions using modern technology, CT imaging upon initial presentation is unlikely to unduly delay other diagnostic or treatment options, and accordingly, there is little downside to using CT before further investigation or treatment with other modalities. In

general, reports in the literature have suggested relatively high sensitivities and specificities for CT in the diagnosis of acute GI bleeding, with sensitivities ranging from 79 to 100% and specificities ranging from 85 to 100%.[8,9,10,11,12,13]

Although CT certainly has a significant, and growing, role in the diagnosis and evaluation of lower GI bleeding, there are currently no convincing data supporting the use of CT for upper GI bleeding (defined as bleeding proximal to the ligament of Treitz). In patients with symptoms clearly suggestive of upper GI bleeding (or symptoms that might possibly represent upper GI bleeding), upper endoscopy should be the primary test of choice.[6]

As mentioned earlier, proper technique is of the utmost importance in studies performed for suspected GI bleeding, as poorly designed protocols will make diagnosis (particularly of active extravasation) nearly impossible. Specifically, positive oral contrast agents cannot be used for this indication, as high-density contrast agents will obscure sites of active extravasation. In general, neutral agents such as water or VoLumen can be used but are not absolutely necessary, particularly given that these studies are often performed in acutely ill patients who may not be able to tolerate drinking contrast. Although there is some argument that the ingestion of water or VoLumen may actually dilute sites of active extravasation, making their identification more difficult, we have used water as a contrast agent at our institution for several years and have not experienced any significant problems in identifying sites of bleeding.[1,2]

Sites of active bleeding are visible as high-density material within the bowel lumen, with attenuation identical to that of the blood pool on any given phase of contrast (▶ Fig. 2.1, ▶ Fig. 2.2, ▶ Fig. 2.3, ▶ Fig. 2.4, ▶ Fig. 2.5). The morphology of this active extravasation will depend on the rapidity of the bleed, with rapid bleeds often demonstrating a linear or "jet-like" morphology (or even resulting in a contrast level within the bowel lumen) and slower bleeds demonstrating a more ill-defined or amorphous pooling of contrast.[1,2] In addition, active bleeding in the bowel (particularly the small bowel) may induce hyperperistalsis, causing the actively extravasated contrast to move more distally in the bowel lumen between the arterial and venous phases. Any suspected site of bleeding must be confirmed on both the arterial and venous phase images, with a true active bleed demonstrating a change in both size and shape/morphology (▶ Fig. 2.1, ▶ Fig. 2.2, ▶ Fig. 2.4). Alternatively, the site of bleeding can be contrasted with intrinsically high-density material within the bowel lumen, which should

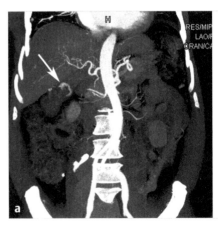
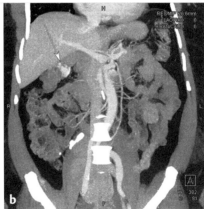

Fig. 2.1 Active extravasation in the hepatic flexure of the colon. Coronal MIP CT images in the arterial (a) and venous (b) phases demonstrate a site of active extravasation (*arrows*) in the hepatic flexure of the colon. Note that the bleed increases in size and changes in morphology in the two phases, allowing a true bleed to be distinguished from intrinsically high-attenuation material.

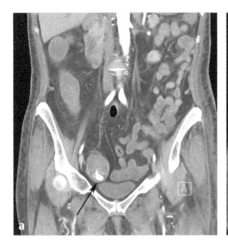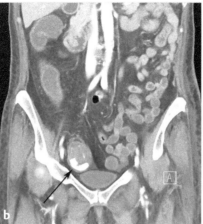

Fig. 2.2 Active bleed in the colon. Coronal arterial (**a**) and venous (**b**) phase CT images demonstrate an active bleed (*arrows*) in the colon, which changes in size and shape between the two phases.

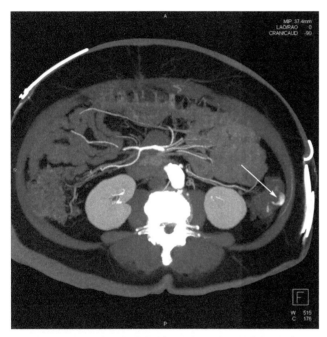

Fig. 2.3 Active bleed in the left colon within a diverticulum. Axial arterial phase CT image demonstrates an active bleed (*arrow*) in the left colon occurring within a diverticulum.

remain identical in both size and morphology between the arterial and venous phase images. If noncontrast images are acquired, this phase can serve as a valuable means of differentiating between intrinsically high-density material and a true bleed, as intrinsically high-density material (unlike bleeding) should be seen on noncontrast images.[2,3,11,14,15] In some cases, even though frankly extravasated contrast may not be visible, a high-density clotted blot (measuring 40–70 HU) may be seen within the bowel lumen, providing a clue as to the site of bleeding ("sentinel clot" sign) (▶ Fig. 2.6).[3] Although this is not as specific as active extravasation, this sentinel clot sign may still prove valuable for helping to guide the endoscopist or interventional radiologist.

In addition to identifying sites of active extravasation, the true value of MDCT relative to other imaging modalities and colonoscopy is its ability to diagnose multiple potential causes of GI bleeding, even in the absence of active extravasation. One area of diagnosis in which MDCT particularly excels is in the diagnosis of a range of vascular abnormalities that can cause GI bleeding such as angiodysplasia, varices in patients with portal hypertension (particularly rectal varices), and arteriovenous malformations (AVMs) (▶ Fig. 2.7, ▶ Fig. 2.8). Angiodysplasia, a relatively common diagnosis in elderly patients, is often visible as an unusual tangle of vessels within the submucosal layer of the bowel (particularly the right colon), often with a dilated feeding artery and an early draining vein.[3] Bowel AVMs are a relatively uncommon finding on imaging but may represent the source of bleeding in a sizable percentage of patients with occult lower GI bleeds. Bowel AVMs are most commonly identified in the proximal small bowel but can be seen anywhere within the GI tract.[2] Finally, varices around the rectum are not

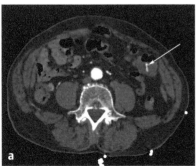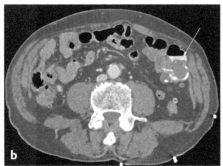

Fig. 2.4 Active bleed in the left colon. Axial arterial (**a**) and venous (**b**) phase CT images demonstrate an active bleed (*arrows*) in the left colon, which changes in size and shape between the two phases. Notice the linear morphology of the bleed in the arterial phase, a common appearance for brisk or rapid bleeds.

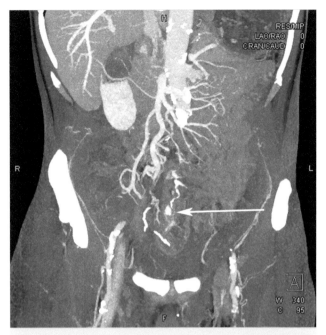

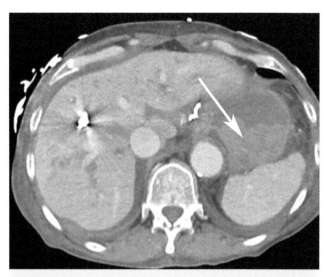

Fig. 2.6 Sentinel clot sign. Axial venous phase CT image demonstrates the sentinel clot sign in the stomach. Although no active extravasation is noted, the presence of high-attenuation clotted blood in the stomach (*arrow*) suggests that the stomach is the source of the patient's bleeding.

Fig. 2.5 Active bleed in the small bowel. Coronal MIP arterial phase CT image demonstrates an active bleed (*arrow*) in the small bowel. Active extravasation is often easiest to appreciate on MIP reconstructions.

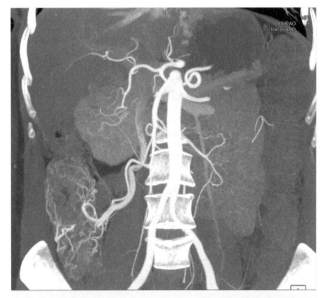

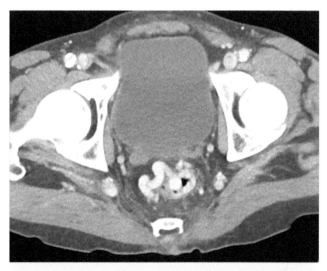

Fig. 2.8 Rectal varices. Axial venous phase CT image demonstrates a tangle of dilated veins both within and surrounding the rectum in a patient with known cirrhosis and portal hypertension, compatible with rectal varices.

Fig. 2.7 Angiodysplasia of the right colon. Coronal MIP arterial phase CT image demonstrates angiodysplasia of the right colon, with an unusual tangle of vessels in the bowel wall, a dilated feeding artery, and an early draining vein.

uncommon in patients with portal hypertension, and although these varices are usually asymptomatic, they can sometimes cause slow, intermittent bleeding (▶ Fig. 2.8).

In addition to vascular abnormalities, MDCT also offers the advantage of a complete evaluation of the small and large bowel for a number of other inflammatory, infectious, and ischemic causes of GI bleeds, including mesenteric ischemia, inflammatory bowel disease (either ulcerative colitis or Crohn's disease), a variety of small and large bowel tumors, Meckel's diverticulum, and fecal impaction.[3] Although diverticular disease (in the absence of frank diverticulitis) is an incredibly common incidental finding in a large percentage of asymptomatic patients, it is a finding that should not be ignored in the setting of unexplained lower GI bleeding. In particular, diverticulosis may account for up to 40% of all cases of lower GI bleeding as well as approximately 50% of patients admitted for rebleeding. Diverticular bleeds are not uncommonly arterial in nature and can produce substantial bleeding with evidence of active extravasation on CT. If no other etiology is identified, the presence of significant diverticulosis (even without evidence of active extravasation) should be noted in the radiologist's dictated report.[8]

2.4 Acute Mesenteric Ischemia

Acute mesenteric ischemia represents an extraordinarily morbid diagnosis in the emergency setting, carrying mortality rates as high as 80%. Unfortunately, clinical examination and laboratory markers for this condition can be relatively nonspecific, making imaging absolutely critical for accurate and timely diagnosis. Laboratory markers that are classically associated with bowel ischemia, such as lactic acid level, leukocytosis, and anion gap, are not consistently identified in all patients with acute mesenteric ischemia. Additionally, elevated lactate levels are not necessarily specific for ischemia. Given that the clinical presentation of these patients may be relatively nonspecific, it is believed that only one-third of all patients are accurately clinically diagnosed with mesenteric ischemia.[16]

The causes of acute mesenteric ischemia can be broadly divided into four major categories, including arterial occlusion, venous occlusion, nonocclusive mesenteric ischemia (NOMI), and complicated bowel obstructions. Arterial occlusion accounts for the vast majority of cases (up to 70%). Arterial occlusion is most often embolic in nature, with sources of embolism including cardiac thrombus (such as patients with atrial fibrillation or prior myocardial infarctions) and heavily ulcerated atherosclerotic plaque in the abdominal aorta or major branch vessels. Arterial occlusion can also result from thrombosis of a branch vessel, particularly in patients with hypercoagulable states and patients with underlying heavy atherosclerotic disease; arterial thrombosis can also occur in the setting of aortic dissection, atherosclerotic aneurysms, and vasculitis.[17] Patients with acute mesenteric ischemia caused by arterial embolus typically have an extremely abrupt onset of symptoms (e.g., severe abdominal pain, diarrhea, GI bleeding), whereas patients with mesenteric ischemia caused by arterial thrombosis tend to have a slightly less abrupt onset of symptoms, likely due to collaterals at sites of preexisting atherosclerosis.[18] Arterial occlusion can occur at any point in the superior mesenteric artery (SMA) distribution, and although emboli are most often identified in the proximal aspect of the SMA (usually the most proximal 3–8 cm as a result of its orientation), emboli can also extend into the smaller branches of the SMA (and sometimes still be visible on imaging).[17,19] Accordingly, arterial occlusion caused by an embolus can involve either the entirety of the SMA distribution (when an embolus is lodged in the proximal SMA) or just a small portion of the SMA distribution (when an embolus extends into a smaller branch). Arterial thrombosis secondary to atherosclerotic plaque most often occurs in the most proximal 2 to 3 cm of the SMA and consequently tends to involve a large portion of the SMA territory.[17,19] Most patients with mesenteric ischemia caused by arterial

occlusion are elderly (>70 years old), with atrial fibrillation serving as a major risk factor in younger patients.[16]

Venous occlusion is much less common, accounting for only 10% of all cases of mesenteric ischemia, although these patients tend to have relatively poor outcomes (with mortality rates up to 40%) as a result of typically indolent, subacute presentations leading to delayed diagnosis. Venous occlusion (i.e., superior mesenteric vein [SMV] thrombosis) can be seen in a number of different settings, including patients with an underlying hypercoagulable syndrome (either diagnosed or undiagnosed, such as sickle cell disease, polycythemia vera, or antiphospholipid antibody syndrome), patients with septic thrombophlebitis caused by a GI tract infection, and patients who have recently undergone hepatobiliary surgery.[16,17] Pregnancy and the use of hypercoagulable medications (such as oral contraceptives) are also considered potential (although uncommon) risk factors for this condition.

NOMI results from poor blood flow to the small bowel (which is quite sensitive to variations in blood flow) and can occur in a number of different settings, including hypotension secondary to myocardial infarction, sepsis, vasoconstriction due to drug use (including cocaine or digitalis), dialysis, and shock physiology. NOMI results from vasoconstriction of the mesenteric arteries in the setting of hypotension, with resultant diversion of blood flow to the brain and heart (and consequently, away from the bowel).[16] NOMI may comprise up to 30% of all cases of mesenteric ischemia. In fact, some have argued that the overall incidence of NOMI is likely greater than the incidence suggested in the literature, and NOMI is overwhelmingly the most common cause of mesenteric ischemia in the intensive care setting. Given that these patients have multiple severe medical comorbidities (some of which account for their mesenteric ischemia), mortality rates for this disorder are quite high, ranging from 30 to 93%.

Complicated bowel obstructions result in strangulation and occlusion of both the arterial and venous blood supply to the bowel and are most commonly diagnosed in the setting of either severe conventional small bowel obstructions or closed-loop small bowel obstruction/volvulus with twisting and strangulation of the bowel's blood supply. Bowel ischemia in the setting of obstruction is relatively uncommon, however, accounting for only approximately 10% of all small bowel obstructions.[16,17]

Although it is easy to simply conflate bowel wall thickening with ischemia, it is worth noting that the imaging findings in these patients can be significantly more subtle; for instance, many patients with bowel ischemia do not demonstrate significant bowel wall thickening. The imaging manifestations of ischemia on MDCT can vary quite dramatically depending on the underlying cause. Arterial occlusion does not typically result in significant bowel wall thickening; in fact, the bowel wall may actually become thinned in appearance over time as a result of transmural ischemia and infarction (so-called "paper-thin" bowel). One should not be too dogmatic about this point, however, as arterial occlusion can rarely result in very mild bowel wall thickening (typically <15 mm).[16]

The key finding in acute mesenteric ischemia is the presence of abnormal bowel wall hypoenhancement, a finding that can be difficult to diagnose confidently, particularly if the entirety of the small bowel distribution demonstrates uniform hypoenhancement (▶ Fig. 2.9, ▶ Fig. 2.10).[20] Sometimes, this bowel wall

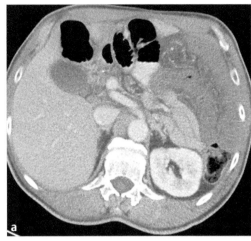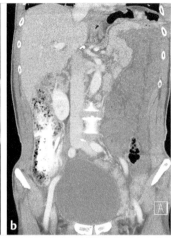

Fig. 2.9 Acute mesenteric ischemia caused by arterial occlusion. Axial (**a**) and coronal (**b**) venous phase CT images demonstrate diffuse hypoenhancement of multiple bowel loops throughout the left hemiabdomen. Thrombus was identified within the SMA (not shown). This constellation of findings is compatible with acute mesenteric ischemia caused by arterial occlusion.

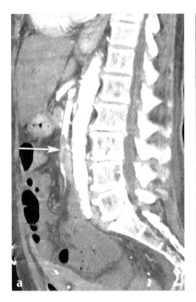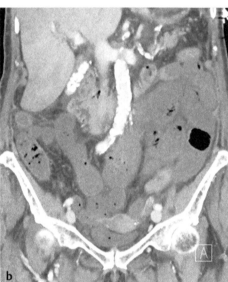

Fig. 2.10 Mesenteric ischemia caused by arterial occlusion. Sagittal arterial phase CT image (**a**) demonstrates extensive occlusive thrombus within the mid to distal aspect of the SMA (*arrow*). Coronal arterial phase CT image (**b**) demonstrates multiple mildly dilated loops of small bowel throughout the midabdomen, particularly on the left, all of which demonstrate diffuse wall hypoenhancement, compatible with mesenteric ischemia caused by arterial occlusion.

hypoenhancement may be more evident on one contrast phase compared to the other. In our experience, identifying sites of abnormal bowel wall enhancement can often be easier in the coronal plane, as this plane more readily allows comparison of the degree of enhancement of different portions of the bowel at the same time. It is conceivable that dual-energy CT may soon serve as a valuable aid for better delineating abnormal bowel wall enhancement, particularly through the use of iodine maps and quantification of iodine uptake using iodine-selective images. Dual-energy CT may help readers improve their diagnostic confidence when abnormal bowel wall enhancement is suspected on the basis of standard axial image review.[5]

One of the difficulties in identifying mesenteric ischemia secondary to arterial occlusion is the relative lack of abnormality in the mesentery. There is often virtually no mesenteric edema, stranding, hemorrhage, or inflammatory change, features that are generally used for the diagnosis of other common bowel disorders.[21] In general, arterial occlusion does not result in bowel dilatation or ileus, although the bowel can dilate once the ischemia progresses to true transmural infarction. Particularly when located in the proximal aspect of the SMA (rather than a smaller branch), the primary embolus may be directly visualized occluding the SMA lumen on arterial phase images. Moreover, when occurring in the acute setting, the lack of any apparent collaterals and the presence of relatively poor flow distal to the embolus (in conjunction with the patient's acute onset of symptoms) should strongly suggest an acute episode.[16]

Venous ischemia is typically a much easier imaging diagnosis, as there is almost always substantial adjacent mesenteric edema, stranding, or even hemorrhage. The bowel wall is often quite dramatically thickened (commonly > 1–1.5 cm) and may be either hypodense (as a result of submucosal edema) or hyperdense (as a result of intramural hemorrhage) in appearance (▶ Fig. 2.11).[21] The juxtaposition of submucosal edema against mucosal and subserosal hyperenhancement is frequently described as the "halo" sign. Typically, particularly on arterial phase images, there may be prominent mucosal hyperenhancement. Even in the absence of true transmural infarction, the small bowel may appear dilated (without evidence of obstruction). In our experience, although the bowel abnormality is easily diagnosed by most radiologists, misdiagnosis in these cases most often results from lack of recognition of the presence of thrombus in the SMV. For any patient who presents with acute abdominal pain, it is critical to consistently evaluate

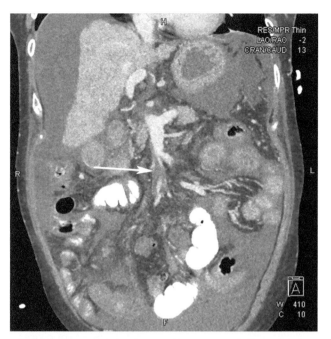

Fig. 2.11 Mesenteric ischemia caused by venous occlusion. Coronal venous phase CT image demonstrates thrombus within the SMV (*arrow*). Additionally, note the presence of multiple thickened loops of small bowel throughout the left hemiabdomen and portions of the pelvis, likely representing mesenteric ischemia caused by venous occlusion.

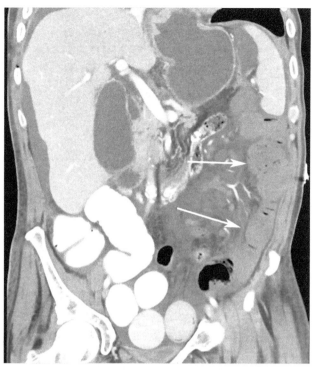

Fig. 2.13 Mesenteric ischemia. Axial venous phase CT image demonstrates diffusely thick-walled, hyperenhancing small bowel throughout the abdomen (*arrows*) in a patient with hypotension in the intensive care setting, compatible with mesenteric ischemia.

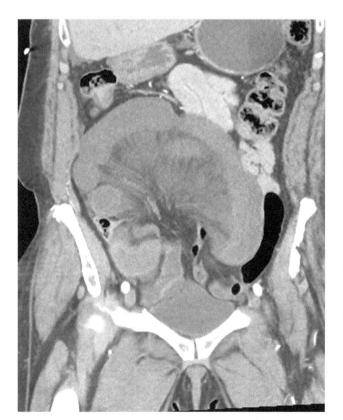

Fig. 2.12 Nonocclusive mesenteric ischemia. Coronal arterial phase CT image demonstrates diffusely hypoenhancing bowel with extensive mesenteric edema and stranding in a patient with known severe hypotension in the intensive care setting. These findings are compatible with nonocclusive mesenteric ischemia.

the SMV in every case, and it is worth noting that the SMV can often be best evaluated in the coronal plane.[1]

NOMI can be quite difficult to diagnose based on imaging alone, with imaging features resembling those of either arterial occlusion or venous occlusion (▶ Fig. 2.12, ▶ Fig. 2.13). In many cases, the only sign of NOMI may be nonspecific bowel wall thickening. The key to diagnosis lies in the combination of imaging findings and the patient's clinical history. These patients are critically ill, are almost always found in the acute care or intensive care settings, and nearly always have a history of hypotension or shock physiology.[1,21]

Ischemia in the setting of complex bowel obstruction can demonstrate imaging features of both arterial occlusion and venous occlusion, given that the obstruction results in strangulation and occlusion of both the arterial and venous blood supply to the involved segment of bowel. Certain segments of bowel may demonstrate features of arterial ischemia, including bowel wall hypoenhancement, whereas other segments of bowel may demonstrate features of venous occlusion, with prominent bowel wall edema/hemorrhage and mesenteric edema/hemorrhage. It is critical in these cases for a radiologist to differentiate these complex bowel obstructions from simple, routine bowel obstructions. Closed-loop obstructions often demonstrate a unique tethered, radiating appearance of the dilated small bowel loops, quite different from the configuration of the bowel in conventional obstructions. In some cases of closed-loop small bowel obstructions or volvulus, the twist in

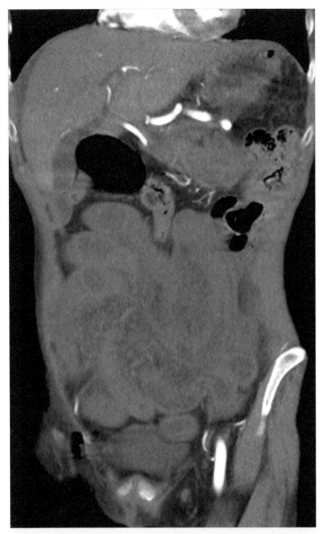

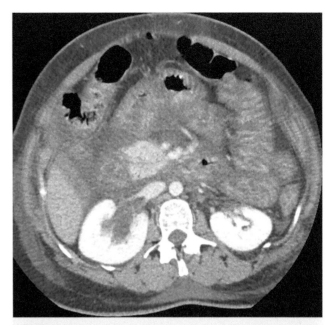

Fig. 2.15 Bowel ischemia. Coronal venous phase CT image demonstrates dilated loops of small bowel in the left hemiabdomen, all of which demonstrate wall hypoenhancement, with extensive mesenteric edema and stranding identified medial to these bowel loops, compatible with bowel ischemia. These findings were determined to be secondary to an internal hernia at surgery.

Fig. 2.14 Closed-loop obstruction and bowel ischemia. Coronal arterial phase CT image demonstrates multiple dilated loops of small bowel in the right hemiabdomen, all of which demonstrate an unusual tethered or radiating appearance, with extensive mesenteric edema, stranding, and inflammatory change at the center of these bowel loops. Note that these bowel loops demonstrate diffuse wall hypoenhancement. This constellation of findings is compatible with a closed-loop obstruction and bowel ischemia, findings which were confirmed at surgery.

the mesentery can be directly visualized on CT (i.e., "whorl" sign), although this imaging sign is somewhat nonspecific, as a mild twist in the mesentery can sometimes be seen in healthy patients, as well. An additional helpful imaging feature is the "venous cutoff" sign, in which the mesenteric venous vasculature is seen to become compressed and occluded as a result of the twisting of the mesentery (▶ Fig. 2.14, ▶ Fig. 2.15).[16,21,22,23]

The presence of interloop ascites should always raise concern about the possibility of a complex or complicated bowel obstruction and should prompt closer clinical attention. Other features that have been described as most specific for bowel ischemia in the setting of a strangulated bowel obstruction include diminished bowel wall enhancement and immediately adjacent mesenteric fat stranding. CT is thought to be relatively sensitive and specific for ischemia related to bowel obstruction,

with sensitivities ranging up to 100% and specificities ranging up to 93%.[16]

The presence of pneumatosis and portal venous gas can be seen with any of the previously mentioned underlying causes of mesenteric ischemia; both of these factors are highly sensitive and specific signs for bowel ischemia (although portal venous gas has a greater specificity than pneumatosis) (▶ Fig. 2.16).[1,16] The presence of both pneumatosis and portal venous gas in the same patient considerably increases the specificity for bowel ischemia. Although both imaging findings are most often visualized in the setting of ischemia, it is worth noting that these imaging findings (particularly pneumatosis) can also be seen in patients without ischemia, particularly in patients who have undergone bowel-related procedures (such as placement of a gastrostomy tube or jejunostomy) and in patients with severe bowel inflammation or infection (▶ Fig. 2.17, ▶ Fig. 2.18). In rare instances, trauma to the bowel can also result in pneumatosis without necessarily indicating underlying ischemia. Nevertheless, although these findings can theoretically be benign, the presence of pneumatosis or portal venous gas in any patient should be considered indicative of ischemia until proven otherwise and should prompt urgent clinical evaluation for potential mesenteric ischemia. Pneumatosis, which represents the presence of gas truly within the wall of the bowel (i.e., extending between the layers of the bowel wall), should, however, be differentiated from the common finding of nondependent gas closely abutting the bowel wall and gas trapped within fecal material abutting the dependent portion of the bowel wall. Similarly, portal venous gas is typically represented by small linear foci of gas extending toward the extreme periphery of the liver and should be differentiated

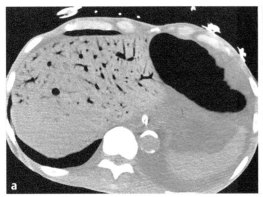
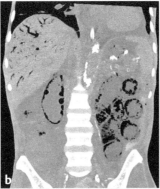

Fig. 2.16 Severe portal venous gas and pneumatosis. Axial noncontrast CT image **(a)** demonstrates extensive branching gas throughout the liver extending to the liver capsular surface, compatible with severe portal venous gas. Coronal noncontrast CT **(b)** image demonstrates extensive branching portal venous gas in the liver. There is also extensive pneumatosis involving multiple small bowel loops in both the right and left hemiabdomen, compatible with mesenteric ischemia.

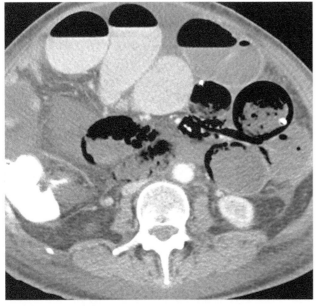

Fig. 2.17 Benign pneumatosis. Axial venous phase contrast-enhanced CT image in a patient who had recently undergone jejunostomy placement demonstrates pneumatosis involving multiple small bowel loops. The patient was asymptomatic, and this finding was determined to represent benign pneumatosis related to the previous procedure.

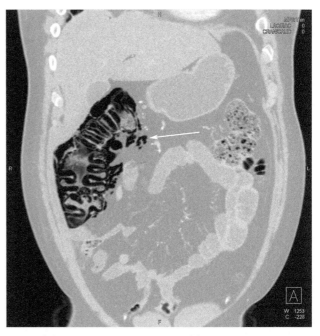

Fig. 2.18 Extensive pneumatosis in the right colon. Coronal contrast-enhanced venous phase CT image demonstrates extensive pneumatosis in the right colon, as well as a few foci of free air extending from the colon into the mesentery medially (*arrow*). These findings were determined to reflect benign pneumatosis in this asymptomatic patient who was receiving steroids for another medical condition.

from pneumobilia, which tends to be more central and clearly within biliary tree branches.[16]

2.5 Conclusion

MDCT now plays a vital role in the diagnosis and risk stratification of a number of different vascular disorders of the small and large bowel, including acute mesenteric ischemia and acute GI bleeding. However, in order for imaging to be maximally accurate for these diagnoses, adherence to proper CT technique is critical, and the proper protocols must be implemented. In cases of acute mesenteric ischemia and acute GI bleeding, the use of outdated or incorrect protocols can make diagnosis much more difficult or potentially preclude a correct diagnosis.

References

[1] Raman SP, Fishman EK. Computed tomography angiography of the small bowel and mesentery. Radiol Clin North Am. 2016; 54(1):87–100

[2] Raman SP, Horton KM, Fishman EK. MDCT and CT angiography evaluation of rectal bleeding: the role of volume visualization. AJR Am J Roentgenol. 2013; 201(3):589–597

[3] Soto JA, Park SH, Fletcher JG, Fidler JL. Gastrointestinal hemorrhage: evaluation with MDCT. Abdom Imaging. 2015; 40(5):993–1009

[4] Sun H, Hou XY, Xue HD, et al. Dual-source dual-energy CT angiography with virtual non-enhanced images and iodine map for active gastrointestinal bleeding: image quality, radiation dose and diagnostic performance. Eur J Radiol. 2015; 84(5):884–891

[5] Fulwadhva UP, Wortman JR, Sodickson AD. Use of dual-energy CT and iodine maps in evaluation of bowel disease. Radiographics. 2016; 36(2):393–406

[6] Lee SS, Park SH. Computed tomography evaluation of gastrointestinal bleeding and acute mesenteric ischemia. Radiol Clin North Am. 2013; 51(1): 29–43

[7] Jacovides CL, Nadolski G, Allen SR, et al. Arteriography for lower gastro-intestinal hemorrhage: role of preceding abdominal computed tomographic angiogram in diagnosis and localization. JAMA Surg. 2015; 150(7):650–656

[8] Moss AJ, Tuffaha H, Malik A. Lower GI bleeding: a review of current management, controversies and advances. Int J Colorectal Dis. 2016; 31(2):175–188

[9] Kim J, Kim YH, Lee KH, Lee YJ, Park JH. Diagnostic performance of CT angiography in patients visiting emergency department with overt gastrointestinal bleeding. Korean J Radiol. 2015; 16(3):541–549

[10] Yoon W, Jeong YY, Shin SS, et al. Acute massive gastrointestinal bleeding: detection and localization with arterial phase multi-detector row helical CT. Radiology. 2006; 239(1):160–167

[11] Artigas JM, Martí M, Soto JA, Esteban H, Pinilla I, Guillén E. Multidetector CT angiography for acute gastrointestinal bleeding: technique and findings. Radiographics. 2013; 33(5):1453–1470

[12] Martí M, Artigas JM, Garzón G, Alvarez-Sala R, Soto JA. Acute lower intestinal bleeding: feasibility and diagnostic performance of CT angiography. Radiology. 2012; 262(1):109–116

[13] Kennedy DW, Laing CJ, Tseng LH, Rosenblum DI, Tamarkin SW. Detection of active gastrointestinal hemorrhage with CT angiography: a 4(1/2)-year retrospective review. J Vasc Interv Radiol. 2010; 21(6):848–855

[14] Laing CJ, Tobias T, Rosenblum DI, Banker WL, Tseng L, Tamarkin SW. Acute gastrointestinal bleeding: emerging role of multidetector CT angiography and review of current imaging techniques. Radiographics. 2007; 27(4): 1055–1070

[15] Steiner K, Gollub F, Stuart S, Papadopoulou A, Woodward N. Acute gastrointestinal bleeding: CT angiography with multi-planar reformatting. Abdom Imaging. 2011; 36(2):115–125

[16] Dhatt HS, Behr SC, Miracle A, Wang ZJ, Yeh BM. Radiological evaluation of bowel ischemia. Radiol Clin North Am. 2015; 53(6):1241–1254

[17] Shih MC, Hagspiel KD. CTA and MRA in mesenteric ischemia: part 1, Role in diagnosis and differential diagnosis. AJR Am J Roentgenol. 2007; 188(2):452–461

[18] Stone JR, Wilkins LR. Acute mesenteric ischemia. Tech Vasc Interv Radiol. 2015; 18(1):24–30

[19] Sandstrom CK, Ingraham CR, Monroe EJ, Johnson GE. Beyond decreased bowel enhancement: acute abnormalities of the mesenteric and portal vasculature. Abdom Imaging. 2015; 40(8):2977–2992

[20] Chen YC, Huang TY, Chen RC, et al. Comparison of ischemic and nonischemic bowel segments in patients with mesenteric ischemia: multidetector row computed tomography findings and measurement of bowel wall attenuation changes. Mayo Clin Proc. 2016; 91(3):316–328

[21] Furukawa A, Kanasaki S, Kono N, et al. CT diagnosis of acute mesenteric ischemia from various causes. AJR Am J Roentgenol. 2009; 192(2):408–416

[22] Makar RA, Bashir MR, Haystead CM, et al. Diagnostic performance of MDCT in identifying closed loop small bowel obstruction. Abdom Radiol (NY). 2016; 41(7):1253–1260

[23] Gore RM, Silvers RI, Thakrar KH, et al. Bowel obstruction. Radiol Clin North Am. 2015; 53(6):1225–1240

3 Portal Hypertension

Robert O'Shea and Rachel Abou Mrad

3.1 Introduction

The term "portal hypertension" was first credited to Gilbert and Villaret in 1906 in research studies performed to investigate the etiology of ascites, gastrointestinal bleeding, and hepatofugal collateral development.[1] The normal hepatic venous pressure typically ranges from approximately 5 to 10 mm Hg[2]; portal hypertension represents an increase in pressure in the portal venous system to a level that exceeds the pressure in the inferior vena cava by more than 5 mm Hg.[3] However, the clinical manifestations of portal hypertension typically do not occur until this pressure difference is considerably higher, and thresholds at which patients typically develop bleeding or ascites have been established.

For many patients with cirrhosis, portal hypertension represents the clinical manifestation of liver disease—the actual signs and symptoms that patients with end-stage liver disease experience. Portal hypertension is the final common pathway of many forms of chronic liver disease, and its development is the turning point in the course of a chronic liver disease, a threshold event that signifies the transition from asymptomatic liver disease to decompensated cirrhosis. Portal hypertension can also occur in patients with acute severe liver disease, and the signs and symptoms in these cases may be indistinguishable from those in cases of chronic liver disease. Clinically, portal hypertension is recognized by the development of variceal bleeding, ascites, or hepatic encephalopathy. In early clinical studies, the prognosis of patients who presented with these forms of decompensation was invariably grim.[4] Before advances such as liver transplant were available, these studies reported 1-year survival rates of less than 40% when patients presented with either varices or ascites and 5-year survival rates of approximately 10%.[4]

Liver disease was previously classified as either compensated or decompensated. Liver disease, however, is more intuitively thought of as a spectrum, with implications for patients with advanced liver disease who are asymptomatic—classified as chronic liver failure or acute-on-chronic liver failure in patients who have developed acute decompensation (ascites, hemorrhage, encephalopathy, and/or bacterial infections).[5,6] When patients are stratified by this method, it is still clear that those who have developed decompensation are at an increased mortality risk, but it is also clear that the symptomatic presentation of decompensation more typically represents the end stage of a patient's evolution through the course of his or her disease (▶ Table 3.1).[7] Thus, patients who are diagnosed with cirrhosis while asymptomatic are at a very low risk of short-term mortality, which is manifestly not the case once patients become symptomatic (▶ Fig. 3.1).[7] It is clear from natural history studies that there is also a hierarchy of decompensation events that may culminate in mortality, and that as a patient experiences more of these events, the risks increase. Thus, patients with cirrhosis may be further subclassified more discretely into separate stages of disease. ▶ Fig. 3.2 shows an example of this progression risk based on a cohort of patients followed in a liver unit; the cases have been subclassified into five discrete stages, and transition rates have been calculated.[8]

3.2 Anatomy of Portal Hypertension

Portal hypertension develops as a complication of resistance to portal blood flow (▶ Fig. 3.3). This resistance most often occurs within the liver (as in cases of cirrhosis) but can also be prehepatic (as in cases of portal vein thrombosis) or posthepatic, in which an obstruction to outflow of the liver exists (as in cases of Budd–Chiari syndrome) (▶ Table 3.2).[9] Portal hypertension can be further subdivided into presinusoidal, sinusoidal, and postsinusoidal pressure elevations.

3.3 Noncirrhotic Portal Hypertension

Although considerably less common than portal hypertension in the setting of cirrhosis, noncirrhotic portal hypertension can occur in patients with certain vascular disorders. These cases can be classified by the site of blood flow obstruction (prehepatic, hepatic, or posthepatic). In patients with noncirrhotic portal hypertension, the hepatic venous pressure gradient (HVPG) is typically normal or minimally increased and liver function is usually preserved.

The incidence of noncirrhotic portal hypertension varies across the globe. For instance, this condition is very common among men in their second and third decades of life in India and is possibly responsible for almost one-third of all variceal bleeding episodes in this population,[10] whereas in Japan it is more common among women in their fourth decade of life.

A number of etiologies for noncirrhotic portal hypertension have been proposed, including chronic infections, exposure to certain medications or toxins, the presence of a hypercoagulable condition such as thrombophilia, and the presence of immunological or genetic disorders.[9] In Europe and the United States, other etiologies include congenital hepatic fibrosis and nodular regenerative hyperplasia, often seen in patients who have been treated with a number of chemotherapeutic agents or immunosuppressants.[11] Regardless of the inciting event, these injuries are thought to result in obstruction of the

Table 3.1 Survival in patients with cirrhosis by stage of liver disease[7]

	Compensated cirrhosis		Decompensated cirrhosis	
	Stage 1	Stage 2	Stage 3	Stage 4
Clinical features	No varices, no ascites	Varices, no ascites	Ascites with or without varices	Bleeding with or without ascites
1-year mortality rate	1%	3%	20%	57%
1-year rate of progression	7%	6.6%	7.6%	

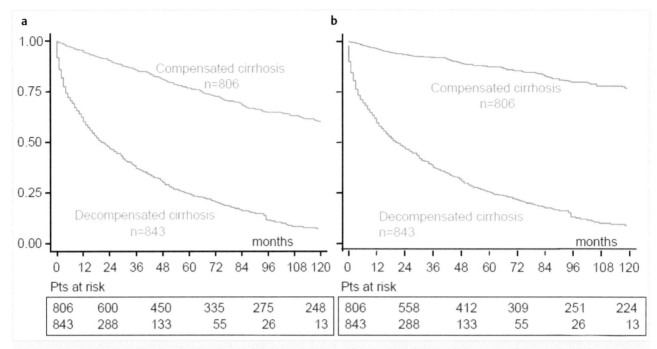

Fig. 3.1 Survival according to degree of symptoms (compensated vs. decompensated cirrhosis). **(a)** At initial diagnosis. **(b)** Among patients remaining in a compensated vs. decompensated state.[7] Survival based on presence or absence of decompensation. **(a)** divides patients by the presence of symptoms at initial presentation; **(b)** divides patients into those who remained asymptomatic vs. those who developed decompensation over the course of follow-up.

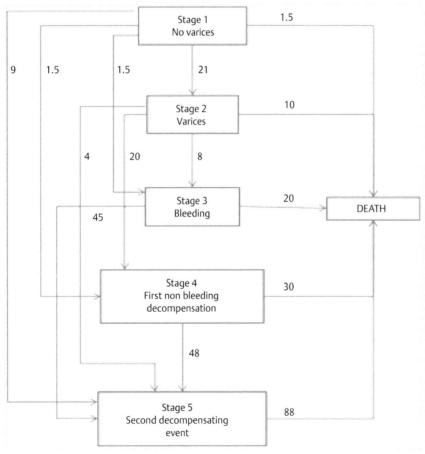

Fig. 3.2 Rates over 5 years of developing progressive liver disease among patients with cirrhosis. This was derived from the long-term follow-up of almost 500 patients with various stages of cirrhosis who were diagnosed between 1981 and 1984, broken down by clinical stages. The arrows represent the progression of liver disease, and the numbers the percentage of patients progressing to the stage over 5 years of follow-up.[8]

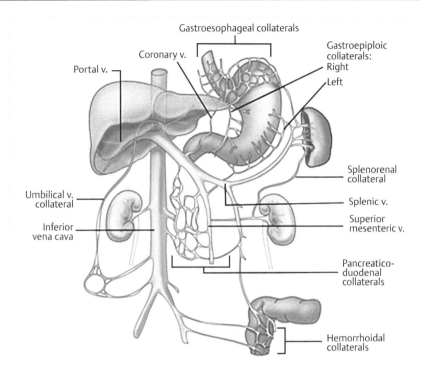

Gastroesophageal collaterals

Coronary v.

Portal v.

Gastroepiploic collaterals: Right Left

Splenorenal collateral

Splenic v.

Superior mesenteric v.

Umbilical v. collateral

Inferior vena cava

Pancreatico-duodenal collaterals

Hemorrhoidal collaterals

Fig. 3.3 Normal and abnormal portal venous anatomy. (Reproduced with permission from Middleton WD, Robinson KA. Ultrasound assessment of the hepatic vasculature. Available online at: https://radiologykey.com/ultrasound-assessment-of-the-hepatic-vasculature/.)

Table 3.2 Causes of portal hypertension[9]

Prehepatic	Congenital portal vein atresia
	Intraluminal obstruction (thrombus, neoplasia)
	Thrombosis
	Malignancy
	Myeloproliferative disorders
	Genetic prothrombotic predisposition
	Inflammatory event (pancreatitis)
	Intra-abdominal infection
	Extraluminal vascular compression
	Pancreatic malignancy
	Retroperitoneal fibrosis
Intrahepatic	Presinusoidal such as early schistosomiasis, or primary biliary cirrhosis
	Idiopathic portal hypertension
	Cystic fibrosis
	Sinusoidal
	Acute/chronic viral hepatitis
	Acute alcoholic hepatitis
	Nodular regenerative hyperplasia
	Infiltrative disorders (e.g., lymphoproliferative and myeloproliferative diseases)
	Postsinusoidal such as veno-occlusive disease (sinusoidal obstruction syndrome), graft versus host disease, chemotherapeutic agents used before hematopoietic stem transplant including 6-mercaptopurine, oxaliplatin, tacrolimus, and azathioprine
Posthepatic	Budd–Chiari syndrome
	Myeloproliferative disorders leading to thrombosis
	Genetic prothrombotic predisposition (JAK2, antiphospholipid syndrome, factor 5 Leiden, prothrombin gene mutation)
	Congenital webs
	Vena cava syndrome
	Extraluminal vascular compression
	Congestion from right heart failure, constrictive pericarditis, or pulmonary hypertension

extrahepatic portal vein or microinfarction of the small- or medium-sized portal veins.

Clinicians must be able to distinguish between cirrhotic and noncirrhotic portal hypertension, as the approaches to treatment and prognosis are different for each entity. For example, patients with portal vein thrombosis (a presinusoidal cause of portal hypertension) are at high risk of developing bleeding but tend to have entirely preserved hepatic synthetic function; as a result, these patients tend to have a much better chance of surviving a variceal bleed than patients with decompensated alcoholic cirrhosis.[12,13,14]

3.4 Normal Anatomy/Physiology

To understand the derangements of the portal circulation, one must first understand normal liver histology, particularly the spaces between the hepatocytes and the liver sinusoids, in which much of the molecular transport into the hepatocytes takes place and where the hepatic stellate cells are found.[15] These cells store fat-soluble vitamins but also have the ability to transform into activated cells that play a key role in chronic liver injury.

The liver receives approximately 25% of the total resting cardiac output and has a dual blood supply: the hepatic artery supplies approximately 25% of the total and the portal vein supplies the remainder. This blood is passed to the sinusoids, composed of one discontinuous layer of fenestrated endothelial cells, which are meant to function as low-pressure vascular channels, allowing blood to percolate across the hepatocytes before being delivered to the central veins. The total hepatic blood flow from both sources is typically 800 to 1,200 mL/min, or approximately 100 mL/min per 100 g of liver weight.[16,17] These two distinct sources of blood (oxygen-rich arterial blood from the hepatic artery and nutrient-rich blood from the portal vein) blend in

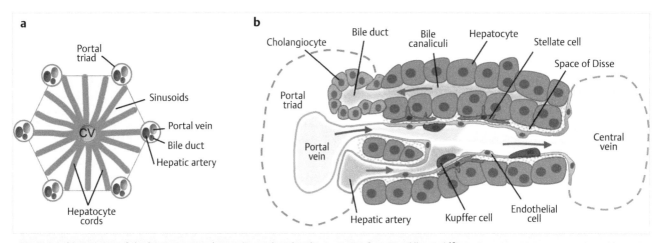

Fig. 3.4 (a,b) Anatomy of the liver microcirculation. (Reproduced with permission from Gordillo et al.[18])

the sinusoids, and the overall perfusion pressure is maintained by the hepatic arterial buffer response (▶ Fig. 3.4).[18]

The space between the sinusoidal endothelium and hepatocytes is the space of Disse, where the resident macrophages of the liver (Kupffer cells) and the hepatic stellate cells (Ito cells) are located. Because of the presence of fenestrae between the sinusoidal endothelial cells, there is free flow of sinusoidal blood into the space of Disse. This arrangement has important consequences; in the healthy liver, plasma that collects in the space of Disse flows back toward the portal tracts, collecting in lymphatic vessels and forming a large fraction of the body's lymph. However, in case of cirrhosis, the obstruction to flow results in overaccumulation of lymph, which presents as ascites. The stellate cells, which are typically quiescent cells that store vitamin A, may respond to injury by transforming into an activated form, proliferating and causing contraction and secretion of collagen. These stellate cells are therefore central to the development and maintenance of portal hypertension.[19]

3.5 Definition and Measurement

The pressure in the portal vein is difficult to measure directly. A close estimate, however, can be obtained by measuring the wedged hepatic venous pressure, which estimates the sinusoidal pressure. This technique was described in 1951 by Myers and Taylor.[20]

In this procedure, a balloon-tipped catheter is introduced via a transjugular approach and advanced into the hepatic veins, effectively occluding hepatic flow; this results in a continuous column of fluid between the catheter and the sinusoid, which can be measured. The gradient that exists between the wedged hepatic venous pressure and the free hepatic venous pressure, reflected in the intra-abdominal vena caval pressure, represents the resistance to flow across the liver.[21,22] Portal hypertension is diagnosed when the resistance to blood flow across the liver, defined as the difference between the wedged hepatic venous pressure (a measure of the flow into the liver from the portal vein) and the free hepatic pressure, is more than 5 mm Hg.[23] Clinically significant portal hypertension typically does not become manifest until the gradient is at least twice that.[24,25]

This indirect measurement of portal pressure can be performed at the same time as a transjugular biopsy. In patients with suspected advanced liver disease, this approach is helpful not only in establishing a histologic diagnosis but also in assessing prognosis. Some have described this technique as a "splanchnic sphygmomanometer" that can be used to monitor the effect of therapy and assess the risk of bleeding. As this field has evolved, it has become increasingly clear that a threshold HVPG exists that may predict the likelihood of a patient developing variceal bleeding (initial or recurrent), ascites, or other end points that define decompensation.[26] The importance of the HVPG, which is a function of both the fixed and dynamic elements in cirrhosis, has been widely accepted, as this measurement conveys important prognostic information for patients with compensated cirrhosis, variceal bleeding, or decompensation. The HVPG has been recommended as a validated surrogate outcome measure for clinical trials in portal hypertension.[27] Moreover, direct measurement of the HVPG has been used to predict the risk of development of esophageal varices,[25] to predict outcomes in cases of acute variceal bleeding,[28] and to assess the prognosis of patients with recurrent hepatitis C after liver transplant.[29] Several authorities have recommended the routine use of HVPG measurement to help manage portal hypertension. However, HVPG measurement is invasive, expensive, and associated with a small but real incidence of complications.

3.6 Overview of Physiology/ Pathophysiology of Cirrhosis/ Portal Hypertension

At the macro level, portal hypertension can be understood in terms of the laws of physics governing flow, or Ohm's law: pressure = vascular resistance × blood flow. The first event that occurs in the pathway to portal hypertension is an increase in resistance to flow, in part as a result of the disruption of the normal venous channels with the accumulation of progressive fibrosis.[30]

The resistance to flow is proportional to the length of the blood vessel and the viscosity of the blood and inversely proportional to the radius to the fourth power. Because vessel length and blood viscosity are essentially fixed, the radius of the blood vessels becomes the most important driver of portal pressure, and changes in a blood vessel's diameter—or by extension, cumulatively throughout the whole liver—are the biggest drivers of resistance since the radius term is raised to the fourth power. Thus, if a vessel's size were reduced by half, there would be a 16-fold increase in resistance. Blood flow, however, is also markedly altered in cirrhosis.

As pressure increases across the portal venous system, an extensive network of portosystemic collaterals develops, diverting a large fraction of portal blood to the systemic circulation and bypassing the liver. Cirrhosis also tends to be accompanied by an increase in the presence of vasodilators. These vasodilators perpetuate a hyperkinetic systemic circulation, with reduced arterial pressure and peripheral resistance and increased cardiac output. This was first described in detail by Kowalski and Abelmann,[31] who reported that patients with cirrhosis typically presented with the signs and symptoms of "warm extremities, cutaneous vascular spiders, wide pulse pressure, and capillary pulsations in the nail beds." This set of symptoms is sometimes referred to as "warm shock" and is now considered one of the hallmarks of cirrhosis.

A secondary event that occurs in all forms of portal hypertension is the emergence of an expanded plasma volume. This expansion of plasma volume is caused by renal sodium retention, which precedes the increase in cardiac output. The expanded blood volume represents a negative feedback loop and serves to further increase portal pressure.

Portal venous inflow is itself driven by the hyperdynamic circulation of cirrhosis and by increased plasma volume (▶ Fig. 3.5).[32,33]

Historically, two theories regarding the evolution of portal hypertension were proposed, referred to as the "backward flow theory" and the "forward flow theory."[34] The former theory speculated that the progressive increase in resistance across the portal venous stem would lead to a relatively hypodynamic circulation in the mesentery, which is seen in early cirrhosis.[35] However, in later stages, there is strong evidence of a hyperdynamic splanchnic circulation, with an increase in portal inflow driving the development of portal hypertension[33,36] (hence the "forward flow" theory).

Splanchnic vasodilatation itself can be explained by the combination of increased local vasodilator production and increased systemic vasodilators in the circulation, both of which lead in turn to a decreased response to vasoconstrictors.[37] Both the amount of portal venous inflow to the liver and the degree of resistance to flow can be modified.[38] The recognition that this was the case greatly influenced our current understanding of how patients with cirrhosis should be cared for clinically.

3.7 Hepatic Resistance

Although most forms of cirrhosis encompass aspects of both increased resistance to blood flow and increased splanchnic flow, increased intrahepatic resistance to flow is the critical element in most cases of portal hypertension. This may occur at a presinusoidal, sinusoidal, or postsinusoidal level. Cirrhosis is often thought of as a fixed obstruction, based on deposition of scar and development of regenerative nodules that distort normal patterns of blood flow. In support of this concept, histologic studies that have compared the extent of fibrosis with measurements of portal hypertension have demonstrated specific features, including small nodularity and septal thickness, to be independently predictive of clinically significant portal hypertension.[39]

However, research has shown all of intrahepatic resistance is not fixed. Early seminal studies demonstrated that there was a

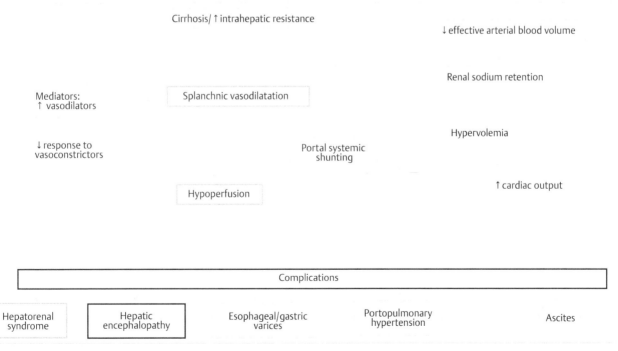

Cirrhosis/ ↑ intrahepatic resistance

↓ effective arterial blood volume

Renal sodium retention

Mediators:
↑ vasodilators

Splanchnic vasodilatation

↓ response to vasoconstrictors

Portal systemic shunting

Hypervolemia

↑ cardiac output

Hypoperfusion

Complications

| Hepatorenal syndrome | Hepatic encephalopathy | Esophageal/gastric varices | Portopulmonary hypertension | Ascites |

Fig. 3.5 Portal hypertension: pathophysiology.

dynamic component involved in the total resistance to flow across the liver, as the blood flow in an isolated rat liver in this research was responsive to vasodilators.[40] These vasodilators were thought to be acting on the myofibroblasts in perivenous and perisinusoidal locations. The extent of vasodilatation, moreover, is substantial and therefore has clinical implications, accounting for as much as 40% of the total resistance across the liver.[41]

A large body of work has shown that the hepatic stellate cells play a major role in the physiologic control of portal flow. Because of the contractile properties and perisinusoidal location of these cells, they may regulate sinusoidal blood flow and resistance and thus may serve as a potentially modifiable target in portal hypertension. The microenvironment that regulates hepatic stellate cell contractility is a control point that determines the relative degree of relaxation or constriction. Several studies have shown that vascular mediators (e.g., angiotensin II) may act to stimulate proliferation of hepatic stellate cells and increase their ability to contract.[42] Moreover, stellate cells likely participate in the immunologic response to injury, both as targets and as sources of a number of autocrine and paracrine signals for other cells of the immune response.[19]

Although multiple components of the normal hemodynamics of the liver are deranged in portal hypertension, it is likely that the hyperdynamic circulation of cirrhosis is driven primarily by abnormalities in vasodilatation, with relative imbalance in nitric oxide (NO) as the primary effector; this was first postulated in 1991 by Vallance and Moncada.[43] Multiple studies have since demonstrated the central role of NO in creating and sustaining the hyperdynamic circulation. This fact takes on particular significance in cirrhosis because of the possibility that NO may be a modifiable factor that could affect the outcome of portal hypertension. Extensive studies have investigated the control of NO synthesis and the potential counter-regulatory agents that promote constriction.[44,45,46,47,48]

3.8 Mechanisms of Portal Hypertension

The resistance to flow and the amount of flow through the portal venous system can be envisioned as a two-compartment model, each of which has its own modifiers of circulatory hemodynamics: (1) the intrahepatic circulation, which reflects the longstanding injury related to chronic liver disease in terms of the accumulation of endothelial injury and scar tissue, and (2) the changes in splanchnic blood flow, which feeds the portal system. Each of these is modified by a number of mechanisms and agents that interact with these pathways (▶ Table 3.3,

Table 3.3 Factors affecting intrahepatic flow

Vasoconstrictors	Vasodilators
Norepinephrine	Nitric oxide
Thrombin	Carbon monoxide
Angiotensin II	Heme oxygenase
Endothelin	Hydrogen sulfide
Prostanoids	
Leukotrienes	
Thromboxane A2	

Table 3.4 Factors affecting splanchnic inflow[49,50,51,52]

Enhanced angiogenic factors	Antagonists
Vascular endothelial growth factor	Sorafenib/sunitinib
Platelet-derived growth factor	Vasohibin
Reduced nicotinamide adenine dinucleotide phosphate (NADPH) oxidase	
Cannabinoids	
Cyclooxygenase	
Apelin (endogenous ligand of angiotensinlike receptor 1)	
Microparticles	
Placental growth factor	

▶ Table 3.4, ▶ Table 3.5). The cumulative effect of these pathways is what can be seen clinically.

By far, the most important mediator of intrahepatic resistance is NO. NO is a gas that diffuses across the cell membranes and can therefore act in an autocrine or paracrine fashion. It is produced from the amino acid L-arginine by a family of NO synthases, including an endothelial NO synthase (eNOS) responsible for most of the physiologic production of NO, a neuronal form of synthase (nNOS), and an inducible form of NO synthase (iNOS). When produced, NO binds to soluble guanylate cyclase, resulting in increased levels of cyclic guanosine monophosphate, which in turn results in an increase in cytosolic Ca^{++} and leads to relaxation of the vascular wall.[55]

The regulation of NO is primarily controlled by regulation of the synthases; synthesis is activated by increases in intracellular calcium or by fluid shear stress and insulinlike growth factor.

Phosphorylation of eNOS by the serine/threonine protein kinase Akt activates the enzyme, leading to NO production.[56] NO in turn is inhibited by caveolin 1, which acts as a molecular

Table 3.5 Factors affecting splanchnic vasodilation[53,54]

Vascular endothelial growth factor

Nitric oxide

Prostacyclin

Carbon monoxide

Endocannabinoids

Endothelium-derived hyperpolarizing factor

Hydrogen sulfate

Glucagon

Adrenomedullin

Calcitonin gene-related peptide

Cyclooxygenase-derived prostanoids (prostaglandin H2, thromboxane A2)

Vasoactive intestinal peptide

Tumor necrosis factor/bacterial translocation → endotoxin

Substance P

Estrogen

Cholecystokinin

Adenosine

Bile acids

Ammonia

Histamine

chaperone and serves to regulate production and drive inactivation of NO.[57]

eNOS is regulated by complex protein–protein interactions and posttranslational modification.[58] Among positive regulator proteins, Hsp9062 and serine/threonine kinases Akt/protein kinase B contribute to the activation of eNOS in the splanchnic arterial circulation.[59] Akt/protein kinase B directly phosphorylates eNOS at Ser1177 (human) or Ser1179 (bovine) and enhances its ability to generate NO.[56,60,61,62]

Although NO synthesis does take place in cirrhotic livers (with normal levels of eNOS mRNA and protein), several mechanisms have been proposed to explain the differences in NO produced in cirrhotic liver: there is an increased expression of the proteins responsible for inactivation (caveolin), and the overall production of NO is not sufficient to overcome the increase in inflow and powerful mechanisms of vasoconstriction in these patients.

Another important vasodilator is carbon monoxide (CO), which is produced by heme oxygenases (HOs) in the process of breaking down heme to biliverdin and serves as an activator of guanylate cyclase. Two isoforms of HO have been identified: HO-1 and HO-2. HO-1 is inducible by multiple agents, whereas HO-2 is constitutively expressed.[63,64] HO levels tend to be higher in patients with liver disease (particularly in those with cirrhosis), leading to high CO levels, which correlate with increases in cardiac output and inversely with systemic vascular resistance.[65] Portal inflow is dictated by the degree of splanchnic vasodilation, the other vascular bed central to the clinical syndromes brought on by portal hypertension[38]; this in turn is fueled by the hyperdynamic circulation and the increase in intravascular volume.

The same mediators that drive vascular resistance and vasodilatation are active in the splanchnic circulation, including NO, which is produced in relative excess. Studies have demonstrated that metabolites of NO are relatively increased in patients with cirrhosis,[66] which is thought to result from increases in shear stress (perhaps through upregulation of vascular endothelial growth factor [VEGF] expression) and from bacterial translocation and portosystemic shunting, all of which characterize cirrhosis. A number of studies have also suggested an association between the levels of NO (or its metabolites) and the degree of decompensation of liver disease, finding, for example, higher levels in patients with Child–Pugh class C cirrhosis than in patients with earlier stages of liver disease and in patients with peritonitis versus those with ascites but without peritonitis. Many of these same mediators are also involved in angiogenesis,[37] which plays a major role in the development of portal systemic shunts but also contributes to the progression of fibrosis within the liver.[67,68]

Other major players in this system include the vasodilator prostacyclin (PGI2), which acts by stimulating adenylyl cyclase and increasing the generation of cyclic adenosine monophosphate.[69] Glucagon also plays a central role in splanchnic vasodilatation, acting to relax vascular smooth muscle and decrease the effect of endogenous vasoconstrictors. Glucagon levels in turn are relatively high because of overproduction and decreased clearance. Hydrogen sulfide (H_2S) may also be important in vasodilatation. Preliminary studies have found that patients with portal hypertension had significantly lower serum H_2S concentrations and that disease severity and the portal vein diameter (a proxy for the degree of portal hypertension) were inversely correlated with H_2S concentration.[70]

Endocannabinoids may also be important mediators of the hyperkinetic circulation, partly through activation of NO production. Endocannabinoid levels are increased in patients with cirrhosis, and studies using blockade of the cannabinoid receptors in vascular smooth muscle have demonstrated improvements in systemic blood pressure.[71] Unfortunately, these receptor blockers have not yet become available clinically.

Increased levels of tumor necrosis factor alpha (TNFα) have been found in multiple liver diseases and are thought to reflect the interaction between endotoxin from the gut and immune function (via the pathogen-associated molecular pattern molecules and damage-associated molecular patterns) by their effects on mononuclear cells. In alcoholic hepatitis, the presence of detectable TNF conveys a poor prognosis, but the overall levels are elevated in liver diseases associated with portal hypertension.[72,73,74] The mechanism by which TNFα induces NO is unclear but may be via increasing the gene expression and activity of one of the key cofactors of NO synthesis, tetrahydrobiopterin BH4 GTP-cyclohydrolase I, in endothelial cells,[75,76] as enhanced BH4 production directly increases eNOS-derived NO bioavailability.

Adrenomedullin is another vasodilator that may act via effects on NO production; it phosphorylates and activates Akt and increases cGMP production and has been found to circulate in increased levels in patients with cirrhosis.[77]

Other agents that have been tested based on the pathophysiologic understanding of portal hypertension include angiotensin receptor antagonists,[78] which have been shown to improve the generation of NO and hepatic endothelial dysfunction, perhaps via an effect on developing hepatic fibrosis.[79,80]

Balancing these changes in vasodilator levels is an accompanying increase in the relative amounts of circulating vasoconstrictors. A number of physiologic mediators have been implicated in this process, most notably endothelin 1 (ET-1) and ET-3, both of which are produced in the splanchnic circulation and found in increased concentration in cirrhotic livers,[81] as are their receptors. ET-1 has been shown to increase intrahepatic resistance, as have a number of other mediators, including norepinephrine, cysteinyl leukotrienes, thromboxane A2, and angiotensin, as well as the sympathetic nervous system.[82,83]

3.9 Prognostic Scoring Systems

Although it would seem intuitive that the optimal mechanisms to monitor the development and progression of end-stage liver disease would use specific markers for fibrosis, or liver histology, the science of quantitative fibrosis measurement is still in development.[84,85] Markers of fibrosis and fibrinolysis, both singly and jointly (including a vast array of markers, such as amino terminal propeptide of type III collagen, matrix metalloproteinase, tissue inhibitor of matrix metalloproteinase, hyaluronic acid, type IV collagen, serum osteopontin, TGF beta, and YKL-40), have been studied and their levels correlated with liver disease, particularly in patients with advanced disease.[86]

A number of fibrosis panels have been developed and validated in several populations, including the ELF panel,[87] FibroTest/FibroSure,[88,89] and HepaScore (▶ Table 3.6). These panels may be useful in estimating the degree of fibrosis, but

Table 3.6 Combination panels of biologic markers to estimate fibrosis[86]

Elf panel	FibroMeter	FibroTest/FibroSure	HepaScore
Hyaluronic acid	Platelet count	Alpha-2-globulin	Age
Amino terminal propeptide of type III procollagen	Alpha-2-macroglobulin	Alpha-2-macroglobulin	Sex
Tissue inhibitor of metalloproteinases-1	Aspartate aminotransferase	Gamma globulin	Total bilirubin
	Age	Apolipoprotein A	Gamma-glutamyl transferase
	Prothrombin time index	Gamma-glutamyl transferase	Hyaluronic acid
	Hyaluronic acid	Total bilirubin	Alpha-2-macroglobulin
	Blood urea nitrogen		

their utility may be disease specific,[90,91] and their role in estimating clinical outcomes is not yet clear.[92] Additionally, the serologic scoring systems tend to be more effective in identifying cases at the extremes of the histologic spectrum (e.g., separating patients with no significant fibrosis from those with cirrhosis) but less useful in distinguishing finer gradations across the histologic spectrum.

Multiple scoring systems that rely on clinical characteristics and routinely collected laboratory data have been used to classify patients with liver disease. The best known and longest used is the Child–Turcotte–Pugh (CTP) score, which was originally derived as an estimator of prognosis in patients undergoing shunt surgery and was later modified to estimate prognosis in patients who presented with variceal bleeding. The original Child–Turcotte score incorporated a measure of nutritional status ("excellent" vs. "good" vs. "poor, wasting"),[93] which was replaced in Pugh's modification with prothrombin time. The severity of a patient's disease is established by adding the points for each factor; the sum is used to separate patients into three distinct classes: CTP class A (5–6 points), CTP class B (7–9 points), and CTP class C, the most severely ill group (10–15 points) (▶ Table 3.7). The overall likelihood of survival (even in patients who did not present with acute decompensation) can also be estimated based on the CTP score (▶ Fig. 3.6).[7]

Although the CTP score is useful, it was clear from the outset that other factors, including renal function, may have prognostic significance and may allow for better estimates of short- and long-term outcomes.[95,96,97] Therefore, another prognostic score, devised initially to estimate prognosis in patients undergoing placement of a transjugular intrahepatic portosystemic shunt (TIPS) and later generalized to all patients with liver disease, was developed: the Model for End-Stage Liver Disease (MELD) score. This score combines the values for creatinine, total

bilirubin, and international normalized ratio (INR) into the following formula[98]:

$$MELD = 3.8 \ln (\text{bilirubin mg/dL}) + 11.2 \ln (INR) \\ + 9.6 \ln (\text{creatinine mg/dL}),$$

where ln = natural logarithm. The initial version[99] also included a variable for the etiology of liver disease.

The MELD score has several distinct advantages over other estimators of prognosis: it is linear, unlike the CTP score (which is categorical), and thereby allows a more nuanced view of an individual patient's risk. For instance, some patients with Child–Pugh class C disease are clearly sicker than others. A patient with a bilirubin level of 12 mg/dL is more appropriately recognized as being more ill than a patient with a bilirubin level of 4 mg/dL—yet no recognition of this is incorporated into the CTP score. The MELD score also removes the subjective nature of some elements of the physical examination from the equation (e.g., degree of ascites or hepatic encephalopathy), thus making it a more easily generalizable score (▶ Fig. 3.7).[100,101] These manifestations of decompensation may add independent information to the prognosis, but with their removal, the MELD score can be adopted for other uses, such as determining the allocation of organs for possible liver transplant candidates (which has been the case in the United States since 2002). Serum sodium levels have recently been added to the MELD score for this purpose.

Both the CTP and the MELD score have been tested extensively in a number of clinical circumstances, and each has distinct advantages; overall, when considering the case of an individual patient, they are both useful.[102] Multiple attempts have been made to better understand the course of patients with cirrhosis and to improve the prognostic ability of these early scoring systems. Multiple clinical variables are frequently included in these prognostic determinations (▶ Table 3.8).

Several nonliver-specific scores have been suggested for critically ill patients with cirrhosis (e.g., the APACHE score or the Sequential Organ Failure Assessment score).[103] A separate score has recently been proposed for patients with acute-on-chronic liver failure who are hospitalized in the intensive care unit: the Chronic Liver Failure-Sequential Organ Failure Assessment score, which includes the variables of age and white blood cell count. This score also includes laboratory data (including bilirubin level, creatinine level, and INR), clinical parameters, the presence of hepatic encephalopathy, mean arterial pressure, and oxygenation level.

Table 3.7 Factors included in Child–Turcotte–Pugh score[94]

	Score		
	1	2	3
Encephalopathy	None	1–2	3–4
Ascites	None	Mild	Moderate
Bilirubin, mg/dL	1–2	2–3	>3
Albumin, g/dL	>3.5	2.8–3.5	<2.8
Prothrombin time, s	1–4 (1.7)	4–6 (1.7–2.3)	>6 (>2.3)

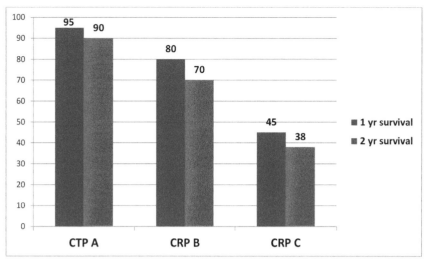

Fig. 3.6 One- and two-year survival rates in patients with Child–Pugh class A, B, or C disease.[7] These are drawn from a review of 118 studies evaluating predictors of mortality in patients with mortality.

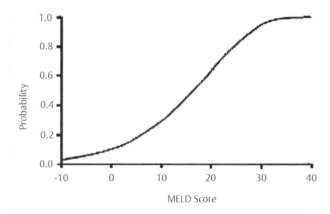

Fig. 3.7 Survival curve for MELD vs. mortality.[101] Three-month mortality among patients with cirrhosis, classified by MELD score.

Table 3.8 Clinical predictors of outcomes in patients with cirrhosis[7]

Compensated cirrhosis	Decompensated cirrhosis
Age	Child–Turcotte–Pugh score
Albumin level	Presence of hepatic encephalopathy
Total bilirubin level	Presence of hepatocellular carcinoma
Platelet count	Presence of bleeding
Sex	Creatinine level
Prothrombin time	Prothrombin time
Child–Turcotte–Pugh score	Albumin level
Presence of vascular spiders	Blood urea nitrogen level/ presence of azotemia
Spleen size	Presence of ascites
Presence of varices	Total bilirubin level
Gamma globulin	Age

More recently, there has been an attempt to measure HVPG directly as a prognostic marker.[104] The concept that the degree of portal hypertension might improve the prognostic ability of the CTP score was first recognized in an early study of the concept of "preprimary prophylaxis" of esophageal varices (i.e., the possibility that medical therapy might not just delay the onset of bleeding but might even halt the development of varices that would place a patient at risk of bleeding).[25] In this study, a baseline measurement of HVPG > 10 or those who had a decrease in HVPG by > 10% at 1 year were shown to predict the likelihood of a patient developing varices or variceal bleeding, even among patients followed for as long as 6 years (▶ Fig. 3.8).

Similar findings were noted in a study evaluating outcomes in patients who were treated for hepatitis C and had a sustained virologic response, which typically is associated with a substantially improved prognosis and a lower likelihood of liver-related mortality. Unfortunately, for patients with cirrhosis and clinically significant portal hypertension (defined as HVPG > 10), there was still a strong and disproportionate risk of decompensation at 1, 5, and 7 years of 3, 19, and 22%, respectively.[105] These data suggest that even after controlling for other risk factors for mortality in liver disease, HVPG is a useful predictor of outcome.

Although the direct measurement of HVPG represents the gold standard for prognosis, this technique is inconvenient, expensive, and invasive, leading researchers to investigate other methods to estimate portal pressures noninvasively, including transient elastography.[106,107] Some preliminary data have demonstrated that these measurements of liver stiffness may be useful not just for assessing fibrosis but also for predicting the natural history of liver decompensation.[108,109]

The HVPG has been most strongly linked to the risk of developing esophageal varices and ascites,[110] and interventions that decrease HVPG have been shown to reduce the risk of these hemodynamic complications.[38] Surprisingly, however, a large body of evidence suggests that measurements of HVPG can also be used to predict other outcomes that might be less anticipated,[111] such as the development of hepatocellular carcinoma.[112] The data regarding the association between HVPG and outcomes are probably most clearly defined by evidence relating the association of the hemodynamic response to interventions, as measured by serial HVPG measurements and outcomes.[113]

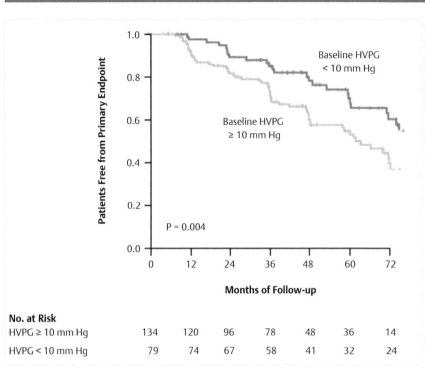

Fig. 3.8 Probability of not developing either esophageal varices or variceal bleeding, according to the HVPG.[25] Patients were followed for more than 5 years in a clinical trial of timolol to prevent the development of varices, and had documented portal hypertension (with measurements of HVPG of at least 6 mm Hg) on entry into the study—subdivided by their baseline HVPG.

No. at Risk

HVPG ≥ 10 mm Hg	134	120	96	78	48	36	14
HVPG < 10 mm Hg	79	74	67	58	41	32	24

3.10 Clinical Complications of Cirrhosis

Ascites is the most common manifestation of cirrhosis, occurring in 50% of patients over 10 years of follow-up.[114] Ascites itself may be further complicated by downstream consequences, including spontaneous bacterial peritonitis, hepatorenal syndrome, and hepatic hydrothorax. Other clinical manifestations of portal hypertension include gastrointestinal bleeding from several etiologies, most notably esophageal varices or gastric varices, as well as portal hypertensive gastropathy.

In many ways, portal hypertension reflects widespread vascular dysfunction, and other complications of cirrhosis (including hepatic encephalopathy, portopulmonary hypertension, and hepatopulmonary syndrome) should be considered part of this spectrum.

Although most studies of patients with portal hypertension have demonstrated a slow, almost inexorable, decline and inevitable progression to the development of clinical decompensation, it is important to bear in mind that some interventions to treat the underlying cause of liver disease, even at the point of cirrhosis, may also have a large effect on the eventual outcome. This was first demonstrated in a study of patients with alcoholic liver disease, in which large differences were seen between those who were able to become abstinent versus those who continued to drink (▶ Fig. 3.9).[115]

Similar rates of improvement in prognosis have been observed in patients with other chronic liver diseases that can be successfully treated, including chronic hepatitis B,[116] hepatitis C,[117] and autoimmune hepatitis.[118]

3.10.1 Gastrointestinal Bleeding from Esophageal Varices

Esophageal varices often develop in patients with liver disease and portal hypertension, usually once the HVPG is higher than 10 mm Hg, and the likelihood of developing varices increases with worsening severity of liver disease; some studies have found that esophageal varices are present in 50% of patients with cirrhosis at diagnosis. These varices tend to enlarge in 10 to 20% of patients within 2 years.[119,120] In addition, the likelihood of bleeding increases with increasing severity of liver disease; patients with more severe liver disease as measured by the CTP score are more likely to bleed than those with earlier stage cirrhosis—even when the size of varices and other stigmata are similar.[121] Among all patients with liver disease, 20 to 30% will develop bleeding over a 2-year time frame.[32]

The primary source supplying blood to the esophageal varices is the left gastric vein, which divides into a posterior branch (which drains into the azygous vein) and an anterior branch (from which varices arise). Anatomic studies of the gastroesophageal junction have defined four distinct areas of venous drainage: the gastric zone; the palisade zone with parallel vessels in groups, mainly within the lamina propria; the perforating zone, where blood is channeled into extrinsic veins; and the truncal zone (▶ Fig. 3.10).[122,123] Flow within the palisade zone can be bidirectional, perhaps related to changes in pressure during the respiratory cycle, and is thought to serve as a buffering or watershed area between the portal and azygous system; this may also be the site at which there is maximal resistance to the increased flow of portal blood in patients with portal hypertension. Turbulent flow in the perforating veins may explain the frequency of bleeding at that point in the esophagus.[124]

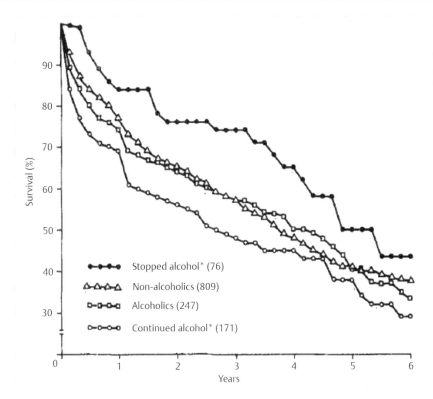

Fig. 3.9 Survival of patients with cirrhosis— divided into those with nonalcoholic and those with alcoholic liver disease. Survival among alcoholics was further divided into those who continued or stopped alcohol abuse.

Legend:
- Stopped alcohol* (76)
- Non-alcoholics (809)
- Alcoholics (247)
- Continued alcohol* (171)

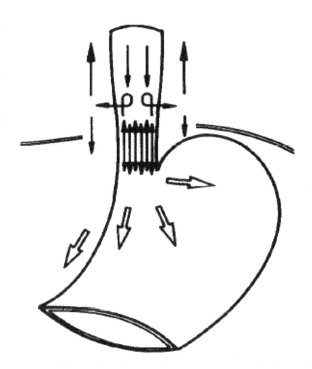

Fig. 3.10 Normal venous circulation of the gastroesophageal junction.[122]

The risk of variceal bleeding varies depending on the etiology of the patient's liver disease, with a higher likelihood of bleeding among patients with alcoholic cirrhosis than among those with viral hepatitis leading to cirrhosis.[125] Acute variceal bleeding can be catastrophic, with a very high mortality rate; mortality rates of 25 to 35% have been reported even in more recent studies.[126] A number of studies have attempted to identify predictors of first variceal bleeding among patients with esophageal varices; not surprisingly, the severity of a patient's underlying liver disease, as measured by the Child–Pugh score, has been shown to consistently predict the likelihood of bleeding.[121] In addition, the endoscopic appearance of varices has been shown to predict the likelihood of variceal bleeding,[127] with several endoscopic stigmata correlated with an increased risk of bleeding. Larger varices are also more likely to bleed than smaller ones, which may reflect the intravariceal pressure.[121,128,129,130] Studies that have measured variceal pressure have also demonstrated a significant correlation between increasing pressures and increased risk of bleeding.[131] This physiology may be understood by examining a modification of Laplace's law, which defines the tension in the wall of the varix as being proportional to the pressure gradient between the variceal and intraesophageal pressures and the radius of the varix, and inversely proportional to the thickness of the variceal wall.[132]

Outcomes in patients with variceal bleeding have been shown to depend on a number of factors, including: the patient's age; etiology and severity of liver disease; the presence of associated conditions, including renal failure and hepatocellular carcinoma; the presence of infection or shock; the presence of portal vein thrombosis; hematocrit level; aminotransferase levels; and HVPG value.[28,133,134,135,136,137,138] An HVPG higher than 20 has been shown to have a sensitivity and specificity for predicting endoscopic treatment failure of 62 and 81%, respectively.[139] Several of these predictors have been combined into prognostic scores, including MELD scores.[140,141,142] One of the strongest predictors of rebleeding is the presence of active bleeding at the time of index endoscopy, with a 10-fold increased risk of mortality among patients with a MELD score higher than 18 compared to those not experiencing bleeding.[133]

Most recent studies suggest that initial treatment will successfully stop bleeding in approximately 90% of patients.[142,143] On average, 50% of patients will stop bleeding spontaneously, but approximately one-third of patients will develop rebleeding within 6 weeks; most of these cases will occur within 5 days of the initial bleed.[144] Each episode of bleeding is associated with significant morbidity and mortality, although these rates have improved dramatically with the introduction of better treatment options, decreasing from approximately 65 to 40%[145] and to nearly 0% in patients with CTP A or B cirrhosis. This has been attributed to decreased rebleeding rates and decreased bacterial infection rates.[126]

Interventions for patients with acute variceal bleeding include endoscopic therapy (variceal ligation or sclerotherapy), early TIPS placement, or interventional radiologic treatment, along with vasoactive drugs. Antibiotics will also decrease the risk of rebleeding[146]; the mechanism for this is not clear but likely reflects the flux of endotoxin through the portal venous flow and the downstream effects on portal pressure and liver circulation.

Vasoactive drugs that have been the most extensively evaluated include terlipressin, a derivative of vasopressin (not available in the United States), and somatostatin and its analogues (octreotide or vapreotide).[147] Various endoscopic options have been extensively evaluated and are highly effective; however, endoscopic variceal ligation or banding is associated with a lower rate of complications than endoscopic sclerotherapy and is therefore the endoscopic intervention of choice.[148,149] Endoscopic stents have been used successfully in patients with refractory bleeding, but this option is typically reserved for particularly difficult situations.[150] Combination therapy (e.g., both endoscopic and pharmacologic treatment) has also been tested, and this research has demonstrated that combined modalities are more effective than single approaches.[151,152]

The likelihood of treatment success depends on a number of factors, including the degree of portal hypertension. A number of studies evaluating the role of early TIPS placement have demonstrated a better outcome in patients with a high risk of endoscopic treatment failure, defined as those with an HVPG higher than 20 mm Hg, those with Child–Pugh class B disease and active bleeding, or those with Child–Pugh class C disease and a CTP score lower than 13.[139,153]

3.11 Conclusion

Portal hypertension is the ultimate clinical end point of most chronic liver diseases, and management of its signs and symptoms of decompensation represents a major focus for physicians caring for this challenging group of patients. The major manifestations of portal hypertension—ascites, renal dysfunction, variceal bleeding, and hepatic encephalopathy—are associated with increased morbidity and mortality, and are useful variables that allow better prognostication for individual patients. Improvements in clinical monitoring and care have resulted in some improvement in outcomes for these patients, but the molecular mechanisms and pathways that are responsible for the initiation and progression of portal hypertension are imperfectly understood. Expanding basic science advances in endothelial function and physiology are gradually being translated into applied research that holds the promise of benefit for these patients.

References

[1] Gilbert A, Villaret M. Contribution à l'étude du syndrome d'hypertension portale: cytologie des liquides d'ascite dans les cirrhoses. Compt Rend Soc Biol. 1906; 60:820–823

[2] Myers JD, Taylor WJ. Occlusive hepatic venous catheterization in the study of the normal liver, cirrhosis of the liver and noncirrhotic portal hypertension. Circulation. 1956; 13(3):368–380

[3] Vorobioff JD. Hepatic venous pressure in practice: how, when, and why. J Clin Gastroenterol. 2007; 41 Suppl 3:S336–S343

[4] Garceau AJ, Chalmers TC. The natural history of cirrhosis. I. Survival with esophageal varices. N Engl J Med. 1963; 268:469–473

[5] Bernal W, Jalan R, Quaglia A, Simpson K, Wendon J, Burroughs A. Acute-on-chronic liver failure. Lancet. 2015; 386(10003):1576–1587

[6] Jalan R, Gines P, Olson JC, et al. Acute-on chronic liver failure. J Hepatol. 2012; 57(6):1336–1348

[7] D'Amico G, Garcia-Tsao G, Pagliaro L. Natural history and prognostic indicators of survival in cirrhosis: a systematic review of 118 studies. J Hepatol. 2006; 44(1):217–231

[8] D'Amico G, Pasta L, Morabito A, et al. Competing risks and prognostic stages of cirrhosis: a 25-year inception cohort study of 494 patients. Aliment Pharmacol Ther. 2014; 39(10):1180–1193

[9] Schouten JN, Garcia-Pagan JC, Valla DC, Janssen HL. Idiopathic noncirrhotic portal hypertension. Hepatology. 2011; 54(3):1071–1081

[10] Sarin SK, Kumar A, Chawla YK, et al. Members of the APASL Working Party on Portal Hypertension. Noncirrhotic portal fibrosis/idiopathic portal hypertension: APASL recommendations for diagnosis and treatment. Hepatol Int. 2007; 1(3):398–413

[11] Khanna R, Sarin SK. Non-cirrhotic portal hypertension - diagnosis and management. J Hepatol. 2014; 60(2):421–441

[12] García-Pagán JC, Gracia-Sancho J, Bosch J. Functional aspects on the pathophysiology of portal hypertension in cirrhosis. J Hepatol. 2012; 57(2): 458–461

[13] Bosch J. Vascular deterioration in cirrhosis: the big picture. J Clin Gastroenterol. 2007; 41 Suppl 3:S247–S253

[14] Blendis L, Wong F. The hyperdynamic circulation in cirrhosis: an overview. Pharmacol Ther. 2001; 89(3):221–231

[15] Wisse E, De Zanger RB, Charels K, Van Der Smissen P, McCuskey RS. The liver sieve: considerations concerning the structure and function of endothelial fenestrae, the sinusoidal wall and the space of Disse. Hepatology. 1985; 5(4): 683–692

[16] Greenway CV, Stark RD. Hepatic vascular bed. Physiol Rev. 1971; 51(1):23–65

[17] Rappaport AM. Hepatic blood flow: morphologic aspects and physiologic regulation. Int Rev Physiol. 1980; 21:1–63

[18] Gordillo M, Evans T, Gouon-Evans V. Orchestrating liver development. Development. 2015; 142(12):2094–2108

[19] Friedman SL. Hepatic stellate cells: protean, multifunctional, and enigmatic cells of the liver. Physiol Rev. 2008; 88(1):125–172

[20] Myers JD, Taylor WJ. An estimation of portal venous pressure by occlusive catheterization of a hepatic venule. J Clin Invest. 1951; 30:662–663

[21] Groszmann RJ, Glickman M, Blei AT, Storer E, Conn HO. Wedged and free hepatic venous pressure measured with a balloon catheter. Gastroenterology. 1979; 76(2):253–258

[22] Groszmann RJ, Wongcharatrawee S. The hepatic venous pressure gradient: anything worth doing should be done right. Hepatology. 2004; 39(2):280–282

[23] Sharara AI, Rockey DC. Gastroesophageal variceal hemorrhage. N Engl J Med. 2001; 345(9):669–681

[24] Berzigotti A, Gilabert R, Abraldes JG, et al. Noninvasive prediction of clinically significant portal hypertension and esophageal varices in patients with compensated liver cirrhosis. Am J Gastroenterol. 2008; 103(5):1159–1167

[25] Groszmann RJ, Garcia-Tsao G, Bosch J, et al. Portal Hypertension Collaborative Group. Beta-blockers to prevent gastroesophageal varices in patients with cirrhosis. N Engl J Med. 2005; 353(21):2254–2261

[26] D'Amico G, Garcia-Pagan JC, Luca A, Bosch J. Hepatic vein pressure gradient reduction and prevention of variceal bleeding in cirrhosis: a systematic review. Gastroenterology. 2006; 131(5):1611–1624

[27] Gluud C, Brok J, Gong Y, Koretz RL. Hepatology may have problems with putative surrogate outcome measures. J Hepatol. 2007; 46(4):734–742

[28] Moitinho E, Escorsell A, Bandi JC, et al. Prognostic value of early measurements of portal pressure in acute variceal bleeding. Gastroenterology. 1999; 117(3):626–631

[29] Blasco A, Forns X, Carrión JA, et al. Hepatic venous pressure gradient identifies patients at risk of severe hepatitis C recurrence after liver transplantation. Hepatology. 2006; 43(3):492–499

[30] Bosch J, Groszmann RJ, Shah VH. Evolution in the understanding of the pathophysiological basis of portal hypertension: How changes in paradigm are leading to successful new treatments. J Hepatol. 2015; 62(1) Suppl: S121–S130

[31] Kowalski HJ, Abelmann WH. The cardiac output at rest in Laennec's cirrhosis. J Clin Invest. 1953; 32(10):1025–1033

[32] de Franchis R, Primignani M. Natural history of portal hypertension in patients with cirrhosis. Clin Liver Dis. 2001; 5(3):645–663

[33] Iwakiri Y, Groszmann RJ. The hyperdynamic circulation of chronic liver diseases: from the patient to the molecule. Hepatology. 2006; 43(2) Suppl 1: S121–S131

[34] Murray JF, Dawson AM, Sherlock S. Circulatory changes in chronic liver disease. Am J Med. 1958; 24(3):358–367

[35] Benoit JN, Womack WA, Hernandez L, Granger DN. "Forward" and "backward" flow mechanisms of portal hypertension. Relative contributions in the rat model of portal vein stenosis. Gastroenterology. 1985; 89(5): 1092–1096

[36] Vorobioff J, Bredfeldt JE, Groszmann RJ. Increased blood flow through the portal system in cirrhotic rats. Gastroenterology. 1984; 87(5):1120–1126

[37] Abraldes JG, Iwakiri Y, Loureiro-Silva M, Haq O, Sessa WC, Groszmann RJ. Mild increases in portal pressure upregulate vascular endothelial growth factor and endothelial nitric oxide synthase in the intestinal microcirculatory bed, leading to a hyperdynamic state. Am J Physiol Gastrointest Liver Physiol. 2006; 290(5):G980–G987

[38] Bosch J, García-Pagán JC. Complications of cirrhosis. I. Portal hypertension. J Hepatol. 2000; 32(1) Suppl:141–156

[39] Nagula S, Jain D, Groszmann RJ, Garcia-Tsao G. Histological-hemodynamic correlation in cirrhosis-a histological classification of the severity of cirrhosis. J Hepatol. 2006; 44(1):111–117

[40] Bhathal PS, Grossman HJ. Reduction of the increased portal vascular resistance of the isolated perfused cirrhotic rat liver by vasodilators. J Hepatol. 1985; 1(4):325–337

[41] Rodríguez-Vilarrupla A, Fernández M, Bosch J, García-Pagán JC. Current concepts on the pathophysiology of portal hypertension. Ann Hepatol. 2007; 6(1):28–36

[42] Bataller R, Ginès P, Nicolás JM, et al. Angiotensin II induces contraction and proliferation of human hepatic stellate cells. Gastroenterology. 2000; 118 (6):1149–1156

[43] Vallance P, Moncada S. Hyperdynamic circulation in cirrhosis: a role for nitric oxide? Lancet. 1991; 337(8744):776–778

[44] Wiest R, Das S, Cadelina G, Garcia-Tsao G, Milstien S, Groszmann RJ. Bacterial translocation in cirrhotic rats stimulates eNOS-derived NO production and impairs mesenteric vascular contractility. J Clin Invest. 1999; 104(9):1223–1233

[45] Bories PN, Campillo B, Azaou L, Scherman E. Long-lasting NO overproduction in cirrhotic patients with spontaneous bacterial peritonitis. Hepatology. 1997; 25(6):1328–1333

[46] Battista S, Bar F, Mengozzi G, Zanon E, Grosso M, Molino G. Hyperdynamic circulation in patients with cirrhosis: direct measurement of nitric oxide levels in hepatic and portal veins. J Hepatol. 1997; 26(1):75–80

[47] Garcia-Tsao G, Angulo P, Garcia JC, Groszmann RJ, Cadelina GW. The diagnostic and predictive value of ascites nitric oxide levels in patients with spontaneous bacterial peritonitis. Hepatology. 1998; 28(1):17–21

[48] Such J, Hillebrand DJ, Guarner C, et al. Nitric oxide in ascitic fluid is an independent predictor of the development of renal impairment in patients with cirrhosis and spontaneous bacterial peritonitis. Eur J Gastroenterol Hepatol. 2004; 16(6):571–577

[49] Fernandez M, Mejias M, Garcia-Pras E, Mendez R, Garcia-Pagan JC, Bosch J. Reversal of portal hypertension and hyperdynamic splanchnic circulation by combined vascular endothelial growth factor and platelet-derived growth factor blockade in rats. Hepatology. 2007; 46(4):1208–1217

[50] Angermayr B, Fernandez M, Mejias M, Gracia-Sancho J, Garcia-Pagan JC, Bosch J. NAD(P)H oxidase modulates angiogenesis and the development of portosystemic collaterals and splanchnic hyperaemia in portal hypertensive rats. Gut. 2007; 56(4):560–564

[51] Huang HC, Wang SS, Hsin IF, et al. Cannabinoid receptor 2 agonist ameliorates mesenteric angiogenesis and portosystemic collaterals in cirrhotic rats. Hepatology. 2012; 56(1):248–258

[52] Bocca C, Novo E, Miglietta A, Parola M. Angiogenesis and fibrogenesis in chronic liver diseases. Cell Mol Gastroenterol Hepatol. 2015; 1(5):477–488

[53] Fernández-Rodriguez CM, Prieto J, Quiroga J, et al. Plasma levels of substance P in liver cirrhosis: relationship to the activation of vasopressor systems and urinary sodium excretion. Hepatology. 1995; 21(1):35–40

[54] Colle I, Geerts AM, Van Steenkiste C, Van Vlierberghe H. Hemodynamic changes in splanchnic blood vessels in portal hypertension. Anat Rec (Hoboken). 2008; 291(6):699–713

[55] Wiest R, Groszmann RJ. Nitric oxide and portal hypertension: its role in the regulation of intrahepatic and splanchnic vascular resistance. Semin Liver Dis. 1999; 19(4):411–426

[56] Fulton D, Gratton JP, McCabe TJ, et al. Regulation of endothelium-derived nitric oxide production by the protein kinase Akt. Nature. 1999; 399(6736): 597–601

[57] García-Cardeña G, Martasek P, Masters BS, et al. Dissecting the interaction between nitric oxide synthase (NOS) and caveolin. Functional significance of the nos caveolin binding domain in vivo. J Biol Chem. 1997; 272(41):25437–25440

[58] Sessa WC. eNOS at a glance. J Cell Sci. 2004; 117(Pt 12):2427–2429

[59] Iwakiri Y, Tsai MH, McCabe TJ, et al. Phosphorylation of eNOS initiates excessive NO production in early phases of portal hypertension. Am J Physiol Heart Circ Physiol. 2002; 282(6):H2084–H2090

[60] Dimmeler S, Fleming I, Fisslthaler B, Hermann C, Busse R, Zeiher AM. Activation of nitric oxide synthase in endothelial cells by Akt-dependent phosphorylation. Nature. 1999; 399(6736):601–605

[61] Michell BJ, Griffiths JE, Mitchelhill KI, et al. The Akt kinase signals directly to endothelial nitric oxide synthase. Curr Biol. 1999; 9(15):845–848

[62] Gallis B, Corthals GL, Goodlett DR, et al. Identification of flow-dependent endothelial nitric-oxide synthase phosphorylation sites by mass spectrometry and regulation of phosphorylation and nitric oxide production by the phosphatidylinositol 3-kinase inhibitor LY294002. J Biol Chem. 1999; 274(42):30101–30108

[63] Maines MD, Trakshel GM, Kutty RK. Characterization of two constitutive forms of rat liver microsomal heme oxygenase. Only one molecular species of the enzyme is inducible. J Biol Chem. 1986; 261(1):411–419

[64] Chen YC, Ginès P, Yang J, et al. Increased vascular heme oxygenase-1 expression contributes to arterial vasodilation in experimental cirrhosis in rats. Hepatology. 2004; 39(4):1075–1087

[65] Tarquini R, Masini E, La Villa G, et al. Increased plasma carbon monoxide in patients with viral cirrhosis and hyperdynamic circulation. Am J Gastroenterol. 2009; 104(4):891–897

[66] Guarner C, Soriano G, Tomas A, et al. Increased serum nitrite and nitrate levels in patients with cirrhosis: relationship to endotoxemia. Hepatology. 1993; 18(5):1139–1143

[67] Gana JC, Serrano CA, Ling SC. Angiogenesis and portal-systemic collaterals in portal hypertension. Ann Hepatol. 2016; 15(3):303–313

[68] Thabut D, D'Amico G, Tan P, et al. Diagnostic performance of Baveno IV criteria in cirrhotic patients with upper gastrointestinal bleeding: analysis of the F7 liver-1288 study population. J Hepatol. 2010; 53(6):1029–1034

[69] Sitzmann JV, Campbell K, Wu Y, St Clair C. Prostacyclin production in acute, chronic, and long-term experimental portal hypertension. Surgery. 1994; 115(3):290–294

[70] Wang C, Han J, Xiao L, Jin CE, Li DJ, Yang Z. Role of hydrogen sulfide in portal hypertension and esophagogastric junction vascular disease. World J Gastroenterol. 2014; 20(4):1079–1087

[71] Bátkai S, Járai Z, Wagner JA, et al. Endocannabinoids acting at vascular CB1 receptors mediate the vasodilated state in advanced liver cirrhosis. Nat Med. 2001; 7(7):827–832

[72] Lopez-Talavera JC, Cadelina G, Olchowski J, Merrill W, Groszmann RJ. Thalidomide inhibits tumor necrosis factor alpha, decreases nitric oxide synthesis, and ameliorates the hyperdynamic circulatory syndrome in portal-hypertensive rats. Hepatology. 1996; 23(6):1616–1621

[73] Kilbourn RG, Belloni P. Endothelial cell production of nitrogen oxides in response to interferon gamma in combination with tumor necrosis factor, interleukin-1, or endotoxin. J Natl Cancer Inst. 1990; 82(9):772–776

[74] Lopez-Talavera JC, Merrill WW, Groszmann RJ. Tumor necrosis factor alpha: a major contributor to the hyperdynamic circulation in prehepatic portal-hypertensive rats. Gastroenterology. 1995; 108(3):761–767

[75] Rosenkranz-Weiss P, Sessa WC, Milstien S, Kaufman S, Watson CA, Pober JS. Regulation of nitric oxide synthesis by proinflammatory cytokines in human

umbilical vein endothelial cells. Elevations in tetrahydrobiopterin levels enhance endothelial nitric oxide synthase specific activity. J Clin Invest. 1994; 93(5):2236–2243

[76] Wever RM, van Dam T, van Rijn HJ, de Groot F, Rabelink TJ. Tetrahydrobiopterin regulates superoxide and nitric oxide generation by recombinant endothelial nitric oxide synthase. Biochem Biophys Res Commun. 1997; 237(2):340–344

[77] Genesca J, Gonzalez A, Catalan R, et al. Adrenomedullin, a vasodilator peptide implicated in hemodynamic alterations of liver cirrhosis: relationship to nitric oxide. Dig Dis Sci. 1999; 44(2):372–376

[78] Abraldes JG, Albillos A, Bañares R, et al. Simvastatin lowers portal pressure in patients with cirrhosis and portal hypertension: a randomized controlled trial. Gastroenterology. 2009; 136(5):1651–1658

[79] Bataller R, Sancho-Bru P, Ginès P, Brenner DA. Liver fibrogenesis: a new role for the renin-angiotensin system. Antioxid Redox Signal. 2005; 7(9–10): 1346–1355

[80] Tandon P, Abraldes JG, Berzigotti A, Garcia-Pagan JC, Bosch J. Renin-angiotensin-aldosterone inhibitors in the reduction of portal pressure: a systematic review and meta-analysis. J Hepatol. 2010; 53(2):273–282

[81] Møller S, Gülberg V, Henriksen JH, Gerbes AL. Endothelin-1 and endothelin-3 in cirrhosis: relations to systemic and splanchnic haemodynamics. J Hepatol. 1995; 23(2):135–144

[82] Graupera M, García-Pagán JC, Titos E, et al. 5-lipoxygenase inhibition reduces intrahepatic vascular resistance of cirrhotic rat livers: a possible role of cysteinyl-leukotrienes. Gastroenterology. 2002; 122(2):387–393

[83] Graupera M, García-Pagán JC, Abraldes JG, et al. Cyclooxygenase-derived products modulate the increased intrahepatic resistance of cirrhotic rat livers. Hepatology. 2003; 37(1):172–181

[84] Chevallier M, Guerret S, Chossegros P, Gerard F, Grimaud JA. A histological semiquantitative scoring system for evaluation of hepatic fibrosis in needle liver biopsy specimens: comparison with morphometric studies. Hepatology. 1994; 20(2):349–355

[85] Calvaruso V, Burroughs AK, Standish R, et al. Computer-assisted image analysis of liver collagen: relationship to Ishak scoring and hepatic venous pressure gradient. Hepatology. 2009; 49(4):1236–1244

[86] Boursier J, Bacq Y, Halfon P, et al. Improved diagnostic accuracy of blood tests for severe fibrosis and cirrhosis in chronic hepatitis C. Eur J Gastroenterol Hepatol. 2009; 21(1):28–38

[87] Rosenberg WM, Voelker M, Thiel R, et al. European Liver Fibrosis Group. Serum markers detect the presence of liver fibrosis: a cohort study. Gastroenterology. 2004; 127(6):1704–1713

[88] Imbert-Bismut F, Ratziu V, Pieroni L, Charlotte F, Benhamou Y, Poynard T, MULTIVIRC Group. Biochemical markers of liver fibrosis in patients with hepatitis C virus infection: a prospective study. Lancet. 2001; 357(9262): 1069–1075

[89] Smith JO, Sterling RK. Systematic review: non-invasive methods of fibrosis analysis in chronic hepatitis C. Aliment Pharmacol Ther. 2009; 30(6):557–576

[90] Fontana RJ, Goodman ZD, Dienstag JL, et al. HALT-C Trial Group. Relationship of serum fibrosis markers with liver fibrosis stage and collagen content in patients with advanced chronic hepatitis C. Hepatology. 2008; 47(3):789–798

[91] Fontana RJ, Dienstag JL, Bonkovsky HL, et al. HALT-C Trial Group. Serum fibrosis markers are associated with liver disease progression in non-responder patients with chronic hepatitis C. Gut. 2010; 59(10):1401–1409

[92] Crossan C, Tsochatzis EA, Longworth L, et al. Cost-effectiveness of non-invasive methods for assessment and monitoring of liver fibrosis and cirrhosis in patients with chronic liver disease: systematic review and economic evaluation. Health Technol Assess. 2015; 19(9):1–409, v–vi

[93] Child CG, Turcotte JG. Surgery and portal hypertension. Major Probl Clin Surg. 1964; 1:1–85

[94] Pugh RN, Murray-Lyon IM, Dawson JL, Pietroni MC, Williams R. Transection of the oesophagus for bleeding oesophageal varices. Br J Surg. 1973; 60(8): 646–649

[95] Abad-Lacruz A, Cabré E, González-Huix F, et al. Routine tests of renal function, alcoholism, and nutrition improve the prognostic accuracy of Child-Pugh score in nonbleeding advanced cirrhotics. Am J Gastroenterol. 1993; 88(3):382–387

[96] Fernández-Esparrach G, Sánchez-Fueyo A, Ginès P, et al. A prognostic model for predicting survival in cirrhosis with ascites. J Hepatol. 2001; 34(1):46–52

[97] Maroto A, Ginès A, Saló J, et al. Diagnosis of functional kidney failure of cirrhosis with Doppler sonography: prognostic value of resistive index. Hepatology. 1994; 20(4 Pt 1):839–844

[98] Malinchoc M, Kamath PS, Gordon FD, Peine CJ, Rank J, ter Borg PC. A model to predict poor survival in patients undergoing transjugular intrahepatic portosystemic shunts. Hepatology. 2000; 31(4):864–871

[99] Wiesner R, Edwards E, Freeman R, et al. United Network for Organ Sharing Liver Disease Severity Score Committee. Model for end-stage liver disease (MELD) and allocation of donor livers. Gastroenterology. 2003; 124(1):91–96

[100] Kamath PS, Wiesner RH, Malinchoc M, et al. A model to predict survival in patients with end-stage liver disease. Hepatology. 2001; 33(2):464–470

[101] Wiesner RH, McDiarmid SV, Kamath PS, et al. MELD and PELD: application of survival models to liver allocation. Liver Transpl. 2001; 7(7):567–580

[102] Durand F, Valla D. Assessment of the prognosis of cirrhosis: Child-Pugh versus MELD. J Hepatol. 2005; 42(1) Suppl:S100–S107

[103] Galbois A, Das V, Carbonell N, Guidet B. Prognostic scores for cirrhotic patients admitted to an intensive care unit: which consequences for liver transplantation? Clin Res Hepatol Gastroenterol. 2013; 37(5):455–466

[104] Ripoll C, Groszmann R, Garcia-Tsao G, et al. Portal Hypertension Collaborative Group. Hepatic venous pressure gradient predicts clinical decompensation in patients with compensated cirrhosis. Gastroenterology. 2007; 133(2):481–488

[105] Lens S, Rincón D, García-Retortillo M, et al. Association between severe portal hypertension and risk of liver decompensation in patients with hepatitis C, regardless of response to antiviral therapy. Clin Gastroenterol Hepatol. 2015; 13(10):1846–1853.e1

[106] Zykus R, Jonaitis L, Petrenkienė V, Pranculis A, Kupčinskas L. Liver and spleen transient elastography predicts portal hypertension in patients with chronic liver disease: a prospective cohort study. BMC Gastroenterol. 2015; 15:183

[107] Colecchia A, Marasco G, Taddia M, et al. Liver and spleen stiffness and other noninvasive methods to assess portal hypertension in cirrhotic patients: a review of the literature. Eur J Gastroenterol Hepatol. 2015; 27(9):992–1001

[108] Vergniol J, Foucher J, Terrebonne E, et al. Noninvasive tests for fibrosis and liver stiffness predict 5-year outcomes of patients with chronic hepatitis C. Gastroenterology. 2011; 140(7):1970–1979, 1979.e1–1979.e3

[109] Klibansky DA, Mehta SH, Curry M, Nasser I, Challies T, Afdhal NH. Transient elastography for predicting clinical outcomes in patients with chronic liver disease. J Viral Hepat. 2012; 19(2):e184–e193

[110] Bosch J, Abraldes JG, Berzigotti A, García-Pagan JC. The clinical use of HVPG measurements in chronic liver disease. Nat Rev Gastroenterol Hepatol. 2009; 6(10):573–582

[111] Ripoll C. Hepatic venous pressure gradient and outcomes in cirrhosis. J Clin Gastroenterol. 2007; 41 Suppl 3:S330–S335

[112] Kim MY, Baik SK, Yea CJ, et al. Hepatic venous pressure gradient can predict the development of hepatocellular carcinoma and hyponatremia in decompensated alcoholic cirrhosis. Eur J Gastroenterol Hepatol. 2009; 21 (11):1241–1246

[113] Villanueva C, Aracil C, Colomo A, et al. Acute hemodynamic response to beta-blockers and prediction of long-term outcome in primary prophylaxis of variceal bleeding. Gastroenterology. 2009; 137(1):119–128

[114] Ginés P, Quintero E, Arroyo V, et al. Compensated cirrhosis: natural history and prognostic factors. Hepatology. 1987; 7(1):122–128

[115] D'Amico G, Morabito A, Pagliaro L, Marubini E. Survival and prognostic indicators in compensated and decompensated cirrhosis. Dig Dis Sci. 1986; 31(5):468–475

[116] Villeneuve JP, Condreay LD, Willems B, et al. Lamivudine treatment for decompensated cirrhosis resulting from chronic hepatitis B. Hepatology. 2000; 31(1):207–210

[117] Singal AG, Volk ML, Jensen D, Di Bisceglie AM, Schoenfeld PS. A sustained viral response is associated with reduced liver-related morbidity and mortality in patients with hepatitis C virus. Clin Gastroenterol Hepatol. 2010; 8(3):280–288, 288.e1

[118] Dufour JF, DeLellis R, Kaplan MM. Reversibility of hepatic fibrosis in autoimmune hepatitis. Ann Intern Med. 1997; 127(11):981–985

[119] D'Amico G, Luca A. Natural history. Clinical-haemodynamic correlations. Prediction of the risk of bleeding. Baillieres Clin Gastroenterol. 1997; 11(2): 243–256

[120] Berzigotti A, Escorsell A, Bosch J. Pathophysiology of variceal bleeding in cirrhotics. Ann Gastroenterol. 2001; 14:150–157

[121] North Italian Endoscopic Club for the Study and Treatment of Esophageal Varices. Prediction of the first variceal hemorrhage in patients with cirrhosis of the liver and esophageal varices. A prospective multicenter study. N Engl J Med. 1988; 319(15):983–989

[122] Vianna A, Hayes PC, Moscoso G, et al. Normal venous circulation of the gastroesophageal junction. A route to understanding varices. Gastroenterology. 1987; 93(4):876–889

[123] Kitano S, Terblanche J, Kahn D, Bornman PC. Venous anatomy of the lower oesophagus in portal hypertension: practical implications. Br J Surg. 1986; 73(7):525–531

[124] McCormack TT, Rose JD, Smith PM, Johnson AG. Perforating veins and blood flow in oesophageal varices. Lancet. 1983; 2(8365–8366):1442–1444

[125] Le Moine O, Hadengue A, Moreau R, et al. Relationship between portal pressure, esophageal varices, and variceal bleeding on the basis of the stage and cause of cirrhosis. Scand J Gastroenterol. 1997; 32(7): 731–735

[126] Carbonell N, Pauwels A, Serfaty L, Fourdan O, Lévy VG, Poupon R. Improved survival after variceal bleeding in patients with cirrhosis over the past two decades. Hepatology. 2004; 40(3):652–659

[127] Beppu K, Inokuchi K, Koyanagi N, et al. Prediction of variceal hemorrhage by esophageal endoscopy. Gastrointest Endosc. 1981; 27(4):213–218

[128] Garcia-Tsao G, Groszmann RJ, Fisher RL, Conn HO, Atterbury CE, Glickman M. Portal pressure, presence of gastroesophageal varices and variceal bleeding. Hepatology. 1985; 5(3):419–424

[129] Rigau J, Bosch J, Bordas JM, et al. Endoscopic measurement of variceal pressure in cirrhosis: correlation with portal pressure and variceal hemorrhage. Gastroenterology. 1989; 96(3):873–880

[130] Lebrec D, De Fleury P, Rueff B, Nahum H, Benhamou JP. Portal hypertension, size of esophageal varices, and risk of gastrointestinal bleeding in alcoholic cirrhosis. Gastroenterology. 1980; 79(6):1139–1144

[131] Nevens F, Bustami R, Scheys I, Lesaffre E, Fevery J. Variceal pressure is a factor predicting the risk of a first variceal bleeding: a prospective cohort study in cirrhotic patients. Hepatology. 1998; 27(1):15–19

[132] Polio J, Groszmann RJ. Hemodynamic factors involved in the development and rupture of esophageal varices: a pathophysiologic approach to treatment. Semin Liver Dis. 1986; 6(4):318–331

[133] Bambha K, Kim WR, Pedersen R, Bida JP, Kremers WK, Kamath PS. Predictors of early re-bleeding and mortality after acute variceal haemorrhage in patients with cirrhosis. Gut. 2008; 57(6):814–820

[134] Cerqueira RM, Andrade L, Correia MR, Fernandes CD, Manso MC. Risk factors for in-hospital mortality in cirrhotic patients with oesophageal variceal bleeding. Eur J Gastroenterol Hepatol. 2012; 24(5):551–557

[135] Burroughs AK, Triantos CK, O'Beirne J, Patch D. Predictors of early rebleeding and mortality after acute variceal hemorrhage in patients with cirrhosis. Nat Clin Pract Gastroenterol Hepatol. 2009; 6(2):72–73

[136] Abraldes JG, Villanueva C, Bañares R, et al. Spanish Cooperative Group for Portal Hypertension and Variceal Bleeding. Hepatic venous pressure gradient and prognosis in patients with acute variceal bleeding treated with pharmacologic and endoscopic therapy. J Hepatol. 2008; 48(2): 229–236

[137] Ready JB, Robertson AD, Goff JS, Rector WG, Jr. Assessment of the risk of bleeding from esophageal varices by continuous monitoring of portal pressure. Gastroenterology. 1991; 100(5, Pt 1):1403–1410

[138] Patch D, Armonis A, Sabin C, et al. Single portal pressure measurement predicts survival in cirrhotic patients with recent bleeding. Gut. 1999; 44 (2):264–269

[139] Monescillo A, Martínez-Lagares F, Ruiz-del-Arbol L, et al. Influence of portal hypertension and its early decompression by TIPS placement on the outcome of variceal bleeding. Hepatology. 2004; 40(4):793–801

[140] Reverter E, Tandon P, Augustin S, et al. A MELD-based model to determine risk of mortality among patients with acute variceal bleeding. Gastroenterology. 2014; 146(2):412–19.e3

[141] Augustin S, Muntaner L, Altamirano JT, et al. Predicting early mortality after acute variceal hemorrhage based on classification and regression tree analysis. Clin Gastroenterol Hepatol. 2009; 7(12):1347–1354

[142] D'Amico G, De Franchis R, Cooperative Study Group. Upper digestive bleeding in cirrhosis. Post-therapeutic outcome and prognostic indicators. Hepatology. 2003; 38(3):599–612

[143] Abid S, Jafri W, Hamid S, et al. Terlipressin vs. octreotide in bleeding esophageal varices as an adjuvant therapy with endoscopic band ligation: a randomized double-blind placebo-controlled trial. Am J Gastroenterol. 2009; 104(3):617–623

[144] Graham DY, Smith JL. The course of patients after variceal hemorrhage. Gastroenterology. 1981; 80(4):800–809

[145] McCormick PA, O'Keefe C. Improving prognosis following a first variceal haemorrhage over four decades. Gut. 2001; 49(5):682–685

[146] Hou MC, Lin HC, Liu TT, et al. Antibiotic prophylaxis after endoscopic therapy prevents rebleeding in acute variceal hemorrhage: a randomized trial. Hepatology. 2004; 39(3):746–753

[147] Ioannou GN, Doust J, Rockey DC. Systematic review: terlipressin in acute oesophageal variceal haemorrhage. Aliment Pharmacol Ther. 2003; 17(1):53–64

[148] Villanueva C, Piqueras M, Aracil C, et al. A randomized controlled trial comparing ligation and sclerotherapy as emergency endoscopic treatment added to somatostatin in acute variceal bleeding. J Hepatol. 2006; 45(4):560–567

[149] Laine L, el-Newihi HM, Migikovsky B, Sloane R, Garcia F. Endoscopic ligation compared with sclerotherapy for the treatment of bleeding esophageal varices. Ann Intern Med. 1993; 119(1):1–7

[150] Hubmann R, Bodlaj G, Czompo M, et al. The use of self-expanding metal stents to treat acute esophageal variceal bleeding. Endoscopy. 2006; 38(9): 896–901

[151] Bañares R, Albillos A, Rincón D, et al. Endoscopic treatment versus endoscopic plus pharmacologic treatment for acute variceal bleeding: a meta-analysis. Hepatology. 2002; 35(3):609–615

[152] de Franchis R. Evolving consensus in portal hypertension. Report of the Baveno IV consensus workshop on methodology of diagnosis and therapy in portal hypertension. J Hepatol. 2005; 43(1):167–176

[153] García-Pagán JC, Caca K, Bureau C, et al. Early TIPS (Transjugular Intrahepatic Portosystemic Shunt) Cooperative Study Group. Early use of TIPS in patients with cirrhosis and variceal bleeding. N Engl J Med. 2010; 362(25):2370–2379

4 Management of Complications of Portal Hypertension: Transjugular Intrahepatic Portosystemic Shunt (TIPS)

Anthony M. Esparaz and Nicholas Fidelman

4.1 Introduction

In the more than 20 years of clinical research that has been performed since the transjugular intrahepatic portosystemic shunt (TIPS) intervention was introduced, multiple indications, contraindications, and technical standards for TIPS placement have been described.[1] Originally described by Rösch et al in 1969,[2] TIPS acts as a side-to-side portacaval shunt to decrease the portosystemic pressure gradient by diverting blood from the portal to the systemic circulation.[3] Hepatic sinusoidal pressure is lowered and circulatory flow is increased, decreasing the effects of portal hypertension.[4] TIPS placement has become an established procedure for the treatment of complications related to portal hypertension, including variceal bleeding and ascites.[5,6]

A number of factors have influenced the current application of TIPS, including multiple clinical trials exploring procedural safety and efficacy, as well as the establishment of the Model of End-Stage Liver Disease (MELD) scoring system for assessment of short-term mortality in patients undergoing TIPS placement.[3] Furthermore, long-term shunt patency has markedly improved since the introduction of polytetrafluoroethylene (PTFE)-covered stents.[7]

In this chapter, common indications and contraindications for TIPS are discussed. The standard technique for stepwise TIPS placement is described, as well as common complications and the management of these events. The role of pediatric TIPS and TIPS in unconventional situations such as portal vein occlusion, hepatic vein occlusion, and split-liver transplantation is discussed in a separate chapter.

4.2 History of TIPS

The TIPS procedure was initially described by Rösch et al in 1969.[2] In this study, the authors used a silicone-coated spring coil to create portosystemic shunts in dogs; these shunts remained patent for up to 2 weeks. However, the technique only became reproducible in humans with the later development of endovascular stents.[4] In 1982, Colapinto et al[8] and Gordon et al[9] were the first to create TIPS in 20 patients with variceal bleeding, but long-term results were poor, as most patients had rebleeding and 9 died within 1 month of the procedure. In the mid-1980s, Palmaz et al[10,11] developed expandable metallic stents and demonstrated their long-term patency in cirrhotic livers of dogs. This led to the implantation of metallic Palmaz stents in human patients at the University of Freiburg in 1988.[1] In the following years, numerous randomized studies, consensus conferences, and clinical efforts led to a vast improvement in the TIPS technique, as well as delineation of the most appropriate indications and patient selection for TIPS placement.[12,13,14]

Multiple mechanisms are responsible for shunt dysfunction and occlusion, including acute intrashunt thrombosis, pseudointimal hyperplasia from iatrogenic bile leaks into the shunt, and intimal hyperplasia in the outflow hepatic vein.[4] Several experimental and clinical trials assessed the use of covered stent grafts in achieving long-term shunt patency.[15,16,17,18] Ultimately, the best results were realized with the use of stents covered with PTFE.[18,19,20,21,22] More recent comparisons of covered stents with bare metal stents have shown decreased intimal hyperplasia and prolonged shunt patency with expanded PTFE (ePTFE)-covered stents.[7,23,24,25]

Steady adaptation and incorporation of these results, combined with increasing clinical experience and improved technical facilities, have led to the rapidly increasing acceptance of TIPS placement as an established procedure for the treatment of complications related to portal hypertension.

4.3 Indications

By diverting blood flow from the portal to systemic circulation, TIPS placement results in decreased hepatic sinusoidal pressure and increased circulatory blood flow, successfully reducing the portosystemic pressure in more than 90% of cases.[26,27,28] TIPS efficacy has been established for the secondary prevention of variceal bleeding and the treatment of refractory ascites, as evidenced by multiple randomized controlled trials (RCTs) and meta-analyses of RCTs.[3] Typical indications for TIPS are summarized in ▸ Table 4.1.[3]

4.3.1 TIPS for the Secondary Prevention of Variceal Bleeding

The strongest evidence for the efficacy of TIPS placement exists for the secondary prophylaxis of variceal bleeding.[3,29] Since 1994, a total of 13 RCTs assessing TIPS for this indication have been published, depicting results for 948 patients, 472 of whom underwent TIPS placement.[26,27,28,30,31,32,33,34,35,36,37,38,39] Recent

Table 4.1 Typical indications for TIPS placement

Indication	Best available level of evidence[a]
Secondary prevention of variceal bleeding	1A
Refractory ascites	1A
Budd–Chiari syndrome	4
Hepatic hydrothorax	4
Hepatic veno-occlusive disease	4
Hepatorenal syndromes (types 1 and 2)	2B
Hepatopulmonary syndrome	4
Portal hypertensive gastropathy	2B
Acute refractory variceal bleeding	1B

[a]1A, systematic review of randomized controlled trials; 1B, individual randomized controlled trial; 2B, individual cohort study; 4, case series.

meta-analyses by Burroughs et al[40] and Zheng et al[41] highlighted a greater than threefold decrease in the risk of recurrent variceal bleeding after TIPS placement compared with various forms of endoscopic therapy. Rates of rebleeding after TIPS ranged from 9 to 40.6%, whereas continued endoscopic treatment demonstrated rebleeding rates of 20.5 to 60.6%. All-cause mortality was similar in the two groups, but there was a greater than twofold increase in the rate of development of hepatic encephalopathy (HE) after TIPS placement.[26,27,28,30,31,32,33,34,35,36,37,38,39]

4.3.2 TIPS for the Treatment of Refractory Ascites

A diagnosis of refractory ascites portends a poor prognosis in patients with liver cirrhosis because of the risk of complications (e.g., spontaneous bacterial peritonitis, dilutional hyponatremia, hepatorenal syndrome); this condition is associated with 1-year survival of less than 50%.[4] Despite this high mortality rate, patients with refractory ascites tend to have paradoxically low MELD scores, thus conferring a lower position on the waiting list for a liver transplant.[42]

Although large-volume paracentesis has been shown to be safe and easy to perform for the treatment of refractory ascites, it negatively affects systemic hemodynamics and renal function, limiting its use as a long-term treatment option.[43] TIPS placement, on the other hand, improves renal function and system hemodynamics while treating ascites. In a 2010 review, Rössle and Gerbes[44] found that within 4 weeks of TIPS placement, urinary sodium excretion and serum creatinine levels improved significantly, and within 4 to 6 months, there was an associated increase in serum sodium concentration, glomerular filtration rate, and urinary volume with normalization of plasma renin, aldosterone, and noradrenaline concentrations. These findings suggest that TIPS placement reverses hyperdynamic circulation and amends central underfilling.

A recent analysis that included 16 studies of TIPS placement for refractory ascites demonstrated a complete response in 51% of patients and a complete or partial response not requiring paracenteses in 68%.[45] Furthermore, a meta-analysis by D'Amico et al[46] assessing results from five earlier RCTs demonstrated a 7.1-fold decrease in the risk of recurrent tense ascites after TIPS placement, along with rates of improvement of 38 to 84% with TIPS versus 0 to 43% with large-volume paracentesis. Although four earlier RCTs found no significant difference in survival between TIPS and large-volume paracentesis,[47,48,49,50] two of the more recent studies demonstrated improved survival in patients who underwent TIPS placement compared to patients treated with large-volume paracentesis.[51,52] Finally, in a meta-analysis of four studies,[48,49,50,51] Salerno et al[53] observed a recurrence of tense ascites in 42% of patients who underwent TIPS placement versus 89% of those who underwent paracentesis ($p < 0.0001$), with an associated decrease in the number of paracenteses per patient in those with TIPS (1.6 ± 3.5 vs. 7.1 ± 8.8; $p < 0.0001$). The overall rate of complications related to portal hypertension (gastrointestinal bleed, hepatorenal syndrome, spontaneous bacterial peritonitis) was also significantly lower in the TIPS group than in the paracentesis group (15 vs. 28%, $p = 0.005$).

4.3.3 TIPS for the Treatment of Acute Variceal Bleeding

When variceal bleeding occurs, endoscopic and/or pharmacologic therapies are initially used.[29] For cases in which bleeding is not controlled by conventional methods, TIPS has been used for rescue treatment with good results.

Two RCTs[54,55] and a retrospective surveillance study[56] compared TIPS with medical therapy for acute variceal bleeding. In 2004, Monescillo et al[54] randomized high-risk patients with a measured portosystemic pressure gradient of more than 20 mm Hg within 24 hours of admission to receive either early bare-stent TIPS ($n = 26$) or medical treatment ($n = 26$). Early TIPS placement reduced treatment failure ($p = 0.003$) and in-hospital and 1-year mortality ($p < 0.05$).

In 2010, García-Pagán et al[55] randomly assigned 63 high-risk cirrhotic patients with acute variceal bleeding at index endoscopy within 24 hours after admission to receive either a covered-stent TIPS ($n = 32$) or medical therapy including propranolol or nadolol plus a nitrate followed by endoscopic band ligation if drugs were not effective ($n = 31$). During the median 16-month follow-up, the TIPS group demonstrated a significantly lower rate of rebleeding or failure to control bleeding (3 vs. 45%, $p = 0.001$). Moreover, actuarial survival at 1 year was significantly better in the TIPS group (87.5 vs. 61.3%, $p < 0.001$). These results were corroborated by a post-RCT surveillance study by the same authors,[56] who concluded that early use of TIPS in hospitalized patients with acute variceal bleeding was associated with a significant improvement in rates of failure to control bleeding or rebleeding (7 vs. 47%, $p < 0.001$).

4.3.4 TIPS for the Treatment of Hepatic Hydrothorax

Hepatic hydrothorax occurs when there is direct passage of peritoneal ascitic fluid into the pleural cavity via diaphragmatic leaks. This condition is defined as a significant pleural effusion, usually more than 500 mL, in a cirrhotic patient without primary cardiac or pulmonary disease.[3] Several retrospective case series have described the use of TIPS for hepatic hydrothorax in more than 150 patients.[57,58,59,60] At least, partial improvement in clinical symptoms (dyspnea, rate of thoracenteses) was reported in 68 to 82% of patients, and complete resolution of hepatic hydrothorax was reported in 57 to 71% of patients.[57,58,59,60] One-year survival rates, as described in two studies,[57,58] were 64 and 48%. While TIPS placement was associated with strong long-term survival and response rates in these studies, it is also noteworthy that TIPS is the only therapeutic option that concurrently treats refractory ascites and hepatic hydrothorax.

4.4 Patient Selection and Contraindications

A dynamic collaboration must take place among hepatologists, gastroenterologists, interventional radiologists, and the patients themselves when deciding on TIPS placement as the most appropriate treatment for complications of portal hypertension. Absolute and relative contraindications to TIPS placement are listed in

Table 4.2 Contraindications to TIPS placement

Absolute contraindications	Relative contraindications
Primary prevention of variceal bleeding	Hepatocellular carcinoma (especially if central)
Congestive heart failure	Obstruction of all hepatic veins
Severe tricuspid regurgitation	Portal vein thrombosis
Severe pulmonary hypertension	Moderate pulmonary hypertension
Multiple hepatic cysts	Severe uncorrectable coagulopathy (INR > 5)
Uncontrolled systemic infection or sepsis	Uncorrectable thrombocytopenia of < 20,000 cells/cm^3
Unrelieved biliary obstruction	Hepatic encephalopathy

Abbreviation: INR, international normalized ratio.

▶ Table 4.2.[3] Generally speaking, absolute contraindications include congestive heart failure, severe tricuspid regurgitation, and severe pulmonary arterial hypertension (with mean pulmonary pressure > 45 mm Hg). Relative contraindications include HE (which may worsen after TIPS placement), active sepsis, and anatomical conditions that may complicate creation of the shunt, such as chronic organized portal vein thrombosis, hepatic vein thrombosis, polycystic liver disease, and multiple hepatic masses.[61,62]

Multiple studies have focused on models to predict survival after TIPS placement.[63,64,65,66] Child–Pugh class C disease,[63] variceal hemorrhage requiring emergent TIPS placement, alanine aminotransferase level greater than 100 IU/L, serum bilirubin level greater than 3 mg/dL, and pre-TIPS HE unrelated to bleeding[64] are all associated with an increased risk of post-TIPS mortality. A MELD score higher than 18 predicts a significantly increased 3-month mortality rate after TIPS placement (85 vs. 55%, $p = 0.037$), compared with MELD scores less than or equal to 18.[42,67,68]

Irrespective of the predictors considered, the risks and benefits associated with TIPS creation must be balanced in the context of each patient's clinical scenario. There may be situations in which the added risks of a difficult TIPS procedure are justified (e.g., in patients with hepatocellular carcinoma and refractory variceal bleeding). Predictors can only be used to inform the treating team and the patient about expected outcomes and must always be weighed against the urgency of treatment escalation.[1]

4.5 Preparation for TIPS Placement

As with any procedure, TIPS placement is associated with notable risks that must be weighed against the clinical benefits for the individual patient. A thorough understanding of the patient's history and a detailed physical examination are required. Additionally, laboratory results obtained within 24 hours of the procedure should be reviewed, including complete blood count, coagulation panel, and metabolic panel, to evaluate liver and renal function.[3] Coagulopathy (international normalized ratio [INR] for prothrombin time > 1.5), thrombocytopenia (platelet count < 50,000 cells/mL), and anemia (hematocrit < 25%) should be corrected before initiation of the procedure. Patients with renal insufficiency should receive hydration.

Preprocedural cross-sectional liver imaging must be performed shortly before TIPS placement.[69] Thorough preprocedural planning requires assessment of the size and configuration of the liver, including the patency and anatomical course of the hepatic venous structures in relation to the portal venous structures. In an emergent situation, bedside sonographic liver evaluation is required at the very least to demonstrate hepatic and portal vein patency. In those patients with known cardiac or pulmonary disease, an echocardiogram should be obtained to exclude pulmonary arterial hypertension.[3]

Finally, TIPS placement carries a risk for periprocedural infection or sepsis, including the possibility of infection in the stent itself. Nevertheless, little published evidence exists to support the use of prophylactic antibiotics before TIPS placement.[69] In patients who do not receive prophylactic antibiotics, infection rates range from 3 to 16%.[70] Prophylactic administration of ceftriaxone has been suggested by some authors.[71] Additionally, antibiotic administration may be considered to prevent infection of the stent lumen, termed "endotipsitis"; this condition has a published prevalence of 1.3%.[1,72,73] Overall, acute infection secondary to TIPS placement appears to be infrequent, leaving the argument regarding prophylactic antibiotics unresolved. It is likely that improved technical skills combined with increasing global clinical experience (e.g., fewer catheter exchanges) have lowered the incidence of postprocedure infection. Nevertheless, one must consider the generally poor clinical status and tolerance of infection in patients requiring TIPS when the decision regarding prophylactic antibiotic use is made.

4.6 Conventional TIPS Technique

Commonly used methods for TIPS placement have been reviewed in detail in the literature.[1,69,74] Typically, most practitioners employ general anesthesia with endotracheal intubation.[3] In general, the right internal jugular vein approach is used. After the neck is prepared and draped in the usual sterile fashion, sonographic guidance is used to gain internal jugular venous access. Percutaneous access requires dilation to accept a 10-French (Fr) sheath, the minimum caliber required for later stent placement (Viatorr, W.L. Gore and Associates). Most practitioners prefer to create the shunt from the right hepatic vein approach after access (▶ Fig. 4.1a), as anterior transhepatic puncture of the right portal vein is believed to be the safest approach.[69] However, portal vein access may be obtained from any hepatic vein. Some practitioners prefer to obtain right atrial pressure immediately after sheath insertion to allow early identification of abnormal right-sided heart pressures, which would contraindicate TIPS placement.[69] Although no clinical study has described an absolute right atrial pressure threshold above which TIPS should not be placed, strong consideration against intervention should be made when the right atrial pressure exceeds 20 mm Hg.[75]

Wedged hepatic venography is then performed to delineate the anatomic relationship between the selected hepatic vein and the portal venous system and to select a target for transhepatic needle puncture. Many practitioners use balloon occlusion hepatic venography with carbon dioxide to highlight the course and directional flow in the portal veins (▶ Fig. 4.1b). Direct wedging of a catheter or sheath against the hepatic parenchyma

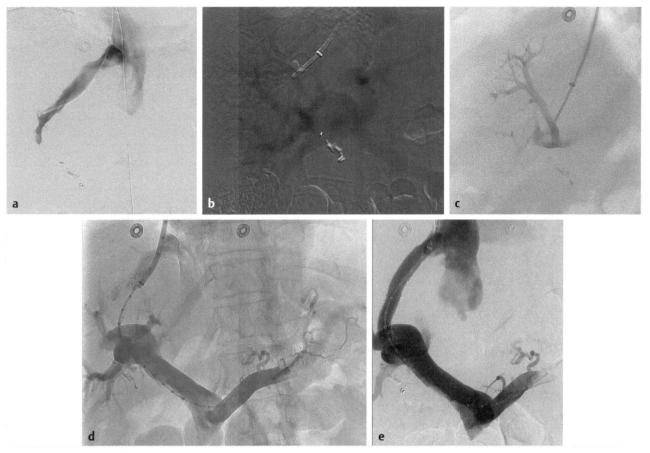

Fig. 4.1 A 54-year-old woman with cirrhosis and refractory ascites underwent TIPS placement. **(a)** Right hepatic venogram. **(b)** Balloon occlusion portal venogram using carbon dioxide. **(c)** Direct right portal venogram obtained through the Colapinto needle after portal vein cannulation. **(d)** Simultaneous portal and hepatic venograms obtained via a 5-French marking catheter (portal vein injection) and via a 10-French TIPS sheath (hepatic vein injection). This technique allows estimation of the length of the hepatic transparenchymal tract. **(e)** Portal venogram after deployment and dilation of the Viatorr stent.

may also be used for venography, but this method may confer a higher risk of direct hepatic parenchymal injury compared with balloon occlusion catheter use.[69] The use of carbon dioxide results in retrograde sinusoidal perfusion and portal opacification with little risk for anaphylaxis and renal toxicity when compared with even dilute iodinated contrast.[76]

Next, fluoroscopically guided needle passes are made through the hepatic parenchyma toward the desired portal vein target. A variety of transjugular access sets are commercially available in the United States, including the Rösch-Uchida (Cook Medical), Ring (Cook Medical), Haskal (Cook Medical), and Hawkins (AngioDynamics) transjugular access sets. Each has its own advantages and shortcomings[69,74]; the individual interventional radiology operator must decide which set to use in each clinical scenario.

The selected portal venous target will affect the direction of the needle throw. For instance, for a right hepatic vein to right portal vein access, an anterior needle throw is required.[69] Aspiration of a flush of blood through a syringe on the TIPS needle indicates the location of the needle tip in a vascular structure. Contrast material can then be injected to determine whether access to the target portal vein structure has been achieved (▶ Fig. 4.1c). If the site of portal vein entry is large enough without severe angulation along the projected course of the shunt, a

0.035-inch guidewire can then be introduced via the needle into the portal vein and through to the splenic or superior mesenteric vein (SMV). Then, a 5-Fr catheter is advanced to the splenic vein or SMV, and a stiff guidewire is left in place. Portal venography and pressure measurements should then be obtained (▶ Fig. 4.1d), and a portosystemic gradient can be calculated as the difference between the measured portal vein and right atrial pressures. An angioplasty balloon is then used to dilate the hepatic parenchymal track and allow passage of the TIPS sheath into the portal vein.

Covered stents, particularly ePTFE stents, are now widely used for TIPS creation (▶ Fig. 4.1e) because of their prolonged patency.[7,23,24,25] As described earlier, catheterization of the portal vein with a 10-Fr TIPS sheath is required to place the Viatorr stent graft. This step may be technically challenging because of "buckling" of the sheath in the right atrium. A variety of maneuvers may be employed to advance the sheath, such as use of a partially deflated angioplasty balloon, stiff plastic tapered-sheath introducer, the TIPS needle, or deployment of a self-expanding bare-metal stent, such as a Wallstent (Boston Scientific, Natick, MA), across the parenchymal tract. The stent graft could then be placed within the bare-metal stent.[3]

Of note, when ePTFE stents are used, the uncovered caudal portion of the stent should be left in the portal vein, while the covered portion should be placed in the hepatic parenchymal tract and hepatic vein. The cranial portion of the stent should extend to the hepatic vein–inferior vena cava (IVC) junction. Typically, a 10- to 12-mm stent is used in adults, and 8-mm stents are used in children.

After deployment of the TIPS stent, trans-TIPS portal venography and pressure measurements should be obtained in the portal vein and right atrium, with calculation of a post-TIPS gradient. To prevent a rebleeding episode in patients with a history of variceal bleeds, a post-TIPS portosystemic gradient of 12 mm Hg or less should be achieved.[77] The Society of Interventional Radiology and American Association for the Study of Liver Disease guidelines recommend a reduction of the portosystemic gradient to less than 8 mm Hg for the treatment of refractory ascites.[78] Others have suggested that a gradient value of less than 12 mm Hg may provide adequate control of ascites.[79] Notably, gradients less than 5 mm Hg have been associated with an increased risk of liver failure or severe HE requiring intervention.[80]

In patients who have a history of variceal bleeding, concurrent embolization of varices identified during TIPS placement may be beneficial. Tesdal et al[81] published a large retrospective study demonstrating that patients who underwent concurrent variceal embolization at the time of TIPS placement were significantly less likely to develop variceal rebleeding compared with those who underwent TIPS placement alone (61 vs. 84% at 2 years; 53 vs. 81% at 4 years; p = 0.02). In a prospective trial of 106 cirrhotic patients with recurrent variceal bleeding, 52 were randomized to undergo TIPS placement alone, and 54 underwent TIPS placement with embolotherapy for coronary vein varices. At 6 months, the rate of variceal rebleeding was significantly lower in the patients who received concurrent variceal embolization (5.7 vs. 20%, p = 0.029).[82] Similarly, in a recent meta-analysis of six RCTs or nonrandomized comparative studies, Qi et al[83] reported a significantly lower incidence of variceal rebleeding in those receiving concurrent variceal embolization with TIPS placement versus those undergoing TIPS placement alone (odds ratio [OR] = 2.02; 95% confidence interval [CI], 1.29–3.17; p = 0.002).

After the procedure, patients are usually monitored for at least 6 hours in an appropriately equipped unit. Urine output, mental status, and laboratory values, including complete blood count, coagulation panel, serum creatinine, and liver function tests, should be checked regularly. Shunt patency is usually demonstrated by liver ultrasound with Doppler on the day after TIPS placement. However, because of the retention of small air bubbles in the ePTFE graft material after placement, flow in covered stents is often difficult to detect sonographically within 72 hours of TIPS placement.[3]

4.7 Complications of TIPS

Gaba et al[69] have reviewed the technical complications of TIPS placement in great detail, as well as the methods for prevention and management of such complications. Several specific issues raised by these authors are discussed below.

4.7.1 Wedged Venography–Related Liver Injury

Liver laceration is a rare complication of wedged hepatic venography that can be avoided by use of the balloon-occlusion catheter technique with slow hand injection of carbon dioxide.[84] Maleux et al[85] reported a 1.8% risk of contrast extravasation during wedged venography with carbon dioxide in a series of 163 patients, without clinical consequence. On the other hand, Bookstein et al[86] reported a 7.5% incidence of contrast extravasation with iodinated contrast material. Use of carbon dioxide allows the pressure from the injection to be dissipated over a larger hepatic surface area. If laceration does occur, initial management should include monitoring of vital signs, with consideration of balloon tamponade or embolization of the bleeding vessel.[69] Furthermore, some authors advocate for therapeutic paracentesis before TIPS placement, as the presence of ascites impairs localized tamponade and increases the risk of significant bleeding from venography-induced liver capsular injury.[84]

4.7.2 Hepatic Arterial, Nontarget Organ, and Biliary Injuries

Inadvertent hepatic arterial puncture is uncommon, occurring with an incidence of approximately 6%.[87,88] When it does occur, the rate of symptomatic injury is less than 2%,[69] although potential complications include pseudoaneurysm formation, hemorrhage, vascular dissection or occlusion, and arterioportal fistula. These, in turn, may worsen preexisting portal hypertension.

Nontarget organ injury, particularly to the gallbladder, right kidney, duodenum, and colonic hepatic flexure, is rare.[69] However, as the number of needle passes required for portal venous access increases, so too does the incidence of nontarget organ injury.[87]

Biliary puncture with resultant fistula formation is also infrequent, occurring with an incidence of less than 5%.[87] However, fistulous communication between the biliary and vascular systems can result in hemobilia, sepsis, stent infection, and cholangitis, leading to significant morbidity.[89,90]

Careful preprocedural planning, analysis of prior cross-sectional imaging results, and knowledge of the anatomic relationship between the hepatic and portal venous systems are crucial to correctly direct needle punctures and reduce the risk of nontarget injury.[69] In most cases, nontarget injury is well tolerated. However, additional intervention such as arteriography and embolization may be required in some cases. In the case of biliary-vascular fistulas, internal or internal–external biliary diversion may be necessary.

4.7.3 Shunt Malposition

Appropriate positioning of the covered TIPS stent is crucial for long-term patency and optimal function.[69] At the proximal (inflow) end of the stent, the covered portion should begin at the junction of the portal vein with the hepatic parenchymal tract. Deployment of the covered portion within the portal vein can reduce intrahepatic portal venous perfusion. The distal (outflow) portion of the stent should extend to or within 1 cm of the hepatic vein–IVC confluence. Failure to position the stent this way can result in outflow stenosis and dysfunction.[91] Furthermore, a shunt that is too long and terminates in the hepatic level IVC or right atrium can complicate future liver transplantation, leaving insufficient room for caval cross-clamping at the time of surgery.[69] Therefore, judicious attention to proper shunt length measurement and deployment is vital to avoid stent malposition. Proper shunt length is best determined by measuring the hepatic parenchymal tract during the procedure using a catheter with radiopaque markers.[69]

4.7.4 Shunt Occlusion

The most frequent technical complications related to TIPS placement are shunt stenosis and occlusion. However, with the introduction of ePTFE Viatorr covered stents, long-term patency has significantly increased, with 1-year patency rates of up to 86%.[92,93] Early stent occlusion and dysfunction are often related to technical factors, including shortening and migration.[69] Bile-related factors, such as transection leading to biliary fistula formation, have also been implicated in shunt occlusion.[94] Additionally, stenosis has been associated with pseudointimal hyperplasia.[95] However, incidence of biliary fistula and pseudointimal hyperplasia has been greatly reduced with the use of covered stents. Often, duplex ultrasound evaluation provides clues to suggest stenosis.

4.7.5 Hepatic Dysfunction

A postprocedural increase in serum bilirubin concentration is observed frequently because of decreased hepatic perfusion from diversion of portal venous flow.[1] True liver failure after TIPS placement is thought to be due to sudden changes in the portosystemic gradient and hepatic sinusoidal underperfusion after shunt placement, but hepatic ischemia and infarction are infrequent because of the hepatic arterial buffer or reserve.[88] This concept describes an immediate physiologic increase in hepatic arterial flow to compensate for reduced portal perfusion caused by TIPS placement.[96]

Developing liver ischemia often manifests as persistent or worsening right upper quadrant abdominal pain, worsening HE, and worsening hepatic dysfunction.[69] Computed tomography (CT) or magnetic resonance imaging (MRI) may be used to delineate the extent of hepatic ischemic injury in such cases. To prevent TIPS-induced hepatic failure, critically low portosystemic gradients should be avoided after TIPS placement.[80] True hepatic ischemia or failure related to TIPS placement may require treatment with shunt reduction.[3]

4.7.6 Hepatic Encephalopathy

Diversion of blood via portacaval shunting in TIPS reduces the first-pass clearance of ammonia in the liver, leading to hyperammonemia.[97] Excess ammonia leads to swelling of astrocytes and can induce cytokine-mediated neuroinflammation through an excessively permeable blood–brain barrier in cirrhosis.[98] Ultimately, this leads to altered neurotransmission and function.

The incidence of HE after TIPS ranges from 15 to 48%.[99,100,101] Predicting whether HE will occur after TIPS is difficult; however, increased age, increased serum bilirubin, history of pre-TIPS HE, and low serum sodium concentration have been found to be associated with post-TIPS HE.[63,99,100,101]

Treatment options for HE depend on the severity and clinical presentation. For episodic HE, treatment should be focused on identification, prevention, and treatment of precipitating events, including general support and appropriate nutritional management.[102] The mainstay of treatment for HE is lactulose (a nonabsorbable disaccharide) because of its purgative effect as an osmotic agent and secondary effect of increasing stool acidity, thus limiting the intestinal absorption of additional ammonium ions.[98] Supplementing lactulose with rifaximin (a nonabsorbable antibiotic) has been shown to reduce the incidence of breakthrough episodes of HE, decrease the frequency of hospitalizations and length of stay for HE, and, most notably, improve the rate of survival.[103,104,105]

Unfortunately, despite these medical measures, 3 to 7% of patients with TIPS develop recurrent or persistent HE.[105] Management of refractory HE requires a multidisciplinary approach, with the ultimate treatment of liver transplantation. Nevertheless, newer techniques for shunt reduction are being developed and may serve as a "bridge" therapy to liver transplantation.[3,98]

Endovascular techniques for shunt reduction, including intrinsic, intramural, and extrinsic methods, have been comprehensively described in a recent review by Pereira et al.[98] For patients who require TIPS occlusion, the Amplatzer Vascular Plug (AVP; AGA Medical, Golden Valley, MN) is used to occlude large-diameter high-flow vessels. The main advantages of this device are its resistance to migration and the ease of placement. Shunt reduction techniques narrow the diameter of the shunt by stents and consequently diminish the blood flow through it. There are several feasible methods for deploying a stent graft.

- Intrinsic or luminal reduction: This can be performed using balloons or balloon-expandable stents with varying degrees of dilation giving the stent an hourglass shape.
- Intramural reduction: This can be achieved using sutures to alter the stent wall.
- Extrinsic or parallel reduction: This is accomplished by inflating a balloon to varying degrees, placed parallel to a reducing stent graft within the TIPS stent.[98]

4.8 Conclusion

TIPS placement has become an established method of treatment for complications related to portal hypertension, with the strongest available evidence supporting its use in refractory ascites and secondary prevention of variceal bleeding. Technical advancements and growing international clinical experience over the past several years have resulted in improved long-term shunt patency and decreased complication rates. Post-TIPS HE remains the major obstacle, requiring careful patient selection and medical treatment, and sometimes also requiring shunt reduction as a bridge to liver transplantation. Potential technical challenges related to TIPS placement have further led to the development of endovascular portosystemic shunt variants, such as the direct intrahepatic portacaval shunt. Unconventional clinical situations, such as patients with portal vein or hepatic vein occlusion, pediatric patients, and patients with split-liver transplant grafts, have resulted in alterations of the traditional TIPS technique. These scenarios are the subject of another chapter and demonstrate the important role that interventional radiologists play in adapting the TIPS technique to a variety of patient populations.

References

[1] Rössle M. TIPS: 25 years later. J Hepatol. 2013; 59(5):1081–1093

[2] Rösch J, Hanafee WN, Snow H. Transjugular portal venography and radiologic portacaval shunt: an experimental study. Radiology. 1969; 92(5): 1112–1114

[3] Fidelman N, Kwan SW, LaBerge JM, Gordon RL, Ring EJ, Kerlan RK, Jr. The transjugular intrahepatic portosystemic shunt: an update. AJR Am J Roentgenol. 2012; 199(4):746–755

[4] Fanelli F. The evolution of transjugular intrahepatic portosystemic shunt: Tips. ISRN Hematol. 2014; 2014:762096

[5] Colapinto RF, Stronell RD, Gildiner M, et al. Formation of intrahepatic portosystemic shunts using a balloon dilatation catheter: preliminary clinical experience. AJR Am J Roentgenol. 1983; 140(4):709–714

[6] Boyer TD. Transjugular intrahepatic portosystemic shunt in the management of complications of portal hypertension. Curr Gastroenterol Rep. 2008; 10(1):30–35

[7] Bureau C, Garcia Pagan JC, Layrargues GP, et al. Patency of stents covered with polytetrafluoroethylene in patients treated by transjugular intrahepatic portosystemic shunts: long-term results of a randomized multicentre study. Liver Int. 2007; 27(6):742–747

[8] Colapinto RF, Stronell RD, Birch SJ, et al. Creation of an intrahepatic portosystemic shunt with a Grüntzig balloon catheter. Can Med Assoc J. 1982; 126(3):267–268

[9] Gordon JD, Colapinto RF, Abecassis M, et al. Transjugular intrahepatic portosystemic shunt: a nonoperative approach to life-threatening variceal bleeding. Can J Surg. 1987; 30(1):45–49

[10] Palmaz JC, Sibbitt RR, Reuter SR, Garcia F, Tio FO. Expandable intrahepatic portacaval shunt stents: early experience in the dog. AJR Am J Roentgenol. 1985; 145(4):821–825

[11] Palmaz JC, Garcia F, Sibbitt RR, et al. Expandable intrahepatic portacaval shunt stents in dogs with chronic portal hypertension. AJR Am J Roentgenol. 1986; 147(6):1251–1254

[12] Rössle M, Siegerstetter V, Huber M, Ochs A. The first decade of the transjugular intrahepatic portosystemic shunt (TIPS): state of the art. Liver. 1998; 18(2):73–89

[13] Boyer TD, Haskal ZJ, American Association for the Study of Liver Diseases. The role of transjugular intrahepatic portosystemic shunt (TIPS) in the management of portal hypertension: update 2009. Hepatology. 2010; 51(1): 306

[14] Dariushnia SR, Haskal ZJ, Midia M, et al. Society of Interventional Radiology Standards of Practice Committee. Quality improvement guidelines for transjugular intrahepatic portosystemic shunts. J Vasc Interv Radiol. 2016; 27(1):1–7

[15] Bloch R, Pavcnik D, Uchida BT, et al. Polyurethane-coated Dacron-covered stent-grafts for TIPS: results in swine. Cardiovasc Intervent Radiol. 1998; 21 (6):497–500

[16] Otal P, Rousseau H, Vinel JP, Ducoin H, Hassissene S, Joffre F. High occlusion rate in experimental transjugular intrahepatic portosystemic shunt created with a Dacron-covered nitinol stent. J Vasc Interv Radiol. 1999; 10(2, Pt 1): 183–188

[17] Tanihata H, Saxon RR, Kubota Y, et al. Transjugular intrahepatic portosystemic shunt with silicone-covered Wallstents: results in a swine model. Radiology. 1997; 205(1):181–184

[18] Haskal ZJ. Improved patency of transjugular intrahepatic portosystemic shunts in humans: creation and revision with PTFE stent-grafts. Radiology. 1999; 213(3):759–766

[19] Nishimine K, Saxon RR, Kichikawa K, et al. Improved transjugular intrahepatic portosystemic shunt patency with PTFE-covered stent-grafts: experimental results in swine. Radiology. 1995; 196(2):341–347

[20] Saxon RR, Timmermans HA, Uchida BT, et al. Stent-grafts for revision of TIPS stenoses and occlusions: a clinical pilot study. J Vasc Interv Radiol. 1997; 8 (4):539–548

[21] Haskal ZJ, Brennecke LH. Transjugular intrahepatic portosystemic shunts formed with polyethylene terephthalate-covered stents: experimental evaluation in pigs. Radiology. 1999; 213(3):853–859

[22] Andrews RT, Saxon RR, Bloch RD, et al. Stent-grafts for de novo TIPS: technique and early results. J Vasc Interv Radiol. 1999; 10(10):1371–1378

[23] Yang Z, Han G, Wu Q, et al. Patency and clinical outcomes of transjugular intrahepatic portosystemic shunt with polytetrafluoroethylene-covered stents versus bare stents: a meta-analysis. J Gastroenterol Hepatol. 2010; 25 (11):1718–1725

[24] Otal P, Smayra T, Bureau C, et al. Preliminary results of a new expanded-polytetrafluoroethylene-covered stent-graft for transjugular intrahepatic portosystemic shunt procedures. AJR Am J Roentgenol. 2002; 178(1):141–147

[25] Rössle M, Siegerstetter V, Euringer W, et al. The use of a polytetrafluoroethylene-covered stent graft for transjugular intrahepatic portosystemic shunt (TIPS): long-term follow-up of 100 patients. Acta Radiol. 2006; 47(7):660–666

[26] Rössle M, Haag K, Ochs A, et al. The transjugular intrahepatic portosystemic stent-shunt procedure for variceal bleeding. N Engl J Med. 1994; 330(3): 165–171

[27] Cello JP, Ring EJ, Olcott EW, et al. Endoscopic sclerotherapy compared with percutaneous transjugular intrahepatic portosystemic shunt after initial sclerotherapy in patients with acute variceal hemorrhage. A randomized, controlled trial. Ann Intern Med. 1997; 126(11):858–865

[28] Sanyal AJ, Freedman AM, Luketic VA, et al. Transjugular intrahepatic portosystemic shunts compared with endoscopic sclerotherapy for the prevention of recurrent variceal hemorrhage. A randomized, controlled trial. Ann Intern Med. 1997; 126(11):849–857

[29] Loffroy R, Favelier S, Pottecher P, et al. Transjugular intrahepatic portosystemic shunt for acute variceal gastrointestinal bleeding: indications, techniques and outcomes. Diagn Interv Imaging. 2015; 96(7–8):745–755

[30] Groupe d'Etude des Anastomoses Intra-Hepatiques. TIPS vs sclerotherapy + propranolol in the prevention of variceal rebleeding: preliminary results of a multicenter randomized trial. Hepatology. 1995; 22: A297

[31] Cabrera J, Maynar M, Granados R, et al. Transjugular intrahepatic portosystemic shunt versus sclerotherapy in the elective treatment of variceal hemorrhage. Gastroenterology. 1996; 110(3):832–839

[32] Sauer P, Theilmann L, Stremmel W, Benz C, Richter GM, Stiehl A. Transjugular intrahepatic portosystemic stent shunt versus sclerotherapy plus propranolol for variceal rebleeding. Gastroenterology. 1997; 113(5): 1623–1631

[33] Jalan R, Forrest EH, Stanley AJ, et al. A randomized trial comparing transjugular intrahepatic portosystemic stent-shunt with variceal band ligation in the prevention of rebleeding from esophageal varices. Hepatology. 1997; 26(5):1115–1122

[34] Merli M, Salerno F, Riggio O, et al. Transjugular intrahepatic portosystemic shunt versus endoscopic sclerotherapy for the prevention of variceal bleeding in cirrhosis: a randomized multicenter trial. Gruppo Italiano Studio TIPS (G.I.S.T.). Hepatology. 1998; 27(1):48–53

[35] Sauer P, Benz C, Thelmann L, Richter G, Stremmel W, Stiehl A. Transjugular intrahepatic portosystemic stent shunt (TIPS) vs. endoscopic banding in the prevention of variceal rebleeding: final results of a randomized study. Gastroenterology. 1998; 114:A1334

[36] García-Villarreal L, Martínez-Lagares F, Sierra A, et al. Transjugular intrahepatic portosystemic shunt versus endoscopic sclerotherapy for the prevention of variceal rebleeding after recent variceal hemorrhage. Hepatology. 1999; 29(1):27–32

[37] Pomier-Layrargues G, Villeneuve JP, Deschênes M, et al. Transjugular intrahepatic portosystemic shunt (TIPS) versus endoscopic variceal ligation in the prevention of variceal rebleeding in patients with cirrhosis: a randomised trial. Gut. 2001; 48(3):390–396

[38] Narahara Y, Kanazawa H, Kawamata H, et al. A randomized clinical trial comparing transjugular intrahepatic portosystemic shunt with endoscopic sclerotherapy in the long-term management of patients with cirrhosis after recent variceal hemorrhage. Hepatol Res. 2001; 21(3):189–198

[39] Gülberg V, Schepke M, Geigenberger G, et al. Transjugular intrahepatic portosystemic shunting is not superior to endoscopic variceal band ligation for prevention of variceal rebleeding in cirrhotic patients: a randomized, controlled trial. Scand J Gastroenterol. 2002; 37(3):338–343

[40] Borroughs AK, Vangeli M. Transjugular intrahepatic portosystemic shunt versus endoscopic therapy: randomized trials for secondary prophylaxis of variceal bleeding: an updated meta-analysis. Scand J Gastroenterol. 2002; 27:249–252

[41] Zheng M, Chen Y, Bai J, et al. Transjugular intrahepatic porosystemic shunt versus endoscopic therapy in the secondary prophylaxis of variceal rebreeding in cirrhotic patients: meta-analysis update. J Clin Gastroenterol. 2008; 42:507–516

[42] Schepke M, Roth F, Fimmers R, et al. Comparison of MELD, Child-Pugh, and Emory model for the prediction of survival in patients undergoing transjugular intrahepatic portosystemic shunting. Am J Gastroenterol. 2003; 98(5):1167–1174

[43] Ginès P, Tító L, Arroyo V, et al. Randomized comparative study of therapeutic paracentesis with and without intravenous albumin in cirrhosis. Gastroenterology. 1988; 94(6):1493–1502

[44] Rössle M, Gerbes AL. TIPS for the treatment of refractory ascites, hepatorenal syndrome and hepatic hydrothorax: a critical update. Gut. 2010; 59(7):988–1000

[45] Russo MW, Sood A, Jacobson IM, Brown RS, Jr. Transjugular intrahepatic portosystemic shunt for refractory ascites: an analysis of the literature on efficacy, morbidity, and mortality. Am J Gastroenterol. 2003; 98(11):2521–2527

[46] D'Amico G, Luca A, Morabito A, Miraglia R, D'Amico M. Uncovered transjugular intrahepatic portosystemic shunt for refractory ascites: a meta-analysis. Gastroenterology. 2005; 129(4):1282–1293

[47] Lebrec D, Giuily N, Hadengue A, et al. Transjugular intrahepatic portosystemic shunts: comparison with paracentesis in patients with cirrhosis and refractory ascites: a randomized trial. French Group of Clinicians and a Group of Biologists. J Hepatol. 1996; 25(2):135–144

[48] Rössle M, Ochs A, Gülberg V, et al. A comparison of paracentesis and transjugular intrahepatic portosystemic shunting in patients with ascites. N Engl J Med. 2000; 342(23):1701–1707

[49] Ginès P, Uriz J, Calahorra B, et al. Transjugular intrahepatic portosystemic shunting versus paracentesis plus albumin for refractory ascites in cirrhosis. Gastroenterology. 2002; 123(6):1839–1847

[50] Sanyal AJ, Genning C, Reddy KR, et al. North American Study for the Treatment of Refractory Ascites Group. The North American Study for the Treatment of Refractory Ascites. Gastroenterology. 2003; 124(3):634–641

[51] Salerno F, Merli M, Riggio O, et al. Randomized controlled study of TIPS versus paracentesis plus albumin in cirrhosis with severe ascites. Hepatology. 2004; 40(3):629–635

[52] Narahara Y, Kanazawa H, Fukuda T, et al. Transjugular intrahepatic portosystemic shunt versus paracentesis plus albumin in patients with refractory ascites who have good hepatic and renal function: a prospective randomized trial. J Gastroenterol. 2011; 46(1):78–85

[53] Salerno F, Cammà C, Enea M, Rössle M, Wong F. Transjugular intrahepatic portosystemic shunt for refractory ascites: a meta-analysis of individual patient data. Gastroenterology. 2007; 133(3):825–834

[54] Monescillo A, Martínez-Lagares F, Ruiz-del-Arbol L, et al. Influence of portal hypertension and its early decompression by TIPS placement on the outcome of variceal bleeding. Hepatology. 2004; 40(4):793–801

[55] García-Pagán JC, Caca K, Bureau C, et al. Early TIPS (Transjugular Intrahepatic Portosystemic Shunt) Cooperative Study Group. Early use of TIPS in patients with cirrhosis and variceal bleeding. N Engl J Med. 2010; 362(25):2370–2379

[56] Garcia-Pagán JC, Di Pascoli M, Caca K, et al. Use of early-TIPS for high-risk variceal bleeding: results of a post-RCT surveillance study. J Hepatol. 2013; 58(1):45–50

[57] Dhanasekaran R, West JK, Gonzales PC, et al. Transjugular intrahepatic portosystemic shunt for symptomatic refractory hepatic hydrothorax in patients with cirrhosis. Am J Gastroenterol. 2010; 105(3):635–641

[58] Siegerstetter V, Deibert P, Ochs A, Olschewski M, Blum HE, Rössle M. Treatment of refractory hepatic hydrothorax with transjugular intrahepatic portosystemic shunt: long-term results in 40 patients. Eur J Gastroenterol Hepatol. 2001; 13(5):529–534

[59] Wilputte JY, Goffette P, Zech F, Godoy-Gepert A, Geubel A. The outcome after transjugular intrahepatic portosystemic shunt (TIPS) for hepatic hydrothorax is closely related to liver dysfunction: a long-term study in 28 patients. Acta Gastroenterol Belg. 2007; 70(1):6–10

[60] Spencer EB, Cohen DT, Darcy MD. Safety and efficacy of transjugular intrahepatic portosystemic shunt creation for the treatment of hepatic hydrothorax. J Vasc Interv Radiol. 2002; 13(4):385–390

[61] Krajina A, Hulek P, Fejfar T, Valek V. Quality improvement guidelines for Transjugular Intrahepatic Portosystemic Shunt (TIPS). Cardiovasc Intervent Radiol. 2012; 35(6):1295–1300

[62] Haskal ZJ, Martin L, Cardella JF, et al. Society of Cardiovascular & Interventional Radiology, Standards of Practice Committee, SCVIR Standards of Practice Committee. Quality improvement guidelines for transjugular intrahepatic portosystemic shunts. J Vasc Interv Radiol. 2001; 12(2):131–136

[63] Jalan R, Elton RA, Redhead DN, Finlayson ND, Hayes PC. Analysis of prognostic variables in the prediction of mortality, shunt failure, variceal rebleeding and encephalopathy following the transjugular intrahepatic portosystemic stent-shunt for variceal haemorrhage. J Hepatol. 1995; 23(2):123–128

[64] Chalasani N, Clark WS, Martin LG, et al. Determinants of mortality in patients with advanced cirrhosis after transjugular intrahepatic portosystemic shunting. Gastroenterology. 2000; 118(1):138–144

[65] Malinchoc M, Kamath PS, Gordon FD, Peine CJ, Rank J, ter Borg PC. A model to predict poor survival in patients undergoing transjugular intrahepatic portosystemic shunts. Hepatology. 2000; 31(4):864–871

[66] Ferral H, Vasan R, Speeg KV, et al. Evaluation of a model to predict poor survival in patients undergoing elective TIPS procedures. J Vasc Interv Radiol. 2002; 13(11):1103–1108

[67] Kamath PS, Wiesner RH, Malinchoc M, et al. A model to predict survival in patients with end-stage liver disease. Hepatology. 2001; 33(2):464–470

[68] Salerno F, Merli M, Cazzaniga M, et al. MELD score is better than Child-Pugh score in predicting 3-month survival of patients undergoing transjugular intrahepatic portosystemic shunt. J Hepatol. 2002; 36(4):494–500

[69] Gaba RC, Khiatani VL, Knuttinen MG, et al. Comprehensive review of TIPS technical complications and how to avoid them. AJR Am J Roentgenol. 2011; 196(3):675–685

[70] Dravid VS, Gupta A, Zegel HG, Morales AV, Rabinowitz B, Freiman DB. Investigation of antibiotic prophylaxis usage for vascular and nonvascular interventional procedures. J Vasc Interv Radiol. 1998; 9(3):401–406

[71] Gülberg V, Deibert P, Ochs A, Rossle M, Gerbes AL. Prevention of infectious complications after transjugular intrahepatic portosystemic shunt in cirrhotic patients with a single dose of ceftriaxone. Hepatogastroenterology. 1999; 46(26):1126–1130

[72] Brown RS, Jr, Brumage L, Yee HF, Jr, Lake JR, Roberts JP, Somberg KA. Enterococcal bacteremia after transjugular intrahepatic portosystemic shunts (TIPS). Am J Gastroenterol. 1998; 93(4):636–639

[73] Bouza E, Muñoz P, Rodríguez C, et al. Endotipsitis: an emerging prosthetic-related infection in patients with portal hypertension. Diagn Microbiol Infect Dis. 2004; 49(2):77–82

[74] Clark TW. Stepwise placement of a transjugular intrahepatic portosystemic shunt endograft. Tech Vasc Interv Radiol. 2008; 11(4):208–211

[75] Valji K. Hepatic, splenic, and portal vascular systems. In: Valji K, ed. Vascular and Interventional Radiology. 2nd ed. Philadelphia, PA: Elsevier; 2006:269–319

[76] Scanlon T, Ryu RK. Portal vein imaging and access for transjugular intrahepatic portosystemic shunts. Tech Vasc Interv Radiol. 2008; 11(4):217–224

[77] Garcia-Tsao G, Groszmann RJ, Fisher RL, Conn HO, Atterbury CE, Glickman M. Portal pressure, presence of gastroesophageal varices and variceal bleeding. Hepatology. 1985; 5(3):419–424

[78] Boyer TD, Haskal ZJ. American Association for the Study of Liver Diseases Practice Guidelines: the role of transjugular intrahepatic portosystemic shunt creation in the management of portal hypertension. J Vasc Interv Radiol. 2005; 16(5):615–629

[79] Casado M, Bosch J, García-Pagán JC, et al. Clinical events after transjugular intrahepatic portosystemic shunt: correlation with hemodynamic findings. Gastroenterology. 1998; 114(6):1296–1303

[80] Chung HH, Razavi MK, Sze DY, et al. Portosystemic pressure gradient during transjugular intrahepatic portosystemic shunt with Viatorr stent graft: what is the critical low threshold to avoid medically uncontrolled low pressure gradient related complications? J Gastroenterol Hepatol. 2008; 23(1):95–101

[81] Tesdal IK, Filser T, Weiss C, Holm E, Dueber C, Jaschke W. Transjugular intrahepatic portosystemic shunts: adjunctive embolotherapy of gastroesophageal collateral vessels in the prevention of variceal rebleeding. Radiology. 2005; 236(1):360–367

[82] Chen S, Li X, Wei B, et al. Recurrent variceal bleeding and shunt patency: prospective randomized controlled trial of transjugular intrahepatic portosystemic shunt alone or combined with coronary vein embolization. Radiology. 2013; 268(1):900–906

[83] Qi X, Liu L, Bai M, et al. Transjugular intrahepatic portosystemic shunt in combination with or without variceal embolization for the prevention of variceal rebleeding: a meta-analysis. J Gastroenterol Hepatol. 2014; 29(4):688–696

[84] Semba CP, Saperstein L, Nyman U, Dake MD. Hepatic laceration from wedged venography performed before transjugular intrahepatic portosystemic shunt placement. J Vasc Interv Radiol. 1996; 7(1):143–146

[85] Maleux G, Nevens F, Wilmer A, et al. Early and long-term clinical and radiological follow-up results of expanded-polytetrafluoroethylene-covered stent-grafts for transjugular intrahepatic portosystemic shunt procedures. Eur Radiol. 2004; 14(10):1842–1850

[86] Bookstein JJ, Appelman HD, Walter JF, Foley WD, Turcotte JG, Lambert M. Histological-venographic correlates in portal hypertension. Radiology. 1975; 116(3):565–573

[87] Freedman AM, Sanyal AJ, Tisnado J, et al. Complications of transjugular intrahepatic portosystemic shunt: a comprehensive review. Radiographics. 1993; 13(6):1185–1210

[88] Haskal ZJ, Cope C, Shlansky-Goldberg RD, et al. Transjugular intrahepatic portosystemic shunt-related arterial injuries: prospective comparison of large- and small-gauge needle systems. J Vasc Interv Radiol. 1995; 6(6):911–915

[89] LaBerge JM, Ring EJ, Gordon RL, et al. Creation of transjugular intrahepatic portosystemic shunts with the wallstent endoprosthesis: results in 100 patients. Radiology. 1993; 187(2):413–420

[90] Rösch J, Antonovic R, Dotter CT. Transjugular approach to the liver, biliary system, and portal circulation. Am J Roentgenol Radium Ther Nucl Med. 1975; 125(3):602–608

[91] Clark TW, Agarwal R, Haskal ZJ, Stavropoulos SW. The effect of initial shunt outflow position on patency of transjugular intrahepatic portosystemic shunts. J Vasc Interv Radiol. 2004; 15(2, Pt 1):147–152

[92] Cura M, Cura A, Suri R, El-Merhi F, Lopera J, Kroma G. Causes of TIPS dysfunction. AJR Am J Roentgenol. 2008; 191(6):1751–1757

[93] Charon JP, Alaeddin FH, Pimpalwar SA, et al. Results of a retrospective multicenter trial of the Viatorr expanded polytetrafluoroethylene-covered stent-graft for transjugular intrahepatic portosystemic shunt creation. J Vasc Interv Radiol. 2004; 15(11):1219–1230

[94] LaBerge JM, Ferrell LD, Ring EJ, Gordon RL. Histopathologic study of stenotic and occluded transjugular intrahepatic portosystemic shunts. J Vasc Interv Radiol. 1993; 4(6):779–786

[95] Nazarian GK, Ferral H, Castañeda-Zúñiga WR, et al. Development of stenoses in transjugular intrahepatic portosystemic shunts. Radiology. 1994; 192(1):231–234

[96] Gülberg V, Haag K, Rössle M, Gerbes AL. Hepatic arterial buffer response in patients with advanced cirrhosis. Hepatology. 2002; 35(3):630–634

[97] Fanelli F, Salvatori FM, Rabuffi P, et al. Management of refractory hepatic encephalopathy after insertion of TIPS: long-term results of shunt reduction with hourglass-shaped balloon-expandable stent-graft. AJR Am J Roentgenol. 2009; 193(6):1696–1702

[98] Pereira K, Carrion AF, Salsamendi J, Doshi M, Baker R, Kably I. Endovascular management of refractory hepatic encephalopathy complication of transjugular intrahepatic portosystemic shunt (TIPS): comprehensive review and clinical practice algorithm. Cardiovasc Intervent Radiol. 2016; 39(2):170–182

[99] Somberg KA, Riegler JL, LaBerge JM, et al. Hepatic encephalopathy after transjugular intrahepatic portosystemic shunts: incidence and risk factors. Am J Gastroenterol. 1995; 90(4):549–555

[100] Riggio O, Merlli M, Pedretti G, et al. Hepatic encephalopathy after transjugular intrahepatic portosystemic shunt. Incidence and risk factors. Dig Dis Sci. 1996; 41(3):578–584

[101] Riggio O, Angeloni S, Salvatori FM, et al. Incidence, natural history, and risk factors of hepatic encephalopathy after transjugular intrahepatic portosystemic shunt with polytetrafluoroethylene-covered stent grafts. Am J Gastroenterol. 2008; 103(11):2738–2746

[102] Riggio O, Nardelli S, Moscucci F, Pasquale C, Ridola L, Merli M. Hepatic encephalopathy after transjugular intrahepatic portosystemic shunt. Clin Liver Dis. 2012; 16(1):133–146

[103] Laleman W, Simon-Talero M, Maleux G, et al. EASL-CLIF-Consortium. Embolization of large spontaneous portosystemic shunts for refractory hepatic encephalopathy: a multicenter survey on safety and efficacy. Hepatology. 2013; 57(6):2448–2457

[104] Bai M, He C, Yin Z, et al. Randomised clinical trial: L-ornithine-L-aspartate reduces significantly the increase of venous ammonia concentration after TIPSS. Aliment Pharmacol Ther. 2014; 40(1):63–71

[105] Bass NM, Mullen KD, Sanyal A, et al. Rifaximin treatment in hepatic encephalopathy. N Engl J Med. 2010; 362(12):1071–1081

5 Management of Complications of Portal Hypertension: Special Considerations

Rex M. Pillai, Mark J. Sands, and Baljendra S. Kapoor

5.1 Introduction

The role of interventional radiology in managing the complications of portal hypertension continues to evolve. The early days of percutaneous intervention were primarily diagnostic; transhepatic portography and arterioportography were performed to determine the presence and etiology of portal hypertension and to help with surgical planning. In the current era of noninvasive imaging, these early percutaneous diagnostic procedures have largely been supplanted by Doppler sonography, computed tomography (CT), and magnetic resonance (MR) angiography. The focus of interventional radiology has since shifted to therapeutic interventions to reduce and mitigate the sequelae of portal hypertension. Classically, interventional radiology has been associated with the transjugular intrahepatic portosystemic shunt (TIPS) procedure, which was introduced in the 1980s with the advent of metallic stents and is now considered a mainstay in the management of portal hypertension (see Chapter 4).[1]

This chapter focuses on special considerations regarding unique anatomical, technical, and physiological challenges in the percutaneous interventional treatment of portal hypertension.

5.2 Portal Vein Thrombosis

Portal vein thrombosis is a relatively rare condition that can occur in cirrhotic and noncirrhotic livers (▶ Fig. 5.1a,b). Etiologies of portal vein thrombosis include iatrogenic causes (prior portal vein catheterization), hypercoagulable states, trauma, tumors, postinflammatory conditions (pancreatitis), and postsurgical states.

Patients with cirrhosis and portal vein thrombosis are often asymptomatic, with the condition identified incidentally on imaging. Occlusion of the portal vein or its branches in noncirrhotic livers can cause localized alterations in hemodynamics; this occurrence accounts for less than 10% of all cases of portal hypertension.[2] These patients usually present with variceal bleeding, ascites, and abdominal pain.[3] Anticoagulation can be performed in cases of acute thrombosis, but this treatment is generally contraindicated in patients with active bleeding. Recanalization of the occluded portal vein by angioplasty and stenting via a transjugular or a percutaneous transhepatic approach can be performed to alleviate symptoms. Surgical shunting or devascularization is typically avoided in the cirrhotic patient to maintain transplant options in the future.[4]

The technical approach to a thrombosed portal vein recanalization has been described by several authors.[4,5,6,7,8,9,10] These cases are undertaken using a variety of methods, including percutaneous transhepatic, transjugular, trans-splenic, or combined surgical transmesenteric approaches. Thrombosis of a portal vein can increase the technical complexity of creating a TIPS, especially in the setting of chronic occlusion and cavernous transformation.[4]

When used with the results from previous cross-sectional imaging, intraparenchymal CO_2 portography and direct puncture portal venography (▶ Fig. 5.2a) can be extremely useful in cases of portal vein thrombosis.[7] Newer techniques using CT and live fluoroscopic fusion for needle guidance may assist the operator with finding the appropriate orientation and anatomic position of the portal vessels for puncture (▶ Fig. 5.2b,c). The next step is to probe with a stiff guidewire and attempt to direct the wire toward the expected position of the main portal vein. Once the guidewire is advanced to the expected location of the portal vein, an angiographic catheter is inserted and a portogram may be performed (▶ Fig. 5.2d,e). If the occluded portal vein cannot be punctured, the ideal target may be a nonthrombosed intrahepatic portal vein branch or a collateral vein within the cavernoma (▶ Fig. 5.3a). If the portogram confirms

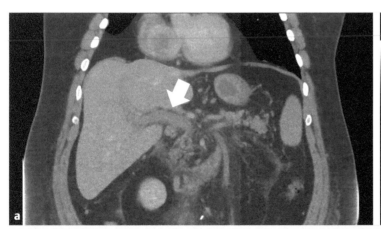
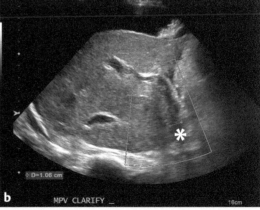

Fig. 5.1 Portal vein thrombus. **(a)** Coronal section from a contrast-enhanced CT image through the liver depicts occlusive thrombus in the main portal vein (*arrow*). **(b)** Color Doppler axial ultrasound (US) image through the liver shows no significant flow through the main portal vein (*). This finding makes creation of a TIPS challenging in this particular patient.

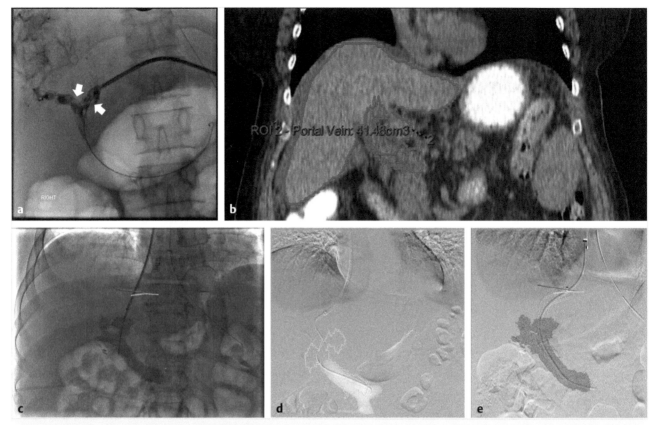

Fig. 5.2 Puncture of an occluded portal vein. (a) Digital subtraction angiography image depicting extensive portal venous thrombosis (*arrows*) during a direct puncture portal venogram. (b) 3D information on the location of the portal vein (*shaded in red*) can be obtained from cross-sectional imaging (CT, MR imaging, cone-beam CT) and (c) fused to a live fluoroscopic image to guide puncture (FlightPlan, GE Healthcare, UK). (d) Digital subtraction angiography image using CO_2 contrast after shunt creation shows the angiographic catheter opacifying the main portal vein, matching the expected position (*yellow outline*). (e) Fluoroscopic spot image of the liver demonstrating completed TIPS creation with the planning overlay of the portal vein (*shaded in red*) for comparison.

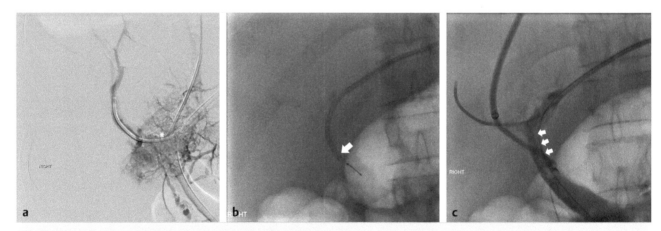

Fig. 5.3 Recanalization of an occluded portal vein through distal portal branches or collateral veins in cavernous transformation. (a) Digital subtraction angiography images depicting access into the portal system via nonthrombosed peripheral portal vein branches (*). (b) Recanalization of the main portal vein using mechanical thrombectomy device (*arrow*) (Indigo CAT8, Penumbra, Alameda, CA). (c) Postintervention digital subtraction angiography images of the portal venous system after balloon angioplasty and mechanical thrombectomy of the occluded portal vein segment show a patent system (*arrows*) appropriate for completion of TIPS creation.

correct positioning within the portal venous system, further intervention can be performed to recanalize the portal vein, including mechanical thrombectomy and pulse-spray thrombolysis, with or without stent placement (▶ Fig. 5.3b,c). The TIPS placement can then be completed in the usual fashion. In all cases, stent graft positioning should be intrahepatic, with the possibility for future transplant kept under consideration.

5.3 Budd–Chiari Syndrome and Veno-occlusive Disease

Budd–Chiari syndrome encompasses all obstructions to the hepatic vein outflow at the level of the hepatic vein and/or the inferior vena cava (IVC), including:
- Hepatic venules.
- Main hepatic veins.
- Hepatic vein orifice–suprahepatic IVC.
- Suprahepatic IVC–right atrium.

This causes symptoms of massive ascites, hepatosplenomegaly, abdominal pain, variceal bleeding, and jaundice from hepatic congestion, which, when left untreated, progresses to hepatic necrosis and fibrosis.[11]

Hepatic venography and cavography should be performed to identify venous drainage. This is achieved by positioning a flush catheter below the infrahepatic IVC and performing a power injection of contrast at a rate of 20 mL/s for a total volume of 40 mL. Patients with Budd–Chiari syndrome may have complete occlusion of the hepatic veins with the classic "spider web" appearance on imaging (▶ Fig. 5.4) due to small draining collateral and recanalized veins.

The aim of treatment in these patients is to restore physiological flow to relieve hepatic congestion and prevent progression to irreversible liver damage. Initial therapy is often systemic anticoagulation. Endovascular options are also available and highly effective if the obstruction occurs over a short segment.[12] Acute thrombosis can be treated with catheter-directed thrombolysis or mechanical thrombectomy.[13] Functional stenosis in the vena cava or hepatic veins should be treated with angioplasty (and/or

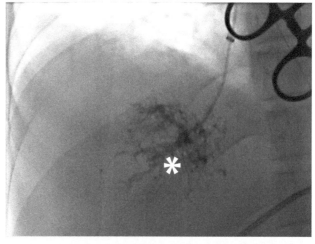

Fig. 5.4 Patient with Budd–Chiari syndrome. Digital subtraction angiography image depicting occlusion of the hepatic veins with "spider web" appearance of venous collaterals (*).

stents) if a significant gradient across the lesion exists (< 4 mm Hg).[14] The use of intravascular ultrasound (IVUS) to plan and evaluate stent placement is helpful and is becoming more accessible to operators as utilization costs decrease.

Longer segments of venous occlusion are more difficult to reopen and are associated with high reocclusion rates. In these patients and those with disease progression despite anticoagulation, TIPS placement may be required to provide adequate outflow.[15,16] These cases present a challenge for interventional radiologists placing a TIPS, as there may not be a suitable vein for placement of the transjugular access sheath. Instead, the access system is preferentially wedged into the small hepatic vein stump for anchoring purposes (▶ Fig. 5.5a). As always, review of cross-sectional imaging is important to determine the anatomy and orientation of the portal vein in relation to the hepatic vein stump. Some radiologists prefer a left internal jugular vein access approach, as this approach may provide favorable working angles.[14] At this point, a small amount of contrast can be injected through the access system to confirm proper

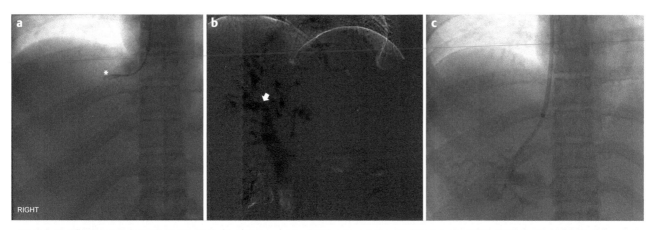

Fig. 5.5 Portal vein access for TIPS creation in Budd–Chiari syndrome. **(a)** Fluoroscopic image of the liver depicts the TIPS sheath wedged in the central hepatic vein stump, and injection of a small amount of iodinated contrast confirms this location with opacification of the hepatic parenchyma (*). **(b)** A wedged hepatic venous portogram using CO_2 contrast depicts the anatomy and orientation of the portal vein (*arrow*). **(c)** Fluoroscopic image of the liver demonstrates successful portal vein puncture.

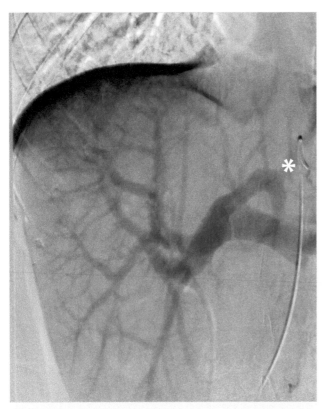

Fig. 5.6 Hepatic arterioportography. The celiac artery was accessed using a Sos configuration catheter (*) from the right common femoral artery. A digital subtraction angiographic image of the liver obtained after an appropriate delay demonstrates the portal venous anatomy.

positioning in the hepatic parenchyma. A CO_2 portogram should be performed to localize the portal vein (▶ Fig. 5.5b), and the needle should be torqued in the correct orientation to perform the transhepatic puncture (▶ Fig. 5.5c). The remainder of the TIPS creation follows the usual steps involving tract dilation and stent graft placement.

In the event that the portal vein cannot be localized with CO_2, which is often the case as the obstruction tends to be postsinusoidal, access guidance with IVUS[15] or arterial portography can be used (▶ Fig. 5.6).

TIPS placement in this setting, as with other causes of portal hypertension, is preferable to surgical methods. Surgical portacaval shunts are often difficult to create in cases of Budd–Chiari syndrome because of overgrowth of the caudate lobe limiting access to the portal vein.[17] Additionally, the surgical shunt uses a high-flow retrohepatic cava because of extrinsic compression from the caudate lobe. Long-term survival after TIPS placement is excellent, with rates exceeding 90% at 5 years.[14]

5.4 Direct Intrahepatic Portosystemic Shunt

Direct puncture of the main portal vein via the IVC (direct intrahepatic portosystemic shunt, or DIPS) is a method used in cases where the anatomy challenges the traditional TIPS placement approach. This can be seen in the setting of unfavorable hepatic or portal vein orientation, venous occlusion, extremely shrunken livers at risk for capsular perforation, and in the presence of hepatic parenchymal lesions. The presence of a tumor in the liver is considered a contraindication to the creation of a portacaval shunt using the traditional approach. This may stem from concerns regarding theoretical endovascular seeding of malignant cells during puncture attempts.[18]

DIPS placement is technically challenging and requires careful planning with evaluation of preprocedural imaging. Review of axial multiphase CT or MR images is extremely useful in this regard. An optimal level for IVC puncture is determined below the level of the hepatic veins. Access is then obtained into the IVC via the jugular vein, and a needle with an exaggerated curve (nearly 90° angle) is used for the puncture (Rösch-Uchida transjugular liver access set, Cook, Bloomington, IN). The use of an IVUS probe from a femoral vein approach is advised to guide the puncture (▶ Fig. 5.7a).[19] The target is the main portal vein proximal to the bifurcation. Once access is obtained into the main portal vein, the rest of the procedure is completed in the typical fashion.

An alternative approach to DIPS creation via a percutaneous transhepatic approach is useful in patients with anatomy precluding them from conventional TIPS placement. With this technique, a 10-French sheath is initially placed in the IVC via jugular vein access. Transhepatic access into a branch of the right portal vein is obtained percutaneously using an 18- or 21-gauge Chiba needle (Cook) under US guidance. The needle is then advanced further into the IVC under imaging guidance (▶ Fig. 5.7b), either US or rotational fluoroscopy (cone-beam CT) with live fluoroscopy fusion. A 0.018- or 0.035-inch wire can then be passed through the transhepatic access and snared into the transjugular sheath. With access obtained between the IVC and portal system (▶ Fig. 5.7c), the shunt can then be created in the typical fashion (▶ Fig. 5.7d). Embolization of the transhepatic portal vein access tract with Gelfoam, coils, glue, and vascular plugs has been shown to decrease the risk of bleeding complications after the procedure (▶ Fig. 5.7e).[18]

A transcaval approach may pose a higher risk of vascular injury and bleeding complications. The use of covered stents is critical in these patients, as extrahepatic puncture of the portal vein is common.

5.5 Liver Transplant

Advances in liver transplantation are allowing patients with liver failure to live longer. As a result, there is an increased incidence of portal hypertension in these patients. This is largely due to recurrence of underlying hepatitis C infection (63%) or graft failure (18%).[20] Still, only a small percentage (< 5%) of TIPS placements are performed in transplant patients.[20]

Technical issues for TIPS placements in transplant patients stem primarily from anatomic considerations (▶ Table 5.1). The radiologist must have extensive knowledge of the posttransplant hepatic and portal venous orientation and surgical anastomoses to perform a successful TIPS placement.

The mechanism by which the cava has been reconstructed must be identified before any intervention, especially if a conventional technique has not been used.[20,21] The piggyback technique in liver transplant differs from conventional reconstruction in that it allows for the preservation of the recipient retrohepatic

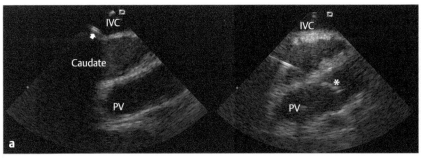

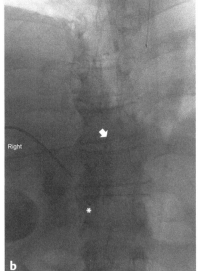
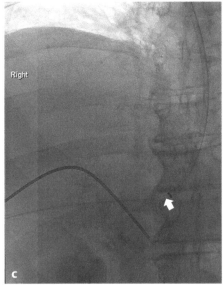

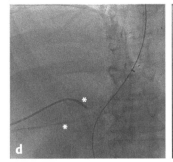
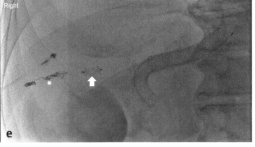

Fig. 5.7 DIPS placement. **(a)** Sagittal image from a side-firing IVUS probe via a transfemoral approach allows real-time visualization of the needle during the puncture of the portal vein (PV). **(b)** Fluoroscopic image of the liver obtained while advancing a 21-gauge Chiba needle (*arrow*) (Cook) toward the 10-French transjugular sheath (*) in the IVC via percutaneous transhepatic portal venous access. **(c)** An 0.035-inch wire was passed through the transhepatic access and snared into the transjugular sheath (*arrow*). **(d)** Fluoroscopic image of the liver depicts the completed DIPS procedure after tract dilation and covered stent placement. The transhepatic portal vein access sheaths (*) are still present and were subsequently removed after tract embolization. **(e)** Percutaneous tract embolization minimizes bleeding complications. Gelfoam (Pfizer), pushable Nester coils (*) (Cook), and an Amplatzer II vascular plug (*arrow*) (St. Jude Medical) were used in this case. (Part a: The image is provided courtesy of Hamed Aryafar, MD, Associate Professor of Clinical Radiology at University of California, San Diego.)

IVC and maintenance of venous return during the procedure. The caval reconstruction involves creating either an end-to-side or side-to-side (cavocaval) anastomosis between the recipient retrohepatic vena cava and the donor hepatic vein stump or donor suprahepatic vena cava, respectively. Technical challenges to creating a TIPS in these patients include stenosis and severe

angulation of the anastomoses. The partially extrahepatic location of the donor stump poses a risk for bleeding if it is punctured.

Left lateral or split liver transplants are common in pediatric practice. The donor left or right hepatic vein is surgically anastomosed to the recipient IVC in an end-to-side fashion. Split liver transplants are associated with further anatomic difficulties, as the relationships between the hepatic veins and portal veins may change as the graft grows. Interventional radiologists typically do not perform a high volume of left-sided TIPS placements; therefore, performing a TIPS placement in a left lobe graft may prove technically challenging.

Clinical outcomes after TIPS placement in transplant patients tend to be poorer compared to outcomes in patients with native livers (77 vs. 93% 5-year survival rates),[22] especially in the treatment of refractory ascites.[20] Overall, the favorable predictors of mortality after TIPS placement tend to be more conservative in transplant livers (Model for End-Stage Liver Disease (MELD) score < 15) than in native livers (MELD < 17).[20,23]

Table 5.1 Hepatic venous anastomoses in liver transplants

Transplant type	Donor-to-recipient IVC	Donor-to-recipient portal vein
Orthotopic	End-to-end (IVC to IVC)	End-to-end
Piggyback	End-to-side (RHV to IVC)	End-to-end
Cavocaval	Side-to-side (IVC to IVC)	End-to-end
Split	End-to-side (LHV to IVC)	End-to-end

Abbreviations: IVC, inferior vena cava; LHV, left hepatic vein; RHV, right hepatic vein.

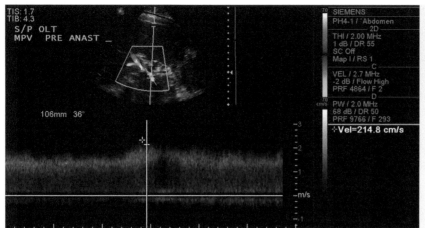

Fig. 5.8 Flow velocity within the main portal vein at the anastomosis. Transverse spectral Doppler US image through the liver depicts turbulent and increased flow velocity within the main portal vein at the anastomosis. Normal flow velocity in the portal vein is approximately 58 cm/s. Peak velocities greater than 125 cm/s indicate significant stenosis.

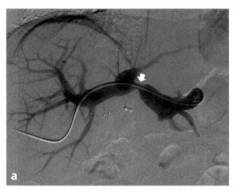
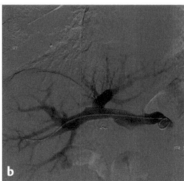

Fig. 5.9 Percutaneous transhepatic portal vein interventions. **(a,b)** Digital subtraction portography demonstrates portal vein stenosis (**a**, *arrow*) before and (**b**) after angioplasty and uncovered stent placement.

Posttransplant portal vein complications occur in a small percentage (<5%) of patients. Acute (occurring <6 months after transplant) issues include anastomotic strictures and thrombosis. Late (occurring >6 months after transplant) portal vein stenosis is typically related to intimal hyperplasia at the anastomosis leading to portal hypertension.[23] A stenosis greater than 50% or gradient greater than 4 mm Hg warrants treatment in most cases. Noninvasive Doppler US imaging of significant portal vein stenosis will demonstrate increased velocities (approximately three- to fourfold) at the anastomosis or peak velocity greater than 125 cm/s (▶ Fig. 5.8).[24,25] Percutaneous access into the portal vein, usually from the right, allows in-line management of the main portal vein anastomosis with angioplasty and noncovered stent placement, if necessary (▶ Fig. 5.9a,b).[26] As with other transhepatic portal venous access procedures, embolization of the tract mitigates bleeding complications.

5.6 Pediatric Transjugular Intrahepatic Portacaval Shunts

As in adults, portal hypertension in pediatric patients can result from cirrhotic and noncirrhotic causes. The causes of cirrhosis in children, however, are vastly different from those in adults and predominantly stem from diseases of cholestasis (biliary atresia, Alagille's syndrome, familial cholestasis syndromes), fibrocystic disease (choledochal cysts, autosomal recessive polycystic disease), autoimmune disease (sclerosing cholangitis, primary biliary cirrhosis, autoimmune hepatitis), congenital

mutations (cystic fibrosis, Wilson's disease, alpha-1-antitrypsin deficiency), and nonalcoholic fatty liver disease. Noncirrhotic causes are less common and primarily related to portal vein obstruction due to thrombosis, mass, trauma, or surgical etiologies. The intrahepatic and extrahepatic causes of portal hypertension in the pediatric population are as follows:
- Intrahepatic:
  - Cryptogenic cirrhosis.
  - Biliary atresia.
  - Familial cholestasis syndromes.
  - Fibrocystic disease (choledochal cysts, autosomal recessive polycystic disease).
  - Wilson's disease.
  - Cystic fibrosis.
  - Alpha-1-antitrypsin deficiency.
  - Autoimmune disease (hepatitis, sclerosing cholangitis, primary biliary cirrhosis).
  - Fatty liver disease.
- Extrahepatic:
  - Portal venous obstruction/occlusion.
  - Splenomegaly.
  - IVC obstruction/occlusion.
  - Right heart failure, tricuspid regurgitation.
  - Restrictive cardiomyopathy.
  - Constrictive pericarditis.

The management of portal hypertension in pediatric patients is largely based on the techniques used in adults. Creation of a TIPS has historically been reserved for patients with variceal

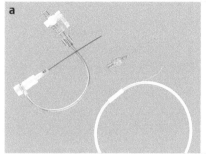 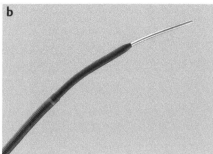 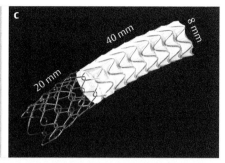

Fig. 5.10 Devices used in pediatric TIPS placements. **(a)** Pediatric micropuncture set (21 gauge, 4 cm, Cook). **(b)** Modified Colapinto needles that can be used through 7-French sheaths (18 gauge, 40-50 cm, Cook). **(c)** Smaller diameter and shorter covered stents (8 mm × 40 mm, VIATORR, Gore Medical, Flagstaff, AZ). (Parts a and b: Reproduced with permission of Cook Medical, Bloomington, IN. Part c: The image is provided courtesy of W. L. Gore and Associates.)

bleeding that is not amenable to endoscopic treatment and those with refractory ascites.[27]

The technical aspects of shunt creation in children are similar to the technical aspects of procedures performed in adults; however, certain issues must be considered when treating pediatric patients. First, these patients will routinely require general anesthesia for adequate sedation and pain control. Awareness of the patient's size will help with procedure planning: the diminutive size of the liver affects the relationship between the hepatic and portal venous system and increases the risk of capsular perforation. Pediatric patients will also tolerate smaller contrast loads during venography and portography.

Pediatric tools available for interventional procedures include shorter micropuncture access needles (21-gauge, 4 cm, Cook), smaller and shorter TIPS modified Colapinto needles (18-gauge, 40–50 cm, Cook) that can be placed through a 7-French sheath, and smaller and shorter stents (8 mm × 40 mm, VIATORR, Gore, Flagstaff, AZ) (▶ Fig. 5.10a–c).

TIPS placement in children is typically performed as a bridge to liver transplant.[27,28,29] Extension of stents into the main portal vein should be avoided to allow for future surgical anastomosis.[27] Continued liver growth in pediatric patients is an important issue, as this growth can affect long-term shunt patency. Diligent surveillance is required as these patients may require stent dilation to accommodate the growing hepatic and portal veins.

The complication rates for TIPS placement in children are similar to those seen in adults (▶ Table 5.2). The risk of post-TIPS encephalopathy appears to be diminished in children for

Table 5.2 TIPS-related complication rates

Complication	Incidence (%)
Mortality	< 1
Hepatic encephalopathy (adults)	20
Renal failure	5
Hepatic failure	5
Infection	2
Stent migration	2
Portal vein thrombosis	2
Puncture of liver capsule	5
Extrahepatic portal vein puncture	2

reasons that are not completely understood. It has been suggested that pediatric patients have robust circulatory compensation and decreased central nervous system susceptibility in the setting of liver failure.[27]

Creation of a TIPS in a pediatric patient can be a useful tool for managing portal hypertension. The decision to place a TIPS is best made in consensus with a multidisciplinary team involving pediatric hepatobiliary surgeons, hepatologists, and interventional radiologists so that appropriate longitudinal care can be provided.

5.7 Splenic Artery Embolization

Partial splenic embolization has been performed in the setting of portal hypertension to improve liver function, treat variceal hemorrhage and encephalopathy, and increase cell counts (notably in cases of thrombocytopenia).[30,31] This technique is not typically used as a primary method to treat the physiological complications of portal hypertension, but it has shown efficacy as an alternative or adjuvant treatment option in these patients.

The technical considerations for this procedure are similar to those of other visceral embolizations. Access is obtained into the celiac artery, typically by a common femoral artery approach, using a suitable visceral artery catheter. Power injection digital subtraction angiography is then performed, typically at a rate of 5 mL/s for a total volume of 15 to 20 mL. Once the splenic arterial and pancreatic branch anatomy is elucidated, the distal main splenic artery or intrasplenic branches are selected with a microcatheter system (▶ Fig. 5.11a). Embolization is then performed using particles in the 500- to 700-μm range (polyvinyl alcohol [PVA] or Embospheres, Merit, South Jordan, UT). The goal is to embolize approximately 50% of the splenic volume (▶ Fig. 5.11b), although some operators prefer lesser initial embolization (30–40%) to reduce the risk of post-procedural complications (pain, pleural effusion, pneumonia, splenic abscess, portal vein thrombosis).[30,31,32,33]

Pre-, intra-, and postprocedural treatment with antibiotics is advocated (Spigos' protocol) to mitigate the complications of splenic abscess (▶ Table 5.3).[33] Broad-spectrum coverage is required as these abscesses tend to be polymicrobial (> 55%).[34] Some authors advocate the administration of Pneumovax,[30] although data supporting this are currently limited.

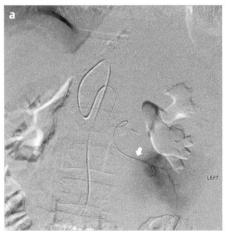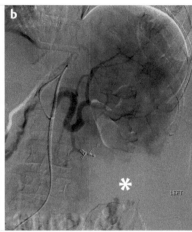

Fig. 5.11 Partial splenic embolization. **(a,b)** Fluoroscopic and digital subtraction angiographic images of the spleen depict selection of distal branches of the main splenic artery using a microcatheter (**a**, *arrow*), allowing for controlled embolization of a splenic volume using microcoils and PVA particles (**b**, *).

The debate between proximal and distal splenic embolization stems largely from the trauma surgery experience. An increased rate of infarction has been reported with distal embolization, whereas an increased rate of infection has been reported with proximal embolization.[30] Use of coils and vascular plug devices (Amplatzer, St. Jude Medical, St. Paul, MN) for proximal embolization has been described, although some operators prefer distal embolization as described earlier or proximal embolization with temporary agents (Gelfoam, Pfizer, New York, NY), as patients may require repeat embolization if the target splenic embolization or desired physiological effects are not achieved during the initial procedure.[31]

The principal mechanism of action for improved liver function with this technique is believed to be related to increasing hepatic and superior mesenteric arterial flow through a reduction in splenic arterial perfusion (▶ Table 5.4).[32] A few studies have demonstrated a 12-month improvement in total protein, prothrombin time, and albumin levels after partial splenic embolization.[31]

The addition of splenic arterial embolization to variceal ligation has been associated with decreased rebleeding rates when compared with ligation alone.[31] A decreased incidence of hepatic encephalopathy has also been described in patients undergoing partial splenic embolization when combined with other treatments such as portacaval shunts and balloon retrograde transvenous obliteration.[31,32]

5.8 Arterioportal Fistulas

Arterioportal fistulas are rarely a cause of portal hypertension. The vast majority of these fistulas are intrahepatic (>75%) and can be congenital or occur secondary to liver tumors, trauma, surgery, or percutaneous procedures such as biopsy or transhepatic cholangiogram.[35]

Most arterioportal fistulas are asymptomatic. Those that are hemodynamically significant can cause portal hypertension and symptoms of decreased liver function (elevated liver enzymes), gastrointestinal bleeding, hemobilia, and pain.[35] Unlike systemic arteriovenous malformations, arterioportal fistulas have not been associated with congestive heart failure.[35]

Arterioportal fistulas can be diagnosed with noninvasive Doppler US and CT angiography:
- Doppler US
  - Turbulent flow with or without aliasing at site of arterioportal fistula.
  - Reduced resistive index of feeding hepatic artery (<0.5 or decreased from baseline).
  - Flow reversal or arterialization of associated portal vein.
- CT or MR angiography
  - Segmental hepatic parenchymal enhancement during arterial phase imaging.
  - Dilated feeding hepatic artery and portal vein.

The gold standard for diagnosis is catheter-based angiography, with visualization of both a hepatic arterial branch and portal venous branch on early phase imaging. If the main portal vein or first-order branch is visualized, the fistula is considered hemodynamically significant (▶ Fig. 5.12).[36]

Arterioportal fistulas can be treated surgically by ligation, segmentectomy, lobectomy, or transplant if necessary. These surgeries can be technically challenging and may result in significant blood loss. In the interest of minimizing invasiveness and mitigating complications, endovascular approaches have gained popularity. These procedures are similar to other visceral embolization procedures, including precise selection of the feeding artery of the fistula with a microcatheter system (▶ Fig. 5.13a). The artery is then embolized using microcoils as proximal to the fistula as possible (▶ Fig. 5.13b). The angiographic end point is reduction of a hemodynamically significant

Table 5.3 Antibiotic administration in partial splenic embolization

Preprocedure	Intraprocedure	Postprocedure
1 M U penicillin G and 3 mg/kg gentamicin 6 h before the procedure	1 M U penicillin G and 80 mg gentamicin solution mixed with the embolic agent	1 M U penicillin G and 3 mg/kg gentamicin for 5 d after the procedure

Source: Data from Spigos et al.[33]

Table 5.4 Alteration of arterial flow in partial splenic embolization

Vessel	Preintervention flow (%)	Postintervention flow (%)
Main splenic artery	19	3
Main hepatic artery	3	15
Superior mesenteric artery	6	19

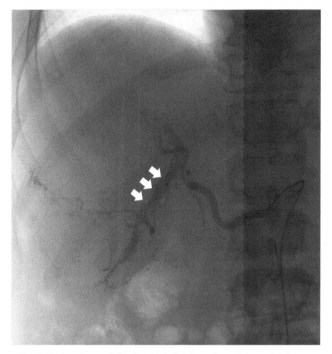

Fig. 5.12 Arterioportal fistulas. Digital subtraction angiographic image obtained during the arterial phase demonstrates early filling of the right portal vein (*arrows*) consistent with an arterioportal fistula. Given that this is a first-order branch, this finding is likely hemodynamically significant.

fistula to one that is not hemodynamically significant (nonvisualization of main portal vein or first-order branch) (▶ Fig. 5.13c).[37] In addition to coils, Gelfoam (Pfizer, New York, NY) or PVA material can be used to help achieve this end point. Approximately 25% of these cases will require repeat embolization to attain technical success.[37]

Embolization of arterioportal fistulas in native livers is far less problematic than embolization in transplanted livers. The hepatic graft is more reliant on hepatic arterial supply and is more susceptible to postembolization ischemia.[37] The larger the arterioportal fistula and more central the feeding artery, the larger the potential zone of ischemia. Embolization procedures have been classified as low risk (peripheral, small) or high risk (central, large) for ischemia based on this experience. Some authors advocate treating small, rapidly growing arterioportal fistulas even if they are asymptomatic, as they can be difficult to treat if they grow too large.[37]

Our knowledge and understanding of portal hypertension and its complications are constantly progressing. The unique challenges faced in treating this disease are matched by the innovative minimally invasive treatments offered by interventional radiology. As percutaneous interventions have become common in order to decrease morbidity in these patients, the role of the interventional radiologist in their management will be increasingly more important.

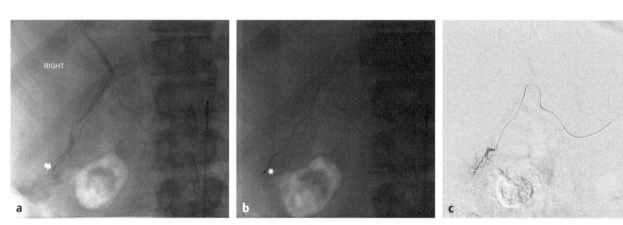

Fig. 5.13 Endovascular treatment of arterioportal fistulas. **(a–c)** Fluoroscopic and digital subtraction angiographic images of the liver depict selection of the hepatic artery branch **(a)** associated with the arterioportal fistula using a microcatheter (*arrow*). The vessel is then embolized using microcoils **(b**, *)** until early phase filling of the adjacent portal vein is no longer visualized **(c)**.

References

[1] Boyer TD, Haskal ZJ, American Association for the Study of Liver Diseases. The role of transjugular intrahepatic portosystemic shunt (TIPS) in the management of portal hypertension: update 2009. Hepatology. 2010; 51(1):306

[2] Okuda K, Ohnishi K, Kimura K, et al. Incidence of portal vein thrombosis in liver cirrhosis. An angiographic study in 708 patients. Gastroenterology. 1985; 89(2):279–286

[3] Amitrano L, Guardascione MA, Brancaccio V, et al. Risk factors and clinical presentation of portal vein thrombosis in patients with liver cirrhosis. J Hepatol. 2004; 40(5):736–741

[4] Senzolo M, Tibbals J, Cholongitas E, Triantos CK, Burroughs AK, Patch D. Transjugular intrahepatic portosystemic shunt for portal vein thrombosis with and without cavernous transformation. Aliment Pharmacol Ther. 2006; 23(6):767–775

[5] Bilbao JI, Longo JM, Rousseau H, et al. Transjugular intrahepatic portocaval shunt after thrombus disruption in partially thrombosed portal veins. Cardiovasc Intervent Radiol. 1994; 17(2):106–109

[6] Bilbao JI, Elorz M, Vivas I, Martínez-Cuesta A, Bastarrika G, Benito A. Transjugular intrahepatic portosystemic shunt (TIPS) in the treatment of venous symptomatic chronic portal thrombosis in non-cirrhotic patients. Cardiovasc Intervent Radiol. 2004; 27(5):474–480

[7] Walser EM, NcNees SW, DeLa Pena O, et al. Portal venous thrombosis: percutaneous therapy and outcome. J Vasc Interv Radiol. 1998; 9(1, Pt 1):119–127

[8] Blum U, Haag K, Rössle M, et al. Noncavernomatous portal vein thrombosis in hepatic cirrhosis: treatment with transjugular intrahepatic portosystemic shunt and local thrombolysis. Radiology. 1995; 195(1):153–157

[9] Ferral H, Bilbao JI. The difficult transjugular intrahepatic portosystemic shunt: alternative techniques and "tips" to successful shunt creation. Semin Intervent Radiol. 2005; 22(4):300–308

[10] Mammen S, Keshava SN, Kattiparambil S. Acute portal vein thrombosis, no longer a contraindication for transjugular intrahepatic porto-systemic shunt (TIPS) insertion. J Clin Exp Hepatol. 2015; 5(3):259–261

[11] Bittencourt PL, Couto CA, Ribeiro DD. Portal vein thrombosis and budd-Chiari syndrome. Hematol Oncol Clin North Am. 2011; 25(5):1049–1066, vi–vii

[12] Walser EM, Soloway R, Raza SA, Gill A. Transjugular portosystemic shunt in chronic portal vein occlusion: importance of segmental portal hypertension in cavernous transformation of the portal vein. J Vasc Interv Radiol. 2006; 17(2, Pt 1):373–378

[13] Uflacker R. Applications of percutaneous mechanical thrombectomy in transjugular intrahepatic portosystemic shunt and portal vein thrombosis. Tech Vasc Interv Radiol. 2003; 6(1):59–69

[14] Kaufman J, Lee M. Vascular and Interventional Radiology: The Requisites. Philadelphia, PA: Saunders; 2014

[15] Hasija RP, Nagral A, Marar S, Bavdekar AR. Transjugular intrahepatic portosystemic shunt (TIPSS) for Budd Chiari syndrome. Indian Pediatr. 2010; 47(6):527–528

[16] Boyvat F, Harman A, Ozyer U, Aytekin C, Arat Z. Percutaneous sonographic guidance for TIPS in Budd-Chiari syndrome: direct simultaneous puncture of the portal vein and inferior vena cava. AJR Am J Roentgenol. 2008; 191(2):560–564

[17] Punamiya SJ. Interventional radiology in the management of portal hypertension. Indian J Radiol Imaging. 2008; 18(3):249–255

[18] Petersen BD, Clark TW. Direct intrahepatic portocaval shunt. Tech Vasc Interv Radiol. 2008; 11(4):230–234

[19] Farsad K, Fuss C, Kolbeck KJ, et al. Transjugular intrahepatic portosystemic shunt creation using intravascular ultrasound guidance. J Vasc Interv Radiol. 2012; 23(12):1594–1602

[20] Saad WE. Transjugular intrahepatic portosystemic shunt before and after liver transplantation. Semin Intervent Radiol. 2014; 31(3):243–247

[21] Patel NH, Patel J, Behrens G, Savo A. Transjugular intrahepatic portosystemic shunts in liver transplant recipients: technical considerations and review of the literature. Semin Intervent Radiol. 2005; 22(4):329–333

[22] Wright TL, Donegan E, Hsu HH, et al. Recurrent and acquired hepatitis C viral infection in liver transplant recipients. Gastroenterology. 1992; 103(1):317–322

[23] Bonnel AR, Bunchorntavakul C, Rajender Reddy K. Transjugular intrahepatic portosystemic shunts in liver transplant recipients. Liver Transpl. 2014; 20(2):130–139

[24] Chong WK, Beland JC, Weeks SM. Sonographic evaluation of venous obstruction in liver transplants. AJR Am J Roentgenol. 2007; 188(6):W515–21

[25] Huang TL, Cheng YF, Chen TY, et al. Doppler ultrasound evaluation of postoperative portal vein stenosis in adult living donor liver transplantation. Transplant Proc. 2010; 42(3):879–881

[26] Woodrum DA, Bjarnason H, Andrews JC. Portal vein venoplasty and stent placement in the nontransplant population. J Vasc Interv Radiol. 2009; 20(5):593–599

[27] Heyman MB, LaBerge JM. Role of transjugular intrahepatic portosystemic shunt in the treatment of portal hypertension in pediatric patients. J Pediatr Gastroenterol Nutr. 1999; 29(3):240–249

[28] Van Ha TG, Funaki BS, Ehrhardt J, et al. Transjugular intrahepatic portosystemic shunt placement in liver transplant recipients: experiences with pediatric and adult patients. AJR Am J Roentgenol. 2005; 184(3):920–925

[29] Lorenz JM. Placement of transjugular intrahepatic portosystemic shunts in children. Tech Vasc Interv Radiol. 2008; 11(4):235–240

[30] Ahuja C, Farsad K, Chadha M. An overview of splenic embolization. AJR Am J Roentgenol. 2015; 205(4):720–725

[31] Koconis KG, Singh H, Soares G. Partial splenic embolization in the treatment of patients with portal hypertension: a review of the english language literature. J Vasc Interv Radiol. 2007; 18(4):463–481

[32] Helaly AZ, Al-Warraky MS, El-Azab GI, Kohla MA, Abdelaal EE. Portal and splanchnic hemodynamics after partial splenic embolization in cirrhotic patients with hypersplenism. APMIS. 2015; 123(12):1032–1039

[33] Spigos DG, Jonasson O, Mozes M, Capek V. Partial splenic embolization in the treatment of hypersplenism. AJR Am J Roentgenol. 1979; 132(5):777–782

[34] Brook I, Frazier EH. Microbiology of liver and spleen abscesses. J Med Microbiol. 1998; 47(12):1075–1080

[35] Saad WE. Arterioportal fistulas in liver transplant recipients. Semin Intervent Radiol. 2012; 29(2):105–110

[36] Saad WE, Davies MG, Rubens DJ, et al. Endoluminal management of arterioportal fistulae in liver transplant recipients: a single-center experience. Vasc Endovascular Surg. 2006; 40(6):451–459

[37] Saad WE, Lin E, Ormanoski M, Darcy MD, Rubens DJ. Noninvasive imaging of liver transplant complications. Tech Vasc Interv Radiol. 2007; 10(3):191–206

6 Management of Complications of Portal Hypertension: Balloon-Occluded Retrograde Transvenous Obliteration, Plug-Assisted Retrograde Transvenous Obliteration, Coil-Assisted Retrograde Transvenous Obliteration, and Balloon-Assisted Antegrade Transvenous Obliteration

Murthy R. Chamarthy and Sanjeeva P. Kalva

6.1 Introduction

Variceal bleeding is the most common complication of portal hypertension. The treatment of varices is dependent on the clinical presentation, the underlying etiology of portal hypertension, and specific characteristics of the varices, such as the size, extent, and location of the varices and the presence of concomitant portosystemic communications. Endoscopic variceal banding is a commonly practiced therapy for symptomatic and asymptomatic esophageal and gastroesophageal varices. Patients in whom endoscopic therapy fails are triaged to portal decompression procedures such as placement of a transjugular intrahepatic portosystemic shunt (TIPS) or other surgical shunts. These therapies are highly effective for esophageal and gastroesophageal varices with low variceal recurrence rates but are less effective in the management of isolated or dominant gastric varices. Gastric varices are treated with endovascular occlusion through a preexisting TIPS, through a new transjugular or transhepatic portal venous approach, or through a systemic venous approach made possible by physiologic portosystemic communications resulting from portal hypertension. The variceal obliterative procedures for gastric variceal occlusion that will be reviewed in this chapter include balloon-occluded retrograde transvenous obliteration (BRTO), plug-assisted retrograde transvenous obliteration (PARTO), coil-assisted retrograde transvenous obliteration (CARTO), and balloon-assisted antegrade transvenous obliteration (BATO).

6.2 Concept of BRTO/PARTO/CARTO

Varices related to portal hypertension are managed through either direct obliteration of the varices or portal decompression. The former approach aims at occluding (through endoscopic therapies) the large submucosal varices, which are prone to bleeding, while sparing the small, nonsubmucosal varices for continued portosystemic shunting. This approach alleviates bleeding and prevents future bleeding from at-risk varices but does little to prevent the development of new varices or alter the progression of portal hypertension. The latter approach aims to decompress the portal vein through the creation of a portosystemic shunt (TIPS or surgical shunt) or the decrease of portal blood flow through splenectomy or splenic embolization. This approach effectively decreases the portal pressure, reduces variceal bleeding, and prevents the development of new varices. However, portosystemic shunt creation may result in hepatic encephalopathy because of portal flow diversion and decreased

hepatic detoxification. Systemic venous variceal obliterative procedures aim at direct obliteration of the varices (similar to that achieved with endoscopic therapies) but differ in that they occlude not only the submucosal varices but also the periadventitial large varices and the concomitant portosystemic shunts. These approaches use balloons, vascular plugs, or coils to occlude the systemic venous outflow of the varices and embolize the varices through retrograde injection of liquid embolic materials. In this process, the physiologic shunt is also obliterated. This has profound hemodynamic effects, including decreased rebleeding, improved hepatic encephalopathy and hepatic function, and progression of portal hypertension. Given the excellent outcomes of endoscopic obliteration of esophageal varices, systemic venous variceal obliterative procedures are practiced mainly for gastric varices.

6.3 Gastric Varices

Gastric varices are less commonly encountered than esophageal varices. The prevalence of gastric varices is approximately 17% in cirrhotic patients.[1] Gastric varices may occur along with esophageal varices (gastroesophageal varices) or may be isolated. Isolated gastric varices occur in the presence of splenic or portal vein occlusion. Sarin et al[1,2] classified gastric varices into four types based on their endoscopic appearance: GOV1, GOV2, IGV1, and IGV2. GOV1 varices are the most common type (75%) and include esophageal varices extending below the gastroesophageal junction along the lesser curvature of the stomach. GOV2 varices include gastroesophageal varices that extend along the cardia (21%). Isolated gastric varices are rare and may involve the fundus of the stomach (IGV1) or may involve the rest of the stomach excluding the fundus (IGV2).

The risk of bleeding from gastric varices is significantly lower compared to the risk from esophageal varices (10–36% vs. 70–80%); however, the morbidity and mortality associated with gastric variceal bleeding are high.[1,2] This is because of the large size and location of gastric varices, which make endoscopic therapies difficult and less effective. Rebleeding rates of gastric varices after endoscopic therapy exceed 70%. In addition, decompression of gastric varices is not effectively achieved with TIPS or surgical shunts because of the low portal pressures associated with gastric varices. The mean portosystemic gradient in the presence of gastric varices is 11.2 compared to 15.5 with esophageal varices.[2,3] These low portal pressures result from the presence of concomitant portosystemic shunts that are associated with gastric varices.

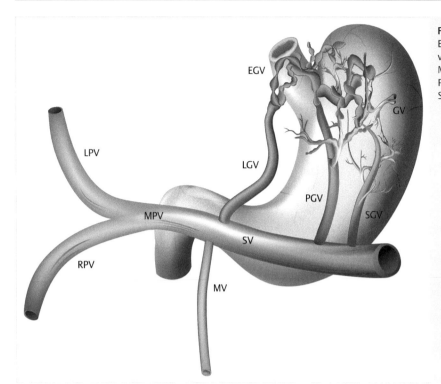

Fig. 6.1 Afferent gastric variceal system. EGV, gastroesophageal varices; GV, gastric varices, LGV, left gastric vein; LPV, left portal vein; MPV, main portal vein; MV, mesenteric vein; PGV, posterior gastric vein; RPV, right portal vein; SGV, short gastric vein; SV, splenic vein.

6.3.1 Anatomy of Gastric Varices

Venous drainage of the stomach is achieved through the left gastric vein, posterior gastric vein, short gastric veins, and gastroepiploic veins. The left gastric vein drains the distal esophagus, fundus, and the lesser curvature of the stomach, courses along the lesser curvature of the stomach, and drains into the portal vein at the portosplenic confluence. The posterior gastric and short gastric veins drain the body of the stomach and empty into the splenic vein. The gastroepiploic veins drain the body and greater curvature of the stomach and the omentum and drain into the splenic vein from the left gastroepiploic vein or the superior mesenteric vein from the right gastroepiploic vein.

In the presence of portal hypertension, the flow in these afferent veins is retrograde (away from the portal vein) and the afferent veins communicate with various systemic veins via enlarged varices. The gastric veins near the esophagus communicate with the submucosal venous plexus of the lower and midesophagus and drain into the azygos and hemiazygos veins. The veins near the bare area of the stomach communicate with the left inferior phrenic vein. The vertical portion of the left inferior phrenic vein (the ascending phrenic vein) forms the gastrorenal shunt and drains into the left renal vein after joining with the left adrenal vein (most common, 98%) or the left gonadal vein (2%). In addition, the medial horizontal portion of the inferior phrenic vein may drain directly into the inferior vena cava or the right inferior phrenic vein. The lateral horizontal portion of the left inferior phrenic vein receives tributaries from the pericardial vein and intercostal veins. Occasionally, the azygos and hemiazygos veins communicate with the medial horizontal portion of the left inferior phrenic vein.

Depending on the flow dynamics, one or more portosystemic communications enlarge and form large shunts. Such shunts include the gastrorenal shunt (gastric varices draining into the left renal vein through the ascending left inferior phrenic vein) and the gastrocaval shunt (gastric varices draining into the medial horizontal left inferior phrenic vein). The former is the most common, occurring in 80 to 85% of patients with gastric varices and in 10 to 15% of patients with portal hypertension.[4] The veins feeding into the varices are often called the "afferents," and the veins draining into the systemic veins are often called the "efferents". This nomenclature is extensively used in various classifications as described below and detailed in ▶ Fig. 6.1 and ▶ Fig. 6.2.

6.3.2 Classification of Gastric Varices

Various classifications have been proposed to address the complex anatomy, hemodynamics, and pathophysiology of gastric varices and their relevance to systemic venous obliterative procedures. Irrespective of the classification used for description purposes, it is important to identify the flow dynamics during the procedure and modify the technique of embolization based on the flow pattern, opacification of the varices, and reflux of contrast material into the systemic and/or portal veins.

Kiyosue Classification

In this classification, Kiyosue et al[5] classified the afferents and the efferents into various types to address the complexity of venous flow into and out of the gastric varices. The afferents are classified into three types. In type 1, there is a single afferent vein communicating with the varices. In types 2 and 3, multiple afferent veins exist, and they may directly contribute to the varices (type 2) or may communicate with other afferent veins before contributing to the varices (type 3). Depending on the flow pattern and hemodynamic changes with ongoing embolization, there is a risk of nontarget spread of embolic

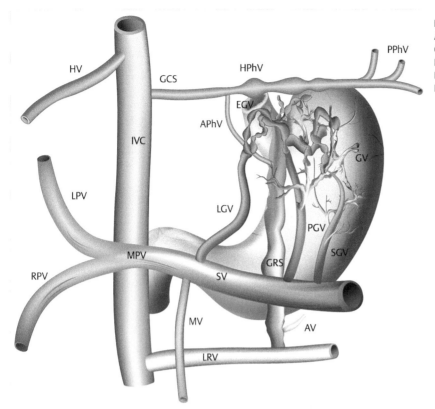

Fig. 6.2 Efferent gastric variceal system. APhV, ascending phrenic vein; AV, adrenal vein; GCS, gastrocaval shunt; GRS, gastrorenal shunt; HPhV, horizontal phrenic vein; HV, hepatic vein; IVC, inferior vena cava; LRV, left renal vein; PPhV, pericardiophrenic vein.

materials into the portal vein with types 2 and 3 afferent systems. An antegrade balloon occlusion or embolization of the afferent veins may allow successful treatment of the varices in these scenarios.

The efferent system is classified into four types depending on the number and caliber of the efferent veins. In type A, there is a single efferent draining vein, commonly a gastrorenal shunt. In type B, multiple efferent draining veins exist, but there is a single large shunt with multiple small efferents that do not pose any significant risk of nontarget systemic embolization during the procedure. Type B is subclassified into B1 (small low flow), B2 (medium-sized low flow), and B3 (large high flow without discrete shunt). In type C, multiple large shunts exist, with a high risk of nontarget systemic embolization unless the shunts are actively occluded before the varices are treated (C1, smaller second shunt; C2, larger sizable second shunt). In type D, there is no sizable systemic venous communication to allow systemic venous variceal obliteration. A recent modification of type D, known as Saad–Kiyosue Type D2, takes into consideration the uncommon portosystemic shunts (through efferents such as the azygos, hemiazygos, pericardial, or intercostal veins) that allow for systemic venous variceal obliterative procedures.

Hirota Classification

In the Hirota classification system, the gastric varices are classified into different types based on the degree of visualization during balloon-occluded retrograde venography (BORV).[6] In grade 1, the gastric varices are well opacified without visualization of any collateral veins. In grade 2, there are a few small collaterals but the gastric varices are adequately opacified for > 3 minutes. In grade 3, the gastric varices demonstrate medium to large

collaterals with only partial opacification and quick disappearance of contrast material (< 3 min). In grade 4, there are large collateral veins without opacification of the gastric varices. Grade 5 indicates a shunt that is not amenable to balloon occlusion; this is the most common cause of technical failure.

Fukuda–Hirota Hemodynamic Classification

In the Fukuda–Hirota hemodynamic classification system, the flow pattern in the gastric and esophageal varices and concomitant portosystemic shunt opacification during arterioportography are taken into consideration.[7] In type 1, there is a predominant left-sided portosystemic shunt resulting in fundal gastric varices without esophageal varices. In type 2, the esophageal varices are opacified but are not connected to and are independent of gastric variceal drainage. Type 3 is represented by complex gastroesophageal varices with a gastrorenal shunt as the primary outflow. Type 4 involves gastric varices supplied by the left gastric vein.

Matsumoto Hemodynamic Classification

Based on left gastric arteriography, Matsumoto et al[8] classified gastric varices into type I and type II based on the presence or absence of communication between the left gastric artery and the gastrorenal shunt, respectively. The varices are subdivided further into a and b groups based on the hepatopetal or hepatofugal blood flow within the left gastric vein. The type Ib group (presence of communication from the left gastric artery to the gastrorenal shunt and presence of hepatofugal flow within the left gastric vein) is associated with the highest risk of worsening esophageal varices subsequent to BRTO.

Saad–Caldwell Classification

The Saad–Caldwell classification is based on the type of varices (gastroesophageal vs. gastric) and the presence of a gastrorenal shunt (type a, without gastrorenal shunt; type b, with gastrorenal shunt).[9] Type I gastric varices correlate with Sarin's GOV1 class, and the management of these varices is similar to that used for esophageal varices. TIPS placement is preferred for type Ia, whereas a TIPS procedure with left gastric vein embolization is suggested for type Ib. Type II gastric varices correlate with Sarin's IGV1 class. TIPS placement with afferent venous embolization is suggested for type IIa; BRTO is suggested for type IIb, as TIPS placement would be less effective in the presence of a high-flow gastrorenal shunt. Type III gastric varices are complex cardiofundic gastric varices associated with esophageal varices. TIPS placement and antegrade variceal embolization are suggested for type IIIa, and BRTO with or without TIPS placement is suggested for type IIIb. Type IV gastric varices occur in the presence of splenic or portal vein thrombosis. BRTO can be considered if the portal vein is patent and a gastrorenal shunt is present. Otherwise, splenic artery embolization is recommended.

6.4 BRTO

6.4.1 Indications and Contraindications

The indications and contraindications for BRTO procedures in the management of gastric varices are summarized in ▶ Table 6.1 and ▶ Table 6.2.[10] The main indication for BRTO/PARTO/CARTO is the presence of large gastric or gastroesophageal varices that are at risk of bleeding or have already bled and are recalcitrant to other therapies. The presence of refractory hepatic encephalopathy secondary to a large gastrorenal or gastrocaval shunt is another indication for this procedure. Gastroesophageal varices with predominant afferent supply from the left gastric vein might benefit from a TIPS placement, which can be performed in conjunction with a BRTO/BATO procedure, especially in the setting of predominant esophageal varices, refractory hydrothorax, and ascites.[11] Splenic artery embolization is performed in combination with BRTO or alone (for type

D varices) to decrease the portal pressure in cases with splenic vein thrombosis and splenomegaly.

The BRTO procedure is contraindicated when the main portal vein is occluded and the gastrorenal shunt is the sole pathway for physiologic portal decompression. Occlusion of the gastrorenal shunt in this setting would result in portal flow stagnation and mesenteric venous thrombosis. In these circumstances, the varices may be obliterated if an additional portal decompression surgery is performed. The ability of cavernous transformation of the portal vein to handle the increased portal circulation from a BRTO procedure is unknown and debatable. Partial thrombosis of the portal vein may in fact benefit from the procedure, with increased flow and decreased stasis. Splenic vein thrombosis is a partial contraindication; BRTO can be performed in conjunction with splenic artery embolization to address the problem of portal hypertension. Coexisting esophageal varices or refractory hydrothorax or ascites are relative contraindications; in such cases, combination therapy with TIPS placement might be considered. A conventional BRTO procedure cannot be performed in the absence of a gastrorenal shunt. In this setting, BATO (type D1) or a nonconventional venous access (type D2) is needed for obliteration. The procedure is also contraindicated when there is a high risk of nontarget embolization of systemic or portal veins.

6.4.2 BRTO versus TIPS for the Treatment of Gastric Varices

Since its introduction by Olson et al and Kanagawa et al,[12,13] obliterative therapies with balloon or coil/plug occlusion have been extensively used throughout the eastern hemisphere for the treatment of gastric varices and are now gaining widespread recognition throughout the western hemisphere.[14] Obliterative therapy is advantageous in that it directly addresses the problem of gastric varices in the setting of normal or low portal pressure. BRTO is ideal for the management of gastric varices, especially in the presence of abnormal liver function or hepatic encephalopathy wherein TIPS is contraindicated. The risk of rebleeding after treatment of gastric varices is less with BRTO compared to TIPS

Table 6.1 Indications for BRTO

Primary indications

Bleeding gastric varices (emergent or elective setting)

High-risk gastric varices (primary prophylaxis, elective setting)

Refractory hepatic encephalopathy (emergent or elective setting)

Liver transplant patients with steal phenomenon from portal vein or augmentation of portal vein stenosis (emergent or elective setting)

Gastroesophageal variceal bleeding amenable to TIPS but model for end-stage liver disease > 18 or hepatocellular carcinoma lesions precluding TIPS placement

Adjunctive indications

BRTO + TIPS placement: gastric variceal bleeding in presence of significant ascites, hydrothorax, uncontrolled esophageal varices, or coexisting portal vein thrombosis

BRTO + splenic artery embolization: gastric variceal bleeding in presence of splenic vein thrombosis, hypersplenism, and esophageal varices

Abbreviations: BRTO, balloon-occluded retrograde transvenous obliteration; TIPS, transjugular intrahepatic portosystemic shunt.

Table 6.2 Contraindications for BRTO

Complete portal vein thrombosis or cavernous transformation (consider transhepatic or trans-TIPS portal venous interventions with or without TIPS placement/BRTO)

Splenic vein thrombosis (consider splenic artery embolization with or without BRTO)

Lack of gastrorenal shunt, type D1 (consider BATO or TIPS)

Refractory hydrothorax, ascites, and esophageal varices (consider TIPS placement with or without BRTO)

Inadequate balloon occlusion of gastrorenal shunt or incomplete occlusion of collaterals (consider CARTO, PARTO, or BATO and TIPS placement)

Abbreviations: BATO, balloon-assisted antegrade transvenous obliteration; BRTO, balloon-occluded retrograde transvenous obliteration; CARTO, coil-assisted retrograde transvenous obliteration; PARTO, plug-assisted retrograde transvenous obliteration; TIPS, transjugular intrahepatic portosystemic shunt.

Table 6.3 BRTO versus TIPS

	BRTO	TIPS
Indication	Bleeding gastric varices	Bleeding gastroesophageal varices
Objective	Obliteration of gastric varices via sclerosis of gastrorenal shunt	Portal decompression through creation of a portacaval shunt
Portal pressures	Usually low or normal	More effective at high portal pressures
Complications	Worsening portal hypertension, ascites, splenomegaly, and esophageal varices	Worsening hepatic encephalopathy and liver function
Advantages	Preserved hepatic function, decreased hepatic encephalopathy	Addresses portal hypertension and associated sequelae

Abbreviations: BRTO, balloon-occluded retrograde transvenous obliteration; TIPS, transjugular intrahepatic portosystemic shunt.

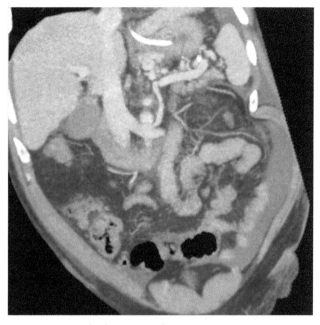

Fig. 6.3 Preprocedural imaging workup. Maximum intensity projection reconstruction images in a patient presenting with gastric variceal bleeding confirm gastric varices and the presence of a gastrorenal shunt. Smaller collaterals and the presence of a gastrocaval shunt might be difficult to identity on anatomic imaging; these entities would need to be evaluated on balloon-occluded retrograde venography. The portal and splenic veins are noted to be patent. The patient is a candidate for BRTO.

(0–2% vs. 15–20%); however, the benefit–risk ratio must be considered on a case-by-case basis.[4]

The creation of TIPS results in decompression of portal hypertension and improvement of gastric varices by directing flow away from gastrorenal or gastrocaval shunts. However, in a setting of low or normal portal pressures with posterior gastric or short gastric afferents, the benefit from TIPS placement might be limited. TIPS placement is the procedure of choice (either alone or in combination with an obliterative procedure) in the management of gastric varices in the presence of coexisting esophageal varices (especially GOV1 type) or refractory hydrothorax and ascites. TIPS placement can also be performed when BRTO is contraindicated or cannot be performed. An indwelling TIPS stent provides easy access for antegrade obliteration. Worsening liver function with a high MELD (Model for End-Stage Liver Disease) score, hepatic encephalopathy, and right heart failure are relative contraindications for TIPS. ▶ Table 6.3 describes the relative advantages and disadvantages of TIPS and BRTO procedures in the management of gastric varices.

6.4.3 Workup and Management

Patients with cirrhosis and portal hypertension might present in an emergent or elective setting with upper gastrointestinal bleeding from gastric varices or hepatic encephalopathy. In an emergent setting, the first steps should be toward stabilization and maintenance of the airway, breathing, and circulation.[15] Emergent gastric tube inflation might be needed. Nonaggressive careful volume resuscitation is recommended to prevent portal hypertension. The initial workup should involve endoscopic evaluation to assess the presence, location, and size of esophageal and gastric varices, assess the risk of bleeding, and treat varices that are bleeding or at risk of bleeding. If the initial endoscopic intervention demonstrates gastric varices or fails to control the bleeding, endovascular interventions can be undertaken. Imaging evaluation is of paramount importance when BRTO is considered. Contrast-enhanced computed tomography (CT) or magnetic resonance (MR) imaging of the abdomen should be performed to assess the patency of portal and splenic veins and the presence of gastrorenal and gastrocaval shunts

and to determine the size, location, course, and multiplicity of the venous efferents (▶ Fig. 6.3). This information is needed to plan venous access (jugular vs. femoral) and to determine the size of the balloon and the appropriate location for occlusion of the efferents.[16] Laboratory evaluation should be performed to detect anemia and to assess platelet count, kidney and liver function, and baseline ammonia level. A multidisciplinary, patient-centered approach is helpful in identifying suitable candidates for BRTO. It is important to individualize therapy based on clinical presentation, imaging findings, and available resources and expertise.

6.4.4 BRTO Technique

BRTO involves balloon occlusion of the gastrorenal shunt and administration of sclerosant material into the efferent vein in a retrograde fashion to obliterate the shunt, varices, and possibly the afferent system. Various strategies exist to access and occlude the collaterals, thereby allowing adequate stagnation of the sclerosant while preventing nontarget migration. A detailed technique has been described by Saad et al.[10] With this technique, femoral or jugular venous access is obtained (▶ Fig. 6.4), and a long 50- to 70-cm, 7- to 12-Fr sheath is positioned in the inferior vena cava. The left renal vein is catheterized with a Cobra or Simmons 2 catheter, and the adrenal–phrenic venous trunk is cannulated. The catheter is then exchanged for a compliant balloon occlusion catheter over a wire. The balloon is inflated at the base (caudal segment) of the vertical portion of the inferior phrenic vein (the efferent vein of the shunt). Contrast material is injected to assess whether the balloon was

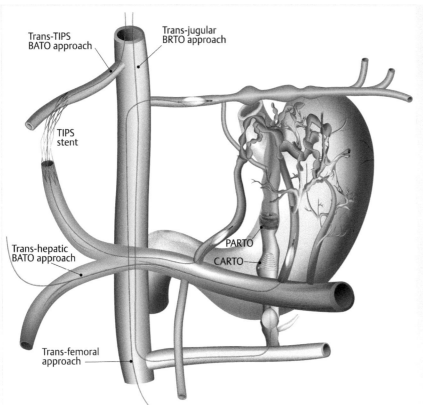

Fig. 6.4 Approaches for BRTO, BATO, CARTO, and PARTO. BATO, balloon-occluded antegrade transvenous obliteration; BRTO, balloon-occluded retrograde transvenous obliteration; CARTO, coil-assisted retrograde transvenous obliteration; PARTO, plug-assisted retrograde transvenous obliteration; TIPS, transjugular intrahepatic portosystemic shunt.

occlusive enough to prevent reflux of the contrast material into the renal vein. If there is reflux, the balloon is exchanged for a larger balloon. Contrast material injection allows detection of the varices, collaterals, and competing shunts (▶ Fig. 6.5a). Any significant collaterals and competing shunts that would result in nontarget embolization are occluded with coils or vascular plugs after selective cannulation (▶ Fig. 6.5b).

The volume of sclerosant that is required for adequate obliteration of the varices is calculated with contrast material injection. The sclerosant materials commonly used are Sotradecol (sodium tetradecyl sulfate; Bioniche Pharma USA LLC, Lake Forest, IL) and ethanolamine oleate (EO; Oldamin, ASKA Pharmaceutical, Tokyo, Japan; and QOL Medical, Vero Beach, FL). The sclerosant solution is prepared by mixing one part of Lipiodol, two parts of 3% Sotradecol, and three parts of air or carbon dioxide to form a foam, which is then injected into the varices while the balloon is kept inflated. Foam administration provides maximum surface area contact and better distribution to the nondependent tortuous submucosal portions of the gastric varices and reduces the total required sclerosant volume. Inadequate occlusion of the shunt results in an increased risk of toxicity and embolization, especially in patients with known right-to-left shunt. Outside of the United States, 10% EO is mixed with nonionic contrast material in a 1:1 ratio and used as a sclerosant. The limited availability of EO and haptoglobin (an antidote for EO-induced hemoglobinuria) restricted the use of EO in the United States, whereas extensive experience with Sotradecol and its well-known safety profile have resulted in its widespread acceptance. Dose-reduction strategies may include aiming for staged sclerosis, decreasing the target volume with balloon advancement, and using other sclerosant solutions such as absolute alcohol, 50% dextrose, and polidocanol, as well as liquid embolic materials such as *N*-acetyl cyanoacrylate and ethylene vinyl copolymer.[10]

Adequate occlusion of the collaterals is necessary to trap and achieve adequate stagnation of the sclerosant. The occlusion balloon is left inflated for 6 to 24 hours to allow for adequate sclerosis, thrombus formation, and obliteration. Low-flow gastric shunts might sclerose with shorter indwelling times; however, balloon inflation is recommended for at least a few hours to prevent mobilization of variceal thrombus. Aspiration of any remaining sclerosant should be performed for cases in which shorter indwelling times are used before balloon deflation. A radiograph can be used to confirm sustained inflation of the balloon before bedside deflation. Posttreatment renal venogram can be used to demonstrate renal vein patency, and an intraprocedural cone-beam CT scan or postprocedural CT scan can confirm appropriate distribution of contrast material within the varices (▶ Fig. 6.5c).

6.4.5 CARTO and PARTO

The balloon used in the BRTO procedure can be replaced with coils (CARTO) or a vascular plug (PARTO) (▶ Fig. 6.4). The use of a vascular plug or coils obviates the need for prolonged balloon inflation times, thereby decreasing the hospital stay/observation times. In addition, the embolic material may be replaced with a mixture of Sotradecol, contrast material, and Gelfoam or a mixture of Gelfoam and contrast material. When a Gelfoam mixture is used as the embolic material, occlusion of small collateral venous channels may not be required, as the risk of systemic or portal embolization of sclerosant is low.

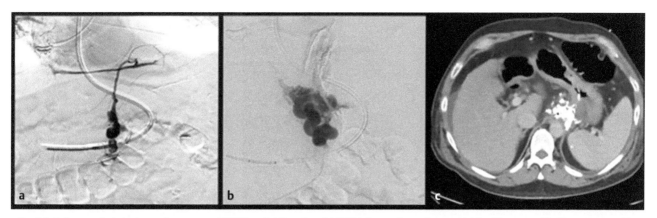

Fig. 6.5 Balloon-occluded retrograde venogram (BORV) and obliteration. **(a)** BORV via transfemoral approach identifies a type C1 efferent system. The ascending portion of the inferior phrenic vein was coil embolized. **(b)** Repeat BORV demonstrates adequate occlusion to allow for stagnation of the sclerosant without collaterals; an approximate volume of the sclerosants was calculated. **(c)** Post-BRTO CT scan demonstrates distribution of the Lipiodol within the gastric varices, consistent with good obliterative result. Cone-beam CT can also provide this information during the procedure.

6.4.6 BATO

BATO is an antegrade technique for obliteration of the gastric varices, wherein access to the gastric varices is commonly obtained through TIPS (trans-TIPS BATO) or through a transhepatic approach (percutaneous transhepatic obliteration) (▶ Fig. 6.4).[17] Indications for BATO include failed catheterization, absence of gastrorenal shunt, and incomplete gastrorenal shunt occlusion (BATO bailout). Approach via an existing TIPS shunt provides easy access for obliteration of the gastric varices and also prevents complications from possible leakage of sclerosants into the portal venous circulation. A combination of BRTO with BATO increases the success rate of gastric variceal obliteration from 94–98% to 98–100%.[18,19]

6.4.7 Outcomes

Technical success of BRTO, defined as complete obliteration of gastric varices, ranges from 77 to 100%.[20] Multiple studies have reported a gastric variceal rebleeding rate of 0 to 15% after successful BRTO.[21,22] On intent-to-treat analysis, the risk of gastric variceal rebleeding rates has ranged from 0 to 31.6%.[23] Results comparing different treatment modalities for the management of gastric varices are limited and variable, but outcomes might be superior with BRTO compared to TIPS and endoscopic management (▶ Table 6.4).[24,25,26,27,28,29,30,31] BRTO can also result in increased portal venous flow, leading to short-term improvement in liver function.[22,32,33] An increased benefit is seen in patients with relatively preserved liver function before the procedure.[33] BRTO is also associated with a reduction in hepatic encephalopathy from shunt occlusion and increased hepatopetal flow.[21,32] However, the long-term continued benefit from increased portal flow needs to be evaluated further. Patient survival after BRTO procedure is 83 to 98% at 1 year and 36 to 69% at 5 years; hepatic synthetic reserve and the presence of hepatocellular carcinoma are the two most important prognostic factors for predicting survival benefit.[23,34]

6.4.8 Complications

Complications from BRTO might be grouped into those resulting from the procedure/technique and those expected from alteration of the portal hemodynamics.[32,35,36] Nausea and vomiting (21%), chest and abdominal pain (56–76%), transient fever (26–33%), transient systemic hypertension (35%), transient hematuria (53%), bacterial peritonitis (8%), and pulmonary infarction (2%) can occur secondary to occlusion. Portal and renal vein thrombosis (approximately 5%) can occur if there is spillage of the sclerosant material into the portal and renal venous circulations; the clinical significance of this event is uncertain. There is a risk of pulmonary edema and pulmonary embolism due to nontarget embolization/migration of the sclerosant material from inadequate occlusion or balloon rupture. Rupture of the balloon has been reported in 2.3 to 16% of patients in different series, with the clinical effect dependent on the timing of the rupture and flow dynamics of the gastrorenal shunt.[37,38] Coil migration and nontarget embolization are also concerns with BRTO. Coil embolization very close to the varices or ischemia from the procedure itself can result in gastric ulcers (9%). Use of EO can result in hemoglobinuria and renal toxicity (49%). There is also a transient spike in liver dysfunction secondary to variceal obliteration and hemolysis. Renal failure and hepatorenal syndrome can develop secondary to hemolysis and contrast nephropathy. Rupture of the retroperitoneal portion of the gastrorenal shunt is usually

Table 6.4 Outcomes: TIPS versus endoscopic treatment versus BRTO for gastric varices

Study	Rebleeding rates		
	TIPS (%)	Endoscopic treatment (%)	BRTO (%)
Mahadeva et al (2003)[24]	15	30	
Choi et al (2003)[25]	15		0
Ninoi et al (2004)[26]	20		2
Lo et al (2007)[27]	11	38	
Procaccini et al (2009)[28]	25	10	
Hong et al (2009)[29]		71.4	15.4
Min et al (2011)[30]		18	6.7
Kochhar et al (2015)[31]	17.4	17.2	

Abbreviations: BRTO, balloon-occluded retrograde transvenous obliteration; TIPS, transjugular intrahepatic portosystemic shunt.

self-limiting, although care must be taken to prevent spasm and rupture precluding the BRTO procedure.[16] Although rare, cerebrovascular accidents in patients with right-to-left shunting and life-threatening bleeding immediately after balloon inflation and before injection of sclerosants are severe complications with high morbidity and mortality.

Increased portal flow results in increased portal hypertension and, thereby, development of esophageal varices (40%), ascites (7%), or hydrothorax (12%). There is an increase in the size of the esophageal varices with time (aggravation rate at 1 year, 7.3–35%; at 2 years, 45–66%; at 3 years, 45–91%),[22] and 36 to 57% of these varices bleed.[39] Portal hypertensive gastropathy is noted in 2 to 13% of cases. A rare complication of paradoxical liver failure subsequent to BRTO necessitating liver transplant or resulting in death has also been reported.[23]

6.4.9 Follow-Up

There are no specific guidelines or recommendations for follow-up after BRTO. A chest radiograph should be obtained on the day after the BRTO procedure to exclude any pulmonary complications. Laboratory evaluation should include follow-up of liver and renal functions. Careful attention should be paid to fluid levels and volume status. Endoscopic ultrasound evaluation 1 to 2 days after BRTO can confirm sclerosis and occlusion of the varices and presents an opportunity to treat any persistent varices. Endoscopy and cross-sectional imaging surveillance should be performed every 3 to 6 months to monitor for worsening gastric or esophageal varices.[40]

6.5 Conclusion

Treatment of gastric varices requires adequate understanding of their location and size, concomitant portosystemic communications, and portal flow dynamics. Systemic venous techniques for variceal obliteration including BRTO, CARTO, and PARTO aim at occluding the varices and portosystemic shunt while improving the portal flow. These techniques are highly effective both in isolation and in conjunction with portal decompression (TIPS) or splenic embolization. A multidisciplinary, patient-centered approach is required to achieve the best outcomes.

References

[1] Sarin SK, Lahoti D, Saxena SP, Murthy NS, Makwana UK. Prevalence, classification and natural history of gastric varices: a long-term follow-up study in 568 portal hypertension patients. Hepatology. 1992; 16(6):1343–1349

[2] Ryan BM, Stockbrugger RW, Ryan JM. A pathophysiologic, gastroenterologic, and radiologic approach to the management of gastric varices. Gastroenterology. 2004; 126(4):1175–1189

[3] Chao Y, Lin HC, Lee FY, et al. Hepatic hemodynamic features in patients with esophageal or gastric varices. J Hepatol. 1993; 19(1):85–89

[4] Saad WE, Darcy MD. Transjugular intrahepatic portosystemic shunt (TIPS) versus balloon-occluded retrograde transvenous obliteration (BRTO) for the management of gastric varices. Semin Intervent Radiol. 2011; 28(3):339–349

[5] Kiyosue H, Mori H, Matsumoto S, Yamada Y, Hori Y, Okino Y. Transcatheter obliteration of gastric varices. Part 1. Anatomic classification. Radiographics. 2003; 23(4):911–920

[6] Hirota S, Matsumoto S, Tomita M, Sako M, Kono M. Retrograde transvenous obliteration of gastric varices. Radiology. 1999; 211(2):349–356

[7] Fukuda T, Hirota S, Sugimoto K, Matsumoto S, Zamora CA, Sugimura K. "Downgrading" of gastric varices with multiple collateral veins in balloon-occluded retrograde transvenous obliteration. J Vasc Interv Radiol. 2005; 16 (10):1379–1383

[8] Matsumoto A, Hamamoto N, Nomura T, et al. Balloon-occluded retrograde transvenous obliteration of high risk gastric fundal varices. Am J Gastroenterol. 1999; 94(3):643–649

[9] Saad WE. Vascular anatomy and the morphologic and hemodynamic classifications of gastric varices and spontaneous portosystemic shunts relevant to the BRTO procedure. Tech Vasc Interv Radiol. 2013; 16(2):60–100

[10] Saad WE, Kitanosono T, Koizumi J, Hirota S. The conventional balloon-occluded retrograde transvenous obliteration procedure: indications, contraindications, and technical applications. Tech Vasc Interv Radiol. 2013; 16(2):101–151

[11] Saad WE, Wagner CC, Lippert A, et al. Protective value of TIPS against the development of hydrothorax/ascites and upper gastrointestinal bleeding after balloon-occluded retrograde transvenous obliteration (BRTO). Am J Gastroenterol. 2013; 108(10):1612–1619

[12] Olson E, Yune HY, Klatte EC. Transrenal-vein reflux ethanol sclerosis of gastroesophageal varices. AJR Am J Roentgenol. 1984; 143(3):627–628

[13] Kanagawa H, Mima S, Kouyama H, Gotoh K, Uchida T, Okuda K. Treatment of gastric fundal varices by balloon-occluded retrograde transvenous obliteration. J Gastroenterol Hepatol. 1996; 11(1):51–58

[14] Saad WE. The history and evolution of balloon-occluded retrograde transvenous obliteration (BRTO): From the United States to Japan and back. Semin Intervent Radiol. 2011; 28(3):283–287

[15] Al-Osaimi AM, Sabri SS, Caldwell SH. Balloon-occluded retrograde transvenous obliteration (BRTO): preprocedural evaluation and imaging. Semin Intervent Radiol. 2011; 28(3):288–295

[16] Saad WE, Nicholson DB. Optimizing logistics for balloon-occluded retrograde transvenous obliteration (BRTO) of gastric varices by doing away with the indwelling balloon: concept and techniques. Tech Vasc Interv Radiol. 2013; 16(2):152–157

[17] Saad WE, Sze DY. Variations of balloon-occluded retrograde transvenous obliteration (BRTO): balloon-occluded antegrade transvenous obliteration (BATO) and alternative/adjunctive routes for BRTO. Semin Intervent Radiol. 2011; 28(3):314–324

[18] Arai H, Abe T, Takagi H, Mori M. Efficacy of balloon-occluded retrograde transvenous obliteration, percutaneous transhepatic obliteration and combined techniques for the management of gastric fundal varices. World J Gastroenterol. 2006; 12(24):3866–3873

[19] Saad WE, Kitanosono T, Koizumi J. Balloon-occluded antegrade transvenous obliteration with or without balloon-occluded retrograde transvenous obliteration for the management of gastric varices: concept and technical applications. Tech Vasc Interv Radiol. 2012; 15(3):203–225

[20] Patel A, Fischman AM, Saad WE. Balloon-occluded retrograde transvenous obliteration of gastric varices. AJR Am J Roentgenol. 2012; 199(4):721–729

[21] Cho SK, Shin SW, Lee IH, et al. Balloon-occluded retrograde transvenous obliteration of gastric varices: outcomes and complications in 49 patients. AJR Am J Roentgenol. 2007; 189(6):W365–72

[22] Fukuda T, Hirota S, Sugimura K. Long-term results of balloon-occluded retrograde transvenous obliteration for the treatment of gastric varices and hepatic encephalopathy. J Vasc Interv Radiol. 2001; 12(3):327–336

[23] Saad WE, Sabri SS. Balloon-occluded retrograde transvenous obliteration (BRTO): technical results and outcomes. Semin Intervent Radiol. 2011; 28(3):333–338

[24] Mahadeva S, Bellamy MC, Kessel D, Davies MH, Millson CE. Cost-effectiveness of N-butyl-2-cyanoacrylate (histoacryl) glue injections versus transjugular intrahepatic portosystemic shunt in the management of acute gastric variceal bleeding. Am J Gastroenterol. 2003; 98(12):2688–2693

[25] Choi YH, Yoon CJ, Park JH, Chung JW, Kwon JW, Choi GM. Balloon-occluded retrograde transvenous obliteration for gastric variceal bleeding: its feasibility compared with transjugular intrahepatic portosystemic shunt. Korean J Radiol. 2003; 4(2):109–116

[26] Ninoi T, Nakamura K, Kaminou T, et al. TIPS versus transcatheter sclerotherapy for gastric varices. AJR Am J Roentgenol. 2004; 183(2):369–376

[27] Lo GH, Liang HL, Chen WC, et al. A prospective, randomized controlled trial of transjugular intrahepatic portosystemic shunt versus cyanoacrylate injection in the prevention of gastric variceal rebleeding. Endoscopy. 2007; 39(8):679–685

[28] Procaccini NJ, Al-Osaimi AM, Northup P, Argo C, Caldwell SH. Endoscopic cyanoacrylate versus transjugular intrahepatic portosystemic shunt for

gastric variceal bleeding: a single-center U.S. analysis. Gastrointest Endosc. 2009; 70(5):881–887

[29] Hong CH, Kim HJ, Park JH, et al. Treatment of patients with gastric variceal hemorrhage: endoscopic N-butyl-2-cyanoacrylate injection versus balloon-occluded retrograde transvenous obliteration. J Gastroenterol Hepatol. 2009; 24(3):372–378

[30] Min SK, Kim SG, Kim YS, et al. Comparison among endoscopic variceal obliteration, endoscopic band ligation, and balloon-occluded retrograde transvenous obliteration for treatment of gastric variceal bleeding [in Korean]. Korean J Gastroenterol. 2011; 57(5):302–308

[31] Kochhar GS, Navaneethan U, Hartman J, et al. Comparative study of endoscopy vs. transjugular intrahepatic portosystemic shunt in the management of gastric variceal bleeding. Gastroenterol Rep (Oxf). 2015; 3(1):75–82

[32] Kumamoto M, Toyonaga A, Inoue H, et al. Long-term results of balloon-occluded retrograde transvenous obliteration for gastric fundal varices: hepatic deterioration links to portosystemic shunt syndrome. J Gastroenterol Hepatol. 2010; 25(6):1129–1135

[33] Saad WE, Wagner CC, Al-Osaimi A, et al. The effect of balloon-occluded transvenous obliteration of gastric varices and gastrorenal shunts on the hepatic synthetic function: a comparison between Child-Pugh and model for end-stage liver disease scores. Vasc Endovascular Surg. 2013; 47(4):281–287

[34] Saad WE. Endovascular management of gastric varices. Clin Liver Dis. 2014; 18(4):829–851

[35] Hiraga N, Aikata H, Takaki S, et al. The long-term outcome of patients with bleeding gastric varices after balloon-occluded retrograde transvenous obliteration. J Gastroenterol. 2007; 42(8):663–672

[36] Shimoda R, Horiuchi K, Hagiwara S, et al. Short-term complications of retrograde transvenous obliteration of gastric varices in patients with portal hypertension: effects of obliteration of major portosystemic shunts. Abdom Imaging. 2005; 30(3):306–313

[37] Saad WE, Nicholson D, Lippert A, et al. Balloon-occlusion catheter rupture during balloon-occluded retrograde transvenous obliteration of gastric varices utilizing sodium tetradecyl sulfate: incidence and consequences. Vasc Endovascular Surg. 2012; 46(8):664–670

[38] Park SJ, Chung JW, Kim HC, Jae HJ, Park JH. The prevalence, risk factors, and clinical outcome of balloon rupture in balloon-occluded retrograde transvenous obliteration of gastric varices. J Vasc Interv Radiol. 2010; 21(4): 503–507

[39] Ninoi T, Nishida N, Kaminou T, et al. Balloon-occluded retrograde transvenous obliteration of gastric varices with gastrorenal shunt: long-term follow-up in 78 patients. AJR Am J Roentgenol. 2005; 184(4):1340–1346

[40] Saad WE, Al-Osaimi AM, Caldwell SH. Pre- and post-balloon-occluded retrograde transvenous obliteration clinical evaluation, management, and imaging: indications, management protocols, and follow-up. Tech Vasc Interv Radiol. 2012; 15(3):165–202

7 Nonvariceal Upper Gastrointestinal Hemorrhage

Eric J. Monroe and Karim Valji

7.1 Introduction

Selective arteriography of the gastrointestinal tract for enteric hemorrhage was an early mainstay in the nascent field of interventional radiology half a century ago.[1,2] Ingenious angiographers soon made the not-so-obvious leap to using this technique for transcatheter management.[3] As the technology and experience with this technique expanded, therapeutic options also evolved, progressing from infusion of vasoconstrictive agents to deployment of a wide range of embolic agents. Mesenteric angiography and intervention soon became a common request for patients with ongoing gastrointestinal bleeding.

As in other arenas of medicine, the multidisciplinary approach to gastrointestinal hemorrhage has evolved substantially in recent decades. Endoscopists have greatly expanded their diagnostic and therapeutic capabilities in this area. Medical therapies also continue to improve, with a wide range of acid-reducing agents and selective cyclooxygenase inhibitors now available. The discovery of and treatment for *Helicobacter pylori* have altered the epidemiology of peptic ulcer disease.[4] However, advances in medical therapy have not convincingly decreased mortality.[5] Gastrointestinal hemorrhage remains a common clinical problem, with an estimated yearly incidence of 100 to 300 per 100,000 people.[6,7,8] This condition also continues to be a leading cause of emergency room visits and hospital admissions, with mortality as high as 10%.[6,9,10] Cases refractory to initial treatment are also common. For these reasons, angiography with catheter-directed therapy remains a critical tool in the management of nonvariceal upper gastrointestinal hemorrhage.[11,12]

7.2 Patient Presentation

Upper gastrointestinal bleeding is defined as bleeding originating from the esophagus to the ligament of Treitz and is far more common than lower gastrointestinal bleeding.[13] Transpapillary bleeding from hepatic and pancreatic sources enters the duodenum and therefore presents as upper gastrointestinal hemorrhage. A wide range of clinical presentations may be encountered, largely dependent on the rate of bleeding. If blood losses have been greater than 500 mL in 24 hours, hemodynamic perturbations such as shock may be present. Conversely, blood losses of less than 100 mL in 24 hours may be asymptomatic and incidentally discovered as anemia.

Hematemesis and bloody aspirate from a nasogastric tube are compelling signs of an upper gastrointestinal source, whereas hematochezia generally suggests a lower source. Melena may result from bleeding anywhere along the length of the gastrointestinal tract, depending on the rate of hemorrhage. The orifice of bleeding alone is an unreliable indicator of pathology.[6] In approximately 10% of cases, brisk bleeding from an upper intestinal tract source may present with bright red blood through the rectum.

A careful review of past medical and surgical history and medication use may favor one source over another. Nonenteric sources of bleeding such as epistaxis or hemoptysis should be reasonably excluded.

7.3 Etiologies

Peptic ulcer disease remains the most common underlying condition causing upper gastrointestinal hemorrhage, manifesting as erosive esophagitis, erosive gastritis, or ulcers of the stomach or duodenum. These manifestations of peptic ulcer disease account for approximately 70% of upper gastrointestinal bleeds.[14] Potentiating factors include *H. pylori* infection, use of nonsteroidal anti-inflammatory medications, and alcohol consumption.

Variceal bleeding and portal hypertensive gastropathy comprise the next largest fraction of cases and are discussed elsewhere in this text.

Mallory–Weiss lesions are focal tears of the distal esophagus and gastroesophageal junction involving the mucosa and underlying vasculature.[15] Bleeding is classically preceded by retching, often associated with alcohol consumption. In the absence of concurrent gastroesophageal variceal bleeding, most of these cases can be managed conservatively. Infrequently, these lesions require endoscopic and/or transcatheter intervention (▶ Fig. 7.1).

Dieulafoy lesions are focal erosions of an otherwise normal submucosal artery found most commonly in the proximal stomach but potentially anywhere along the length of the gastrointestinal tract.[16] Risk factors include antiplatelet agent use

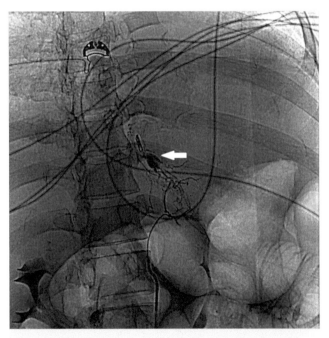

Fig. 7.1 Mallory–Weiss tear. A briskly bleeding gastroesophageal tear was identified at endoscopy and inadequately controlled with clip placement. Selective angiogram of the left gastric artery demonstrates extravasation adjacent to the endoscopically placed clip (*arrow*).

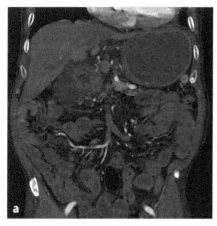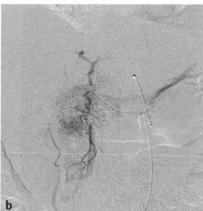

Fig. 7.2 Bleeding gastric adenocarcinoma. (a) Contrast-enhanced CT demonstrates a large, ulcerated mass at the gastric antrum. (b) Digital subtraction angiogram of the distal common hepatic artery. The mass derives its blood supply from branches of the gastroduodenal artery and parasitized hepatic arteries. Neovascularity and tumor blush are present. The gastroduodenal artery is irregular and narrowed.

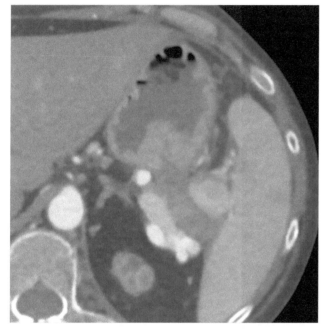

Fig. 7.3 Pancreatitis and spontaneous gastric fistula. A broad fistulous connection between the pancreatic tail and gastric fundus has formed.

gastric bleeding. Hepatic biliary sources are frequently iatrogenic as a result of biopsy or transhepatic biliary drain placement (▶ Fig. 7.5).

An aortoenteric fistula is a rare but life-threatening entity that often results in patient death before further workup can be performed. Although any abnormal fistulous connection between the aorta or branch vessel and the digestive tract meets the broad definition of an aortoenteric fistula, most occur between the transverse duodenum and abdominal aorta. Primary aortoenteric fistulas are most commonly associated with abdominal aortic aneurysms but may also arise as a result of malignancy, peptic ulcer disease, trauma, infection, inflammatory bowel disease, or foreign body ingestion.[19] Secondary aortoenteric fistulas occurring after aortic aneurysm repair or para-aortic surgery are more common. Left untreated, this condition is frequently fatal.

7.4 Initial Management

Patients presenting with hemodynamic instability or obvious active bleeding require admission to the intensive care unit. Management begins with establishment of large-bore intravenous (IV) access followed by resuscitation with crystalloid fluids and/or blood products.[20] A nasogastric tube should be placed, along with an endotracheal tube if airway protection is needed. Nasogastric lavage returning bloody aspirate all but confirms a proximal source of bleeding. A lavage without evidence of bleeding does not exclude an upper gastrointestinal source, however. Approximately 15% of such patients will have high-risk lesions identified at endoscopy.[21]

Reversal of anticoagulation and correction of thrombocytopenia or coagulopathy (when present) should be performed. Empiric therapy with high-dose proton-pump inhibitors should be initiated and continued until the need for acid blockade is excluded. Splanchnic vasoconstrictors such as vasopressin may be initiated to support systemic pressure while decreasing enteric blood flow. Similarly, empiric therapy with a somatostatin analogue (octreotide) may address potential portal hypertensive bleeding but may also reduce the risk of bleeding from nonvariceal etiologies.[22] A wide variety of tests are available to diagnose *H. pylori*, which may then be eradicated with multidrug antibiotic therapy. With medical support established, management can proceed to bleeding localization.

and alcohol consumption. Most lesions identified at endoscopy are successfully managed in that setting[17]; however, bleeding may be intermittent and endoscopically occult.

Both benign and malignant gastrointestinal tumors have the potential to cause gastrointestinal hemorrhage if there is erosion across the mucosal surface. Bleeding in such cases is typically slow and subclinical but may be profound (▶ Fig. 7.2).

Transpapillary bleeding may result from pathology of the liver, gallbladder, or pancreas. Bleeding localized to the pancreatic duct is termed hemosuccus pancreaticus and is typically associated with chronic pancreatitis or pseudocysts.[18] Postpancreatitis pseudoaneurysm of the pancreatic arteries, splenic artery, or gastroduodenal artery and subsequent bleeding may be either retroperitoneal or transpapillary. Less commonly, fistulous connections to the stomach, either spontaneous (▶ Fig. 7.3) or iatrogenic (▶ Fig. 7.4), can lead to postpancreatitis

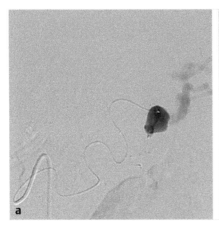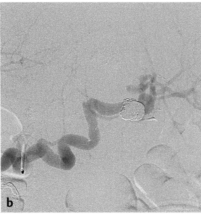

Fig. 7.4 Massive hemorrhage after cyst gastrostomy. **(a)** A large pseudoaneurysm of the distal splenic artery was identified and **(b)** embolized to stasis with coils.

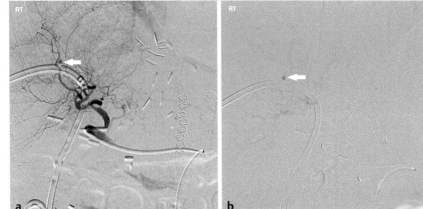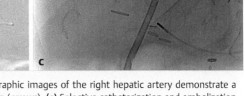

Fig. 7.5 Hemobilia after percutaneous biliary drain placement. **(a)** Early and **(b)** late angiographic images of the right hepatic artery demonstrate a small hepatic arterial pseudoaneurysm immediately adjacent to the percutaneous biliary drain (*arrows*). **(c)** Selective catheterization and embolization with NBCA resulted in immediate cessation of bleeding.

7.5 Diagnosis

7.5.1 Endoscopy

Upper endoscopy is the diagnostic modality of choice for upper gastrointestinal hemorrhage[23,24]; this technique reduces the rate of rebleeding, the need for surgery, and patient mortality compared to medical management.[25] Although many cases of hemorrhage will resolve spontaneously, early endoscopy (within 24 hours) is advocated by many to localize, treat, and prevent the recurrence of bleeding.[23] With this procedure, arterial and portal hypertensive etiologies of bleeding can be readily distinguished. Details of the endoscopic approach are beyond the scope of this text. In general, current prevailing techniques for identifying and treating hemorrhage include ulcer bed irrigation, epinephrine injection, use of clips, thermocoagulation, and sclerosant injection.[4] Despite high initial technical success rates with these techniques, rebleeding occurs in 15 to 20% of cases.[4] Complications of endoscopy include mucosal trauma, aspiration, bowel perforation, and induction of uncontrollable bleeding. Clip localization for uncontrollable bleeding can aid in subsequent angiographic intervention.

7.5.2 Noninvasive Imaging

Nuclear Medicine

Because of the logistics of the examination and image acquisition, scintigraphy is largely reserved for hemodynamically stable patients. This technique remains an invaluable tool for cases of intermittent and/or obscure bleeding, however. The prevailing scintigraphic technique for the evaluation of gastrointestinal bleeding involves autologous red blood cell labeling with technetium-99 m, reinfusion, and subsequent periodic imaging of the abdomen. With this procedure, bleeding rates as low as 0.1 mL/min can be detected.[26] The relatively long half-life of technetium-99 m also allows for delayed imaging and identification of intermittent bleeding occurring over the course of the examination window.

These examinations suffer from poor spatial localization and are not effective at characterizing underlying pathology, but they have the potential to decrease the rate of negative angiograms when used appropriately.[27] Single-photon emission computed tomography (SPECT)/CT offers more conspicuous localization of bleeding compared to planar imaging alone,[28] and so the use of this modality is increasing.

CT Angiography

Similar to scintigraphy, CT angiography has been historically reserved for hemodynamically stable patients with upper gastrointestinal bleeding. As sensitivity for the detection of bleeding has increased, CT has been increasingly applied for the workup of gastrointestinal bleeding. Recent studies have yielded exciting results, particularly in the context of brisk and lower gastrointestinal bleeding.[29,30,31] A recent meta-analysis found CT angiography to be both cost effective and accurate in the detection and localization of gastrointestinal bleeding.[32] Detection of bleeding rates as low as 0.3 mL/min has been demonstrated in an animal model.[33] The seemingly ever-increasing rapidity and quality of CT angiography will almost certainly lead to an increasing role for this modality in the workup of upper gastrointestinal hemorrhage; CT angiography has already supplanted scintigraphy at some institutions. At the authors' institution, the CT angiography protocol for gastrointestinal bleeding includes negative oral contrast and a 100- to 150-mL IV contrast bolus with three-phase acquisition (noncontrast, arterial, and 120-second delay).

7.6 Anatomy

Hemorrhage in the upper gastrointestinal tract originates from branches of either the celiac artery or superior mesenteric artery (SMA). Variation in the mesenteric arterial vasculature is common.[34] The celiac artery arises from the anterior surface of the aorta at the T12–L1 level and classically gives rise to the common hepatic artery, left gastric artery, and splenic artery. Each of these vessels may anomalously originate directly from the aorta; this is most frequently seen with the left gastric artery.[35] The SMA arises from the anterior surface of the aorta approximately 1 cm below the celiac artery. SMA supply to the upper gastrointestinal tract typically occurs via the inferior pancreaticoduodenal artery. The common hepatic artery is replaced to the SMA in approximately 5% of individuals.[36] In less than 1%, the celiac artery and SMA share a common origin from the aorta (▶ Fig. 7.6), termed either the celiomesenteric artery or the celiacomesenteric artery.[37] Rarely, aberrant regression of the embryologic ventral anastomoses leaves a direct connection between the celiac artery and SMA, termed the arc of Buhler.

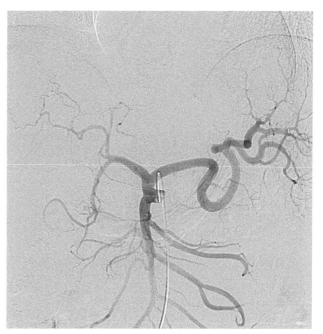

Fig. 7.6 Celiacomesenteric trunk. A common ventral trunk gives rise to both the celiac artery and SMA.

The stomach is richly perfused from the paired gastric arteries, paired gastroepiploic arteries, and short gastric arteries.[38,39,40] The left gastric artery supplies the upper aspects of the lesser curvature and cardia. The right gastric artery collateralizes with the left to supply the lower aspects of the lesser curvature and antrum. The right gastric artery arises from the proper hepatic artery in approximately half of individuals. Variant origins, in decreasing order of frequency, include the left hepatic artery, gastroduodenal artery, common hepatic artery, right hepatic artery, and middle hepatic artery.[41] The right gastroepiploic artery is the terminal branch of the gastroduodenal artery and supplies the greater curvature of the stomach. The short gastric and left gastroepiploic arteries arise from the splenic artery to supply the fundus and lateral aspects of the greater curvature, respectively. This rich and redundant blood supply of the stomach allows for safe empiric embolization in cases of angiographically occult bleeding. However, brisk gastric bleeds may need to be approached from several vessels as collateral flow perfuses the culprit vessel (▶ Fig. 7.7).

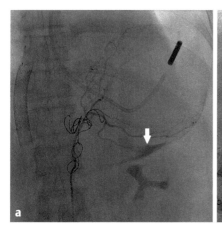
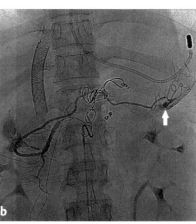

Fig. 7.7 Gastric collateral circulation. **(a)** Injection of the left gastric artery revealed fundal pseudoaneurysm with adjacent pooling of contrast into the gastric lumen (*white arrow*). A coil is present from a prior coronary vein embolization for bleeding varices. **(b)** After multiple branches of the left gastric artery have been coiled, selective angiogram of the right gastroepiploic artery reveals the same pseudoaneurysm (*white arrow*) with ongoing brisk bleeding perfused from collateral flow.

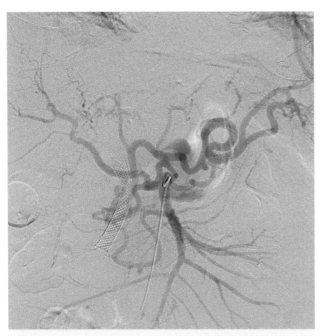

Fig. 7.8 Celiac artery occlusion. The SMA supplies the celiac artery distribution via robust pancreatic collaterals, allowing "backdoor" catheterization.

Arterial supply of the duodenum can be roughly approximated by the duodenal segment.[42] The duodenal bulb is perfused by branches of the right gastric and right gastroepiploic arteries. Named branches of the gastroduodenal artery to this region include the supraduodenal artery and retroduodenal artery; the latter is also called the posterior pancreaticoduodenal arcade. The superior pancreaticoduodenal arterial branches supply the lower aspects of the bulb to the midaspect of the descending duodenum. The remaining duodenum receives blood primarily via the inferior pancreaticoduodenal arterial branches.

The pancreatic arterial anatomy must also be briefly described because of its role in transpapillary bleeding. The superior and inferior pancreaticoduodenal arteries perfuse the head and uncinate process. Typically, the largest of the pancreatic arteries, the dorsal pancreatic artery, has a highly variable origin anywhere posterior to the pancreatic neck. The distal body and tail are supplied by the pancreatic magna and caudal pancreatic arteries, which arise from the mid- and distal splenic artery, respectively. Each of these vessels may collateralize via the transverse pancreatic artery, which follows the long axis of the pancreatic body and tail.[43]

The rich and redundant supply of the upper abdominal visceral organs permits robust collateralization in cases of severe narrowing or occlusion due to atherosclerosis, prior surgery, or other causes. In such cases, a "backdoor" approach to catheterizing a given vascular territory may be required (▸ Fig. 7.8).

7.7 Arteriography and Intervention

7.7.1 Technique and Equipment

A 5-French vascular sheath is placed via the common femoral artery. Rarely, brachial or radial arterial access may be necessary

in cases of occlusive aortoiliac disease or extreme angulation of the mesenteric arterial origins. From the transfemoral route, a wide variety of catheter configurations may be used to selectively catheterize the celiac axis and SMA. Reverse curve catheters provide stable catheterization from the aorta in the majority of cases. Cobra and angled catheters are more readily advanced deeper into the parent mesenteric artery when increased base catheter stability is needed. Selective digital subtraction angiograms of the celiac axis and SMA are acquired with typical flow rates and volumes of 4 to 6 mL/s and 20 to 30 mL, respectively. Frame rates of three to four frames per second are adequate for the arterial phase. Imaging should be continued into the venous phase with the frame rate reduced to one frame per second. Breath hold in the cooperative patient or ventilatory pause in the intubated patient should be requested to optimize angiographic sensitivity. IV administration of glucagon 1 mg may improve imaging when peristalsis causes excessive motion artifact.

Selective catheterization and arteriography of the gastroduodenal, splenic, and left gastric arteries are advised when parent vessel angiograms fail to reveal the source of bleeding. Common hepatic and splenic arterial catheterizations may be achieved with Cobra or angled catheters. In many patients, the left gastric artery can be selectively catheterized by gently withdrawing a reverse curve catheter, causing the catheter tip to seek the cephalad surface of the celiac artery and left gastric arterial origin. Angiography of the splenic artery is acquired with typical flow rates and volumes of 4 to 6 mL/s and 20 to 30 mL, respectively. Flow rates and volumes of 3 to 4 mL/s and 6 to 12 mL, respectively, are sufficient for selective angiograms of the left gastric and gastroduodenal arteries. Often, however, catheterization beyond the celiac artery is best achieved by coaxial introduction of a microcatheter and wire. Microcatheters are capable of achieving flow rates of 2 to 4 mL/s depending on lumen size and catheter length. Hand injections are typically sufficient for deep catheterizations.

The choice of microcatheter size is broadly a tradeoff between facilitating small vessel catheterization and achieving injection rates sufficient to detect pathology. Relatively large (≥ 2.7 French) microcatheters may enable subtle undulation of microcoils in the catheter lumen and occasional loss of coil pushability. Late recognition of coil and microcatheter incompatibility requires recatheterization of the culprit vessels and leads to a delay in treatment. At our institution, microcatheters in the range of 2.0 to 2.3 French are believed to offer the best balance of features for cases of gastrointestinal hemorrhage. More specifically, 0.018-inch coils should be deployed via microcatheters with a 0.021-inch inner diameter.[44]

Imaging should be performed in at least the anteroposterior projection. Repeat injection in more than one imaging plane may be needed for improved localization. This is particularly useful for differentiating the pylorus from the proximal duodenum and separating the anterior and posterior aspects of the pancreaticoduodenal arcade.

The vast majority of angiograms are performed with nonionic iodinated contrast media. Relative contraindications to these agents must be balanced against case urgency. Carbon dioxide and gadolinium-based contrast agents may be used when there are absolute contraindications to iodinated contrast.[45,46]

7.7.2 Findings

Approximately one-half of patients undergoing angiography for upper gastrointestinal bleeding will exhibit direct signs of extravasation.[47,48,49] Visualization typically requires a bleeding rate greater than 0.5 mL/min. Extravasation is recognized as nontubular pooling of contrast, which expands and fails to wash out over the course of the angiogram. Brisk extravasation may outline the adjacent mucosal pattern or source of pathology, such as pooling within a gastric ulcer. Contrast collecting into an enteric fold or along a luminal clot may transiently resemble a vein (▶ Fig. 7.9). When the collection of contrast persists beyond the venous phase, this "pseudovein" finding of arterial extravasation must be considered.[50]

Causes for nonvisualized arterial bleeding are numerous, including intermittent bleeding and a decrease in systemic pressure as a result of massive blood losses.[51,52] Absence of angiographic extravasation does not exclude a life-threatening arterial bleed. Surrogate markers of bleeding include vessel truncation, spasm (▶ Fig. 7.10), pseudoaneurysm (▶ Fig. 7.11), tumor blush (▶ Fig. 7.2), and luminal irregularity. An early draining vein may be the only evidence of a bleeding vascular malformation.

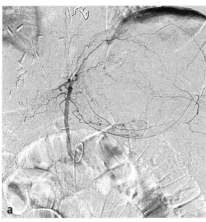
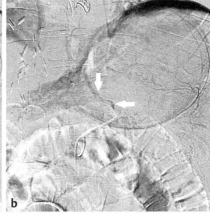

Fig. 7.9 Pseudovein. **(a)** Early and **(b)** delayed angiogram of the left gastric artery demonstrates tubular accumulation of contrast within a gastric fold (*arrows*).

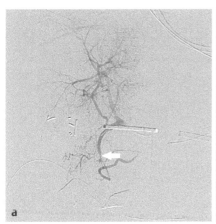
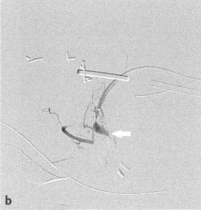

Fig. 7.10 Gastroduodenal artery spasm. **(a)** Angiogram from the proximal gastroduodenal is notable only for spasm of the gastroduodenal artery (*arrow*). **(b)** Angiogram after deeper catheterization confirmed the source of bleeding (*arrow*). Catheter and wire manipulations likely provoked the extravasation.

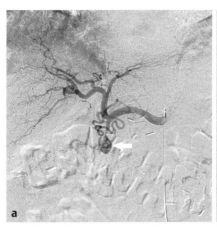
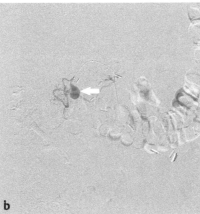

Fig. 7.11 Gastroduodenal artery pseudoaneurysm. **(a)** Nonselective (celiac artery) and **(b)** selective (gastroduodenal artery) angiograms with a conspicuous saccular pseudoaneurysm (*white arrow*) of the inferior aspect of the gastroduodenal artery.

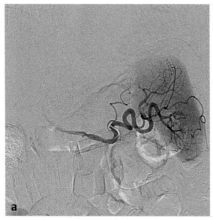
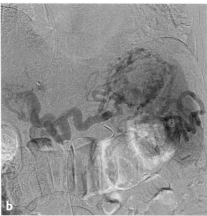

Fig. 7.12 Gastric varices on arteriography. **(a)** Early and **(b)** delayed angiogram of the splenic artery reveals occlusion of the splenic vein. Although no extravasation is identified, collateral drainage through large gastric varices and the coronary vein essentially confirmed left-sided portal hypertension as the etiology of gastric bleeding.

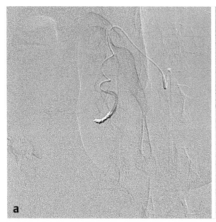
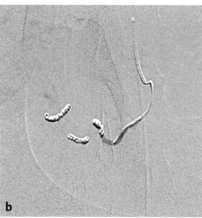

Fig. 7.13 Sandwich embolization of the gastroduodenal artery. A bleeding duodenal mass embolized with coils from **(a)** above via the celiac artery and **(b)** below from the SMA.

Venous bleeding is rarely identified, but late-phase imaging may identify sequelae of portal hypertension; this information can be used to direct additional management (▶ Fig. 7.12).

7.7.3 Endovascular Intervention

Vasopressin Infusion Therapy

The goal of vasopressin infusion is to control hemorrhage by inducing mesenteric vasoconstriction and smooth muscle contraction. Infusion begins at a dose of 0.2 U/min. Repeat angiography is obtained every 20 to 30 minutes until bleeding has stopped, with increasing doses up to 0.4 U/min as needed. Potential complications of this treatment include mesenteric and coronary ischemia. Rebleeding after cessation of infusion is also common.[53] A large series demonstrated that transcatheter vasopressin infusion is efficacious in the treatment of gastric bleeding[54]; however, with improved microcatheter technology offering the ability to select small culprit vessels, as well as increased confidence in the safety and efficacy of empiric embolization, vasoconstrictive agent infusion has almost no role in the current management of upper gastrointestinal hemorrhage.

Embolotherapy

Vascular occlusion involves a balance between target hemostasis and nontarget ischemia. As a general rule, embolization should be performed from the most selective position achievable. Technological advancements have afforded angiographers greater ability to catheterize small vessels, and a wide variety of embolic materials are now available to occlude those vessels. Coils, the standard embolic agent used in the upper gastrointestinal tract, are available in a wide variety of configurations and deployment mechanisms. Aside from appropriate sizing to the target vessel, coil selection is largely a matter of user familiarity. If the discrete feeding vessel can be catheterized, coiling of that vessel alone is typically sufficient. For empiric coil embolization of the left gastric artery, coils are placed in the proximal to midsegment of the artery. For the gastroduodenal artery, empiric embolization is performed by coiling the entire artery. If a bleeding vessel cannot be catheterized, coiling above and below or across the origin is recommended. If dual supply to a bleeding focus is observed and deeper catheterization cannot be obtained, coiling both feeding vessels in a "sandwich" technique is conceptually similar (▶ Fig. 7.13). Gelatin slurry placed in addition to coils expedites hemostasis.

Liquid embolic agents such as *n*-butyl cyanoacrylate (NBCA) "glue" are very effective in rapidly achieving hemostasis, with flow directing the agent to the site of bleeding before polymerization. NBCA is particularly useful for cases of vascular occlusion distal to the site of microcatheter advancement (▶ Fig. 7.14) and for lesions with multiple supplying vessels. NBCA can be delivered through ultramicrocatheters that are not suitable for microcoil delivery. Polymerization begins after contact with ionic

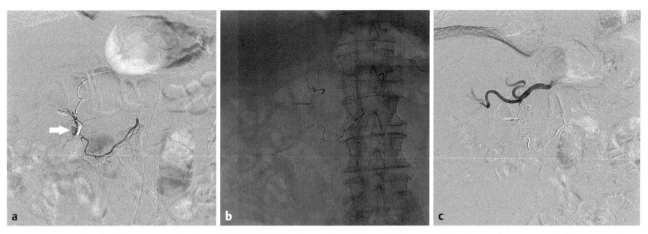

Fig. 7.14 Gastroduodenal artery embolization with NBCA. **(a)** Selective angiogram from the gastroduodenal artery demonstrates brisk extravasation (*arrow*). **(b)** Pancreaticoduodenal arcade embolized with NBCA. **(c)** Postpolymerization angiogram confirms stasis and no further extravasation.

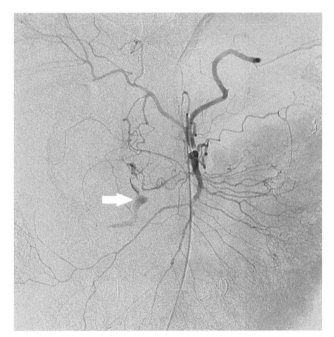

Fig. 7.15 Celiac artery occlusion. SMA supplies the celiac artery territory via an enlarged gastroduodenal artery with extravasation (*arrow*). Brisk cephalad flow in the gastroduodenal artery made it unsuitable for empiric liquid or particulate embolization.

solutions such as blood, resulting in rapid and permanent vascular occlusion that is largely independent of the coagulation cascade.

NBCA is mixed with iodized oil (Lipiodol; Andre Guerbet, Aulnay-Sous-Bois, France) to supply radiopacity and adjust the rate of polymerization. The degree of vessel penetration is controlled by both the injection rate and the NBCA:Lipiodol dilution ratio, typically ranging from 1:1 to 1:4. Delivery via a small syringe (1 or 3 mL) helps to maintain a controlled delivery rate. Iodized oil will begin to degrade polycarbonate syringes within minutes; this agent should therefore be kept in a glass container until embolization is imminent.

A great deal of experience is required to achieve the full benefit of NBCA and avoid pitfalls specific to this embolic agent.

Meticulous technique is needed to prevent premature polymerization, which would spoil the embolic agent and may result in loss of vascular access. A separate preparation table free of ionic solutions and blood is mandatory, and soiled gloves should be changed. A 5% dextrose solution should be used to rinse gloves and the catheter hub. The catheter itself should be loaded with this same solution immediately before delivery of NBCA. Slow infusion may result in premature polymerization, whereas overexuberant delivery can result in nontarget embolization or adherence of the microcatheter tip to the vessel wall.

In certain regions, NBCA remains expensive compared to other embolic agents. Microcatheters must be discarded after a single delivery of glue, adding additional costs to the procedure if a single treatment site is insufficient. Despite these potentially increased costs and technical pitfalls, NBCA has been shown to be a highly effective embolic agent for nonvariceal upper gastrointestinal hemorrhage, with low complication rates.[55]

Gelatin in the form of pledgets or a contrast-enhanced slurry is introduced as a single agent or in combination with coils. Vessels embolized with gelatin slurry alone are likely to recanalize in several weeks. Nonetheless, this agent is effective in cases of self-limited disease such as bleeding after endoscopic biopsy. Particulate embolic agents such as polyvinyl alcohol and trisacryl gelatin may be used in a similar fashion to gelatin slurry and are most appropriate for progressive lesions such as tumors. Tissue necrosis is less likely to occur when relatively large particles (>700 μm) are used. Liquid sclerosing agents such as absolute alcohol have no role in the treatment of nonvariceal upper gastrointestinal hemorrhage.

Brisk unilateral flow in the gastroduodenal artery and pancreaticoduodenal arcade resulting from either celiac or SMA stenosis should be recognized and respected (▶ Fig. 7.15). Delivery of particulate or liquid agents in these cases may quickly result in nontarget embolization and should be avoided if flow is unpredictable or occurs preferentially into nontarget territories.

7.7.4 Empiric Embolization

When bleeding is endoscopically attributed to a specific site in the stomach or duodenum yet angiography fails to reveal the source, empiric embolization of the left gastric artery or gastroduodenal artery, respectively, is safe and effective.[56,57,58,59] This treatment is accomplished with coils alone or in combination with gelatin sponge. Results from the radioembolization literature suggest that recanalization of the gastroduodenal artery is possible, particularly when the cephalad aspect of the coil pack is relatively far from the gastroduodenal arterial origin,[60] but this has not been extensively studied in the context of recurrent gastrointestinal bleeding after embolization. Similarly, empiric embolization for angiographically occult bleeding attributed to a tumor has been associated with cessation of hemorrhage and low complication rates.[61] If collateral pathways are disrupted by atherosclerotic occlusion, compression, or postoperative states, the safety of empiric embolization in such scenarios should be carefully considered (▶ Fig. 7.16).

7.7.5 Special Considerations

Aortoenteric Fistulas

Aortoenteric fistulas caused by aortic prostheses are definitively addressed with surgical graft excision and reconstruction. In emergent situations, endovascular management may be requested for rapid control of bleeding of both primary and secondary aortoenteric fistulas (▶ Fig. 7.17). Endovascular management alone may be considered for patients without an associated infection. In patients with bleeding accompanied by sepsis or other frank infection, stent grafts are associated with a high rate of graft infection and recurrent bleeding.[19,62,63] Endovascular management in this scenario is typically regarded as a temporizing measure and a bridge to open repair. However, the

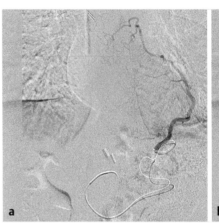
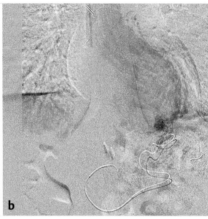

Fig. 7.16 Disrupted collateral circulation after esophagectomy and gastric pull-through. **(a)** Early and **(b)** delayed images demonstrate dominant supply to the gastric pull-through from the right gastroepiploic artery. The left and right gastric arteries had been ligated. No bleeding was identified, and empiric embolization was felt to be unsafe.

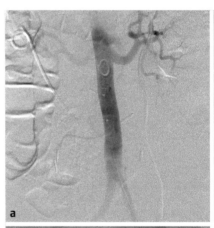
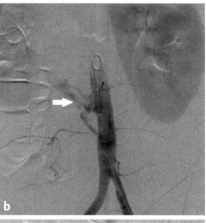
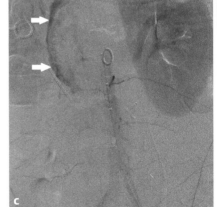
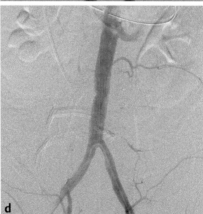

Fig. 7.17 Aortoenteric fistula. Massive upper gastrointestinal bleeding developed after irradiation and resection of a retroperitoneal mass. **(a–c)** Brisk aortic extravasation fills the duodenum (*arrows*). **(d)** An aortic stent graft was placed across the aortic defect with resultant cessation of angiographic extravasation.

use of stent grafts plus long-term antibiotic therapy is becoming an acceptable definitive treatment for infected mycotic aneurysms, and the similar pathogenesis of these entities may allow this therapy to be extrapolated to the treatment of aortoenteric fistulas in patients who are not candidates for surgery.

Hemobilia

Hemobilia following biopsy or transhepatic biliary drain placement may be portal venous or arterial in origin, with or without an arterioportal fistulous component. The indwelling biliary drain may produce a partial tamponade effect, which can lead to a false-negative study; repeat arteriography after the drain has been withdrawn over a wire helps to avoid this pitfall (▶ Fig. 7.18). All arteries supplying the traversed parenchyma should be investigated. Maximal selectivity before embolization reduces nontarget embolization and minimizes the risk of unnecessary parenchymal necrosis. Central arterial injuries can be treated with stent placement to preserve perfusion to large volumes of downstream hepatic parenchyma (▶ Fig. 7.19), although stent patency in this particular circumstance is not well studied.

7.8 Outcomes

With respect to transcatheter treatment of nonvariceal upper gastrointestinal hemorrhage, the interventional radiology literature is limited to uncontrolled trials, which have demonstrated largely favorable results. Cases refractory to endoscopic

management should proceed to angiography and transcatheter intervention.[23] Technical success rates for these procedures range from 52 to 100%.[47,49,64,65,66,67,68] Controlled trials comparing surgery with angiographic intervention have demonstrated at least similar rates of rebleeding, morbidity, and mortality.[69,70] Compared to surgery, angiography and transcatheter intervention reduce the need for subsequent surgical intervention and are associated with fewer complications.[70,71] In most instances, surgery is reserved for lesions refractory to endoscopic and catheter-directed therapies.

Rebleeding after angiography and intervention may occur in up to 30% of patients[72] and is more likely to occur in coagulopathic patients or when coils are used as the sole embolic agent.[49] Patients with a negative angiogram have been shown to have lower rates of early rebleeding than those with bleeding identified at endoscopy or angiography.[73] Bleeding on angiography that cannot be controlled by endovascular means is associated with a particularly poor prognosis.[48]

7.8.1 Complications of Angiography and Embolotherapy

The overall major complication rates of mesenteric angiography and transcatheter embolization generally do not exceed 6%.[74] Risks specific to upper gastrointestinal embolotherapy, including infarction and perforation, are rare. Duodenal stenosis after embolization of bleeding duodenal ulcers occurs more frequently with terminal vessel embolization.[75]

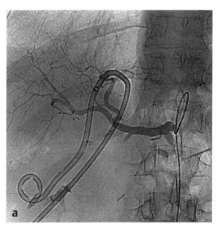
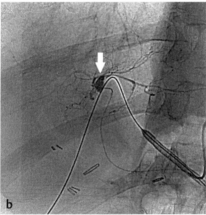

Fig. 7.18 Biliary drain tamponade. (a) Angiogram of the common hepatic artery for hemobilia with a biliary drain in place fails to reveal the source of hemorrhage. (b) With the drain withdrawn over a wire, left hepatic artery angiogram confirms the presence and location of a pseudoaneurysm (*arrow*).

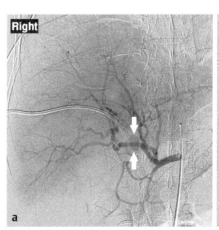
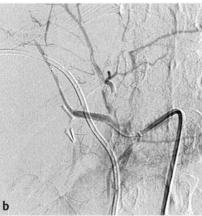

Fig. 7.19 Biliary drain and a central hepatic arterial injury. A common hepatic artery angiogram demonstrates (a) a large pseudoaneurysm surrounding the central right hepatic artery (*arrows*) (b) subsequently treated with a stent.

7.9 Conclusion

Despite continuing advances in medical therapy, nonvariceal upper gastrointestinal hemorrhage is and will continue to be a frequent and serious clinical presentation. Mesenteric angiography has evolved into a more focused but nonetheless critical aspect of the modern interdisciplinary approach. Accordingly, knowledge of relevant anatomy and disease and also skill in transcatheter management remain critical components of the interventionalist's armamentarium.

References

[1] Nusbaum M, Baum S. Radiographic demonstration of unknown sites of gastrointestinal bleeding. Surg Forum. 1963; 14:374–375

[2] Baum S, Roy R, Finkelstein AK, Blakemore WS. Clinical application of selective celiac and superior mesenteric arteriography. Radiology. 1965; 84(2):279–295

[3] Rösch J, Dotter CT, Brown MJ. Selective arterial embolization. A new method for control of acute gastrointestinal bleeding. Radiology. 1972; 102(2):303–306

[4] Simoens M, Rutgeerts P. Non-variceal upper gastrointestinal bleeding. Best Pract Res Clin Gastroenterol. 2001; 15(1):121–133

[5] Rollhauser C, Fleischer DE. Nonvariceal upper gastrointestinal bleeding. Endoscopy. 2004; 36(1):52–58

[6] Fallah MA, Prakash C, Edmundowicz S. Acute gastrointestinal bleeding. Med Clin North Am. 2000; 84(5):1183–1208

[7] Conrad SA. Acute upper gastrointestinal bleeding in critically ill patients: causes and treatment modalities. Crit Care Med. 2002; 30(6) Suppl:S365–S368

[8] Blocksom JM, Tokioka S, Sugawa C. Current therapy for nonvariceal upper gastrointestinal bleeding. Surg Endosc. 2004; 18(2):186–192

[9] Burke SJ, Golzarian J, Weldon D, Sun S. Nonvariceal upper gastrointestinal bleeding. Eur Radiol. 2007; 17(7):1714–1726

[10] Longstreth GF. Epidemiology of hospitalization for acute upper gastrointestinal hemorrhage: a population-based study. Am J Gastroenterol. 1995; 90(2):206–210

[11] Loffroy R, Rao P, Ota S, De Lin M, Kwak BK, Geschwind JF. Embolization of acute nonvariceal upper gastrointestinal hemorrhage resistant to endoscopic treatment: results and predictors of recurrent bleeding. Cardiovasc Intervent Radiol. 2010; 33(6):1088–1100

[12] Millward SF. ACR Appropriateness Criteria on treatment of acute nonvariceal gastrointestinal tract bleeding. J Am Coll Radiol. 2008; 5(4):550–554

[13] Zuckerman GR, Prakash C. Acute lower intestinal bleeding. Part II: etiology, therapy, and outcomes. Gastrointest Endosc. 1999; 49(2):228–238

[14] Lee EW, Laberge JM. Differential diagnosis of gastrointestinal bleeding. Tech Vasc Interv Radiol. 2004; 7(3):112–122

[15] Fisher RG, Schwartz JT, Graham DY. Angiotherapy with Mallory-Weiss tear. AJR Am J Roentgenol. 1980; 134(4):679–684

[16] Durham JD, Kumpe DA, Rothbarth LJ, Van Stiegmann G. Dieulafoy disease: arteriographic findings and treatment. Radiology. 1990; 174(3)(,)(Pt 2):937–941

[17] Schmulewitz N, Baillie J. Dieulafoy lesions: a review of 6 years of experience at a tertiary referral center. Am J Gastroenterol. 2001; 96(6):1688–1694

[18] Lermite E, Regenet N, Tuech JJ, et al. Diagnosis and treatment of hemosuccus pancreaticus: development of endovascular management. Pancreas. 2007; 34(2):229–232

[19] Leonhardt H, Mellander S, Snygg J, Lönn L. Endovascular management of acute bleeding arterioenteric fistulas. Cardiovasc Intervent Radiol. 2008; 31(3):542–549

[20] Khamaysi I, Gralnek IM. Acute upper gastrointestinal bleeding (UGIB) - initial evaluation and management. Best Pract Res Clin Gastroenterol. 2013; 27(5):633–638

[21] Aljebreen AM, Fallone CA, Barkun AN. Nasogastric aspirate predicts high-risk endoscopic lesions in patients with acute upper-GI bleeding. Gastrointest Endosc. 2004; 59(2):172–178

[22] Imperiale TF, Birgisson S. Somatostatin or octreotide compared with H2 antagonists and placebo in the management of acute nonvariceal upper gastrointestinal hemorrhage: a meta-analysis. Ann Intern Med. 1997; 127(12):1062–1071

[23] Barkun AN, Bardou M, Kuipers EJ, et al. International Consensus Upper Gastrointestinal Bleeding Conference Group. International consensus recommendations on the management of patients with nonvariceal upper gastrointestinal bleeding. Ann Intern Med. 2010; 152(2):101–113

[24] Savides TJ, Jensen DM. Therapeutic endoscopy for nonvariceal gastrointestinal bleeding. Gastroenterol Clin North Am. 2000; 29(2):465–487, vii

[25] Gralnek IM, Jensen DM, Gornbein J, et al. Clinical and economic outcomes of individuals with severe peptic ulcer hemorrhage and nonbleeding visible vessel: an analysis of two prospective clinical trials. Am J Gastroenterol. 1998; 93(11):2047–2056

[26] Alavi A. Detection of gastrointestinal bleeding with 99mTc-sulfur colloid. Semin Nucl Med. 1982; 12(2):126–138

[27] Gunderman R, Leef J, Ong K, Reba R, Metz C. Scintigraphic screening prior to visceral arteriography in acute lower gastrointestinal bleeding. J Nucl Med. 1998; 39(6):1081–1083

[28] Bentley BS, Tulchinsky M. SPECT/CT helps in localization and guiding management of small bowel gastrointestinal hemorrhage. Clin Nucl Med. 2014; 39(1):94–96

[29] Sabharwal R, Vladica P, Chou R, Law WP. Helical CT in the diagnosis of acute lower gastrointestinal haemorrhage. Eur J Radiol. 2006; 58(2):273–279

[30] Yoon W, Jeong YY, Shin SS, et al. Acute massive gastrointestinal bleeding: detection and localization with arterial phase multi-detector row helical CT. Radiology. 2006; 239(1):160–167

[31] Jaeckle T, Stuber G, Hoffmann MH, Jeltsch M, Schmitz BL, Aschoff AJ. Detection and localization of acute upper and lower gastrointestinal (GI) bleeding with arterial phase multi-detector row helical CT. Eur Radiol. 2008; 18(7):1406–1413

[32] Wu LM, Xu JR, Yin Y, Qu XH. Usefulness of CT angiography in diagnosing acute gastrointestinal bleeding: a meta-analysis. World J Gastroenterol. 2010; 16(31):3957–3963

[33] Kuhle WG, Sheiman RG. Detection of active colonic hemorrhage with use of helical CT: findings in a swine model. Radiology. 2003; 228(3):743–752

[34] Uflacker R. Atlas of Vascular Anatomy: An Angiographic Approach. Philadelphia, PA: Lippincott Williams & Wilkins; 1997

[35] Song SY, Chung JW, Yin YH, et al. Celiac axis and common hepatic artery variations in 5002 patients: systematic analysis with spiral CT and DSA. Radiology. 2010; 255(1):278–288

[36] Covey AM, Brody LA, Maluccio MA, Getrajdman GI, Brown KT. Variant hepatic arterial anatomy revisited: digital subtraction angiography performed in 600 patients. Radiology. 2002; 224(2):542–547

[37] Kalra M, Panneton JM, Hofer JM, Andrews JC. Aneurysm and stenosis of the celiomesenteric trunk: a rare anomaly. J Vasc Surg. 2003; 37(3):679–682

[38] Lin PH, Chaikof EL. Embryology, anatomy, and surgical exposure of the great abdominal vessels. Surg Clin North Am. 2000; 80(1):417–433, xiv

[39] Michels NA. Blood Supply and Anatomy of the Upper Abdominal Organs with a Descriptive Atlas. Philadelphia, PA: Lippincott; 1955:7

[40] Daseler EH, Anson BJ, et al. The cystic artery and constituents of the hepatic pedicle; a study of 500 specimens. Surg Gynecol Obstet. 1947; 85(1):47–63

[41] Van Damme JP, Bonte J. Vascular Anatomy in Abdominal Surgery. New York, NY: Thieme; 1990

[42] Butler P, Mitchell AW, Ellis H, eds. Applied Radiological Anatomy. Cambridge: Cambridge University Press; 1999

[43] Mosca S, Di Gregorio F, Regoli M, Bertelli E. The superior horizontal pancreatic artery of Popova: a review and an anatomoradiological study of an important morphological variant of the pancreatica magna artery. Surg Radiol Anat. 2014; 36(10):1043–1049

[44] Frisoli JK, Sze DY, Kee S. Transcatheter embolization for the treatment of upper gastrointestinal bleeding. Tech Vasc Interv Radiol. 2004; 7(3):136–142

[45] Sandhu C, Buckenham TM, Belli AM. Using CO2-enhanced arteriography to investigate acute gastrointestinal hemorrhage. AJR Am J Roentgenol. 1999; 173(5):1399–1401

[46] Spinosa DJ, Matsumoto AH, Hagspiel KD, Angle JF, Hartwell GD. Gadolinium-based contrast agents in angiography and interventional radiology. AJR Am J Roentgenol. 1999; 173(5):1403–1409

[47] Toyoda H, Nakano S, Takeda I, et al. Transcatheter arterial embolization for massive bleeding from duodenal ulcers not controlled by endoscopic hemostasis. Endoscopy. 1995; 27(4):304–307

[48] Dempsey DT, Burke DR, Reilly RS, McLean GK, Rosato EF. Angiography in poor-risk patients with massive nonvariceal upper gastrointestinal bleeding. Am J Surg. 1990; 159(3):282–286

[49] Aina R, Oliva VL, Therasse E, et al. Arterial embolotherapy for upper gastrointestinal hemorrhage: outcome assessment. J Vasc Interv Radiol. 2001; 12(2):195–200

[50] Ring EJ, Athanasoulis CA, Waltman AC, Baum S. The pseudo-vein: an angiographic appearance of arterial hemorrhage. J Can Assoc Radiol. 1973; 24 (3):242–244

[51] Walsh RM, Anain P, Geisinger M, et al. Role of angiography and embolization for massive gastroduodenal hemorrhage. J Gastrointest Surg. 1999; 3(1):61–65, discussion 66

[52] Miller M, Jr, Smith TP. Angiographic diagnosis and endovascular management of nonvariceal gastrointestinal hemorrhage. Gastroenterol Clin North Am. 2005; 34(4):735–752

[53] Gomes AS, Lois JF, McCoy RD. Angiographic treatment of gastrointestinal hemorrhage: comparison of vasopressin infusion and embolization. AJR Am J Roentgenol. 1986; 146(5):1031–1037

[54] Eckstein MR, Kelemouridis V, Athanasoulis CA, Waltman AC, Feldman L, van Breda A. Gastric bleeding: therapy with intraarterial vasopressin and transcatheter embolization. Radiology. 1984; 152(3):643–646

[55] Jae HJ, Chung JW, Jung AY, Lee W, Park JH. Transcatheter arterial embolization of nonvariceal upper gastrointestinal bleeding with N-butyl cyanoacrylate. Korean J Radiol. 2007; 8(1):48–56

[56] Arrayeh E, Fidelman N, Gordon RL, et al. Transcatheter arterial embolization for upper gastrointestinal nonvariceal hemorrhage: is empiric embolization warranted? Cardiovasc Intervent Radiol. 2012; 35(6):1346–1354

[57] Padia SA, Geisinger MA, Newman JS, Pierce G, Obuchowski NA, Sands MJ. Effectiveness of coil embolization in angiographically detectable versus non-detectable sources of upper gastrointestinal hemorrhage. J Vasc Interv Radiol. 2009; 20(4):461–466

[58] Ichiro I, Shushi H, Akihiko I, Yasuhiko I, Yasuyuki Y. Empiric transcatheter arterial embolization for massive bleeding from duodenal ulcers: efficacy and complications. J Vasc Interv Radiol. 2011; 22(7):911–916

[59] Dixon S, Chan V, Shrivastava V, Anthony S, Uberoi R, Bratby M. Is there a role for empiric gastroduodenal artery embolization in the management of patients with active upper GI hemorrhage? Cardiovasc Intervent Radiol. 2013; 36(4):970–977

[60] Enriquez J, Javadi S, Murthy R, et al. Gastroduodenal artery recanalization after transcatheter fibered coil embolization for prevention of hepaticoenteric flow: incidence and predisposing technical factors in 142 patients. Acta Radiol. 2013; 54(7):790–794

[61] Tandberg DJ, Smith TP, Suhocki PV, et al. Early outcomes of empiric embolization of tumor-related gastrointestinal hemorrhage in patients with advanced malignancy. J Vasc Interv Radiol. 2012; 23(11):1445–1452

[62] Antoniou GA, Koutsias S, Antoniou SA, Georgiakakis A, Lazarides MK, Giannoukas AD. Outcome after endovascular stent graft repair of aortoenteric fistula: a systematic review. J Vasc Surg. 2009; 49(3):782–789

[63] Burks JA, Jr, Faries PL, Gravereaux EC, Hollier LH, Marin ML. Endovascular repair of bleeding aortoenteric fistulas: a 5-year experience. J Vasc Surg. 2001; 34(6):1055–1059

[64] Kim SK, Duddalwar V. Failed endoscopic therapy and the interventional radiologist: non-variceal upper gastrointestinal bleeding. Tech Gastrointest Endosc. 2005; 7:148–155

[65] Ljungdahl M, Eriksson LG, Nyman R, Gustavsson S. Arterial embolisation in management of massive bleeding from gastric and duodenal ulcers. Eur J Surg. 2002; 168(7):384–390

[66] Defreyne L, Vanlangenhove P, De Vos M, et al. Embolization as a first approach with endoscopically unmanageable acute nonvariceal gastrointestinal hemorrhage. Radiology. 2001; 218(3):739–748

[67] Defreyne L, De Schrijver I, Decruyenaere J, et al. Therapeutic decision-making in endoscopically unmanageable nonvariceal upper gastrointestinal hemorrhage. Cardiovasc Intervent Radiol. 2008; 31(5):897–905

[68] Mirsadraee S, Tirukonda P, Nicholson A, Everett SM, McPherson SJ. Embolization for non-variceal upper gastrointestinal tract haemorrhage: a systematic review. Clin Radiol. 2011; 66(6):500–509

[69] Ripoll C, Bañares R, Beceiro I, et al. Comparison of transcatheter arterial embolization and surgery for treatment of bleeding peptic ulcer after endoscopic treatment failure. J Vasc Interv Radiol. 2004; 15(5):447–450

[70] Eriksson LG, Ljungdahl M, Sundbom M, Nyman R. Transcatheter arterial embolization versus surgery in the treatment of upper gastrointestinal bleeding after therapeutic endoscopy failure. J Vasc Interv Radiol. 2008; 19 (10):1413–1418

[71] Wong TC, Wong KT, Chiu PW, et al. A comparison of angiographic embolization with surgery after failed endoscopic hemostasis to bleeding peptic ulcers. Gastrointest Endosc. 2011; 73(5):900–908

[72] Shin JH. Refractory gastrointestinal bleeding: role of angiographic intervention. Clin Endosc. 2013; 46(5):486–491

[73] Sildiroglu O, Muasher J, Arslan B, et al. Outcomes of patients with acute upper gastrointestinal nonvariceal hemorrhage referred to interventional radiology for potential embolotherapy. J Clin Gastroenterol. 2014; 48(8): 687–692

[74] Angle JF, Siddiqi NH, Wallace MJ, et al. Society of Interventional Radiology Standards of Practice Committee. Quality improvement guidelines for percutaneous transcatheter embolization: Society of Interventional Radiology Standards of Practice Committee. J Vasc Interv Radiol. 2010; 21 (10):1479–1486

[75] Lang EK. Transcatheter embolization in management of hemorrhage from duodenal ulcer: long-term results and complications. Radiology. 1992; 182 (3):703–707

8 Transcatheter Management of Nonvariceal Lower Gastrointestinal Hemorrhage

Richard A. Baum and Stanley Baum

8.1 Introduction

Bleeding from the lower gastrointestinal (GI) tract has always presented a major challenge to clinicians as they attempt to identify the site of hemorrhage and treat the condition. If the bleeding is massive, colonoscopy is usually unsuccessful in identifying the source. If the site can be identified, surgery on an unprepared bowel presents another major obstacle. This chapter will discuss various causes of arterial acute and chronic lower GI bleeding such as diverticulosis, angiodysplasia, neoplasm, postoperative anastomoses, and inflammation.

The transcatheter management of lower GI bleeding is a procedure that has stood the test of time. This life-saving procedure has been performed successfully for more than 50 years by two generations of interventional radiologists. What began with a rogue group of radiologists in the 1960s trying to control lower GI bleeding with direct intra-arterial injection of vasoactive drugs[1,2,3,4] has blossomed into a medical specialty with thousands of practitioners worldwide. Indeed, the beginning of angiography and interventional radiology as a subspecialty can be traced back to the need to develop techniques for the diagnosis and subsequent treatment of GI bleeding. Although the tools of the trade have changed over the past 50 years,[5] the basic approach and techniques remain the same (▶ Fig. 8.1).

The goals of transcatheter treatment of lower GI bleeding can be characterized by the type of bleeding and the durability of treatment. The ultimate goal of treatment is the permanent cessation of bleeding. Even for patients in whom durability of treatment cannot be achieved, a temporary result is acceptable, as this will allow patients to undergo elective surgery rather than an emergent procedure without proper bowel preparation.

8.2 History of Transcatheter Treatment of Lower GI Bleeding

In 1963, Nusbaum and Baum[6] demonstrated the feasibility of identifying experimentally created bleeding sites in the GI tract of dogs. Bleeding sites were created at various points of the GI tract by means of a catheter placed in a small segmental artery and passed through an enterotomy directly into the lumen of the intestine. After selective arteriography of the superior mesenteric artery was performed, the bleeding site was identified. By varying the diameter of the catheter used, different bleeding rates could be obtained. This technique was successful in demonstrating bleeding rates as low as 0.5 mL/min (▶ Fig. 8.2).[7]

When selective mesenteric angiography was initially introduced for clinical use, it was used exclusively to establish a diagnosis of GI bleeding (▶ Fig. 8.3). The selective infusion of vasoconstricting drugs through the same catheter used for the diagnostic angiogram evolved as a natural outgrowth of diagnostic arteriography. The progression from diagnosis to a

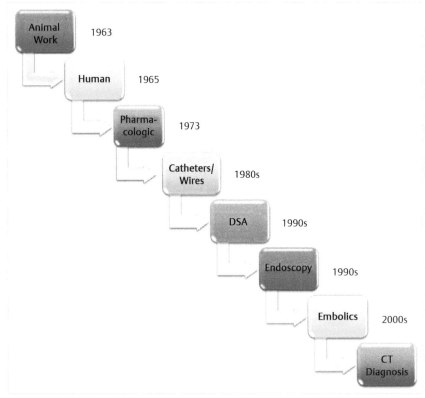

Fig. 8.1 Timeline of major advances in diagnosis and transcatheter treatment of GI bleeding.

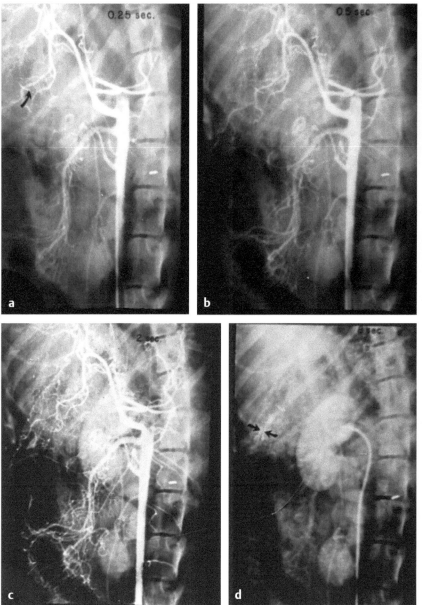

Fig. 8.2 Experimentally created and angiographically identified bleeding sites. **(a–c)** A small catheter was placed in a small segmental branch of the superior mesenteric artery of a dog and advanced through an enterotomy (surgical clip, *arrow*) into the lumen of the small intestine. **(d)** Several seconds after arteriography was performed, extravasation could be seen in the intestine (*double arrows*). Before the insertion of the catheter through the enterotomy, bleeding through the catheter was occurring at a rate of 0.5 mL/min.

therapeutic application of the procedure heralded the beginnings of interventional radiology (▶ Fig. 8.4, ▶ Fig. 8.5).

Advances in catheters and wires over the years have also allowed for more expeditious catheterization of the mesenteric vessels, with catheters specifically designed to atraumatically cannulate the superior and inferior mesenteric arteries. The imaging chain has also seen dramatic improvement over the past half century. Static cut film imaging was replaced with rapid film changers in the 1970s. Digital subtraction angiography revolutionized the way vascular images were obtained in the mid-1980s and 1990s.[8] Image intensifiers were ultimately replaced with flat-panel digital detectors in the 2000s, greatly reducing ionizing radiation exposure to both patients and operators. Iodinated contrast agents have also seen great improvements over the years, greatly reducing their toxic effects.

The development of microcatheters has been particularly beneficial for the transcatheter treatment of lower GI bleeding.

Before this development, pharmacologic treatment was useful if direct access to the bleeding site could not be obtained. Vasoconstrictors were applied to the upstream vasculature, and the resulting splanchnic vasoconstriction resulted in cessation of GI hemorrhage. With coaxial microcatheters, direct access to the injured artery is possible, allowing for a more varied and customizable treatment (▶ Fig. 8.6).[9]

Unlike the stomach and duodenum, which have a redundant vascular supply, the large bowel mucosa is supplied by end arteries from the superior and inferior mesenteric arteries. Although there is collateral flow between medium-sized mesenteric and rectal vasculature, the colonic mucosa is fed by a delicate network of small arteries. This is why particulate embolization is not typically appropriate for managing hemorrhage in the lower GI tract.[10] Direct coil embolization of the injured vessel has become the standard treatment for most colonic bleeding.[10,11,12,13,14,15]

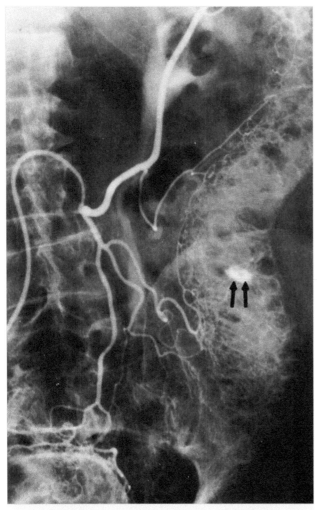

Fig. 8.3 Demonstration of bleeding in a patient with a bleeding descending colon diverticulum. Bleeding diverticulum in the descending colon in a 73-year-old man with lower gastrointestinal hemorrhage. Selective inferior mesenteric arteriography shows extravasation of contrast material in the sigmoid colon (*arrows*). (Reproduced with permission from Baum S, Pentecost MJ, eds. Abrams' Angiography: Interventional Radiology. 2nd ed. Philadelphia, PA: Lippincott Williams 2006:507.)

8.3 Causes of Lower GI Bleeding

8.3.1 Diverticulosis

Bleeding occurs in approximately 10 to 30% of patients with colonic diverticulosis.[16,17,18] The blood loss in most patients is minimal and usually stops when the patient is placed on bed rest. If the bleeding is persistent and severe, an emergency surgical intervention is usually required. Because the disease involves the elderly and the surgery is on an unprepared bowel, morbidity and mortality rates are high (▶ Fig. 8.3, ▶ Fig. 8.4, ▶ Fig. 8.5, ▶ Fig. 8.6, ▶ Fig. 8.7).[19] Before the advent of selective angiography, the diagnosis of diverticular bleeding was made by exclusion.

Emergency arteriography performed at the time of bleeding can pinpoint the location of the bleeding lesion and prevent blind colectomies. This is important, as it has been shown that the bleeding site is more often seen in the ascending and transverse colon despite a higher incidence of diverticulosis in the descending and sigmoid colon (▶ Fig. 8.8). Once the site of bleeding is identified on the arteriogram, superselective embolization can be performed after the catheter is advanced into the bleeding vessel. If this is not successful, the superior or inferior mesenteric artery can be selectively infused with the vasoconstrictor vasopressin.

8.3.2 Angiodysplasia

A frequent cause of lower GI bleeding in the elderly is colonic vascular ectasia or angiodysplasia. These lesions tend to be very small and are usually located in the cecum and ascending colon. They can be seen on colonoscopy and selective arteriography (▶ Fig. 8.8); additionally, some studies have reported the use of preoperative multidetector computed tomography (CT) scans to identify these lesions.[20,21,22] During laparotomy, the surgeon can almost never find these lesions, and even after partial colectomy, the pathologist has difficulty identifying them unless guided by preliminary specimen injection (▶ Fig. 8.9, ▶ Fig. 8.10, ▶ Fig. 8.11).

The cause of angiodysplasia remains unclear. Because the lesions are seen more often in adults and elderly patients, they

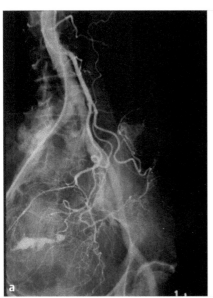
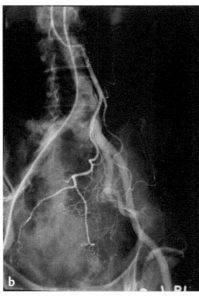

Fig. 8.4 Pharmacological control of a bleeding left-sided colonic diverticulum. **(a)** Selective inferior mesenteric arteriogram demonstrates extravasation of contrast in the sigmoid colon. This was later shown to be at the site of a bleeding diverticulum. **(b)** During the infusion of vasopressin, the extravasation and bleeding stopped.

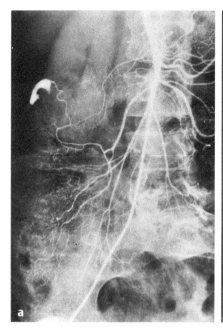
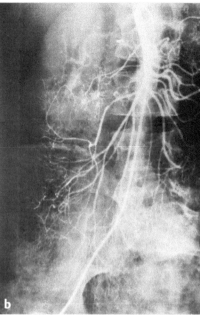

Fig. 8.5 Pharmacological control of a bleeding right-sided diverticulum: bleeding diverticulum in the hepatic flexure in an 80-year-old man presenting with massive lower gastrointestinal bleeding. **(a)** Selective superior mesenteric arteriogram shows extravasation of contrast material from a branch of the right colic artery in the area of the hepatic flexure. **(b)** Repeat selective superior mesenteric arteriogram during the infusion of 0.2 unit per minute of vasopressin shows complete cessation of the bleeding. The patient was infused with vasopressin for 72 hours at decreasing doses, and the catheter was removed at the end of the third day. Bleeding did not recur, and the patient was discharged from the hospital without surgery. (Reproduced with permission from Baum S, Pentecost MJ, eds. Abrams' Angiography: Interventional Radiology. 2nd ed. Philadelphia, PA: Lippincott Williams 2006:507.)

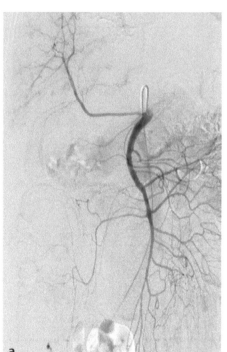
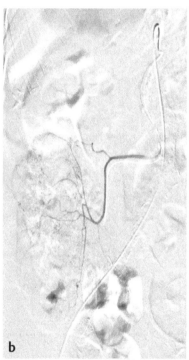
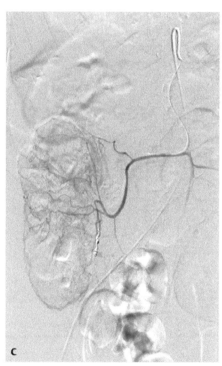

Fig. 8.6 Successful coil embolization of a bleeding diverticulum in the ascending colon. **(a)** Selective and **(b)** superselective superior mesenteric angiography demonstrates a focal right colonic bleed. **(c)** The feeding mesenteric artery is embolized with a coil.

are assumed to be acquired. Some authors have compared them to localized varicosities[23] or have suggested a degenerative etiology.[24] Pathological examination of angiodysplasia suggests that the lesions develop as a result of increased angiogenesis. The basement membrane of the GI tract produces an antiangiogenesis factor; one hypothesis is that with aging, the basement membrane of the colon becomes damaged and no longer produces this protective antiangiogenesis factor.[25] The increased diameter of the right colon and cecum and the resultant high pressure in the wall as a result of peristalsis could damage the basement membrane and would explain why these lesions are more often found in the right colon.

8.3.3 Inflammation

Rectal bleeding may be the first manifestation of colitis; therefore, the diagnosis of bleeding colitis is usually first made by the angiographer. Catheter control of actively bleeding colitis can convert an emergency colectomy to an elective one that allows for better bowel preparation (▶ Fig. 8.12, ▶ Fig. 8.13).

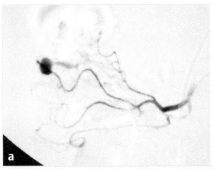
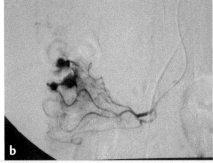
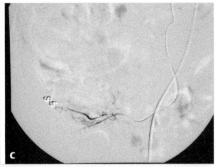

Fig. 8.7 Cecal diverticulum in a 50-year-old man treated by embolization with microcoils. **(a)** Superselective injection into a branch of the ileocecal artery demonstrates massive extravasation of contrast material. **(b)** Several seconds later, the extravasation extends into the cecum. **(c)** Extravasation stops after the microcoils are deposited in the bleeding vessel. (Reproduced with permission from Baum S, Pentecost MJ, eds. Abrams' Angiography: Interventional Radiology. 2nd ed. Philadelphia, PA: Lippincott Williams 2006:508.)

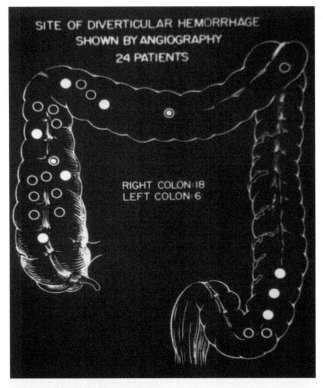

Fig. 8.8 Diverticular hemorrhage.

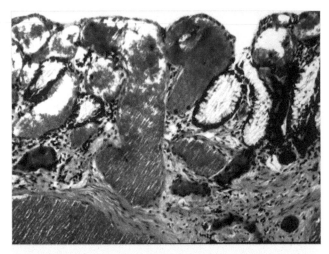

Fig. 8.9 Histology of a right colonic angiodysplasia showing vascular venules extending into the mucosal surface of the colon. The pathologist was able to identify the area for sections because of prior injection of Microfil.

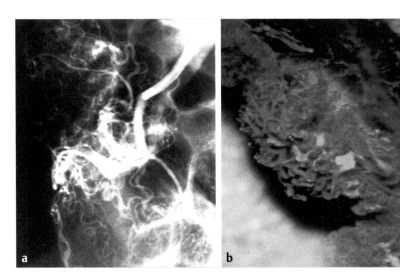

Fig. 8.10 Angiodysplasia in the cecum. **(a)** Superior mesenteric arteriogram demonstrating arteriovenous shunting in the cecum. **(b)** Longitudinal section through the lesion that was previously identified by the injection of Microfil in the resected specimen.

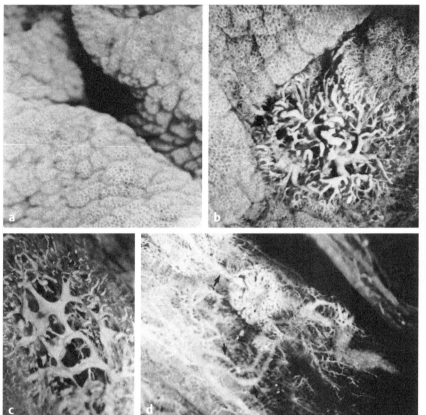

Fig. 8.11 Microvascular anatomy of angiodysplasia of the cecum and ascending colon on pathologic specimens. **(a)** Photograph (×40) of normal colonic mucosa viewed with a dissecting microscope after silicone rubber injection in right colic and ileocolic arteries and tissue clearing using absolute alcohol followed by methyl salicylate. **(b–d)** Specimens of colonic angiodysplasia as viewed under the dissecting microscope following the tissue-clearing technique. The angiodysplasias appear as clusters of tortuous and dilated vessels against a homogeneous background of normal colonic mucosa. Histologically, these vessels are primarily venules extending from the submucosa into the mucosa. Occasionally, as in d (*arrows*), the feeding arteries and draining veins can be identified. (Reproduced with permission from Baum S, Pentecost MJ, eds. Abrams' Angiography: Interventional Radiology. 2nd ed. Philadelphia, PA: Lippincott Williams 2006:511.)

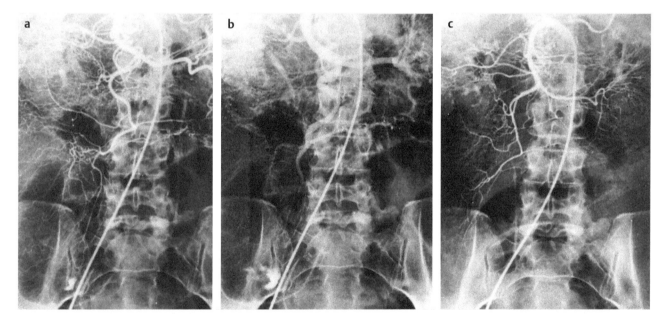

Fig. 8.12 Chronic ulcerative colitis with massive lower gastrointestinal bleeding. **(a)** Selective superior mesenteric arteriogram shows extravasation from a cecal branch of the ileocecal artery. **(b)** The extravasated contrast material persists well in the venous phase of the arteriogram. **(c)** Bleeding stopped during the infusion into the superior mesenteric artery of 0.2 unit per minute of vasopressin. Control of the acute bleeding episode allowed the patient to be adequately prepared and to have a successful elective right colectomy several weeks later. (Reproduced with permission from Baum S, Pentecost MJ, eds. Abrams' Angiography: Interventional Radiology. 2nd ed. Philadelphia, PA: Lippincott Williams 2006:509.)

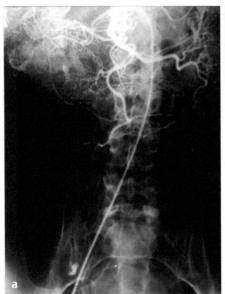
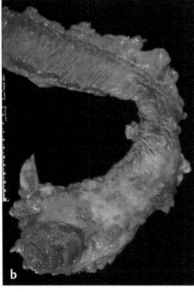

Fig. 8.13 (a,b) Resected specimen of the colon (same patient from ▶ Fig. 8.12). A granulomatous ulcerative colitis mass can be seen in the cecum.

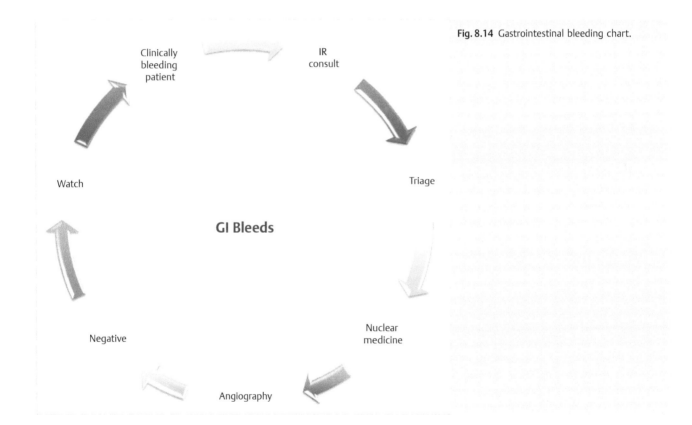

Fig. 8.14 Gastrointestinal bleeding chart.

Clinically bleeding patient

IR consult

Watch

Triage

GI Bleeds

Negative

Nuclear medicine

Angiography

8.4 Logistics of Transcatheter Management

No discussion of the transcatheter treatment of acute lower GI hemorrhage would be complete without a discussion of the logistics of the procedure. In addition to technical challenges, the intermittent nature of lower GI bleeding creates logistical hurdles that need to be overcome. The "door-to-embolization time" varies depending on the patient's rate of bleeding and clinical status. Far too often, delays in treatment result in negative angiograms, greatly limiting the treatment options. Oftentimes, the patient is labeled "too unstable" to travel to angiography for definitive treatment. Far too often, the bleeding has stopped by the time the patient has arrived in the interventional radiology suite (▶ Fig. 8.14).

A multidisciplinary approach involving diagnostic radiologists, nuclear medicine physicians, anesthesiologists, critical care physicians, and nurses can improve the time it takes to transport and begin a procedure in a patient with active bleeding. Patients should never be returned to their rooms after a positive scan. Recently, CT diagnosis of GI bleeding has been found to streamline the logistics of embolic treatment.[26,27] These scans are performed in seconds, eliminating the need for time-consuming nuclear medicine studies in many patients.

8.4.1 Provocative Angiography

Provocative angiography is a technique that some have used to improve the sensitivity of contrast angiography. Pharmacoangiography is performed using a combination of vasodilators and thrombolytics infused directly into the splanchnic vasculature. Patients are also typically fully anticoagulated at the time of the provocative angiogram. It has been reported that this technique increases the sensitivity of contrast angiography by approximately 30%.[28]

Because of the potential risk for creating hemodynamic instability, provocative angiography is a technique that requires pre-planning and a multidisciplinary approach. The patient and/or family must fully understand the risks and potential benefits of the procedure.[29]

8.5 Conclusion

There are very few procedures in all of medicine that have a half-century history. The transcatheter treatment of lower GI bleeding not only has stood the test of time but also has evolved, and is now being performed by a second generation of interventional radiologists. Diagnostic angiography gave rise to pharmacologic treatment, which then evolved to embolotherapy. Specific tools and imaging techniques have been developed to rapidly identify the location and then treat active lower GI hemorrhage. The entire specialty of interventional radiology can trace its roots back to this single procedure.

References

[1] Nusbaum M, Baum S, Blakemore WS, Tumen H. Clinical experience with selective intra-arterial infusion of vasopressin in the control of gastrointestinal bleeding from arterial sources. Am J Surg. 1972; 123(2):165–172

[2] Baum S, Nusbaum M. The control of gastrointestinal hemorrhage by selective mesenteric arterial infusion of vasopressin. Radiology. 1971; 98(3):497–505

[3] Baum S, Nusbaum M, Tumen HJ. Gastrointestinal bleeding. Lancet. 1970; 1 (7663):106–107

[4] Nusbaum M, Baum S, Blakemore WS. Clinical experience with the diagnosis and management of gastrointestinal hemorrhage by selective mesenteric catheterization. Ann Surg. 1969; 170(3):506–514

[5] Baum S, Nusbaum M, Kuroda K, Blakemore WS. Direct serial magnification arteriography as an adjuvant in the diagnosis of surgical lesions in the alimentary tract. Am J Surg. 1969; 117(2):170–176

[6] Nusbaum M, Baum S. Radiographic demonstration of unknown sites of gastrointestinal bleeding. Surg Forum. 1963; 14:374–375

[7] Alavi A, McLean GK. Studies of GI bleeding with scintigraphy and the influence of vasopressin. Semin Nucl Med. 1981; 11(3):216–223

[8] Rees CR, Palmaz JC, Alvarado R, Tyrrel R, Ciaravino V, Register T. DSA in acute gastrointestinal hemorrhage: clinical and in vitro studies. Radiology. 1988; 169(2):499–503

[9] Gordon RL, Ahl KL, Kerlan RK, et al. Selective arterial embolization for the control of lower gastrointestinal bleeding. Am J Surg. 1997; 174(1):24–28

[10] Bandi R, Shetty PC, Sharma RP, Burke TH, Burke MW, Kastan D. Superselective arterial embolization for the treatment of lower gastrointestinal hemorrhage. J Vasc Interv Radiol. 2001; 12(12):1399–1405

[11] Beggs AD, Dilworth MP, Powell SL, Atherton H, Griffiths EA. A systematic review of transarterial embolization versus emergency surgery in treatment of major nonvariceal upper gastrointestinal bleeding. Clin Exp Gastroenterol. 2014; 7:93–104

[12] Tan KK, Strong DH, Shore T, Ahmad MR, Waugh R, Young CJ. The safety and efficacy of mesenteric embolization in the management of acute lower gastrointestinal hemorrhage. Ann Coloproctol. 2013; 29(5):205–208

[13] Tan KK, Wong D, Sim R. Superselective embolization for lower gastrointestinal hemorrhage: an institutional review over 7 years. World J Surg. 2008; 32(12):2707–2715

[14] d'Othée BJ, Surapaneni P, Rabkin D, Nasser I, Clouse M. Microcoil embolization for acute lower gastrointestinal bleeding. Cardiovasc Intervent Radiol. 2006; 29(1):49–58

[15] Lefkovitz Z, Cappell MS, Lookstein R, Mitty HA, Gerard PS. Radiologic diagnosis and treatment of gastrointestinal hemorrhage and ischemia. Med Clin North Am. 2002; 86(6):1357–1399

[16] Behringer GE, Albright NL. Diverticular disease of the colon. A frequent cause of massive rectal bleeding. Am J Surg. 1973; 125(4):419–423

[17] Welch CE, Athanasoulis CA, Galdabini JJ. Hemorrhage from the large bowel with special reference to angiodysplasia and diverticular disease. World J Surg. 1978; 2(1):73–83

[18] Welch CE, Hedberg S. Gastrointestinal hemorrhage. I. General considerations of diagnosis and the rapy. Adv Surg. 1973; 7:95–148

[19] Rigg BM, Ewing MR. Current attitudes on diverticulitis with particular reference to colonic bleeding. Arch Surg. 1966; 92(3):321–332

[20] Junquera F, Quiroga S, Saperas E, et al. Accuracy of helical computed tomographic angiography for the diagnosis of colonic angiodysplasia. Gastroenterology. 2000; 119(2):293–299

[21] Ettorre GC, Francioso G, Garribba AP, Fracella MR, Greco A, Farchi G. Helical CT angiography in gastrointestinal bleeding of obscure origin. AJR Am J Roentgenol. 1997; 168(3):727–731

[22] Ettorre GC, Francioso G, Garribba AP, Fracella MR, Greco A, Farchi G. Spiral computed tomography with arteriography in the diagnosis of digestive system hemorrhages of obscure origin [in Italian]. Radiol Med (Torino). 1995; 90(6):726–733

[23] Boley SJ, Sammartano R, Adams A, DiBiase A, Kleinhaus S, Sprayregen S. On the nature and etiology of vascular ectasias of the colon. Degenerative lesions of aging. Gastroenterology. 1977; 72(4, Pt 1):650–660

[24] Foutch PG. Colonic angiodysplasia. Gastroenterologist. 1997; 5(2):148–156

[25] Baum S. Arteriographic diagnosis and treatment of gastrointestinal bleeding. In: Baum S, Pentecost M, eds. Abrams' Angiography: Interventional Radiology. Philadelphia, PA: Lippincott Williams & Wilkins, 2006:487–515

[26] Chan V, Tse D, Dixon S, et al. Outcome following a negative CT angiogram for gastrointestinal hemorrhage. Cardiovasc Intervent Radiol. 2015; 38(2):329–335

[27] Geffroy Y, Rodallec MH, Boulay-Coletta I, Jullès MC, Ridereau-Zins C, Zins M. Multidetector CT angiography in acute gastrointestinal bleeding: why, when, and how. Radiographics. 2011; 31(3):E35–E46

[28] Kim CY, Suhocki PV, Miller MJ, Jr, Khan M, Janus G, Smith TP. Provocative mesenteric angiography for lower gastrointestinal hemorrhage: results from a single-institution study. J Vasc Interv Radiol. 2010; 21(4):477–483

[29] Bloomfeld RS, Smith TP, Schneider AM, Rockey DC. Provocative angiography in patients with gastrointestinal hemorrhage of obscure origin. Am J Gastroenterol. 2000; 95(10):2807–2812

9 Interventional Management of Benign Refractory Ascites

Louis G. Martin

9.1 Introduction

Those of us who saw the movie *Amadeus* will never forget the opening scene of the carriage traveling through a cold, late-night thunderstorm, bringing the priest to the deathbed of Antonio Salieri, who confesses his role in the death of Wolfgang Amadeus Mozart. Mozart actually died at home on a calm, mild day in Vienna after a short illness—and without Salieri's intervention. A much more dramatic demise actually belonged to Ludwig van Beethoven, who died in a hepatic coma during a violent thunderstorm with snow flurries and hail. According to the case notes of Anton Wawruch, the physician caring for Beethoven at the time of his death in 1827, "Beethoven opened his eyes for the first time in 2 days, raised his right hand in a clenched fist, and stared up into the heavens with a grim and threatening look on his face, and then expired."[1,2] Beethoven is undoubtedly the most celebrated patient to have suffered from refractory ascites (RA). He received paracentesis at least four times during the 2 months that preceded his death (reportedly up to 20 L per session). Beethoven's paracentesis was performed without anesthesia by the introduction of a glass tube through a surgical incision, as was typical practice at the time.[3,4]

Abdominal paracentesis is one of the oldest surgical procedures recorded. It was described in a single passage of the *Hippocratic Writings*, in which the author says "that a puncture of the abdomen near the umbilicus or in the region of the flank should be made either by knife or cautery and that only a small amount of fluid should be allowed to flow at a time."[5] This is a very sophisticated passage despite its brevity; the methodology described lessens the likelihood of trauma to the recanalized umbilical vein, other collateral veins on the surface of the abdomen, and the branches of the superficial epigastric artery and vein. Additionally, this technique reduces the possibility of causing vasomotor instability. In his extant work *De Medicina*, Aulus Cornelius Celsus (c. 25 BC to c. 50 AD) described in detail the technique of paracentesis, recommending the use of a bronze tube with a flange collar to prevent the tube from slipping into the patient's peritoneal cavity. He noted that Erasistratus of Alexandria opposed paracentesis because of its hazards. Six centuries later, Paul of Aegina warned that sudden evacuations have "immediately killed the patient."[6]

Large-volume paracentesis (LVP) was the only treatment available for ascites for more than 2,000 years. Salt restriction was not attempted or even suggested until the early 1900s. Although mercury was advocated as a diuretic in the sixteenth century, there is no record of mercury being used to treat ascites until organic mercurial agents were introduced after World War II. The discovery of sulfanilamide-induced sodium bicarbonate diuresis in the late 1940s ushered in a new age of clinically effective diuretics, which began in the 1950s with the introduction of chlorothiazide and spironolactone, the first orally effective agents to mobilize sodium chloride.[3,7]

In this chapter, we will review the pathogenesis of cirrhotic RA and the differences between compensated and uncompensated cirrhosis. We will discuss the many treatment options available for RA and summarize their benefits, contraindications, and complications. Finally, we will propose a treatment algorithm that meets the needs of the patient and satisfies the goals of the interventional radiologist, hepatologist, and transplant surgeon. References to malignant ascites will be included only when they serve to clarify issues pertaining to cirrhotic ascites.

9.2 Pathogenesis of Cirrhosis

The elements active in the pathogenesis of cirrhosis are not completely known. Its present state of understanding has progressed through: the backward flow theory, the forward flow theory, and the vasodilatation-hyperdynamic circulation theory. Each of these theories has added information to previous theories but has not supplanted them. The backward flow theory postulates that portal hypertension is due solely to increased resistance caused by hepatic sinusoidal fibrosis. This is observed in early cirrhosis before portal flow is diverted into the collateral circulation. The forward flow theory acknowledges the role of increased portal resistance but recognizes the equal importance of increased splanchnic blood flow, providing a rationale for the use of vasoconstrictors in this patient population. The vasodilatation-hyperdynamic circulation theory postulates that the "trigger" of the hyperdynamic syndrome is in the action of multiple vasodilators, primarily nitric oxide and endothelial growth factor, in the splanchnic bed and is activated by the initial increase in portal pressure related to sinusoidal hypertension[8,9,10] (▶ Fig. 9.1).

9.3 Compensated versus Decompensated Cirrhosis

Normally, there is only 50 to 150 mL of fluid in the peritoneum; increased fluid as a result of trauma, infection, neoplasia, or portal hypertension is initially drained via the lymphatics. When this drainage is insufficient, dietary and medicinal assistance may be required. Biliary cirrhosis is usually an indolent process, often taking 8 to 10 years to progress from a compensated to decompensated state. Early clinical signs and manifestations of compensated cirrhosis are pruritus, persistent fatigue, and pain in the right upper quadrant of the abdomen.[11] The onset of decompensation is defined as the presence of one or more of the following complications: jaundice, ascites, spontaneous bacterial peritonitis (SBP), hepatic encephalopathy (HE), hepatorenal syndrome (HRS), variceal hemorrhage, and cancer.[12]

Cirrhosis is the most common cause of ascites, accounting for nearly 85% of all cases. Similarly, ascites is the most frequent decompensating event, occurring in 60% of cirrhotic patients within 10 years of disease onset. The presence of ascites is associated with 50% mortality within 3 years and 50% mortality within 1 year once the ascites has become refractory to diuretics.[13] An increase in hepatic sinusoidal fibrosis, increase in portal vein pressure, and formation of a hyperdynamic splanchnic circulation are important factors involved in the formation of ascites. Rupture of either the liver capsule and/or its surface

Pathogenesis and sequelae of portal hypertension

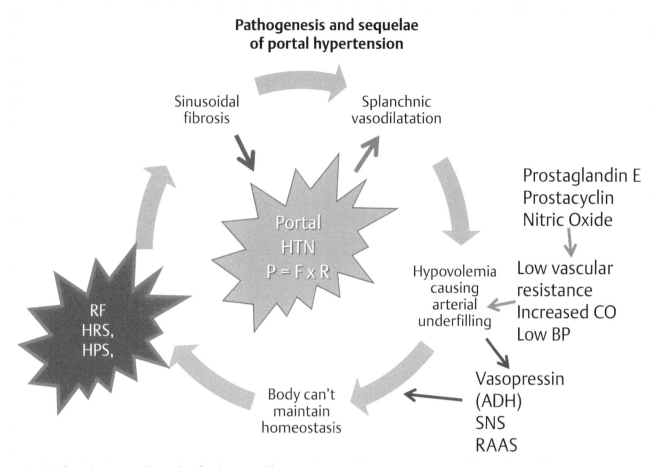

Fig. 9.1 The pathogenesis and sequelae of cirrhotic portal hypertension.

lymphatics allows for high protein fluid leak into the peritoneal space, which is the crucial event in the formation of ascites. In the setting of progressive vasodilatation, the intravascular volume and cardiac output increase to maintain arterial perfusion pressure. With progression of the disease, vasodilatation is accentuated, and cardiac output continues to increase. Eventually, the cardiac response is not enough to maintain perfusion pressure, the renal blood flow drops, and renal failure develops.[8] The additional increase in levels of endogenous vasoactive compounds such as renin, angiotensin, aldosterone, norepinephrine, vasopressin, and antidiuretic hormone results in increased ascites accumulation and sodium retention.[14,15]

The most important markers of decompensated cirrhosis are bleeding and ascites. Additional complications of cirrhosis can include edema, SBP, HE, HRS, hepatopulmonary syndrome, hypersplenism, and liver cancer (hepatocellular carcinoma [HCC], which is the third leading cause of cancer mortality worldwide). The 5-year cumulative risk for the development of HCC in patients with cirrhosis ranges from 5 to 30%.[16,17,18,19]

Survival of cirrhosis depends on the degrees of portal hypertension, liver insufficiency, and circulatory dysfunction. Prognostic factors for survival include the Model for End-Stage Liver Disease (MELD) score,[20] portosystemic pressure gradient ≥ 10 mm Hg,[21] and increased body mass index.[22]

Successful treatment of ascites is dependent on accurate diagnosis of its cause. Because sodium and water retention is the basic abnormality leading to ascites formation, restricting sodium intake and enhancing sodium excretion are the mainstays of ascites treatment. Patients with cirrhosis and ascites must limit sodium intake to 2 g/d. Enhancement of sodium excretion can be accomplished with oral diuretics. The recommended initial dose is spironolactone 100 to 200 mg/d and furosemide 20 to 40 mg/d; the dosages of these medications can be increased if the response is not adequate to control ascites. The usual maximum doses are spironolactone 400 mg/d and furosemide 160 mg/d. The recommended weight loss in patients without peripheral edema is 300 to 500 g/d. There is no limit to the daily weight loss of patients with edema. Approximately 90% of patients respond well to medical therapy for ascites.

9.4 Refractory Ascites

Approximately 5 to 10% of patients with cirrhosis develop RA. Once the diagnosis of RA is established, the expected 1-year survival is approximately 50%. Predictors of poorer survival in patients with RA include low protein levels in the ascitic fluid, elevated Child–Pugh score, previous SBP, heavy alcohol consumption (> 80 g/d in men and > 40 g/d in women), older age, the presence of HCC, and the presence of diabetes.[13,23,24,25,26]

The diagnostic criteria for RA as established by the International Ascites Club[27] and accepted by the American Association for the Study of Liver Disease[28] are as follows: RA is defined as fluid overload that is unresponsive to a sodium-restricted diet

(≤ 50 mEq/d) and diuretic treatment or that recurs rapidly after therapeutic paracentesis. Diuretic-resistant RA is defined as ascites accumulation that is not controlled by a sodium-restricted diet plus maximum doses of spironolactone and furosemide (other alternatives include bumetanide 4 mg/d or an equivalent dose of other loop diuretics for at least 1 week). Diuretic-intractable RA is defined as RA that cannot be treated with the maximal dose of diuretics because of diuretic-induced complications.

Lack of response in patients with RA is defined as weight loss less than 200 g/d during the last 4 days of intensive diuretic treatment and urinary sodium excretion less than 50 mEq/d. Early ascites recurrence is defined as the reappearance of moderate (grade 2) to massive or tense (grade 3) ascites within 4 weeks of initial mobilization. Reaccumulation of ascites within 2 to 3 days of paracentesis should not be considered early ascites because it represents a shift of interstitial fluid to the intraperitoneal space.[27]

Diuretic-induced complications are a frequent occurrence even in hospitalized patients. These complications include the development of HE in the absence of other precipitating factors (25% of patients), increase of serum creatinine to more than 2 mg/dL and/or by more than double the base value (20% of patients), decrease in serum sodium concentration by more than 10 mEq/L to a level lower than 125 mEq/L (30% of patients), and diuretic-induced hypokalemia (decrease of serum potassium to < 3 mEq/L) or hyperkalemia (increase of serum potassium to > 6 mEq/L) despite the use of appropriate measures to correct serum potassium levels.[27,29]

RA is not only a problem in patients with decompensated cirrhosis; one single-center retrospective study found that RA occurred in 62 (5.6%) of 1,058 patients who underwent orthotopic liver transplant (OLT).[30] Successful treatment of RA in the posttransplant patient resulted in significantly improved survival ($p = 0.00001$). Therefore, the interventionalist must search for and correct treatable causes of RA in this patient cohort. Anastomotic stenosis of the inferior vena cava, hepatic veins, and portal veins may also occur in 3 to 7% of patients after OLT. Technical success rates of 94 to 100% and a clinical success rate of 73% have been reported after percutaneous treatment of post-OLT anastomotic strictures.[31,32] In the absence of anastomotic stenosis, transjugular intrahepatic portosystemic shunt (TIPS) placement[33] and splenic artery embolization[34] have been shown to have benefit in the treatment of RA and as a bridge to retransplantation.

9.5 Conditions Coexisting with or Complicating Refractory Ascites

9.5.1 Spontaneous Bacterial Peritonitis

SBP is the most frequent infection to occur in patients with RA affecting 3.5% of outpatients and 12% of hospitalized patients. As many as 65% of patients with borderline renal function, ascitic fluid protein level ≤ 1.5 g/dL, Child–Pugh score ≥ 9, and bilirubin level ≥ 3 mg/dL may experience SBP within 1 year of interventional treatment.[35] The 1-year probability of SBP recurrence is 70%, with a corresponding survival rate of 50 to 80%.[23,36,37] SBP is caused by gut bacteria or bacterial products crossing from the intestinal lumen into the blood or ascitic fluid. This bacterial translocation occurs as a result of overgrowth of intestinal bacteria in an immunologically impaired patient with cirrhosis and with increased intestinal permeability.[38]

A routine cell count of fluid obtained from diagnostic or therapeutic paracentesis should always be performed to rule out SBP. The presence of an ascitic fluid polymorphonuclear leukocyte count ≥ 250 cells/mm^3 without evidence of a surgically correctable source of infection confirms the diagnosis of SBP. A dipstick specifically designed for ascitic fluid and calibrated to 250 cells/mm^3 is reported to have a 95% sensitivity and 79.6% specificity for SBP detection; however, this test is not effective in bloody, chylous, or bilious fluid.[39] Delaying treatment until bacteria grow in ascitic fluid culture may result in the death of the patient. Empiric intravenous administration of a third-generation cephalosporin antibiotic (2 g twice daily) should be initiated immediately, and the antibiotic should be replaced when necessary (depending on the results of ascitic fluid culture and sensitivity tests). Additionally, the high risk of SBP reinfection can be significantly reduced by prophylactic oral administration of norfloxacin 400 mg/d ($p = 0.0063$).[40]

9.5.2 Hepatorenal Syndrome

HRS is defined as the occurrence of renal failure in a patient with advanced liver disease in the absence of an identifiable cause of renal failure; thus, the diagnosis is one of exclusion.[29] However, recent evidence suggests that HRS is preceded and intimately related to cardiac dysfunction. A low cardiac index (CI) has been identified as an independent predictor of the development of HRS.[41] In a study of patients with cirrhosis and ascites but without HRS, patients with a CI lower than 1.5 L/min/m^2 demonstrated significant reductions in stroke volume, stroke volume index, heart rate, systemic vascular resistance, renal blood flow, glomerular filtration rate, and serum aldosterone and an increase in serum creatinine versus patients with a CI higher than 1.5 L/min/m^2. Mortality at 3, 6, and 9 months was also significantly higher in patients with a lower CI, a result not predicted by differences in MELD scores.[42]

The inability to excrete sodium is not apparent until ascitic fluid accumulates in the peritoneal cavity. The renal circulatory bed attempts to compensate for the hyperdynamic cirrhotic state through reactive vasodilatation, which results in retention of sodium and water. As decompensation progresses, vasodilatation is accentuated, and the cardiac output continues to increase. When the cardiac response is unable to maintain perfusion pressure, renal vasoconstriction occurs and renal failure develops.[8,41] Ginès and Schrier[43] concluded that HRS is probably the final consequence of extreme underfilling of the arterial circulation secondary to arterial vasodilatation in the splanchnic vascular bed. As a result, arterial pressure must be maintained by activation of vasoconstrictor systems (i.e., the renin–angiotensin–aldosterone system, sympathetic nervous system, and, in late stages, nonosmotic antidiuretic hormone). Thus, in patients with HRS, the renal circulation and most extrasplanchnic vascular beds are vasoconstricted.

There are two types of HRS. Type 1 is characterized by rapidly progressive deterioration of renal function, resulting in a 24-hour creatinine clearance of less than 20 mL/min and a serum creatinine level greater than 2.5 mg/dL in less than 2 weeks.

Bacterial infections, gastrointestinal hemorrhage, major surgical procedures, and acute-on-chronic liver failure are the most frequent precipitating events. In patients with type 1 HRS, hospital survival is less than 10%, and the expected median survival time is only 2 weeks.[44] The European Association for the Study of the Liver recommends that terlipressin (1 mg/4–6 h intravenous bolus) plus albumin should be used as first-line therapy for type 1 HRS. This treatment regimen aims to improve renal function sufficiently to decrease the serum creatinine level to less than 1.5 mg/dL. The terlipressin dose should be increased in a stepwise manner to a maximum of 2 mg/4 h if serum creatinine does not decrease by at least 25% in 3 days. Terlipressin is not available in the United States; potential alternatives include norepinephrine or midodrine plus octreotide in combination with albumin.[45] Vasoconstrictors, mainly terlipressin and beta-blockers, have resulted in improved renal function in some patients with HRS type 1; however, these agents should be used with caution as many patients in this population have a reduced CI and so a further decrease in systemic blood flow and oxygen transport may be deleterious.[42]

Type 2 HRS progresses more slowly, with a serum creatinine level ranging from 1.2 to 2.5 mg/dL; median survival in these patients is 6 months. Type 2 HRS is mainly characterized by the presence of RA. Albumin infusion has been shown to prevent type 2 HRS and improve survival, especially in the setting of SBP.[46] Pentoxifylline, a phosphodiesterase inhibitor, has been shown in a randomized trial to be superior to placebo in preventing type 2 HRS in patients with cirrhosis, ascites, and creatinine clearance levels between 41 and 80 mL/min.[47]

During the progression of liver disease, there is concomitant progression of renal perfusion disturbances and renal sympathetic overactivity.[48] Recently, there has been renewed interest in sympathetic denervation as a treatment for the renal vasoconstrictive complications seen in HRS. Selective catheterization and tracer kinetic techniques have demonstrated that the increased circulating norepinephrine in patients with cirrhosis is due to enhanced sympathetic nervous system activity in the kidneys and other organs.[49] Surgical lumbar sympathectomy has led to improvements in renal function in several patients with HRS.[50] Placement of TIPS has also been reported to improve renal function in patients with type 1 HRS; although these data are encouraging, they are inconclusive, and many patients have contraindications to TIPS placement.[51,52] These treatment options will be discussed in more detail later in this chapter.

9.5.3 Hepatic Encephalopathy

HE describes a spectrum of potentially reversible neuropsychiatric abnormalities seen in patients with liver dysfunction and/or portosystemic shunting. Overt HE develops in 30 to 45% of patients with cirrhosis and in 10 to 50% of patients with TIPS placement (▶ Table 9.1).[53,54] The International Society for Hepatic Encephalopathy and Nitrogen Metabolism consensus document defines the onset of disorientation or asterixis as the onset of overt HE.[55] Some patients with HE have subtle findings that may only be detected using specialized tests; this is known as minimal HE and occurs in up to 80% of patients with cirrhosis.[56] Refractory HE is defined as encephalopathy that recurs or persists despite the use of appropriate medical treatment. The

Table 9.1 Modification of the West Haven criteria for hepatic encephalopathy[67]

Stage	Consciousness	Intellect and behavior	Neurological findings
0	Normal	Normal	Normal examination (classified as minimal hepatic encephalopathy if psychomotor testing is impaired)
1	Mild lack of awareness	Shortened attention span; impaired performance of addition or subtraction	Mild asterixis or tremor
2	Lethargic	Disoriented; inappropriate behavior; impaired performance of subtraction	Obvious asterixis; slurred speech
3	Somnolent but arousable	Gross disorientation; bizarre behavior; confusion	Muscular rigidity and clonus; hyperreflexia; asterixis is usually absent
4	Coma	Coma	Decerebrate posturing

prognosis for patients with overt HE is poor; a population-based cohort study reported a 1-year survival rate of 36%.[57] OLT is the ultimate treatment for refractory HE; however, the shortage of available donor organs markedly limits this treatment option. Alternative therapies such as shunt occlusion or reduction can be used to control symptoms and serve as a bridge therapy to OLT.[58]

The pathogenesis of HE is poorly understood. The most widely accepted theory is that the astrocyte, the only cerebral cell capable of metabolizing ammonia, is morphologically altered by hyperammonemia. Ammonia detoxification in astrocytes leads to accumulation of glutamine, which is the main cause of astrocyte swelling. Ammonia is converted to carbamoyl phosphate, which then enters the urea cycle to be either incorporated into amino acids or excreted in the urine. Increased production and decreased excretion of ammonia are associated with portal hypertension. In patients with normal hepatocyte function, 80 to 90% of ammonia is excreted through first-pass metabolism. Although ammonia is released from several tissues, including kidney and muscle tissue, its highest concentration is in the portal vein, where it is derived from colonic bacteria and metabolism of glutamine in the small bowel. There is evidence that elevated intracellular ammonia results in altered neurotransmission by agonizing gamma-aminobutyric acid (GABA) and by causing cerebral energy failure. Among patients with HE, 90% have elevated serum ammonia concentrations; however, there is poor correlation between the venous concentration of ammonia and the grade of HE, lending credence to other theories regarding HE pathogenesis.[59,60] Discussion of these theories is beyond the scope of this review; the reader is encouraged to investigate the relevant references.[61,62,63,64,65]

Up to 80% of patients with cirrhosis have subtle findings of HE that may only be detected using specialized tests. These are considered to have mild HE, which may affect 30 to 70% of patients with cirrhosis.[56,57] Symptomatically overt HE develops in 30 to 45% of patients with cirrhosis and in 10 to 50% of patients treated by placement of a TIPS shunt.[53,54] The International Society for Hepatic Encephalopathy and Nitrogen Metabolism defines the onset of disorientation or asterixis as signaling the onset of overt HE. Refractory HE is defined as a recurrent or persistent encephalopathy despite appropriate medical treatment. HE is reversible; its treatment relies on suppressing the production of the toxic substances in the intestine, which is most commonly achieved with the laxative lactulose or with nonabsorbable antibiotics. Treatment of any reversible underlying conditions such as bleeding, infection, renal failure, constipation, use of psychotropic drugs, and electrolyte abnormalities may improve the symptoms.[59] Surgical approaches to reduce the intestinal production of ammonia, such as colectomy or colon exclusion procedures, were used in the past for patients with HE refractory to other measures. Although these approaches were successful, the operative and postoperative morbidity and mortality rates were high; today, OLT should be considered for these patients.[66,67] There is early evidence that partial splenic artery embolization (PSAE) can have a positive effect on the control of HE. In one study, 25 patients with HE were divided into 2 groups: 14 patients underwent transportal obliteration and/or balloon-occluded retrograde transvenous obliteration of porto-systemic shunts followed by PSAE, and 11 patients underwent only transportal obliteration and/or balloon-occluded retrograde transvenous obliteration of portosystemic shunts without PSAE. Serum ammonia levels and HE grades were lower in patients treated with PSAE than in patients not treated with PSAE at 6, 9, 12, and 24 months after treatment.[68]

9.5.4 Hepatic Hydrothorax

Hepatic hydrothorax most often develops because of diaphragmatic defects that allow passage of fluid from the peritoneal space to the pleural space. This complication can be challenging to treat because as little as 500 mL of fluid in the pleural space can cause respiratory symptoms due to the constraints of the thoracic cavity. Treatments include salt restriction, diuretics, thoracentesis, TIPS, video-assisted thoracoscopy, and pleurodesis. It is important to note that a chest tube is not a potential treatment option unless frank pus or a pneumothorax is present. Hepatic hydrothorax should not be treated by placing a chest tube.[69] Pleural effusions are most often right-sided (73%); the remainder are either left-sided (17%) or bilateral (10%). A total of 9% of patients with hepatic hydrothorax may not have detectable ascites. The overall outcome for patients with hepatic hydrothorax managed by diuretics and/or thoracentesis is poor. In one study, the average time from presentation to death for all patients was 368 days, whereas the average survival for those who underwent TIPS placement was 845 days and no deaths were reported who were bridged to OLT.[70,71]

9.5.5 Spontaneous Bacterial Empyema

Spontaneous bacterial empyema (SBEM) is the infection of a preexisting hydrothorax that is not caused by pneumonia.

Fever, dyspnea, and abdominal pain are the most common clinical manifestations of SBEM. SBP is a known complication in patients with cirrhosis and ascites, and SBEM can occur with hematogenous spread or transdiaphragmatic movement of SBP. The incidence of SBEM is 2% in patients with cirrhosis and 13% in patients with cirrhosis and hydrothorax; up to 53% of SBEM cases were associated with SBP.[72] Because SBEM can occur without simultaneous SBP, both paracentesis and thoracentesis should be performed when an infection is suspected in patients with cirrhosis, ascites, and hydrothorax. Primary treatment is with a third-generation cephalosporin. Chest tube insertion should be reserved for patients with frank pus in the pleural space or a respiratory-limiting pleural effusion.[71,72,73]

9.5.6 Umbilical Hernia

Umbilical hernias occur in up to 20% of patients with RA.[74] Every effort should be made to control ascites before elective repair of hernias, as hernias recur in up to 73% of patients if ascites is present at the time of repair.[75] Strangulation can occur within hours to days after an LVP, a peritoneovenous shunt (PVS) placement, or a TIPS placement.[76,77] Patients should be advised to wear an appropriately sized abdominal binder and be alerted to the possibility of an incarcerated hernia. They should be instructed to manually try to reduce the hernia and to immediately seek medical attention if the hernia is not easily reducible. Elective TIPS placement can be considered in patients with thin-walled umbilical hernias to prevent spontaneous rupture.[78,79]

9.5.7 Paracentesis-Induced Circulatory Dysfunction

Patients with tense ascites are frequently treated by removing 7 to 10 L of ascitic fluid. Removal of such large volumes has been determined to cause paracentesis-induced circulatory dysfunction (PICD), a disorder characterized by marked activation of the renin–angiotensin axis. PICD is a frequent and potentially harmful complication of paracentesis involving more than 6 L. Although PICD may be clinically silent, it has been associated with a rapid recurrence of tense ascites, the development of hyponatremia and renal impairment, and shorter survival. The rate of fluid extraction, use of mechanical modifications (because of abdominal decompression), and release of vasodilator molecules such as nitric oxide from the vascular endothelium are postulated to play a major role in the development of PICD.

The rationale for using plasma expanders such as albumin after paracentesis is to maintain the circulatory status and to prevent the subsequent activation of vasoconstrictor systems. In one prospectively randomized study, the incidence of PICD among patients undergoing total paracentesis was significantly higher ($p = 0.03$) in patients treated with saline than in those treated with albumin; however, no significant difference in the incidence of PICD was observed when less than 6 L of ascitic fluid was evacuated (6.7 vs. 5.6% in the saline and albumin groups, respectively). The incidence of PICD in patients receiving saline in this study was similar to that reported in patients treated with dextran 70 (34%) or polygeline (38%), suggesting that these agents are inferior substitutes for albumin.[80]

Beta-blockers are associated with poor survival in patients with PICD, although the mechanism responsible for this deleterious effect is unknown.[81]

9.6 Tools at the Disposal of the Interventionalist

LVP, TIPS or PVS placement, splenic artery embolization, and placement of a PleurX drain or alfapump are the tools presently available for interventionalists treating patients with RA. These procedures compete with OLT for the treatment of end-stage liver disease, but OLT is the only treatment that will significantly extend survival. However, OLT is not an option for all patients. Patients with active alcohol or substance abuse disorders, HIV or other systemic infections, life-limiting medical conditions, or uncontrolled psychiatric disorders; patients with advanced age; and patients who are unable to comply with pretransplant and posttransplant regimens may not be eligible for OLT.

Interventionalists must understand that making an improvement in the quality of life of a patient will not significantly extend the patient's survival. The patient's quality of life may be significantly improved, but he or she still has a fatal disease that at present has only one cure—OLT. The goal of interventionalists should be to avoid doing anything that might delay or jeopardize the patient's chance of undergoing OLT. It is therefore very important for the interventionalist to work closely with the hepatologist and transplant surgeon.

9.6.1 Large-Volume Paracentesis

The American Association for the Study of Liver Diseases practice guideline suggests performing a single LVP with removal of 4 to 6 L, followed by dietary sodium restriction and diuretic therapy, for patients with tense ascites; for patients with RA, the practice guideline recommends the use of serial LVP sessions as needed. These guidelines consider albumin infusion as optional for LVP sessions in which more than 5 L is removed but do not recommend it for paracentesis of lower volumes. Patients with tense ascites are frequently treated by the removal of 7 to 10 L of ascitic fluid.

Disseminated intravascular coagulation and an acute abdomen are the only absolute contraindications to paracentesis. In two retrospective studies, significant bleeding occurred following LVP in < 0.3% of 5,337 patients with coagulopathy and/or thrombocytopenia. In both studies, an increased bleeding rate was associated with significant renal failure.[82,83] In one study, prophylactic transfusion with fresh frozen plasma did not reduce the bleeding rate.[82]

Ultrasound guidance during the LVP session is mandatory for patients who have undergone OLT or abdominal surgery, as these procedures increase the likelihood of the presence of bowel adhesions and collateral veins on the abdominal wall. The patient should be asked to empty the bladder before the procedure. Tunneling the needle for 7 cm in a zig-zag course through the subcutaneous tissue before entering the peritoneal space is recommended to prevent leakage of residual or accumulated ascitic fluid through the paracentesis puncture site.

Analysis of the ascitic fluid is needed only for the initial paracentesis, and should include cell count, culture, albumin level, total protein level in the ascitic fluid, and serum and ascites albumin levels. The serum–ascites albumin gradient or gap is a calculation used to determine the cause of ascites. A value > 1.1 mg/dL indicates a greater than 97% probability of portal hypertension, whereas a value < 1.1 mg/dL indicates that portal hypertension is very unlikely. Prophylactic antibiotics should be administered to cover the most common organisms (*Escherichia coli*, *Klebsiella pneumoniae*, and pneumococci) pending culture of the causative agent if the polymorphonuclear count is > 250/mm³.

Information about the indications, contraindications, preprocedural testing, and case management for LVP is summarized in ▶ Table 9.2.

Table 9.2 Indications, contraindications, complications, and preprocedural assessments for large-volume paracentesis

Indications, contraindications, and complications	
Diagnostic indications	Fluid evaluation to determine the etiology of new-onset ascites, assessment of suspected spontaneous or secondary bacterial peritonitis, detection of cancer cells
Therapeutic indications	Chest pain, respiratory compromise, anorexia, abdominal pain or pressure (including abdominal compartment syndrome) secondary to ascites
Absolute contraindications	Hyperfibrinolysis, disseminated intravascular coagulopathy, an acute abdomen that requires surgery
Relative contraindications	Abdominal wall cellulitis, intra-abdominal adhesions, distended bowel or bladder, pregnancy
Procedural complications	Hyponatremia, hyperkalemia, renal failure, severe infection, gastrointestinal bleeding, intraperitoneal bleeding, spontaneous bacterial peritonitis, paracentesis-induced circulatory dysfunction, shortened survival

Preprocedural laboratory tests[113]	
International normalized ratio	Routinely recommended for patients with liver disease
Activated partial thromboplastin time	Routinely recommended for patients receiving intravenous unfractionated heparin
Platelet count	Not routinely recommended
Hematocrit	Not routinely recommended

Preprocedural patient management[113]	
International normalized ratio > 2.0	Threshold for treatment (i.e., fresh frozen plasma, vitamin K)
Partial thromboplastin time and hematocrit	No consensus
Platelet count < 50,000/μL	Transfusion recommended
Clopidogrel	Withhold for 5 days before procedure
Aspirin	Do not withhold
Low-molecular-weight heparin	Withhold 1 dose before procedure

9.6.2 Transjugular Intrahepatic Portosystemic Shunt

Reported benefits of TIPS placement in patients with RA include improved renal function, sodium excretion, and general well-being; survival benefits are debatable.[84] TIPS placement has been associated with improved survival compared with repeat LVP in a number of national and international randomized studies[85,86,87]; however, other randomized studies comparing TIPS with repeat paracentesis have demonstrated no survival benefit with TIPS placement,[88,89] and still other studies have demonstrated reduced survival in patients treated with TIPS placement.[90] In a recent Cochrane meta-analysis, there was no significant difference in survival between patients with RA treated with LVP and those treated with TIPS placement.[91] In a study using the United Network for Organ Sharing registries from 2002 to 2013, Berry et al identified 97,063 adults with cirrhosis who were followed from the time of transplant listing until the time of death or OLT. Cox proportional hazards and competing risks analyses were used to compare primary outcomes between patients with a TIPS ($n = 7,475$; 7.7%) and without a TIPS ($n = 9,588$; 92.3%). Patients with a TIPS had a lower risk of death (adjusted subhazard ratio, 0.95; 95% confidence interval, 0.9–0.99) than those without a TIPS. TIPS placement was also associated with a lower risk of transplant and with a lower risk of death or transplant (combined outcome).[92]

Most hepatologists and interventional radiologists believe that TIPS placement offers significant benefit to the patient with RA as a bridge to OLT, for control of RA, and as a means to improve quality of life. The high incidence of HE occurring after TIPS placement is the major deterrent to its routine use in patients with end-stage cirrhosis. The overall incidence of post-TIPS HE is reported to be between 25 and 45%. Age over 65 years, elevated bilirubin level, increased serum creatinine level, reduced serum sodium level, presence of heart failure, low arterial blood pressure, high MELD score, high Child–Pugh score, low portosystemic gradient, failure to embolize portosystemic shunts, placement of large-diameter TIPS, and a history of previous episodes of HE have all been implicated in the increased incidence of HE after TIPS.[84,93,94,95,96] A recent meta-analysis narrowed this list down to three major risk factors: age over 65 years, history of previous episodes of HE, and Child–Pugh score ≥ 10.[97] In another meta-analysis, nearly all patients who had a history of overt HE presented with HE after TIPS.[98] However, a history of a single HE episode, especially one associated variceal bleeding, is not a contraindication to TIPS placement; one study found that a high serum creatinine level was the only parameter independently related to the development of chronic/recurrent post-TIPS HE.[97] Numerous studies have shown that a reduction in TIPS diameter and the resultant increase in portosystemic pressure gradient can reduce the incidence of HE.[98] A recent randomized controlled trial designed to evaluate the efficacy of diameter reduction on the incidence of post-TIPS HE had to be stopped because the smaller diameter stents were not able to control the complications of portal hypertension.[99]

Better patient selection for TIPS placement is needed to decrease the risk of HE. Because patients with minimal HE are more likely to develop overt HE after TIPS, one promising approach is pre-TIPS identification of minimal HE. In one study, 54 consecutive patients treated with TIPS were evaluated by critical flicker frequency tests before and after TIPS placement at months 1, 3, 6, 9, and 12 or until OLT or death. After the TIPS procedure, 19 patients (35%) experienced a total of 64 episodes of overt HE (defined as the occurrence of three or more episodes of overt HE or one episode of HE that lasted more than 15 days). Absence of pre-TIPS minimal HE had a strong negative predictive value (91%) for the risk of overt HE after TIPS placement, and the absence of pre-TIPS history of overt HE and a critical flicker frequency value ≥ 39 Hz had a 100% negative predictive value for overt HE after TIPS placement.[100] There is now a readily accessible and easily administered test for minimal HE: the EncephalApp - Stroop Test, which is a short and recently validated test used to screen and diagnose patients with HE. The test is easy for patients to complete and for clinicians to interpret, and a psychologist is not needed for administration. The Stroop task is a test of psychomotor speed and cognitive flexibility that evaluates the functioning of the anterior attention system and has been found to be sensitive for the detection of cognitive impairment in patients with minimal HE. This test is also available as a smartphone application, which is an attractive option for point-of-care testing.[101]

9.6.3 Peritoneovenous Shunt (Denver Shunt)

Some consider PVS placement as a third line of treatment behind OLT, TIPS placement, and LVP,[102] whereas others contend that there is no role for PVS placement in patients with portal hypertension.[103] In patients with RA and HRS or HE, PVS placement may be the only treatment option that may lead to a reasonably acceptable quality of life.

A major criticism of one PVS, the Denver shunt, is that it requires a great deal of maintenance and has a high complication rate that includes an increased risk of SBP, which may jeopardize the likelihood of successful OLT in the future. Despite this, not all transplant surgeons believe that PVS has no place in the care of the OLT candidate; some endorse PVS as a bridge to OLT.[104] A recent review of 1,491 patients undergoing OLT identified 80 patients (5.4%) who had experienced at least one episode of SBP before OLT. There was no difference in long-term mortality between the two groups during a mean 4-year follow-up.[102]

The Denver shunt has one or two silicone miter (duckbill) valves located in the pump chamber, which permit flow in only one direction. The valves are designed so that their inner surfaces coapt when the pressure gradient between the peritoneal or pleural cavity and the central venous system falls below 3 to 5 cm H_2O, slide against each other when manually pumped to reduce buildup on the valves, and open to allow for continuous flow when the peritoneovenous pressure gradient exceeds 5 cm H_2O. Information about the indications, contraindications, preprocedural testing, and case management for PVS is summarized in ▶ Table 9.3; further information about Denver shunt design, care, and management is available at the manufacturer's web site.[105]

9.6.4 Splenic Artery Embolization

The first splenic artery ligation for the treatment of RA was performed in 1935. In this case, a total splenectomy was aborted because the spleen was found to be adherent to the peritoneum and abdominal wall. Ligation of the splenic artery approximately

Table 9.3 Indications, contraindications, and preprocedural assessments for peritoneovenous shunt

Indications and contraindications	
Diagnostic indications	None
Therapeutic indications	Chest pain, respiratory compromise, anorexia, abdominal pain or pressure (including abdominal compartment syndrome) secondary to ascites, hepatorenal syndrome
Absolute contraindications	Hyperfibrinolysis, disseminated intravascular coagulopathy, an acute abdomen that requires surgery, sepsis, morbid obesity, end-stage renal disease requiring dialysis, septation of the peritoneal cavity due to previous infection or surgery, abdominal wall cellulitis, spontaneous bacterial peritonitis
Relative contraindications	Lack of access to health care provider to oversee daily maintenance of shunt, low likelihood of receiving a liver transplant
Preprocedural laboratory testing[113]	
International normalized ratio	Routinely recommended
Activated partial thromboplastin time	Routinely recommended for patients receiving intravenous unfractionated heparin
Platelet count	Not routinely recommended
Hematocrit	Not routinely recommended
Preprocedural patient management[113]	
International normalized ratio > 2.0	Threshold for treatment (i.e., fresh frozen plasma, vitamin K)
Partial thromboplastin time and hematocrit	No consensus
Platelet count < 50,000 μL	Transfusion recommended
Clopidogrel	Withhold for 5 days before procedure
Aspirin	Do not withhold
Low-molecular-weight heparin	Withhold 1 dose before procedure

9 cm from the hilum resulted in relief of ascites formation and hematologic improvement.[106] More recently, proximal splenic artery embolization has generated renewed interest as a treatment for RA and as an effective procedure for reducing portal hyperperfusion and improving intrahepatic hemodynamics in patients undergoing partial or whole OLT.

In patients with cirrhosis and portal hypertension, splenic artery occlusion causes a significant reduction in the portal pressure gradient (PPG), which is directly related to spleen volume and indirectly related to liver volume. The spleen/liver volume ratio accurately predicts the decrease in PPG and can be used to identify patients who may obtain a significant advantage from surgical and nonsurgical procedures that decrease splenic inflow.[107] The specific contribution of splenic blood inflow to portal hypertension in patients with cirrhosis was investigated in one study by assessing the hemodynamic effects of transient splenic artery occlusion in 15 patients with cirrhosis. PPG was measured just before inserting a TIPS shunt, at

baseline, for 15 minutes after splenic artery occlusion, and 5 minutes after recovery. Splenic artery occlusion caused a significant decrease in PPG (range, 4–38%; median, 20%; $p < 0.001$), which promptly returned to baseline values after recovery of the splenic inflow. The decrease in PPG showed a significant correlation with spleen volume ($r = 0.70$; $p < 0.005$), liver volume ($r = -0.63$; $p < 0.01$), and spleen/liver volume ratio ($r = 0.82$; $p < 0.001$). Seven of eight patients with a spleen/liver volume ratio greater than 0.5 had a > 20% decrease in PPG, whereas none of patients with a ratio lower than 0.5 had a marked PPG response.[107] The results of this study correlate with the results of proximal splenic artery embolization performed in patients with RA after OLT who did not have anastomotic stenosis or portal vein thrombosis.[34]

9.6.5 Indwelling Peritoneal Catheter

There are very few data available regarding the use of indwelling peritoneal catheters in patients with RF due to cirrhosis. One study followed 188 consecutive patients with RF **treated with catheters**: more than 90% of the cases were secondary to malignant disease; only 7 patients (3.7%) had RA due to cirrhosis.[108] The overall complication rate with catheter placement was 0.4 per year, which compared favorably with the complication rate seen with peritoneal dialysis catheters (0.6 per year).[109] Another study followed 227 patients with cirrhotic RA who were treated by placement of PleurX drains. In this study, 12% of patients had bacterial peritonitis at admission, and 22% developed bacterial peritonitis during treatment; 10% of these cases occurred in the first 72 hours. Those who developed bacterial peritonitis had a 50% mortality rate at 5 months compared to a 50% mortality rate at 50 months in those without infection.[110] At present, there appears to be a limited role at best for indwelling peritoneal catheters in patients with RA who are not OLT candidates.

9.6.6 Automated Low-Flow Pump System (alfapump)

The automated low-flow pump system "alfapump" consists of an intraperitoneal catheter connected to a subcutaneously implanted battery-powered device that moves fluid from but not to the peritoneal cavity, and a second catheter that subcutaneously connects the pump to the urinary bladder. Patients with this pump therefore directly urinate the ascites. The system has internal sensors that monitor the pressure in the peritoneal cavity and bladder to prevent continuous pump operation when pressure in the abdomen is low or pressure in the bladder is high. The volume and time of infusion can also be programmed. At present, the pump is implanted through a surgical procedure performed under general anesthesia. It is anticipated that less invasive percutaneous placement will be possible in the future. In one study, the alfapump system was associated with a significant reduction in the number of LVPs; 40% of patients did not require any LVP, and 70% of patients required fewer than one LVP per month after pump implantation.[111,112]

A randomized, controlled clinical trial comparing the alfapump system to LVP and TIPS placement is underway. This trial will further investigate the clinical usefulness of this device in patients with RA.

9.7 Conclusion

- Nothing should be done that will delay or impede the patient from undergoing an OLT. Any procedure performed on a patient on the "Transplant List" must be agreed upon by the transplant surgeon, transplant hepatologist, and interventionalist.
- LVP should be continued until it must be performed more frequently than every 3 weeks or until quality of life is adversely affected.
- TIPS placement is the preferred treatment for RA in patients with no history of HE or end-stage renal disease.
- LVP is the preferred treatment in the patient who has a history of HE.
- PSAE should be considered as an ancillary treatment when LVP and TIPS do not adequately control the patient's RA, especially in the post-transplant patient.
- PVS should be considered when the methods listed above fail.

References

[1] Reuben A. Out came copious water. Hepatology. 2002; 36(1):261–264

[2] London SJ. Beethoven: case report of a titan's last crisis. Arch Intern Med. 1964; 113:442–448

[3] Runyon BA. Historical aspects of treatment of patients with cirrhosis and ascites. Semin Liver Dis. 1997; 17(3):163–173

[4] Kubba AK, Young M. Ludwig van Beethoven: a medical biography. Lancet. 1996; 347(8995):167–170

[5] Renouard PV. Paracentesis Abdominalis. In: Comegys CG, ed. History of Medicine from Its Origin to the Nineteenth Century. Philadelphia, PA: Lindsay & Blakiston; 1867:452–453

[6] Conn HO. The paracentesis pendulum. Hepatology. 1985; 5(3):521–522

[7] Eknoyan G. A history of edema and its management. Kidney Int Suppl. 1997; 59:S118–S126

[8] Iwakiri Y, Groszmann RJ. The hyperdynamic circulation of chronic liver diseases: from the patient to the molecule. Hepatology. 2006; 43(2) Suppl 1: S121–S131

[9] Abraldes JG, Iwakiri Y, Loureiro-Silva M, Haq O, Sessa WC, Groszmann RJ. Mild increases in portal pressure upregulate vascular endothelial growth factor and endothelial nitric oxide synthase in the intestinal microcirculatory bed, leading to a hyperdynamic state. Am J Physiol Gastrointest Liver Physiol. 2006; 290(5):G980–G987

[10] Tsai MH, Iwakiri Y, Cadelina G, Sessa WC, Groszmann RJ. Mesenteric vasoconstriction triggers nitric oxide overproduction in the superior mesenteric artery of portal hypertensive rats. Gastroenterology. 2003; 125 (5):1452–1461

[11] Shi TY, Zhang LN, Chen H, et al. Risk factors for hepatic decompensation in patients with primary biliary cirrhosis. World J Gastroenterol. 2013; 19(7): 1111–1118

[12] Hui AY, Chan HL, Leung NW, Hung LC, Chan FK, Sung JJ. Survival and prognostic indicators in patients with hepatitis B virus-related cirrhosis after onset of hepatic decompensation. J Clin Gastroenterol. 2002; 34(5): 569–572

[13] Pedersen JS, Bendtsen F, Møller S. Management of cirrhotic ascites. Ther Adv Chronic Dis. 2015; 6(3):124–137

[14] Levitt DG, Levitt MD. Quantitative modeling of the physiology of ascites in portal hypertension. BMC Gastroenterol. 2012; 12:26

[15] Casado M, Bosch J, García-Pagán JC, et al. Clinical events after transjugular intrahepatic portosystemic shunt: correlation with hemodynamic findings. Gastroenterology. 1998; 114(6):1296–1303

[16] Ginés P, Quintero E, Arroyo V, et al. Compensated cirrhosis: natural history and prognostic factors. Hepatology. 1987; 7(1):122–128

[17] D'Amico G, Morabito A, Pagliaro L, Marubini E. Survival and prognostic indicators in compensated and decompensated cirrhosis. Dig Dis Sci. 1986; 31(5):468–475

[18] Tao X, Wang N, Qin W. Gut microbiota and hepatocellular carcinoma. Gastrointest Tumors. 2015; 2(1):33–40

[19] El-Serag HB. Hepatocellular carcinoma. N Engl J Med. 2011; 365(12):1118–1127

[20] Kamath PS, Wiesner RH, Malinchoc M, et al. A model to predict survival in patients with end-stage liver disease. Hepatology. 2001; 33(2):464–470

[21] Ripoll C, Groszmann R, Garcia-Tsao G, et al. Portal Hypertension Collaborative Group. Hepatic venous pressure gradient predicts clinical decompensation in patients with compensated cirrhosis. Gastroenterology. 2007; 133(2):481–488

[22] Berzigotti A, Garcia-Tsao G, Bosch J, et al. Portal Hypertension Collaborative Group. Obesity is an independent risk factor for clinical decompensation in patients with cirrhosis. Hepatology. 2011; 54(2):555–561

[23] Salerno F, Gerbes A, Ginès P, Wong F, Arroyo V. Diagnosis, prevention and treatment of hepatorenal syndrome in cirrhosis. Gut. 2007; 56(9):1310–1318

[24] Planas R, Montoliu S, Ballesté B, et al. Natural history of patients hospitalized for management of cirrhotic ascites. Clin Gastroenterol Hepatol. 2006; 4 (11):1385–1394

[25] Guardiola J, Xiol X, Escribá JM, et al. Prognosis assessment of cirrhotic patients with refractory ascites treated with a peritoneovenous shunt. Am J Gastroenterol. 1995; 90(12):2097–2102

[26] Moreau R, Delègue P, Pessione F, et al. Clinical characteristics and outcome of patients with cirrhosis and refractory ascites. Liver Int. 2004; 24(5):457–464

[27] Chutaputti A. Management of refractory ascites and hepatorenal syndrome. J Gastroenterol Hepatol. 2002; 17(4):456–461

[28] Runyon BA, AASLD. Introduction to the revised American Association for the Study of Liver Diseases Practice Guideline management of adult patients with ascites due to cirrhosis 2012. Hepatology. 2013; 57(4):1651–1653

[29] Arroyo V, Ginès P, Gerbes AL, et al. Definition and diagnostic criteria of refractory ascites and hepatorenal syndrome in cirrhosis. International Ascites Club. Hepatology. 1996; 23(1):164–176

[30] Nishida S, Gaynor JJ, Nakamura N, et al. Refractory ascites after liver transplantation: an analysis of 1058 liver transplant patients at a single center. Am J Transplant. 2006; 6(1):140–149

[31] Darcy MD. Management of venous outflow complications after liver transplantation. Tech Vasc Interv Radiol. 2007; 10(3):240–245

[32] Miraglia R, Maruzzelli L, Caruso S, et al. Interventional radiology procedures in adult patients who underwent liver transplantation. World J Gastroenterol. 2009; 15(6):684–693

[33] Saad WE, Darwish WM, Davies MG, et al. Transjugular intrahepatic portosystemic shunts in liver transplant recipients: technical analysis and clinical outcome. AJR Am J Roentgenol. 2013; 200(1):210–218

[34] Quintini C, D'Amico G, Brown C, et al. Splenic artery embolization for the treatment of refractory ascites after liver transplantation. Liver Transpl. 2011; 17(6):668–673

[35] Fernández J, Navasa M, Planas R, et al. Primary prophylaxis of spontaneous bacterial peritonitis delays hepatorenal syndrome and improves survival in cirrhosis. Gastroenterology. 2007; 133(3):818–824

[36] Rimola A, García-Tsao G, Navasa M, et al. Diagnosis, treatment and prophylaxis of spontaneous bacterial peritonitis: a consensus document. International Ascites Club. J Hepatol. 2000; 32(1):142–153

[37] Wong F, Bernardi M, Balk R, et al. International Ascites Club. Sepsis in cirrhosis: report on the 7th meeting of the International Ascites Club. Gut. 2005; 54(5):718–725

[38] Hoefs JC, Canawati HN, Sapico FL, Hopkins RR, Weiner J, Montgomerie JZ. Spontaneous bacterial peritonitis. Hepatology. 1982; 2(4):399–407

[39] Téllez-Ávila FI, Chávez-Tapia NC, Franco-Guzmán AM, Uribe M, Vargas-Vorackova F. Rapid diagnosis of spontaneous bacterial peritonitis using leukocyte esterase reagent strips in emergency department: uri-quick clini-10SG® vs. Multistix 10SG®. Ann Hepatol. 2012; 11(5):696–699

[40] Ginés P, Rimola A, Planas R, et al. Norfloxacin prevents spontaneous bacterial peritonitis recurrence in cirrhosis: results of a double-blind, placebo-controlled trial. Hepatology. 1990; 12(4, Pt 1):716–724

[41] Ruiz-del-Arbol L, Monescillo A, Arocena C, et al. Circulatory function and hepatorenal syndrome in cirrhosis. Hepatology. 2005; 42(2):439–447

[42] Krag A, Bendtsen F, Henriksen JH, Møller S. Low cardiac output predicts development of hepatorenal syndrome and survival in patients with cirrhosis and ascites. Gut. 2010; 59(1):105–110

[43] Ginés P, Schrier RW. Renal failure in cirrhosis. N Engl J Med. 2009; 361(13): 1279–1290

[44] Ginés P, Arroyo V, Rodés J. Treatment of ascites and renal failure in cirrhosis. Baillieres Clin Gastroenterol. 1989; 3(1):165–186

[45] Members ECPG, European Association for the Study of the Liver. EASL clinical practice guidelines on the management of ascites, spontaneous bacterial peritonitis, and hepatorenal syndrome in cirrhosis. J Hepatol. 2010; 53(3):397–417

[46] Sort P, Navasa M, Arroyo V, et al. Effect of intravenous albumin on renal impairment and mortality in patients with cirrhosis and spontaneous bacterial peritonitis. N Engl J Med. 1999; 341(6):403–409

[47] Tyagi P, Sharma P, Sharma BC, Puri AS, Kumar A, Sarin SK. Prevention of hepatorenal syndrome in patients with cirrhosis and ascites: a pilot randomized control trial between pentoxifylline and placebo. Eur J Gastroenterol Hepatol. 2011; 23(3):210–217

[48] Ring-Larsen H. Hepatic nephropathy, related to haemodynamics. Liver. 1983; 3(5):265–289

[49] Henriksen JH, Ring-Larsen H. Hepatorenal disorders: role of the sympathetic nervous system. Semin Liver Dis. 1994; 14(1):35–43

[50] Solis-Herruzo JA, Duran A, Favela V, et al. Effects of lumbar sympathetic block on kidney function in cirrhotic patients with hepatorenal syndrome. J Hepatol. 1987; 5(2):167–173

[51] Guevara M, Ginès P, Bandi JC, et al. Transjugular intrahepatic portosystemic shunt in hepatorenal syndrome: effects on renal function and vasoactive systems. Hepatology. 1998; 28(2):416–422

[52] Brensing KA, Textor J, Perz J, et al. Long term outcome after transjugular intrahepatic portosystemic stent-shunt in non-transplant cirrhotics with hepatorenal syndrome: a phase II study. Gut. 2000; 47 (2):288–295

[53] Romero-Gómez M, Boza F, García-Valdecasas MS, García E, Aguilar-Reina J. Subclinical hepatic encephalopathy predicts the development of overt hepatic encephalopathy. Am J Gastroenterol. 2001; 96(9):2718–2723

[54] Boyer TD, Haskal ZJ, American Association for the Study of Liver Diseases. The role of transjugular intrahepatic portosystemic shunt in the management of portal hypertension. Hepatology. 2005; 41(2):386–400

[55] Bajaj JS, Cordoba J, Mullen KD, et al. International Society for Hepatic Encephalopathy and Nitrogen Metabolism (ISHEN). Review article: the design of clinical trials in hepatic encephalopathy–an International Society for Hepatic Encephalopathy and Nitrogen Metabolism (ISHEN) consensus statement. Aliment Pharmacol Ther. 2011; 33(7):739–747

[56] Nusrat S, Khan MS, Fazili J, Madhoun MF. Cirrhosis and its complications: evidence based treatment. World J Gastroenterol. 2014; 20(18):5442–5460

[57] Bajaj JS. Review article: potential mechanisms of action of rifaximin in the management of hepatic encephalopathy and other complications of cirrhosis. Aliment Pharmacol Ther. 2016; 43 Suppl 1:11–26

[58] Pereira K, Carrion AF, Martin P, et al. Current diagnosis and management of post-transjugular intrahepatic portosystemic shunt refractory hepatic encephalopathy. Liver Int. 2015; 35(12):2487–2494

[59] Cash WJ, McConville P, McDermott E, McCormick PA, Callender ME, McDougall NI. Current concepts in the assessment and treatment of hepatic encephalopathy. QJM. 2010; 103(1):9–16

[60] Poh Z, Chang PE. A current review of the diagnostic and treatment strategies of hepatic encephalopathy. Int J Hepatol. 2012; 2012:480309

[61] Ahboucha S, Butterworth RF. Pathophysiology of hepatic encephalopathy: a new look at GABA from the molecular standpoint. Metab Brain Dis. 2004; 19 (3–4):331–343

[62] Fischer JE, Rosen HM, Ebeid AM, James JH, Keane JM, Soeters PB. The effect of normalization of plasma amino acids on hepatic encephalopathy in man. Surgery. 1976; 80(1):77–91

[63] Lozeva-Thomas V. Serotonin brain circuits with a focus on hepatic encephalopathy. Metab Brain Dis. 2004; 19(3–4):413–420

[64] Marchesini G, Fabbri A, Bianchi G, Brizi M, Zoli M. Zinc supplementation and amino acid-nitrogen metabolism in patients with advanced cirrhosis. Hepatology. 1996; 23(5):1084–1092

[65] Mas A. Hepatic encephalopathy: from pathophysiology to treatment. Digestion. 2006; 73 Suppl 1:86–93

[66] Dagenais MH, Bernard D, Marleau D, et al. Surgical treatment of severe postshunt hepatic encephalopathy. World J Surg. 1991; 15(1):109–113, discussion 113–114

[67] Riordan SM, Williams R. Treatment of hepatic encephalopathy. N Engl J Med. 1997; 337(7):473–479

[68] Yoshida H, Mamada Y, Taniai N, et al. Long-term results of partial splenic artery embolization as supplemental treatment for portal-systemic encephalopathy. Am J Gastroenterol. 2005; 100(1):43–47

[69] Krok KL, Cárdenas A. Hepatic hydrothorax. Semin Respir Crit Care Med. 2012; 33(1):3–10

[70] Badillo R, Rockey DC. Hepatic hydrothorax: clinical features, management, and outcomes in 77 patients and review of the literature. Medicine (Baltimore). 2014; 93(3):135–142

[71] Siqueira F, Kelly T, Saab S. Refractory ascites: pathogenesis, clinical impact, and management. Gastroenterol Hepatol (N Y). 2009; 5:647–656

[72] Alonso JC. Pleural effusion in liver disease. Semin Respir Crit Care Med. 2010; 31(6):698–705

[73] Runyon BA, Greenblatt M, Ming RH. Hepatic hydrothorax is a relative contraindication to chest tube insertion. Am J Gastroenterol. 1986; 81(7):566–567

[74] Belghiti J, Durand F. Abdominal wall hernias in the setting of cirrhosis. Semin Liver Dis. 1997; 17(3):219–226

[75] Runyon BA, Juler GL. Natural history of repaired umbilical hernias in patients with and without ascites. Am J Gastroenterol. 1985; 80(1):38–39

[76] Chu KM, McCaughan GW. Iatrogenic incarceration of umbilical hernia in cirrhotic patients with ascites. Am J Gastroenterol. 1995; 90(11):2058–2059

[77] Trotter JF, Suhocki PV. Incarceration of umbilical hernia following transjugular intrahepatic portosystemic shunt for the treatment of ascites. Liver Transpl Surg. 1999; 5(3):209–210

[78] Telem DA, Schiano T, Divino CM. Complicated hernia presentation in patients with advanced cirrhosis and refractory ascites: management and outcome. Surgery. 2010; 148(3):538–543

[79] Triantos CK, Kehagias I, Nikolopoulou V, Burroughs AK. Surgical repair of umbilical hernias in cirrhosis with ascites. Am J Med Sci. 2011; 341(3):222–226

[80] Sola-Vera J, Miñana J, Ricart E, et al. Randomized trial comparing albumin and saline in the prevention of paracentesis-induced circulatory dysfunction in cirrhotic patients with ascites. Hepatology. 2003; 37(5):1147–1153

[81] Ginès A, Fernández-Esparrach G, Monescillo A, et al. Randomized trial comparing albumin, dextran 70, and polygeline in cirrhotic patients with ascites treated by paracentesis. Gastroenterology. 1996; 111(4):1002–1010

[82] McVay PA, Toy PT. Lack of increased bleeding after paracentesis and thoracentesis in patients with mild coagulation abnormalities. Transfusion. 1991; 31(2):164–171

[83] Pache I, Bilodeau M. Severe haemorrhage following abdominal paracentesis for ascites in patients with liver disease. Aliment Pharmacol Ther. 2005; 21 (5):525–529

[84] Moore KP, Wong F, Gines P, et al. The management of ascites in cirrhosis: report on the consensus conference of the International Ascites Club. Hepatology. 2003; 38(1):258–266

[85] Rössle M, Ochs A, Gülberg V, et al. A comparison of paracentesis and transjugular intrahepatic portosystemic shunting in patients with ascites. N Engl J Med. 2000; 342(23):1701–1707

[86] Salerno F, Merli M, Riggio O, et al. Randomized controlled study of TIPS versus paracentesis plus albumin in cirrhosis with severe ascites. Hepatology. 2004; 40(3):629–635

[87] Narahara Y, Kanazawa H, Fukuda T, et al. Transjugular intrahepatic portosystemic shunt versus paracentesis plus albumin in patients with refractory ascites who have good hepatic and renal function: a prospective randomized trial. J Gastroenterol. 2011; 46(1):78–85

[88] Ginès P, Uriz J, Calahorra B, et al. Transjugular intrahepatic portosystemic shunting versus paracentesis plus albumin for refractory ascites in cirrhosis. Gastroenterology. 2002; 123(6):1839–1847

[89] Sanyal AJ, Genning C, Reddy KR, et al. North American Study for the Treatment of Refractory Ascites Group. The North American Study for the Treatment of Refractory Ascites. Gastroenterology. 2003; 124(3):634–641

[90] Lebrec D, Giuily N, Hadengue A, et al. Transjugular intrahepatic portosystemic shunts: comparison with paracentesis in patients with cirrhosis and refractory ascites: a randomized trial. French Group of Clinicians and a Group of Biologists. J Hepatol. 1996; 25(2):135–144

[91] Saab S, Nieto JM, Lewis SK, Runyon BA. TIPS versus paracentesis for cirrhotic patients with refractory ascites. Cochrane Database Syst Rev. 2006(4): CD004889

[92] Berry K, Lerrigo R, Liou IW, Ioannou GN. Association between transjugular intrahepatic portosystemic shunt and survival in patients with cirrhosis. Clin Gastroenterol Hepatol. 2016; 14(1):118–123

[93] Salerno F, Cammà C, Enea M, Rössle M, Wong F. Transjugular intrahepatic portosystemic shunt for refractory ascites: a meta-analysis of individual patient data. Gastroenterology. 2007; 133(3):825–834

[94] Chung HH, Razavi MK, Sze DY, et al. Portosystemic pressure gradient during transjugular intrahepatic portosystemic shunt with Viatorr stent graft: what is the critical low threshold to avoid medically uncontrolled low pressure gradient related complications? J Gastroenterol Hepatol. 2008; 23(1):95–101

[95] Riggio O, Nardelli S, Moscucci F, Pasquale C, Ridola L, Merli M. Hepatic encephalopathy after transjugular intrahepatic portosystemic shunt. Clin Liver Dis. 2012; 16(1):133–146

[96] Shi Y, Tian X, Hu J, et al. Efficacy of transjugular intrahepatic portosystemic shunt with adjunctive embolotherapy with cyanoacrylate for esophageal variceal bleeding. Dig Dis Sci. 2014; 59(9):2325–2332

[97] Bai M, Qi X, Yang Z, et al. Predictors of hepatic encephalopathy after transjugular intrahepatic portosystemic shunt in cirrhotic patients: a systematic review. J Gastroenterol Hepatol. 2011; 26(6):943–951

[98] Riggio O, Angeloni S, Salvatori FM, et al. Incidence, natural history, and risk factors of hepatic encephalopathy after transjugular intrahepatic portosystemic shunt with polytetrafluoroethylene-covered stent grafts. Am J Gastroenterol. 2008; 103(11):2738–2746

[99] Riggio O, Ridola L, Angeloni S, et al. Clinical efficacy of transjugular intrahepatic portosystemic shunt created with covered stents with different diameters: results of a randomized controlled trial. J Hepatol. 2010; 53(2):267–272

[100] Berlioux P, Robic MA, Poirson H, et al. Pre-transjugular intrahepatic portosystemic shunts (TIPS) prediction of post-TIPS overt hepatic encephalopathy: the critical flicker frequency is more accurate than psychometric tests. Hepatology. 2014; 59(2):622–629

[101] Bajaj JS, Thacker LR, Heuman DM, et al. The Stroop smartphone application is a short and valid method to screen for minimal hepatic encephalopathy. Hepatology. 2013; 58(3):1122–1132

[102] Mounzer R, Malik SM, Nasr J, Madani B, Devera ME, Ahmad J. Spontaneous bacterial peritonitis before liver transplantation does not affect patient survival. Clin Gastroenterol Hepatol. 2010; 8(7):623–628.e1

[103] Wongcharatrawee S, Garcia-Tsao G. Clinical management of ascites and its complications. Clin Liver Dis. 2001; 5(3):833–850

[104] Dumortier J, Pianta E, Le Derf Y, et al. Peritoneovenous shunt as a bridge to liver transplantation. Am J Transplant. 2005; 5(8):1886–1892

[105] http://www.bd.com/en-us/offerings/capabilities/interventional-specialties/drainage/about-the-denver-shunt

[106] Watson RB. Ligation of splenic artery for advanced splenic anaemia. BMJ. 1935; 1(3876):821–822

[107] Luca A, Miraglia R, Caruso S, Milazzo M, Gidelli B, Bosch J. Effects of splenic artery occlusion on portal pressure in patients with cirrhosis and portal hypertension. Liver Transpl. 2006; 12(8):1237–1243

[108] Lungren MP, Kim CY, Stewart JK, Smith TP, Miller MJ. Tunneled peritoneal drainage catheter placement for refractory ascites: single-center experience in 188 patients. J Vasc Interv Radiol. 2013; 24(9):1303–1308

[109] Li PK, Szeto CC, Piraino B, et al. International Society for Peritoneal Dialysis. Peritoneal dialysis-related infections recommendations: 2010 update. Perit Dial Int. 2010; 30(4):393–423

[110] Kathpalia P, Bhatia A, Robertazzi S, et al. Indwelling peritoneal catheters in patients with cirrhosis and refractory ascites. Intern Med J. 2015; 45(10):1026–1031

[111] Bellot P, Welker MW, Soriano G, et al. Automated low flow pump system for the treatment of refractory ascites: a multi-center safety and efficacy study. J Hepatol. 2013; 58(5):922–927

[112] Arroyo V. A new method for therapeutic paracentesis: the automated low flow pump system. Comments in the context of the history of paracentesis. J Hepatol. 2013; 58(5):850–852

[113] Patel IJ, Davidson JC, Nikolic B, et al. Standards of Practice Committee, with Cardiovascular and Interventional Radiological Society of Europe (CIRSE) Endorsement. Consensus guidelines for periprocedural management of coagulation status and hemostasis risk in percutaneous image-guided interventions. J Vasc Interv Radiol. 2012; 23(6):727–736

10 Mesenteric Ischemia

Guy E. Johnson

10.1 Introduction

Mesenteric ischemia is an unusual clinical entity with several causes. The etiology of acute mesenteric ischemia (AMI) generally falls into one of several categories: acute arterial occlusion (embolic or thrombotic), portomesenteric venous thrombosis (PMVT), or nonocclusive mesenteric ischemia (NOMI). Chronic mesenteric ischemia (CMI) is a different condition with a separate presentation. Less common causes of AMI include vasculitis and collagen vascular diseases, trauma with vascular injury, and mechanical bowel obstruction with torsion of the vasculature.[1]

Because patient presentation, prognosis, and treatment options differ for the various subtypes of mesenteric ischemia, it is important to differentiate among these distinct causes. This chapter will focus on the most common categories of mesenteric ischemia.

10.2 Epidemiology and Significance of AMI

AMI is a relatively rare but often devastating clinical entity. AMI is a rare cause for hospital admission but may be seen in as many as 30% of patients undergoing abbreviated (damage control) laparotomy for acute abdomen.[2] The mortality of AMI varies depending on the cause of the condition but can reach 70% or higher despite aggressive treatment.[3] In all cases, the prognosis is generally poor. The high mortality associated with AMI has not changed significantly over the last several decades.[3] The difficulty in establishing a diagnosis of AMI may contribute to its poor prognosis, as delays in diagnosis and treatment are associated with increased mortality.[4]

10.3 Pathophysiology of Acute Mesenteric Ischemia

The splanchnic circulation receives approximately 25 to 35% of the cardiac output, depending on metabolic demands.[5] Whatever the cause, ischemic compromise of splanchnic blood flow results in a mismatch between the bowel metabolic oxygen requirement and oxygen supply. Initial ischemic changes in the bowel are confined to the metabolically more active superficial mucosa, which receives most of the blood flow to the gut.[1,6] The ischemic mucosa becomes more permeable, allowing passage of macromolecules into the bowel wall and lumen and resulting in fluid distention. This may progress to sloughing of epithelial cells from the tips of the villi.[6] Computed tomography (CT) findings at this stage may include a dilated lumen with wall thickening from edema (▶ Fig. 10.1); hemorrhage and ulcerations may also be present. The amount of bowel wall attenuation seen on imaging is dependent on whether edema (low density) or hemorrhage (high density) predominates. Bowel wall enhancement is also variable and may not reflect adequate perfusion.[1,7] As ischemia continues, changes progress to the bases of the villi and lead to mucosal necrosis; however,

if ischemia is halted, this mucosal necrosis can heal completely.[7] Without correction, the process continues and the deeper layers of the bowel wall become involved. Involvement of the submucosa and muscularis propria ultimately results in transmural bowel infarction and its very high associated mortality rate.

10.4 Imaging Diagnosis of Acute Bowel Ischemia

The use of invasive catheter arteriography to establish the diagnosis of occlusive mesenteric ischemia has largely been replaced by CT evaluation, which is noninvasive and more widely available.[8] In addition to its expedience, CT has the added potential benefit of suggesting an alternative diagnosis in patients with abdominal pain.[9]

Ideally, CT evaluation in mesenteric ischemia is biphasic, with both arterial and venous phases. Multidetector CT allows for

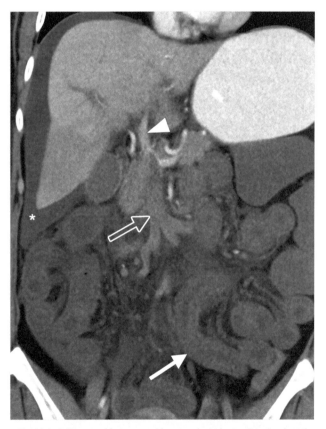

Fig. 10.1 A 51-year-old woman with recent bowel resection developed superior mesenteric vein thrombosis. The thrombus (*open white arrow*) in the superior mesenteric vein is expansile compared to the diminutive portal vein (*arrowhead*) and splenic vein. Note the ascites (*asterisk*) and thick, edematous bowel wall with decreased mucosal enhancement (*solid white arrow*). Despite medical management, the patient's condition progressed to bowel infarction and required extensive bowel resection.

Table 10.1 CT findings of acute mesenteric ischemia

Bowel wall thickening (>3 mm) with:

- Absent mural enhancement
- Mural hyperenhancement
- Mucosal hyperenhancement with submucosal edema (target sign)
- Venous thrombosis
- Solid organ infarction

Superior mesenteric artery occlusion

Mesenteric artery embolism

Celiac artery and inferior mesenteric artery occlusion with distal superior mesenteric artery stenosis

Mesenteric venous cutoff from torsion

Late findings of mesenteric ischemia

- Pneumatosis intestinalis
- Portomesenteric venous gas
- Pneumoperitoneum or retroperitoneal gas
- Bowel wall thinning with absent mural enhancement

Ancillary nonspecific findings of mesenteric ischemia

- Mesenteric fat edema (stranding)
- Ascites
- Portomesenteric venous thrombosis
- Stratification of bowel wall without mural thickening (target sign)
- Dilated bowel
- Focal transition from bowel dilation to collapsed bowel distally

Source: Adapted with permission from Sandstrom et al.[1]

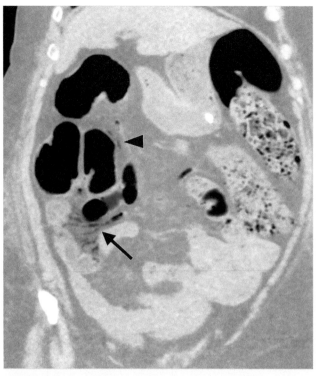

Fig. 10.2 A 61-year-old woman with abdominal pain, vomiting, leukocytosis, and elevated lactate levels. Noncontrast-enhanced coronal CT shows mesenteric venous gas (*arrow*) and minimal pneumatosis intestinalis (*arrowhead*). With supportive care, the patient's pain and CT findings resolved over several days.

multiplanar reformatted images to view mesenteric vessels in multiple planes. This may increase the ability to identify abnormalities such as an embolus lodged within the trunk of the superior mesenteric artery (SMA). CT findings suggestive of mesenteric ischemia are shown in ▶ Table 10.1. Some signs such as bowel wall thickening, luminal dilation, and abnormal enhancement of intestinal mucosa have a lower specificity, whereas other signs such as pneumatosis intestinalis are less ambiguous. However, even though pneumatosis intestinalis and portomesenteric venous gas (▶ Fig. 10.2) are commonly cited as specific and ominous CT signs of mesenteric ischemia, these findings are not absolutely specific for mesenteric ischemia and do not necessarily confer a poor prognosis.[7] Decreased or absent bowel wall enhancement is an ominous sign that can be seen in cases of embolism and mesenteric thrombosis. A detectable occlusion of the mesenteric vasculature is an exquisitely specific sign but has a poor sensitivity. Free intraperitoneal air represents a late sign of perforation from infarcted bowel.[10] In isolation, each finding may be of limited value, but when multiple signs are considered together, the sensitivity and specificity of CT angiography for detecting mesenteric ischemia are 96 and 94%, respectively.[11,12]

Magnetic resonance angiography is quite sensitive and specific for detecting stenosis or occlusion of the SMA origin. Likewise, magnetic resonance angiography can be useful in diagnosing mesenteric venous thrombosis; however, its role is limited by availability and the time required for the examination. Ultrasound can be a useful initial screening tool to identify proximal stenoses of the SMA and celiac arteries, with threshold peak systolic velocities of 200 cm/s for the celiac and 275 cm/s for the SMA, suggesting significant stenoses.[13] The inferior mesenteric artery (IMA) is generally very difficult to identify on ultrasound, however. Doppler ultrasound has good sensitivity and specificity for detecting central mesenteric vascular occlusions, but the accuracy and feasibility of this imaging modality may be limited by the presence of bowel gas. For this reason, Doppler ultrasound is not recommended for the initial evaluation of patients suspected of having AMI.[8]

Imaging signs of embolic occlusion, thrombosis, venous occlusion, and nonocclusive pathologies will be discussed below.

10.4.1 AMI Caused by Arterial Occlusion

Acute SMA occlusion accounts for 67% of all cases of AMI,[14] and acute embolic occlusion is the most common cause of AMI, representing approximately 50% of cases.[5] Most of the remaining cases are caused by mesenteric thrombosis.

Patient Presentation and Diagnosis

Early diagnosis of this condition is essential because it may decrease mortality in patients with AMI.[5,15] A prompt diagnosis itself represents a major challenge in AMI (of any cause) not only because of the rarity of the condition but also because of the relatively nonspecific nature of its presentation. Because the diagnosis is obscure, it is often not considered on initial presentation.[16]

In patients with AMI caused by arterial embolic occlusion, rapid onset of periumbilical abdominal pain is common. The pain may be described as cramplike and continuous, is generally moderate to severe, and may even be resistant to opiates in some patients. In 30 to 50% of patients, the onset of abdominal pain is sudden; in another one-third of patients, the pain begins acutely over less than 1 hour.[16,17] With the severity of the abdominal pain, evidence of peritonitis might be expected on physical examination; however, this is generally not an early finding (hence the classic term *pain out of proportion to the physical examination*).[18] Following the onset of abdominal pain in many patients, a rapid evacuation of the bowel comes in the form of diarrhea (42%), which may be bloody, as well as vomiting (71%).[17] The abdominal pain and gastrointestinal symptoms usually occur as components of a triad of symptoms in these patients: (1) pain out of proportion to the physical examination, (2) vomiting and diarrhea, and (3) an obvious source of an embolus such as atrial fibrillation or recent myocardial infarction.[17] Given the overlap with cardiovascular disease, patients with mesenteric ischemia generally present in their sixth to eighth decade of life.

Because atherosclerosis is generally the cause in patients with AMI caused by arterial thrombosis, the thrombosis generally occurs with longstanding and progressive narrowing of the artery. Therefore, immediate symptoms may occur in the setting of insidious symptoms of CMI (discussed below).

Laboratory abnormalities are nearly always present in patients with this condition. Patients may demonstrate evidence of metabolic acidosis, with high lactate levels and leukocytosis.[19] Assessment of the D-dimer level may be useful, as a normal value may exclude the diagnosis of mesenteric ischemia.[20] Unfortunately, however, there exists no rapid laboratory test that is pathognomonic or sufficient to establish the diagnosis.[12]

In cases of embolic occlusion, the thromboembolus lodges several centimeters past the SMA origin as the vessel narrows distal to the takeoff of the first jejunal branches and middle colic artery. The SMA may be more prone to embolic occlusion because of its relatively acute takeoff from the aorta. CT images in these patients may demonstrate a discrete filling defect (thromboembolus) within the SMA (▶ Fig. 10.3); this filling defect may show a convex proximal surface and can be partially or totally occlusive. Because the jejunal branches and the middle colic artery may be spared, the corresponding bowel may have a normal appearance at CT. Most emboli are cardiogenic; therefore, intracardiac thrombi may also be identified on CT when patients are evaluated for mesenteric ischemia. Synchronous emboli are evident in approximately a quarter of patients.[17]

Treatment

The most common management for acute embolic mesenteric ischemia is surgery. Patients with advanced disease and infarcted bowel who present with peritonitis or shock may proceed to laparotomy even if the diagnosis is not fully established preoperatively. Although invasive, surgical revascularization affords the benefit of direct visual inspection of the bowel to assess for viability. The bowel is evaluated at laparotomy; if the bowel is deemed nonviable, it is resected. In addition to visual inspection and clinical judgment, several other techniques are used for the assessment of viability, including palpation or Doppler ultrasound of distal arterial arcades and injection of

fluorescein. Unfortunately, the sensitivity of such clinical assessment is relatively poor, and "second-look" laparotomy may be necessary to resect more nonviable bowel.[21] Revascularization with a bypass graft can be performed via an antegrade (using the supraceliac aorta as inflow) or retrograde (using the common iliac artery as inflow) approach. Balloon embolectomy is an alternative to bypass that can be performed with or without patch angioplasty of the superior mesenteric arteriotomy.[22] Retrograde stenting after open exposure of the SMA has also been used.[23] Supportive measures may include fluid resuscitation to counteract fluid shifts from third spacing and initiation of broad-spectrum antibiotics to combat bacterial translocation across the ischemic intestinal wall. Anticoagulation with intravenous unfractionated heparin helps to prevent further clot propagation; this medication can be titrated off quickly if surgery becomes necessary.

Endovascular techniques for mesenteric revascularization in acute embolic mesenteric ischemia have gained interest in recent years because of reports of relatively favorable outcomes.[23,24,25] Catheter-directed thrombolysis, aspiration embolectomy, and angioplasty have all been used with good technical success. Vasodilators may be of benefit for cases in which poor flow is compounded by arterial vasospasm (▶ Fig. 10.3d). However, the literature describing the endovascular treatment of acute occlusive mesenteric ischemia remains limited. Relatively few comparative studies have been performed, and none of these studies were randomized.[24,25,26,27] Nonrandomized comparisons between endovascular and open approaches have demonstrated lower rates of complications such as respiratory failure (27 vs. 64%) and renal failure (27 vs. 50%) with endovascular techniques.[27] In one study, mortality was significantly lower (36 vs. 50%) in the endovascular cohort if patients were able to avoid surgical revascularization compared to the group initially treated with open surgical revascularization. There is also some evidence that if bowel resection is required, endovascular treatment before resection may decrease the length of bowel resected.[27] However, these results must be interpreted with caution given the quality of the data.

10.4.2 AMI Caused by PMVT

PMVT accounts for 5 to 15% of all cases of AMI. The mortality rate of PMVT has reached 50% in the past but has decreased in recent years.[28] Unlike mesenteric arterial occlusion, which restricts splanchnic blood inflow, PMVT causes mesenteric ischemia by obstructing outflow. This obstruction causes an increase in vascular resistance and a decreased perfusion pressure within the gut. When there is extensive thrombosis, bowel infarction follows.

The venae rectae of the small bowel coalesce into arcades and then join the right, middle, and ileocolic veins to form the superior mesenteric vein. Thrombotic involvement of the superior mesenteric, portal, and splenic veins is frequently seen, whereas the inferior mesenteric vein, which drains the distal colon, is rarely involved with thrombosis.[29] In approximately 50% of patients, more than one major abdominal vein is involved.[30] Thrombosis of the venae rectae and venous arcades is more likely to result in bowel infarction, whereas large vessel thrombosis may initially have a subclinical course that manifests later as portal hypertension.[31]

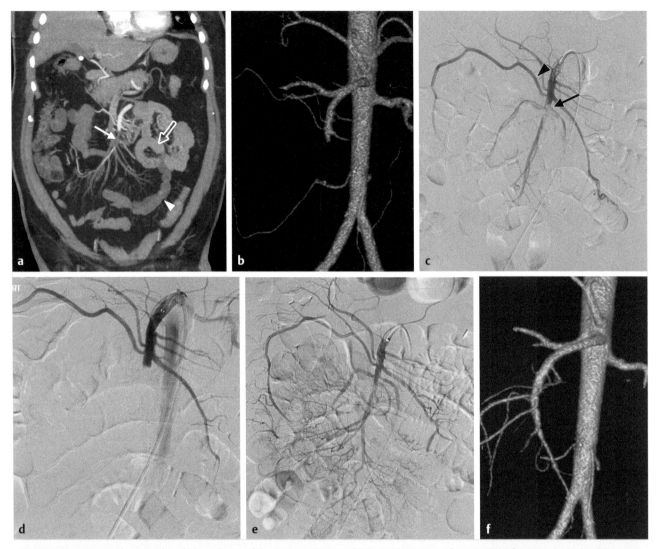

Fig. 10.3 Mesenteric ischemia with embolic occlusion of the SMA in a 68-year-old man with a history of myocardial infarction who had sudden onset of severe abdominal pain. **(a)** A coronal CT image and **(b)** volume-rendered image show embolic occlusion of the proximal SMA trunk (*solid arrow*) with decreased enhancement of the ileum in the right lower abdomen (*arrowhead*) compared to the unaffected jejunum in the left upper quadrant (*open arrow*). **(c)** Initial superior mesenteric arteriogram showing correlative finding to CT with embolus lodged within the trunk of the SMA (*black arrow*) distal to the takeoff of the middle colic artery (*black arrowhead*) and extending into the right colic and several ileal branches of the SMA. **(d)** Vasospasm evident after initial attempts at suction embolectomy, with worsening of perfusion to the affected territories. **(e)** After treatment with a vasodilator, suction embolectomy, and local tPA pulse spray, dramatic improvement can be seen. **(f)** A volume-rendered image from a CT scan obtained later for other reasons shows resolution of the thrombus.

Patient Presentation and Diagnosis

Clinical presentation is determined by the site and degree of venous occlusion and by the acuity of thrombosis. PMVT may be silent if it is nonocclusive or central. However, if the thrombosis is occlusive and acute, the patient presentation can be similar to that seen with other forms of AMI resulting in bowel infarction. As with other types of AMI, the most common symptom is abdominal pain. Although the onset can be sudden, the pain most often begins insidiously. Nausea or vomiting is frequent; melena is not unusual. Because the pain may be less bothersome than in other forms of AMI, patients may not seek medical attention immediately. Some patients with this condition report a personal or family history of venous thromboembolism.

A minority of patients have primary PMVT, in which no cause can be identified. However, most patients have secondary PMVT, in which a risk factor predisposes them to thrombosis. Risk factors include heritable (e.g., factor V Leiden, antithrombin-III deficiency, *JAK2* mutation) or acquired (e.g., malignancy, pregnancy) thrombophilia or an intra-abdominal process such as portal hypertension, pancreatitis, or recent splenectomy. PMVT related to a thrombophilia usually starts in the venae rectae or venous arcades and may progress centrally. In contrast, an intra-abdominal process usually affects the central veins first and may progress into the venae recta.

PMVT may appear on unenhanced CT as a tubular structure filling the vein, hyperdense relative to background blood.[32] Conversely, on contrast-enhanced CT, the thrombus within the

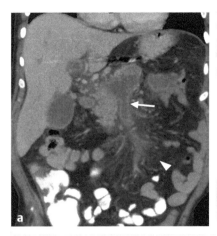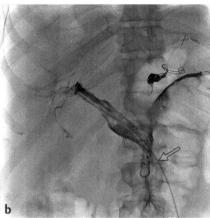

Fig. 10.4 A 60-year-old man with *JAK2* mutation and portomesenteric thrombosis involving the superior mesenteric, splenic, and portal veins. **(a)** Coronal contrast-enhanced CT showing a thrombosed superior mesenteric vein (*arrow*) at the confluence of the splenic vein. There is extensive edema (*arrowhead*) within the mesentery. **(b)** Portal venography was performed 24 hours after initiation of catheter-directed thrombolysis. The catheter (*open arrow*), superimposing the main portal vein, enters from a subxiphoid access point into the left portal vein. Thrombolysis was continued for 48 hours. Despite only partial success, the patient's portomesenteric system was restored to full patency with anticoagulation and time.

vein will appear as a low-density filling defect and may expand the vein (▶ Fig. 10.4). The mesenteric veins may become engorged in PMVT; this is most conspicuous in the small veins of the venae recta. Mesenteric fat edema (stranding) is more pronounced in PMVT than in arterial occlusion.

Treatment

As with other sites of venous thromboembolism in the body, the mainstay of therapy for symptomatic PMVT is anticoagulation. Generally, this begins with low-molecular-weight heparin or intravenous heparin as soon as the diagnosis is established. Anticoagulation stabilizes the thrombus, stops clot propagation, and favors endogenous fibrinolysis. This permits partial or complete recanalization in many patients and protects from progression or recurrence of thrombosis.[30,33] In a retrospective study of patients with PMVT, anticoagulation alone versus an immediate operative approach demonstrated similar morbidity and mortality rates; nonoperative patients avoided bowel resection and had a shorter hospital stay.[34] However, as with any type of mesenteric ischemia, evidence of peritonitis, bowel infarction, or hemodynamic instability warrants immediate surgical exploration. Although surgical and nonoperative management of PMVT have similar outcomes, mortality may still be high (25% or higher) in nonoperative management. Additionally, some patients initially treated nonoperatively may still require surgical resection, as some patients will progress to transmural bowel infarction with anticoagulation alone. Further, as the portal vein is frequently involved, portal hypertension and its sequela are potential long-term risks. Therefore, the goals of therapy in PMVT are not only to restore venous patency and bowel viability in the short term but also to decrease the risk of rethrombosis and portal hypertension.

The role of endovascular therapies in acute and subacute PMVT remains undefined. Some recommend endovascular intervention in patients without infarction but with severe symptoms or a deteriorating condition despite anticoagulation.[35] Some evidence suggests that in patients with PMVT, adding catheter-directed thrombolysis to anticoagulation may be beneficial. In one study, patients with PMVT received either anticoagulation alone or catheter-directed thrombolysis via a percutaneous transhepatic approach followed by anticoagulation. Although there was no difference in mortality, those who received catheter-directed thrombolysis plus anticoagulation required fewer surgeries and were less likely to develop portal hypertension over 3 years of follow-up.[36]

Mechanical or aspiration thrombectomy and catheter-directed pharmacological thrombolysis have been shown to be relatively safe and feasible. For mechanical thrombolysis or thrombectomy and catheter-directed thrombolysis, access into the portomesenteric system may be achieved via a direct transhepatic route (▶ Fig. 10.4b) or via a transjugular approach (▶ Fig. 10.5), similar to that used in a transjugular intrahepatic portosystemic shunt (TIPS) procedure. Although a transhepatic approach may be more facile and potentially provide favorable working angles for the advancement of devices, a transjugular approach ideally preserves the integrity of the liver capsule and may be more appealing in patients with coagulopathy or ascites, decreasing the risk of intra-abdominal bleeding. With a route across the liver capsule, bleeding risks for transhepatic access are theoretically higher, although there is evidence suggesting that this route is feasible with low rates of bleeding.[37] A transjugular approach provides the option of using the same access for placement of a TIPS (▶ Fig. 10.6) to improve outflow if incomplete thrombolysis is achieved.[38] Both approaches have been used with success. A transfemoral arterial approach may be used to position a catheter in the SMA for indirect pharmacological thrombolysis. This approach may have the theoretical benefit of exposing smaller mesenteric veins to a higher concentration of thrombolytic if the vein is too small or the targets too numerous to reach with direct infusion. The theoretical drawbacks to this method are that the thrombolytic infused into the SMA may be preferentially diverted around the thrombosed veins by better flow in the unaffected veins, and there may be a need for prolonged infusion (associated with a higher bleeding risk). Direct and indirect routes of thrombolytic administration have been used in combination.[39]

Technical success rates for the endovascular treatment of PMVT are generally very good, with restoration of at least partial venous patency and flow in 75 to 100% of patients; clinical success is also very good, with resolution of symptoms in 85 to 100% of patients in several series.[35,37,39,40] Complication rates are quite variable in the literature, ranging from very low to a rate of 60% (major complications, mostly hemorrhage) in a series using a variety of techniques. Nonoperative intervention frequently, but not always, obviates the need for surgical resection.

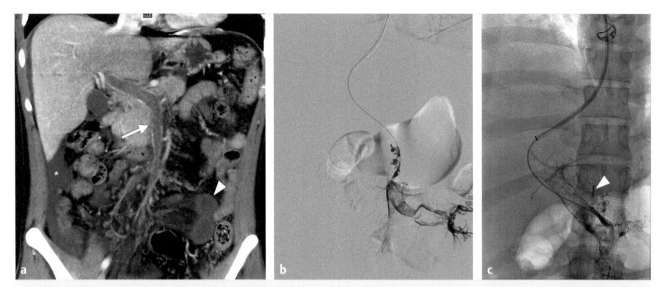

Fig. 10.5 PMVT in a 26-year-old man with inflammatory bowel disease and new abdominal pain and vomiting. **(a)** Coronal oblique CT image shows thrombosis of the mesenteric veins (*arrow*) and portal veins extending into the splenic vein. There is ascites (*asterisk*) with bowel wall thickening (*arrowhead*). Catheter-directed thrombolysis was attempted. **(b)** Initial unsubtracted portal and **(c)** subtracted mesenteric venograms taken after obtaining access into the portal vein via a TIPS approach under intravascular ultrasound (*arrowhead*) guidance show contrast outlining a cast of the portal and mesenteric veins created by thrombus.

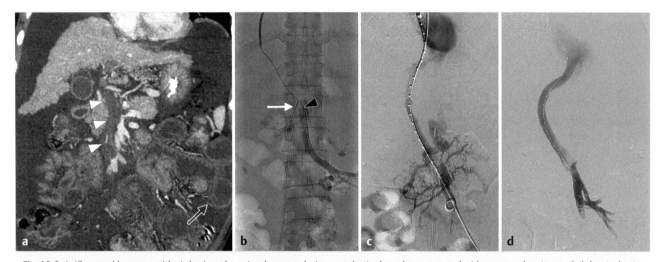

Fig. 10.6 A 45-year-old woman with cirrhosis and previously nonocclusive portal vein thrombus presented with worsened ascites and abdominal pain. **(a)** Coronal-oblique CT shows portomesenteric thrombus (*white arrowheads*) extending into the splenic vein. There is bowel wall edema (*open white arrow*) and large volume ascites. **(b)** A transjugular approach was used to access the portomesenteric vein, guided by intravascular ultrasound (*white arrow*). A venogram shows a "cutoff" (*black arrowhead*) in the mesenteric vein from obstructing clot. **(c)** Partial patency was restored after suction thrombectomy and balloon maceration. **(d)** Ultimately, a TIPS was placed to control portal hypertension and improve outflow of the portomesenteric system. Venogram shows brisk flow.

Although no firm conclusions can be drawn, these outcomes are likely dependent on careful technique and patient selection.

10.4.3 AMI Caused by NOMI

NOMI is distinguished from other causes of AMI by vasoconstriction, rather than embolic or thrombotic occlusion, restricting normal arterial blood flow to the gut. NOMI accounts for approximately 15% of AMI cases, although it is believed to be decreasing in incidence because of the increasing use of vasodilators in intensive care units.[14] In patients with this condition, ischemia is caused by severe, prolonged arterial vasoconstriction with failure of autoregulatory mechanisms. The pathophysiology of NOMI is incompletely understood; however, the macroscopic vessels remain patent and infarction ensues because of insufficient flow of blood. The consequence of the ischemia is the same as with other forms of AMI: if not reversed, the involved gut undergoes necrosis.

Patient Presentation and Diagnosis

Because it occurs in a state of hypoperfusion, NOMI is associated with many different pathological conditions. NOMI can

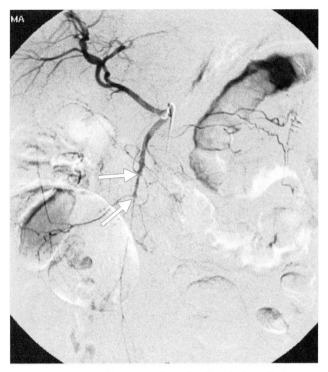

Fig. 10.7 A 70-year-old woman admitted with multiple medical problems and NOMI. Superior mesenteric arteriogram shows narrowing of the origins of the branches of the SMA (*arrows*), diffuse spasm, and no filling of intramural branches.

occur in the setting of shock or other critical illness such as heart or renal failure and is associated with the use of vasopressors or other vasoactive drugs such as digoxin or ergotamine. The prognosis in NOMI is dismal, not only because of the nonspecific presentation of the disease and delays in diagnosis but also because of the critically ill population in which it occurs. Mortality from this disease may be higher than 50%.[41]

As the disease occurs in medically complex situations, patient presentation can be clouded by other comorbid conditions and mental status changes seen in critically ill patients. The classic presentation of AMI may be absent. Instead, patients may complain of vague abdominal pain and bloating, and nausea and vomiting may be present. Because the presentation can be more cryptic, the diagnosis may not be established until the disease has progressed to bowel necrosis and peritonitis.[42]

Although there has been recent interest in the use of CT angiography[43] to diagnose NOMI, catheter angiography remains the modality of choice. Classic findings on angiography (▶ Fig. 10.7) include (1) narrowing of the origins of the branches of the SMA; (2) branch vessel irregularity, with alternating dilation and narrowing ("string of sausages" appearance); (3) spasm of the mesenteric arcades; and (4) impaired or absent filling of intramural branches.[44] Other findings include reflux of injected contrast material from the SMA into the aorta, splaying of the segmental arteries from distention of the subtending bowel, and delayed filling of the portal vein.[41,45] The severity of vasoconstrictive morphologic changes within the SMA and reflux of contrast material from the SMA into the aorta (indicating sluggish flow) have been shown to correlate with 30-day mortality in patients with NOMI.[45]

Treatment

Treatment of NOMI starts with identification and correction of the underlying condition that led to compromised splanchnic perfusion, if possible. Administration of intra-arterial vasodilators such as papaverine directly via a catheter positioned in the SMA may relieve vasospasm. This can be initiated at the time of angiographic diagnosis of NOMI. Alternatively, intravenous prostaglandin E1 may be used, although there is little evidence guiding these therapies.[46,47] There is no role for surgery unless the bowel is infarcted.

10.4.4 Chronic Mesenteric Ischemia

CMI is the result of slowly occlusive disease, most commonly atherosclerosis, affecting the mesenteric vasculature. Other diseases of the arteries such as fibromuscular dysplasia and vasculitis may also cause CMI. Extrinsic compression from the median arcuate ligament can also play a role. CMI is more common in women than in men, and because atherosclerosis is the most common etiology, CMI generally occurs in patients older than 60 years. Because of the collateral network formed by the celiac artery, SMA, and IMA, flow in more than one vessel is generally compromised before the disease manifests. In some cases, CMI may progress to AMI from thrombosis of a critical stenosis of a vessel origin.

Patient Presentation and Diagnosis

Patients with CMI may report a history of dull abdominal pain occurring after eating and lasting for 1 to 2 hours. Resting splanchnic blood flow in patients with underlying stenoses is similar to that in patients without any significant stenosis. However, blood flow in the SMA can double from functional hyperemia in the postprandial state.[48] Therefore, patients with a stenosis may not be able to support the increased flow associated with higher metabolic demand after a meal.[49] This phenomenon is classically described as "intestinal angina." Over time, patients unintentionally lose weight because of a consequent "food fear." Other nonspecific abdominal symptoms may occur, including nausea, vomiting, or diarrhea. Because of the insidious onset and relatively nonspecific presentation of CMI, there may be delays in diagnosis.[50] Patients with CMI may have other risk factors for, or conditions associated with, atherosclerosis such as a history of smoking, hypertension, coronary artery disease, peripheral vascular disease, renal insufficiency, or diabetes.[51] In half of patients, an abdominal bruit is found on physical examination.[52]

In contradistinction to acute embolic occlusion, acute thrombotic occlusion of the SMA often occurs at the origin of the vessel where it is most affected by ostial calcific atherosclerosis (▶ Fig. 10.8). As a result of chronic low-grade ischemia and slowly progressive narrowing, preexisting collateral vessels may be present. However, if this is not the case, or if collaterals are insufficient, the more proximal extent of the thrombosis may jeopardize the jejunum and colon in addition to the ileum.

Treatment

With the goal of reestablishing adequate perfusion to the bowel, surgical revascularization has been the historical treatment of

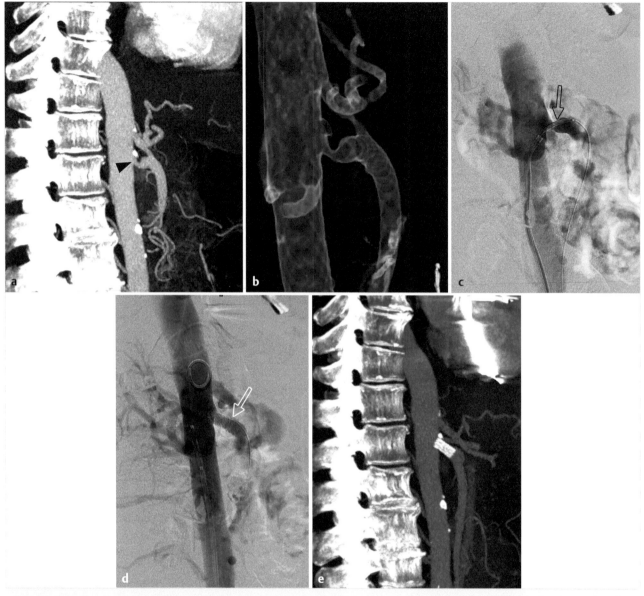

Fig. 10.8 A 64-year-old woman with intestinal angina and "food fear," consistent with CMI. **(a)** Sagittal oblique CT maximum intensity projection image shows a severe atherosclerotic stenosis (*arrowhead*) at the SMA origin. **(b)** Volume-rendered image obtained for planning during angiography shows the lesion to be stented. **(c)** Angiogram completed via the sheath with balloon-expandable stent (*open black arrow*) in position. The unexpanded stent is not yet deployed. **(d)** Aortogram shows precise placement of the stent (*open white arrow*) after deployment, extending to the desired 1 to 2 mm into the aorta. **(e)** Repeat CT performed for another reason confirms good placement of stent.

choice for patients with CMI. Open surgical options for mesenteric revascularization in CMI most commonly involve aortomesenteric bypass, transaortic endarterectomy, or reimplantation of the mesenteric arteries, which may include patch angioplasty.[53] Hybrid techniques, including retrograde stenting after open exposure of the SMA, have also been used.[54]

The use of endovascular techniques for CMI has increased dramatically in recent years. In CMI, the therapeutic target is often the SMA or celiac artery. Interventions involving the IMA are often avoided because of the added difficulty and risk of complications when working with a smaller, potentially more diseased vessel.[55] Because of the rarity of the disease and lack of comparative data to guide optimal technique, practices used for other conditions have been adopted, such as the techniques

used for renal artery stenosis. Generally, for atherosclerotic ostial lesions, primary stenting is favored over primary angioplasty. Balloon-expandable stents can be deployed very precisely, have improved radial force, and are generally favored over self-expanding stents for ostial lesions. There is promising evidence that the use of covered balloon-expandable stents may decrease the rate of intimal hyperplasia causing recurrent stenosis and symptoms as well as repeat interventions.[56]

Complications arising during endovascular therapy for CMI are generally uncommon; however, the consequences of some complications can be significant. Some of the most feared complications involve the SMA itself, including perforation, dissection, distal embolization, or problems with the stent such as migration or thrombosis. These types of complications are associated with the development of additional complications and with significantly higher mortality rates than those seen in patients without mesenteric arterial complications.[55]

Nevertheless, perioperative complications and mortality both occur at a higher rate with open surgery than with endovascular procedures. In a meta-analysis including 1,795 patients from 43 retrospective studies, perioperative morbidity rates for open and endovascular therapy were 33 and 13%, respectively, and perioperative mortality rates were 7.2 and 3.6%, respectively.[57] Additionally, intensive care unit and overall hospital stays may be longer in surgically treated patients. This is true despite the fact that several retrospective comparative studies have shown a bias toward higher rates of comorbid disease in patients treated with endovascular techniques.[53]

Notwithstanding the higher risk of complications and other short-term drawbacks with open revascularization, a long-term benefit may be realized over endovascular therapy. Open surgical revascularization is more durable and associated with less restenosis, a lower risk of recurrent symptoms, and less need for reintervention versus endovascular treatment of CMI.[58] For example, at 5 years, the primary patency rate for open surgery is 81% compared to 49% for endovascular therapy. Secondary patency rates are high for both therapies (98 and 88%, respectively).[57] Further, the benefit of less perioperative mortality with endovascular therapy is lost over time, with no difference at 1 to 5 years. Therefore, thoughtful patient selection is paramount. The choice of therapeutic approach should take into account factors such as lesion anatomy, patient comorbidities, life expectancy, nutritional status, and local experience with the various therapies.

No matter the cause, mesenteric ischemia is an important, albeit rare, disease because of its disastrous consequences. Whether acute or chronic, the nonspecific presentation may cause a diagnostic challenge. Recognition of the disease is important for early, appropriate treatment and improving patient outcomes.

References

[1] Sandstrom CK, Ingraham CR, Monroe EJ, Johnson GE. Beyond decreased bowel enhancement: acute abnormalities of the mesenteric and portal vasculature. Abdom Imaging. 2015; 40(8):2977–2992

[2] Khan A, Hsee L, Mathur S, Civil I. Damage-control laparotomy in nontrauma patients: review of indications and outcomes. J Trauma Acute Care Surg. 2013; 75(3):365–368

[3] Schoots IG, Koffeman GI, Legemate DA, Levi M, van Gulik TM. Systematic review of survival after acute mesenteric ischaemia according to disease aetiology. Br J Surg. 2004; 91(1):17–27

[4] Wadman M, Syk I, Elmståhl S. Survival after operations for ischaemic bowel disease. Eur J Surg. 2000; 166(11):872–877

[5] Oldenburg WA, Lau LL, Rodenberg TJ, Edmonds HJ, Burger CD. Acute mesenteric ischemia: a clinical review. Arch Intern Med. 2004; 164(10):1054–1062

[6] Reilly PM, Wilkins KB, Fuh KC, Haglund U, Bulkley GB. The mesenteric hemodynamic response to circulatory shock: an overview. Shock. 2001; 15(5):329–343

[7] Wiesner W, Khurana B, Ji H, Ros PR. CT of acute bowel ischemia. Radiology. 2003; 226(3):635–650

[8] Oliva IB, Davarpanah AH, Rybicki FJ, et al. ACR Appropriateness Criteria ® imaging of mesenteric ischemia. Abdom Imaging. 2013; 38(4):714–719

[9] Barmase M, Kang M, Wig J, Kochhar R, Gupta R, Khandelwal N. Role of multidetector CT angiography in the evaluation of suspected mesenteric ischemia. Eur J Radiol. 2011; 80(3):e582–e587

[10] Duran R, Denys AL, Letovanec I, Meuli RA, Schmidt S. Multidetector CT features of mesenteric vein thrombosis. Radiographics. 2012; 32(5):1503–1522

[11] Kirkpatrick ID, Kroeker MA, Greenberg HM. Biphasic CT with mesenteric CT angiography in the evaluation of acute mesenteric ischemia: initial experience. Radiology. 2003; 229(1):91–98

[12] Cudnik MT, Darbha S, Jones J, Macedo J, Stockton SW, Hiestand BC. The diagnosis of acute mesenteric ischemia: a systematic review and meta-analysis. Acad Emerg Med. 2013; 20(11):1087–1100

[13] Moneta GL, Lee RW, Yeager RA, Taylor LM, Jr, Porter JM. Mesenteric duplex scanning: a blinded prospective study. J Vasc Surg. 1993; 17(1):79–84, discussion 85–86

[14] Acosta S. Epidemiology of mesenteric vascular disease: clinical implications. Semin Vasc Surg. 2010; 23(1):4–8

[15] Leone M, Bechis C, Baumstarck K, et al. Outcome of acute mesenteric ischemia in the intensive care unit: a retrospective, multicenter study of 780 cases. Intensive Care Med. 2015; 41(4):667–676

[16] Björck M, Acosta S, Lindberg F, Troëng T, Bergqvist D. Revascularization of the superior mesenteric artery after acute thromboembolic occlusion. Br J Surg. 2002; 89(7):923–927

[17] Acosta S, Björck M. Acute thrombo-embolic occlusion of the superior mesenteric artery: a prospective study in a well defined population. Eur J Vasc Endovasc Surg. 2003; 26(2):179–183

[18] Park WM, Gloviczki P, Cherry KJ, Jr, et al. Contemporary management of acute mesenteric ischemia: Factors associated with survival. J Vasc Surg. 2002; 35(3):445–452

[19] Kurland B, Brandt LJ, Delany HM. Diagnostic tests for intestinal ischemia. Surg Clin North Am. 1992; 72(1):85–105

[20] Acosta S, Nilsson TK, Björck M. D-dimer testing in patients with suspected acute thromboembolic occlusion of the superior mesenteric artery. Br J Surg. 2004; 91(8):991–994

[21] Ballard JL, Stone WM, Hallett JW, Pairolero PC, Cherry KJ. A critical analysis of adjuvant techniques used to assess bowel viability in acute mesenteric ischemia. Am Surg. 1993; 59(5):309–311

[22] Herbert GS, Steele SR. Acute and chronic mesenteric ischemia. Surg Clin North Am. 2007; 87(5):1115–1134, ix

[23] Acosta S, Sonesson B, Resch T. Endovascular therapeutic approaches for acute superior mesenteric artery occlusion. Cardiovasc Intervent Radiol. 2009; 32(5):896–905

[24] Block TA, Acosta S, Björck M. Endovascular and open surgery for acute occlusion of the superior mesenteric artery. J Vasc Surg. 2010; 52(4):959–966

[25] Ryer EJ, Kalra M, Oderich GS, et al. Revascularization for acute mesenteric ischemia. J Vasc Surg. 2012; 55(6):1682–1689

[26] Beaulieu RJ, Arnaoutakis KD, Abularrage CJ, Efron DT, Schneider E, Black JH, III. Comparison of open and endovascular treatment of acute mesenteric ischemia. J Vasc Surg. 2014; 59(1):159–164

[27] Arthurs ZM, Titus J, Bannazadeh M, et al. A comparison of endovascular revascularization with traditional therapy for the treatment of acute mesenteric ischemia. J Vasc Surg. 2011; 53(3):698–704, discussion 704–705

[28] Rhee RY, Gloviczki P. Mesenteric venous thrombosis. Surg Clin North Am. 1997; 77(2):327–338

[29] Harnik IG, Brandt LJ. Mesenteric venous thrombosis. Vasc Med. 2010; 15(5):407–418

[30] Amitrano L, Guardascione MA, Scaglione M, et al. Prognostic factors in noncirrhotic patients with splanchnic vein thromboses. Am J Gastroenterol. 2007; 102(11):2464–2470

[31] Kumar S, Kamath PS. Acute superior mesenteric venous thrombosis: one disease or two? Am J Gastroenterol. 2003; 98(6):1299–1304

[32] Goldstein M, Quen L, Jacks L, Jhaveri K. Acute abdominal venous thromboses-the hyperdense CT sign. J Comput Assist Tomogr. 2012; 36(1):8–13

[33] Condat B, Pessione F, Helene Denninger M, Hillaire S, Valla D. Recent portal or mesenteric venous thrombosis: increased recognition and frequent recanalization on anticoagulant therapy. Hepatology. 2000; 32(3):466–470

[34] Brunaud L, Antunes L, Collinet-Adler S, et al. Acute mesenteric venous thrombosis: case for nonoperative management. J Vasc Surg. 2001; 34(4):673–679

[35] Hollingshead M, Burke CT, Mauro MA, Weeks SM, Dixon RG, Jaques PF. Transcatheter thrombolytic therapy for acute mesenteric and portal vein thrombosis. J Vasc Interv Radiol. 2005; 16(5):651–661

[36] Di Minno MN, Milone F, Milone M, et al. Endovascular thrombolysis in acute mesenteric vein thrombosis: a 3-year follow-up with the rate of short and long-term sequaelae in 32 patients. Thromb Res. 2010; 126(4):295–298

[37] Kim HS, Patra A, Khan J, Arepally A, Streiff MB. Transhepatic catheter-directed thrombectomy and thrombolysis of acute superior mesenteric venous thrombosis. J Vasc Interv Radiol. 2005; 16(12):1685–1691

[38] Uflacker R. Applications of percutaneous mechanical thrombectomy in transjugular intrahepatic portosystemic shunt and portal vein thrombosis. Tech Vasc Interv Radiol. 2003; 6(1):59–69

[39] Yang S, Liu B, Ding W, He C, Wu X, Li J. Acute superior mesenteric venous thrombosis: transcatheter thrombolysis and aspiration thrombectomy therapy by combined route of superior mesenteric vein and artery in eight patients. Cardiovasc Intervent Radiol. 2015; 38(1):88–99

[40] Wang MQ, Lin HY, Guo LP, Liu FY, Duan F, Wang ZJ. Acute extensive portal and mesenteric venous thrombosis after splenectomy: treated by interventional thrombolysis with transjugular approach. World J Gastroenterol. 2009; 15(24):3038–3045

[41] Trompeter M, Brazda T, Remy CT, Vestring T, Reimer P. Non-occlusive mesenteric ischemia: etiology, diagnosis, and interventional therapy. Eur Radiol. 2002; 12(5):1179–1187

[42] Howard TJ, Plaskon LA, Wiebke EA, Wilcox MG, Madura JA. Nonocclusive mesenteric ischemia remains a diagnostic dilemma. Am J Surg. 1996; 171(4):405–408

[43] Woodhams R, Nishimaki H, Fujii K, Kakita S, Hayakawa K. Usefulness of multidetector-row CT (MDCT) for the diagnosis of non-occlusive mesenteric ischemia (NOMI): assessment of morphology and diameter of the superior mesenteric artery (SMA) on multi-planar reconstructed (MPR) images. Eur J Radiol. 2010; 76(1):96–102

[44] Siegelman SS, Sprayregen S, Boley SJ. Angiographic diagnosis of mesenteric arterial vasoconstriction. Radiology. 1974; 112(3):533–542

[45] Minko P, Stroeder J, Groesdonk HV, et al. A scoring-system for angiographic findings in nonocclusive mesenteric ischemia (NOMI): correlation with clinical risk factors and its predictive value. Cardiovasc Intervent Radiol. 2014; 37(3):657–663

[46] Wilcox MG, Howard TJ, Plaskon LA, Unthank JL, Madura JA. Current theories of pathogenesis and treatment of nonocclusive mesenteric ischemia. Dig Dis Sci. 1995; 40(4):709–716

[47] Mitsuyoshi A, Obama K, Shinkura N, Ito T, Zaima M. Survival in nonocclusive mesenteric ischemia: early diagnosis by multidetector row computed tomography and early treatment with continuous intravenous high-dose prostaglandin E(1). Ann Surg. 2007; 246(2):229–235

[48] Qamar MI, Read AE. Intestinal blood flow. Q J Med. 1985; 56(220):417–419

[49] Hansen HJ, Engell HC, Ring-Larsen H, Ranek L. Splanchnic blood flow in patients with abdominal angina before and after arterial reconstruction. A proposal for a diagnostic test. Ann Surg. 1977; 186(2):216–220

[50] Björnsson S, Resch T, Acosta S. Symptomatic mesenteric atherosclerotic disease-lessons learned from the diagnostic workup. J Gastrointest Surg. 2013; 17(5):973–980

[51] Moawad J, Gewertz BL. Chronic mesenteric ischemia. Clinical presentation and diagnosis. Surg Clin North Am. 1997; 77(2):357–369

[52] Mateo RB, O'Hara PJ, Hertzer NR, Mascha EJ, Beven EG, Krajewski LP. Elective surgical treatment of symptomatic chronic mesenteric occlusive disease: early results and late outcomes. J Vasc Surg. 1999; 29(5):821–831, discussion 832

[53] Assar AN, Abilez OJ, Zarins CK. Outcome of open versus endovascular revascularization for chronic mesenteric ischemia: review of comparative studies. J Cardiovasc Surg (Torino). 2009; 50(4):509–514

[54] Blauw JT, Meerwaldt R, Brusse-Keizer M, Kolkman JJ, Gerrits D, Geelkerken RH, Multidisciplinary Study Group of Mesenteric Ischemia. Retrograde open mesenteric stenting for acute mesenteric ischemia. J Vasc Surg. 2014; 60(3):726–734

[55] Oderich GS, Tallarita T, Gloviczki P, et al. Mesenteric artery complications during angioplasty and stent placement for atherosclerotic chronic mesenteric ischemia. J Vasc Surg. 2012; 55(4):1063–1071

[56] Oderich GS, Erdoes LS, Lesar C, et al. Comparison of covered stents versus bare metal stents for treatment of chronic atherosclerotic mesenteric arterial disease. J Vasc Surg. 2013; 58(5):1316–1323

[57] Pecoraro F, Rancic Z, Lachat M, et al. Chronic mesenteric ischemia: critical review and guidelines for management. Ann Vasc Surg. 2013; 27(1):113–122

[58] Oderich GS, Bower TC, Sullivan TM, Bjarnason H, Cha S, Gloviczki P. Open versus endovascular revascularization for chronic mesenteric ischemia: risk-stratified outcomes. J Vasc Surg. 2009; 49(6):1472–9.e3

11 Benign Biliary Strictures

Baljendra S. Kapoor and Eunice Moon

11.1 Introduction

Benign biliary strictures can be caused by multiple conditions. Most commonly, benign biliary strictures are associated with surgery, resulting from biliary injury during cholecystectomy, from fibrosis after biliary–enteric anastomosis, or from complications after liver transplant. Benign strictures can also result from chronic pancreatitis, Mirizzi's syndrome, primary and secondary sclerosing cholangitis, autoimmune immunoglobulin G4 (IgG4) cholangitis, and chemotherapy-induced sclerosing cholangitis. Infectious causes of biliary strictures include acquired immunodeficiency syndrome (AIDS)-related cholangiopathy and oriental cholangiohepatitis (pyogenic cholangitis).[1]

11.2 Clinical Presentation

Clinically, benign biliary strictures can be completely asymptomatic. Symptomatic biliary strictures present with clinical and biochemical evidence of biliary obstruction. Typically, the symptoms are related to obstructive jaundice and can include icterus, clay-colored stools, itching, and bradycardia. Biochemical changes include elevation of liver enzyme levels, including total and direct bilirubin and alkaline phosphatase levels. Chronic low-grade biliary obstruction can lead to recurrent cholangitis, stone formation, and even cirrhosis and end-stage liver disease.

11.3 Imaging

The role of imaging in the patient presenting with symptoms of biliary obstruction is to characterize and detect the level of obstruction and to determine the nature of the obstruction. On imaging, benign strictures appear to be smoother, with more symmetric borders and tapered margins, and tend to be shorter than malignant strictures.[2] Malignant strictures of the common bile duct (CBD), on the other hand, demonstrate asymmetry and irregularity with shouldered margins.[2,3]

Ultrasound (US) is usually the first imaging modality used to screen patients presenting with obstructive jaundice. Dilation of the biliary system proximal to the stricture can be identified on US, as well as other pathologies such as biliary stones, intrahepatic abscesses, intra- and extrahepatic masses such as pancreatic pseudocyst, pancreatic mass, and lymph node mass. In patients who have undergone liver transplant, routine duplex US of the hepatic artery may reveal hepatic artery thrombosis or stenosis. US is limited in its ability to identify the underlying cause of the obstructive jaundice and is highly operator dependent.

Contrast-enhanced computed tomography (CT), on the other hand, is not operator dependent and can identify biliary dilation, the level of obstruction, and often the underlying etiology of the obstructive jaundice such as CBD stone, acute pancreatitis, chronic pancreatitis, and pancreatic pseudocyst. Contrast-enhanced CT can also identify malignant changes associated with the obstruction, including wall enhancement, greater degree of proximal dilatation, wall thickness of greater than 1.5 mm, total length of stricture,[2] hilar lymphadenopathy, ascites, and distant metastatic lesions. In addition, CT angiogram can evaluate the patency of the hepatic artery and portal vein in post–liver transplant patients, and aid in diagnosis of post-transplant biliary stricture.

Magnetic resonance imaging (MRI) and magnetic resonance cholangiopancreatography (MRCP) have the distinct advantage of being able to evaluate the biliary system and the biliary enteric anastomosis in the immediate postoperative period. MRCP is highly sensitive for the diagnosis of biliary obstruction and is the imaging modality of choice for identifying the level of obstruction; this modality can also delineate recurrence of the primary pathology (e.g., primary sclerosing cholangitis). However, MRCP has a large range of sensitivity for differentiating between benign and malignant strictures (30–98%).[4,5,6] Furthermore, contrast-enhanced MR angiography (MRA) may be useful in detecting hepatic artery thrombosis or stenosis in patients who have undergone liver transplant. Similar to CT, MRI can detect fluid collections, ascites, and portal vein thrombosis.

Although less commonly used for the diagnosis of malignant biliary strictures, positron emission tomography (PET) with ^{18}F-FDG (fludeoxyglucose) has been shown to be highly sensitive and specific for differentiating between benign and malignant strictures.[7]

Endoscopic retrograde cholangiopancreatography (ERCP) has 90 to 95% sensitivity in detecting biliary complications after liver transplant.[8] These sensitivities are similar to those seen with MRCP, but ERCP is more invasive. ERCP has limited use in patients who have undergone biliary enteric anastomosis, and offers limited visualization of the duct distal to the level of pathology. On the other hand, ERCP is potentially therapeutic as well as diagnostic, allowing decompression of the obstruction with possible balloon dilation and placement of endoscopic stent.[9]

With highly improved cross-sectional imaging techniques, percutaneous transhepatic cholangiography (PTHC) is rarely used only for diagnostic purpose. PTHC is typically performed in combination with percutaneous transhepatic biliary drainage (PTBD) based on the clinical and cross-sectional imaging findings. PTHC/PTBD is usually performed in cases that are unsuitable for endoscopic approach or in which the endoscopic approach has failed. Most interventional radiologists require a platelet count of greater than 50 and an INR (international normalized ratio) of less than 1.4 to 1.5 before performing PTHC. A right mid-axillary approach is the most commonly used approach[10] (▶ Fig. 11.1a). In the right mid-axillary approach, a 20- to 22-gauge needle is advanced in the liver, usually through the right 11th or 10th intercostal space, and directed medially and superiorly. After the stylet is removed, diluted contrast is injected, while the needle is slowly retracted to opacify a bile duct. This step is repeated in different planes, if needed. Entry into the peripheral duct is important to decrease the risk of major vascular complications. However, if the point of duct entry is not satisfactory, initial access may be utilized to opacify the biliary system and a more peripheral access may be

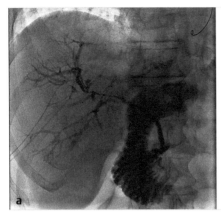 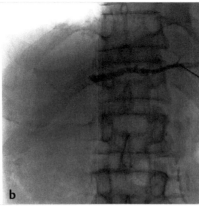

Fig. 11.1 (a) Cholangiogram image of the right-side approach showing opacification of the right-side ducts. **(b)** Cholangiogram image of the left-side approach showing opacification of the left-side duct.

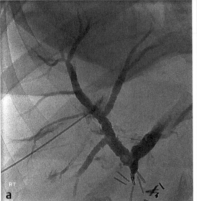 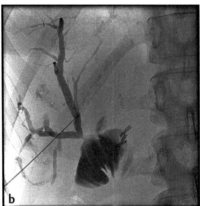 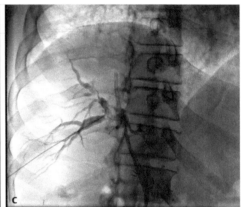

Fig. 11.2 (a) Single fluoroscopic image of percutaneous transhepatic cholangiogram in a 40-year-old woman showing complete occlusion at the level of the common hepatic duct following recent laparoscopic cholecystectomy injury to the common hepatic duct (*arrow*). **(b)** A 57-year-old woman with past medical history of a complex injury to her biliary tree during laparoscopic cholecystectomy that was treated by separate right and left hepaticojejunostomies. Six months later, right upper quadrant ultrasound (not shown) revealed moderately dilated right-sided ducts. A cholangiogram image showing a severe short-segment stenosis involving right hepaticojejunostomy. There is moderate dilatation of the right-sided ducts.
(c) A 63-year-old man who had undergone a liver transplant 1 year previously presented with increasing liver enzyme and bilirubin levels. Gray scale and Doppler ultrasound of the liver demonstrated transplant hepatic artery thrombosis and mild intrahepatic biliary ductal dilatation (not shown). Cholangiogram image showing short-segment central strictures with proximal dilatation involving multiple ducts. Also noted are two endoscopically placed biliary drainage catheters.

obtained by targeting one of the peripheral ducts under fluoroscopic guidance. Imaging is performed in multiple projections to more clearly delineate the biliary stricture and biliary anatomy.

In the event of difficult right mid-axillary approach, a left-sided subxiphoid approach may be used (▶ Fig. 11.1b). Some interventional radiologists prefer the left-sided approach as their initial choice in the appropriate clinical setting. In the left-sided approach, most interventional radiologists prefer to gain initial access under US guidance. PTHC is an invasive procedure and complications include acute hemorrhage, pneumothorax, hemothorax, and/or injury to the hepatic flexure of the colon. Careful review of prior imaging studies and, if available, additional intraprocedural imaging tools can be very useful, particularly in patients with complex biliary anatomy. In addition, three-dimensional (3D) intraprocedural imaging tools such as CBCT (cone-beam computed tomography) may be used to further assess the needle path in difficult or complex cases before placing a large bore sheath or catheter.

PTHC is particularly useful in patients with leak associated with stricture where ductal decompression limits the diagnostic effectiveness of cross-sectional imaging. PTHC, although invasive, can be diagnostic and potentially therapeutic, especially in patients with noninvasive imaging with equivocal results and patients who have undergone biliary enteric anastomoses.

11.4 Causes of Benign Strictures

11.4.1 Iatrogenic

Iatrogenic injuries are by far the most common cause of benign biliary strictures. Up to 70 to 80% of all benign strictures result from iatrogenic injuries. Cholecystectomy and orthotopic liver transplant (OLT) are the most common causes of iatrogenic biliary strictures. Currently, the risk of biliary stricture after open cholecystectomy ranges from 0.1 to 0.2%; the risk after laparoscopic cholecystectomy ranges from 0.4 to 0.6%.[11] Strictures occurring after cholecystectomy usually result from accidental ligation of the common hepatic duct or CBD or from ligation of the cystic duct in close proximity to the common hepatic duct/CBD[12] (▶ Fig. 11.2a).

Strictures that occur after OLT can be anastomotic or nonanastomotic. Anastomotic strictures tend to be more focal and usually due to postoperative fibrosis or secondary to a leak (▸ Fig. 11.2b). Nonanastomotic strictures tend to be multifocal and diffuse in appearance (▸ Fig. 11.2c) and commonly caused by hepatic artery thrombosis but may also be caused by recurrence of the primary disease (e.g., primary sclerosing cholangitis, preservation injury, or infection). Ischemic strictures can involve intra- as well as extrahepatic bile ducts.[13] OLT donors can also develop biliary strictures, most commonly at the junction of the common hepatic duct and intrahepatic ducts.[14]

Treatment of benign biliary strictures is determined primarily by the location of the stricture. The resectability of a benign stricture reflects the anatomic location of the stricture, and is categorized by the Bismuth classification system.[15] In general, biliary surgery can be performed easily in patients with Bismuth type I and II lesions, whereas surgical repair may be considerably more difficult in patients with Bismuth type III, IV, and V lesions.

11.4.2 Chronic Pancreatitis

Approximately 10% of benign biliary strictures are caused by chronic pancreatitis.[16] Long strictures in the distal CBD develop from recurrent pancreaticobiliary inflammation in the head of the pancreas. Furthermore, pseudocyst at the head of the pancreas can cause extrinsic biliary compression.

The clinical presentation of biliary stricture secondary to chronic pancreatitis is variable. Most strictures are asymptomatic. Symptomatic strictures present with abdominal pain, jaundice, abnormal liver enzymes, and fever with or without chills. Biliary obstruction can later progress to secondary biliary cirrhosis and choledocholithiasis.

On imaging, there is smooth tapering of the distal CBD with various degrees of intra- and extrahepatic biliary dilatation (▸ Fig. 11.3). The length of the CBD stricture is reported to range from 1.6 to 5.7 cm, possibly reflecting the variable length of the intrapancreatic portion of the CBD.[17,18] Clinical and radiologic evidence of chronic pancreatitis (i.e., atrophy of the pancreas, calcification, a dilated main pancreatic duct, or pseudocysts) supports the diagnosis of benign strictures related to chronic pancreatitis.

Endoscopic or balloon dilatation with or without stenting is reserved for symptomatic patients with jaundice, cholangitis, or persistently abnormal liver function test results.[19] These strictures may not respond to balloon dilation. Patients with persistent or recurrent jaundice, persistent elevation of alkaline phosphatase, recurrent cholangitis, and liver abscesses may be candidates for biliary–enteric bypass surgery such as choledochoduodenostomy and Roux-en-Y choledochojejunostomy.

11.4.3 Primary Sclerosis Cholangitis

Primary sclerosing cholangitis (PSC) is a rare and chronic inflammatory disorder of unknown etiology. It is characterized by an alternating pattern of biliary stricture and mild dilatation, often described as "beaded" in appearance (▸ Fig. 11.4). PSC is most commonly seen in men in the third and fourth decades of life, often associated with inflammatory bowel disease, most commonly ulcerative colitis. Patients with PSC may remain

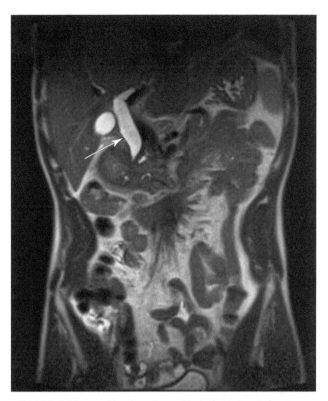

Fig. 11.3 A 30-year-old male patient with alcohol-induced chronic pancreatitis presented with acute abdominal pain and increasing total bilirubin, alkaline phosphatase, and transaminases. A coronal MR (magnetic resonance) HASTE (Half-Fourier-Acquired Single-shot Turbo spin Echo) image showing severely dilated proximal and mid common bile duct (CBD). There is a severe short-segment smooth stricture involving distal CBD (*arrow*) due to chronic pancreatitis.

asymptomatic; alternatively, they can present with nonspecific symptoms such as fever, loss of appetite, fatigue, and weight loss. As the disease progresses, patients present with symptoms related to cholangitis and obstructive jaundice such as itching, icterus, fever with chills, and clay-colored stool. In most patients, PSC results in end-stage liver disease and cirrhosis, necessitating liver transplant.

The MRI findings of PSC correlate with the pathologic appearance of the disease. Findings include periportal edema (high T2 signal around the portal tracts), patchy areas of peripheral arterial hyperenhancement in the early stage of the disease, and changes associated with cirrhosis in the later stage of the disease. On MRCP, PSC is characterized by multifocal intra- and extrahepatic biliary strictures with alternating areas of normal segments or minimally dilated segments. Isolated involvement of the intrahepatic biliary system is seen in approximately one-third of patients, whereas isolated extrahepatic duct involvement is rare. Prominent periportal lymph nodes may also be seen. According to Fulcher et al,[20] the sensitivity of MRCP for the detection of PSC ranges from 80 to 88% and the specificity ranges from 87 to 99%. Imaging also plays a vital role in the detection of complications such as choledocholithiasis and cholangiocarcinoma, which occurs in 3.3 to 36.4% of patients with PSC.

Medical management of PSC involves treatment with ursodeoxycholic acid and immunosuppressants, including steroids. Dominant strictures are treated with balloon dilatation. Eventually, most patients will require a liver transplant, which is

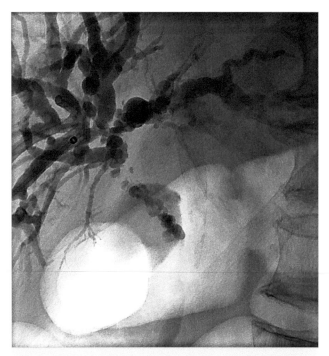

Fig. 11.4 A 32-year-old female patient with known primary sclerosing cholangitis presenting with increasing bilirubin. Ultrasound of the right upper quadrant revealed areas of bilateral ductal dilatation. PTHC and biliary drainage were requested by the hepatology service. Fluoroscopic image of sheath cholangiogram demonstrating beaded appearance of predominantly central biliary tree due to multifocal strictures predominantly involving common hepatic ducts and common bile duct (CBD). Also note intrahepatic ductal dilatation. On previous occasion, due to inability to cross the central strictures, an external biliary drainage catheter was left in place.

associated with excellent 1- and 5-year survival rates of 90 and 85%, respectively.[21]

11.4.4 Chemotherapy-Induced Sclerosing Cholangitis

Chemotherapy-induced sclerosing cholangitis is a form of ischemic cholangitis resulting from hepatic arterial inflammation associated with hepatic arterial infusion therapy of various chemotherapeutic agents including floxuridine, 5-fluorouracil, intrahepatic mitomycin C, formaldehyde, and bevacizumab. Imaging studies will show diffuse or multifocal narrowing of intrahepatic ducts with predominant involvement of the common hepatic duct and sparing of the CBD, due to a separate blood supply from the gastroduodenal arcade.[22] Chemotherapy-induced sclerosing cholangitis may also affect the cystic duct and can result in fistula formation.[22] These ischemic strictures are resistant to endoscopic dilatation alone and often require repeated sessions of balloon dilatation and stenting.[22]

11.4.5 Autoimmune Cholangitis with IgG4-Related Sclerosing Disease

Immune-mediated fibroinflammatory changes can result in sclerosis and narrowing of the bile ducts. In the spectrum of IgG4-related sclerosing diseases, involvement of the biliary system is the second most common manifestation of sclerosing disease after autoimmune pancreatitis.[23] The clinical presentation of IgG4-related sclerosing cholangitis tends to be relatively acute.

Radiologically, IgG4-related sclerosing cholangitis presents as long and continuous strictures of the intrapancreatic segment of the CBD, often with proximal dilatation; multifocal intrahepatic biliary strictures are less common.[24] Cross-sectional imaging that demonstrates a symmetrical, circumferential thick rind of tissue encasing the affected duct is indicative of IgG4-related sclerosing cholangitis.[23] On CT, biliary disease appears as focal or diffuse thickening of the bile duct walls with wall enhancement.[25,26] When the disease affects the hepatic hilar biliary stricture, especially in the presence of an associated soft-tissue mass, its appearance can mimic cholangiocarcinoma.[27]

IgG4-related sclerosing cholangitis responds dramatically to steroid therapy. Stabilization of the patient and decompression along with steroid therapy are strategies for managing this disorder. Stent and drainage can be removed when there is evidence of radiographic and clinical response to the steroid therapy. The patient may require maintenance steroid therapy to prevent future episodes.[28]

11.4.6 Portal Biliopathy

Portal biliopathy refers to pathologic changes in the biliary ducts and gallbladder among patients with portal hypertension.[29,30] These changes most commonly occur secondary to extrahepatic portal vein obstruction. Portal biliopathy is often asymptomatic but sometimes manifests clinically as obstructive jaundice and may lead to the development of choledocholithiasis.

Patients with portal biliopathy often demonstrate enlarged blood vessels surrounding the stenotic bile segments. One proposed mechanism for biliary abnormalities in these patients is peribiliary fibrosis resulting from ischemic or inflammatory changes due to underlying portal thrombosis. However, for patients demonstrating enlarged blood vessels at the level of the biliary stenosis, extrinsic compression is the more likely mechanism.

High-resolution CT and MRI are comparable for providing anatomical detail about the presence and severity of bile duct dilatation, portal vein obstruction, portal cavernoma, and portosystemic collaterals in patients with portal biliopathy.[31] The imaging features of portal biliopathy on MRCP include biliary stenosis, wavy appearance of the bile ducts, angulation of the CBD, and upstream dilatation of the bile ducts.[32]

Portal biliopathy may resolve following decompression of the portal system. In a study by Agarwal et al, decompression of portal hypertension relieved biliary obstruction in 24 of 37 patients (64.9%) and facilitated a second-stage biliary surgery in the remaining 13 patients (35.1%).[33]

11.4.7 Mirizzi Syndrome

Jaundice is a rare clinical presentation in patients with cholelithiasis. Impaction of gallstones in the cystic duct and associated periductal inflammation can cause extrinsic compression of the common hepatic duct, resulting in obstructive jaundice. This finding was first reported by Kehr in 1905[34] and Ruge in 1908[35] and was later highlighted by Mirizzi in 1948.[36]

Mirizzi syndrome occurs in patients with intact gallbladder as well as in those with large cystic duct remnants after a cholecystectomy. Mirizzi syndrome may be associated with low insertion of the cystic duct. This syndrome is classified into two types. Type I lesions typically involve mechanical obstruction without formation of a fistula, whereas type II lesions involve formation of a fistula between the common hepatic duct and the gallbladder due to inflammation and erosion of the impacted stone.

Clinically, patients present with a history of intermittent right upper quadrant pain, chills, fever, and jaundice. The differential diagnosis for this syndrome includes pancreatic cancer and cholangiocarcinoma in the gallbladder neck or proximal common hepatic duct.

US in patients with Mirizzi syndrome may show intra- and extrahepatic biliary ductal dilatation with cholelithiasis. CT, although infrequently used for the diagnosis of cholelithiasis, may demonstrate intra- and extrahepatic biliary ductal dilatation, gallstones, and dilated gallbladder with thickening of the wall. The CBD remains normal in caliber below the obstruction. Percutaneous transhepatic cholangiogram (PTC) may show moderate dilatation of the intrahepatic and common hepatic ducts and a narrowing or curvilinear compression defect along the right lateral aspect of the common hepatic duct, causing complete obstruction of the common hepatic and cystic ducts. The cystic duct and gallbladder are not usually opacified unless they are directly injected during PTC.

The surgical treatment of Mirizzi syndrome depends on the type of lesion and the degree of periductal inflammation. In type I lesions, the major technical challenge is separating the impacted stone from the common hepatic duct and identifying the cystic duct distally for ligation. In type II lesions, the major surgical challenge is the closure of the fistula. A recent study suggested that laparoscopic cholecystectomy may be feasible in patients with type I lesions if the critical view can be demonstrated.[37] However, open cholecystectomy is still recommended in all patients with type II lesions.

11.4.8 Acquired Immunodeficiency Syndrome–Related Cholangitis

AIDS-related cholangitis involves an acalculous inflammation of the biliary tract. Common clinical presentations include right upper quadrant pain, jaundice, and abnormal liver function tests, including a disproportionate elevation of alkaline phosphatase compared to serum transaminases. Biliary abnormalities in patients with AIDS are categorized into two groups: (1) gradual and regular strictures of the terminal portion of the CBD associated with dilatation but without irregularity of the intrahepatic biliary ducts (27%) and (2) distal strictures of the extrahepatic biliary ducts combined with diffuse irregularity of the intrahepatic bile ducts (73%).[20] In the appropriate clinical setting, thickening of the CBD is the finding that most strongly suggests the presence of AIDS-related cholangiopathy.

CT findings for this condition include intrahepatic ductal dilatation and enhancing thickened gallbladder wall. Cholangiographic abnormalities include "brush border" appearance of the bile ducts, pruning of the intrahepatic ducts, focal strictures, and isolated papillary stenosis with CBD dilatation. AIDS cholangiopathy can mimic the appearance of sclerosing cholangitis or periampullary stenosis.

Cytomegalovirus (CMV) or *Cryptosporidium* species was documented in almost all patients presenting with AIDS-related cholangiographic abnormality of the intrahepatic bile ducts. However, anti-CMV therapy has little effect on the course of biliary disease in these patients.[38]

Chronic biliary inflammatory changes may also occur in other locations among patients with AIDS. The most common finding is a nonspecific 4- to 15-mm thickening of the gallbladder wall, thought to be secondary to edema.[39,40]

11.4.9 Oriental Cholangiohepatitis

Also known as recurrent pyogenic cholangitis, oriental cholangiohepatitis is very common in Southeast Asia but is uncommon in the Western hemisphere. However, in recent years, more cases have been reported in the United States, perhaps due to increased immigration from Asia. The pathogenesis of oriental cholangiohepatitis is not clear. Two theories have been postulated: (1) chronic infection with *Clonorchis sinensis* or *Ascaris lumbricoides* causing ductal injury, chronic inflammation, and stricture formation leading to stasis and stone formation and (2) a low-protein diet. Oriental cholangiohepatitis does not have a sex predilection and occurs most frequently in patients aged 20 to 40 years. Symptoms of this condition include recurrent attacks of abdominal pain, along with fevers, chills, nausea, and vomiting.

Patients with recurrent pyogenic cholangitis present with diffuse dilation of the intra- and extrahepatic bile ducts with focal strictures. Marked dilation of the large central ducts is disproportionate to the rapidly tapered peripheral ducts. Ducts are typically filled with soft pigmented stones. Extrahepatic ductal dilation may not correlate with the location of the stone, and strictures are uncommon in this location. However, localized stricture and dilation of the intrahepatic ducts are closely associated with the location of the stones. In the early phase of the disease, the liver may enlarge, but the liver may later atrophy, particularly the lateral segment of the left lobe.

Oriental cholangitis is often difficult to treat. Patients presenting acutely may respond to antibiotics to treat associated cholangitis. If the disease is isolated to a single hepatic lobe, curative hepatic resection can be performed. More commonly, however, definitive treatment is not possible because of diffuse lobar involvement. In such cases, palliative therapy consists of biliary drainage followed by stone removal and stricture dilation, performed percutaneously or endoscopically. Cholangioscopic-assisted stone removal, percutaneous basket retrieval, and ultrasonic lithotripsy may be used to extract and manage the stone burden.[41]

11.5 Management of the Benign Biliary Strictures

Management of benign biliary strictures depends on the underlying etiology and feasibility of the various treatment options including surgery, endoscopy, and percutaneous approaches. Benign biliary strictures, particularly diffuse biliary strictures associated with ischemia or recurrence of underlying disease such as PSC, may require retransplantation of the liver. In patients with underlying focal postsurgical strictures at the biliary enteric anastomosis, surgical revision of the biliary enteric anastomosis is an option but may not be technically feasible or may result in higher morbidity.[42] For patients who are poor surgical candidates, endoscopic or percutaneous dilatation of the stricture and drainage are common alternatives. The percutaneous approach allows placement of large bore catheters or dual catheters to allow drainage of both lobes, resulting in higher success rates.[43,44]

11.5.1 Interventional Radiologic Management of Benign Biliary Strictures

Percutaneous Transhepatic Biliary Drainage

Percutaneous biliary drainage is a well-established clinical indication in the setting of focal and well-defined biliary obstruction (▶ Fig. 11.5). On the other hand, any attempt at biliary drainage in the setting of diffuse multiple biliary strictures without any well-defined segments of obstruction may not provide any benefit to the patient and may unnecessarily predispose the patient to the risk of associated complications.[45] In the presence of acute cholangitis, minimal manipulation of the

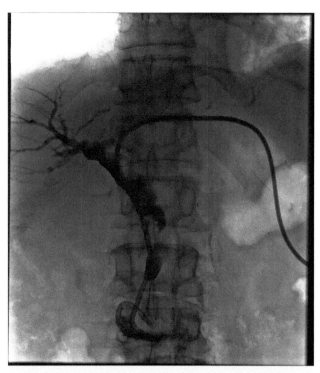

Fig. 11.5 A 61-year-old male patient with severe acute pancreatitis complicated by pseudocyst formation presented with increasing total bilirubin (8.8 mg/dL) and alkaline phosphatase (551 units/L) due to acute cholangitis and was referred from an outside facility for PTHC and biliary drainage. Based on the operator's preference, the left-sided approach was selected. Under ultrasound guidance, the segment 3 duct was accessed. Cholangiogram image showing placement of a 10-Fr internal/external biliary drainage catheter (Boston Scientific Inc.). Note a severe smooth stricture involving distal common bile duct (CBD) due to external compression from pseudocyst and acute pancreatitis.

biliary system is warranted in order to avoid gram-negative septicemia. Therefore, patients presenting with cholangitis may benefit from initial placement of a simple external biliary drainage catheter. Once the acute episode has subsided, the biliary catheter is left in place for a minimum of 4 to 6 weeks for the tract to mature before removal is contemplated. The majority of patients, however, require a longer duration of catheter access for treatment of the stricture. In good surgical candidates, the percutaneous biliary drainage catheter can be used intraoperatively to assist in resection and re-anastomosis. Postoperative cholangiography through the percutaneously placed biliary catheter can also be used to ensure good tube position and patent anastomosis.

Balloon Dilation

Balloon dilation or cholangioplasty of the focal benign biliary strictures is a well-accepted treatment option for focal benign biliary strictures, except in patients with recently created hepaticojejunostomy (< 4 weeks) where narrowing could be the result of postoperative edema (▶ Fig. 11.6). After detailed cholangiographic evaluation of the stricture and biliary system under fluoroscopy, balloon dilation of the stricture using an appropriately sized balloon (5–8 mm for the hepatic ducts and 8–12 mm for the CBD) is attempted. The diameter of the balloon can be oversized by approximately 20%. For the strictures not responding to conventional balloon dilation, a cutting balloon (Boston Scientific Inc., Natick, MA) can be used to dilate the strictures. Oversizing of the diameter is not recommended while using the cutting balloons. Following successful balloon dilation, an external biliary drainage catheter is capped and left in place for a short duration of 1 to 2 weeks. If the patients remain asymptomatic, liver function tests return to normal values, and follow-up cholangiographic evaluation reveals widely patent stricture without any significant proximal ductal dilatation, the external biliary drainage catheter can be removed. Short-term patency of the dilated strictures ranges from 50 to 90%,[46,47,48,49] and long-term patency ranges from 56 to 74%.[47,50,51]

In addition to balloon dilation, gradual dilation of the focal benign biliary strictures by increasing the size of the biliary drainage catheter to 18 to 20 Fr over a prolonged period of time ranging from 6 to 12 months or more has been shown to be an effective treatment.[52] A recently published study using a structured protocol to gradually increase the size of the biliary catheters to 16 to 18 Fr revealed patency rates of 84% at 1 year after treatment, 78% at 2 years, 74% at 5 years, and 67% at 10 years.[53] Another technique described in the literature is the dual-catheter technique, in which a small bore 8 Fr catheter is percutaneously placed via a large bore 14 Fr catheter. The small bore catheter exits from one of the side holes of the larger drain proximal to the site of the stricture and traverses across the stricture parallel to the larger diameter catheter, resulting in larger size dilation without increasing the size of the percutaneous tract.[43]

Stents

In recent years, there has been a significant interest in percutaneous placement of retrievable covered self-expanding metallic stents to improve the patency of biliary strictures. These stents have been shown to provide superior results as compared to

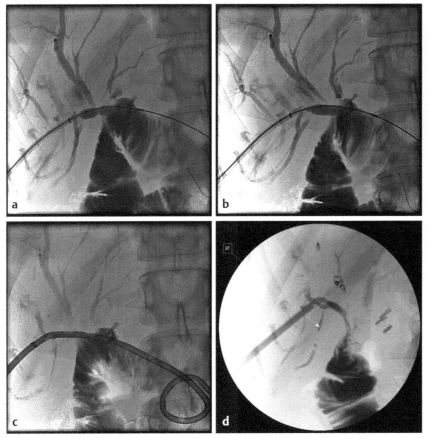

Fig. 11.6 A 57-year-old female patient with past medical history of a complex injury to her biliary tree during laparoscopic cholecystectomy that was treated by separate right and left hepaticojejunostomies. Six months later, right upper quadrant ultrasound (not shown) revealed moderately dilated right-sided ducts. ▶ Fig. 11.2a is a cholangiogram image showing a severe short-segment stenosis involving right hepaticojejunostomy. There is moderate dilatation of the right-sided ducts. **(a,b)** Fluoroscopic images showing balloon dilatation of the right hepaticojejunostomy stricture using a 7 mm × 40 mm balloon (Bard Inc., Tempe, AZ). **(c)** Fluoroscopic image showing placement of a 12-Fr biliary drainage catheter (Boston Scientific Inc.). **(d)** Sheath cholangiogram 6 weeks after balloon dilatation of hepaticojejunostomy stricture showing a widely patent hepaticojejunostomy (*arrow*). The biliary catheter was removed.

balloon dilation for the treatment of benign biliary strictures.[54] The study by Kim et al[54] also demonstrated that the indwelling period of PTBD catheters was significantly reduced when using a temporary stent as compared to balloon dilation. A recently published multicenter study demonstrated the success of biodegradable polydioxanone biliary stents in the management of benign biliary stricture. In this study of 107 patients, estimated stricture recurrence rates at 1, 2, and 3 years were, respectively, 7.2, 26.4, and 29.4%.[55]

11.6 Intraprocedural Imaging and Navigation Tools

11.6.1 Recanalization of the Occluded Segment

Intraprocedural imaging and navigation tools such as CBCT and Syngo (Siemens Healthcare, Forchheim, Germany) can be used in combination with fluoroscopy to delineate the biliary and enteric anatomy prior to image-guided percutaneous reconstruction of severely stenosed or occluded biliary–enteric anastomoses. These newer intraprocedural tools may improve the success rate and operator confidence in these relatively complex procedures[56] (▶ Fig. 11.7).

11.7 Conclusion

Benign biliary strictures are frequently encountered. Correct diagnosis is critical to quickly moving toward an effective treatment. US is an important screening tool, but more definitive diagnosis may not be possible without CT or MRI. However common, benign biliary stricture often requires multidisciplinary management. Depending on the diagnosis, treatment may be minimally invasive or surgical, lengthy, and palliative or definitive with excellent result.

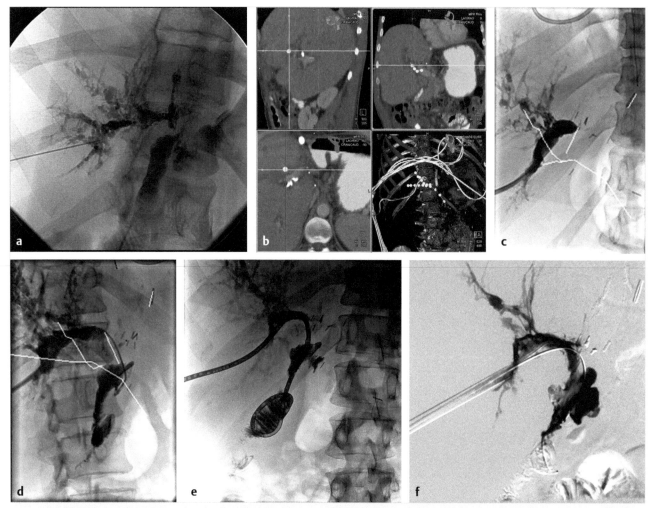

Fig. 11.7 A 34-year-old male patient with known clinical diagnosis of congenital biliary atresia who had undergone left hepatic lobectomy and Kasai procedure presented with repeated episodes of acute cholangitis. Ultrasound revealed intrahepatic biliary ductal dilatation. PTHC and biliary drainage procedure were requested. **(a)** Percutaneous cholangiogram showing markedly irregular intrahepatic biliary ducts compatible with changes consistent with chronic cholangitis. Hepaticojejunostomy demonstrates a near-occlusive stricture at the site of anastomosis. Contrast is seen in the Roux loop of hepaticojejunostomy. **(b)** Multiplanar images of the intraprocedural CBCT fused with prior CT images showing reconstruction path created by Syngo iGuide software (Siemens healthcare; *yellow dots*). **(c)** Fluoroscopic images showing outline of the path (*white lines*) superimposed over fluoroscopy and **(d)** sharp recanalization of the hepaticojejunostomy stricture using pediatric TIPS set (CCOK Inc., Bloomington, IN). **(e)** Cholangiographic image showing placement of a 12-Fr internal–external biliary drainage catheter (Boston Scientific Inc.). **(f)** Sheath cholangiogram after 13 months showing widely patent hepaticojejunostomy. (These images are provided courtesy of Mark Sands, MD, FACR.)

References

[1] Kaffes AJ. Management of benign biliary strictures: current status and perspective. J Hepatobiliary Pancreat Sci. 2015; 22(9):657–663

[2] Choi SH, Han JK, Lee JM, et al. Differentiating malignant from benign common bile duct stricture with multiphasic helical CT. Radiology. 2005; 236(1):178–183

[3] Soto JA, Alvarez O, Lopera JE, Múnera F, Restrepo JC, Correa G. Biliary obstruction: findings at MR cholangiography and cross-sectional MR imaging. Radiographics. 2000; 20(2):353–366

[4] Fulcher AS, Turner MA, Capps GW, Zfass AM, Baker KM. Half-Fourier RARE MR cholangiopancreatography: experience in 300 subjects. Radiology. 1998; 207(1):21–32

[5] Lee MG, Lee HJ, Kim MH, et al. Extrahepatic biliary diseases: 3D MR cholangiopancreatography compared with endoscopic retrograde cholangiopancreatography. Radiology. 1997; 202(3):663–669

[6] Kim MJ, Mitchell DG, Ito K, Outwater EK. Biliary dilatation: differentiation of benign from malignant causes–value of adding conventional MR imaging to MR cholangiopancreatography. Radiology. 2000; 214(1):173–181

[7] Kluge R, Schmidt F, Caca K, et al. Positron emission tomography with [(18)F] fluoro-2-deoxy-D-glucose for diagnosis and staging of bile duct cancer. Hepatology. 2001; 33(5):1029–1035

[8] Seehofer D, Eurich D, Veltzke-Schlieker W, Neuhaus P. Biliary complications after liver transplantation: old problems and new challenges. Am J Transplant. 2013; 13(2):253–265

[9] Thompson CM, Saad NE, Quazi RR, Darcy MD, Picus DD, Menias CO. Management of iatrogenic bile duct injuries: role of the interventional radiologist. Radiographics. 2013; 33(1):117–134

[10] Venbrux AC, Osterman FA, Jr. Percutaneous management of benign biliary strictures. Tech Vasc Interv Radiol. 2001; 4(3):141–146

[11] Vachhani PG, Copelan A, Remer EM, Kapoor B. Iatrogenic hepatopancreaticobiliary injuries: a review. Semin Intervent Radiol. 2015; 32 (2):182–194

[12] Shanbhogue AK, Tirumani SH, Prasad SR, Fasih N, McInnes M. Benign biliary strictures: a current comprehensive clinical and imaging review. AJR Am J Roentgenol. 2011; 197(2):W295–W306

[13] Lorenz JM. The role of interventional radiology in the multidisciplinary management of biliary complications after liver transplantation. Tech Vasc Interv Radiol. 2015; 18(4):266–275

[14] Lee SY, Ko GY, Gwon DI, et al. Living donor liver transplantation: complications in donors and interventional management. Radiology. 2004; 230(2):443–449

[15] Bismuth H, Majno PE. Biliary strictures: classification based on the principles of surgical treatment. World J Surg. 2001; 25(10):1241–1244

[16] Abdallah AA, Krige JE, Bornman PC. Biliary tract obstruction in chronic pancreatitis. HPB (Oxford). 2007; 9(6):421–428

[17] Eckhauser FE, Knol JA, Strodel WE, Achem S, Nostrant T. Common bile duct strictures associated with chronic pancreatitis. Am Surg. 1983; 49(7):350–358

[18] Petrozza JA, Dutta SK. The variable appearance of distal common bile duct stenosis in chronic pancreatitis. J Clin Gastroenterol. 1985; 7(5):447–450

[19] Vitale GC, Reed DN, Jr, Nguyen CT, Lawhon JC, Larson GM. Endoscopic treatment of distal bile duct stricture from chronic pancreatitis. Surg Endosc. 2000; 14(3):227–231

[20] Fulcher AS, Turner MA, Franklin KJ, et al. Primary sclerosing cholangitis: evaluation with MR cholangiography-a case-control study. Radiology. 2000; 215(1):71–80

[21] Karlsen TH, Schrumpf E, Boberg KM. Update on primary sclerosing cholangitis. Dig Liver Dis. 2010; 42(6):390–400

[22] Sandrasegaran K, Alazmi WM, Tann M, Fogel EL, McHenry L, Lehman GA. Chemotherapy-induced sclerosing cholangitis. Clin Radiol. 2006; 61(8):670–678

[23] Vlachou PA, Khalili K, Jang HJ, Fischer S, Hirschfield GM, Kim TK. IgG4-related sclerosing disease: autoimmune pancreatitis and extrapancreatic manifestations. Radiographics. 2011; 31(5):1379–1402

[24] Klöppel G, Lüttges J, Sipos B, Capelli P, Zamboni G. Autoimmune pancreatitis: pathological findings. JOP. 2005; 6(1) Suppl:97–101

[25] Kawamoto S, Siegelman SS, Hruban RH, Fishman EK. Lymphoplasmacytic sclerosing pancreatitis (autoimmune pancreatitis): evaluation with multidetector CT. Radiographics. 2008; 28(1):157–170

[26] Takahashi N, Fletcher JG, Fidler JL, Hough DM, Kawashima A, Chari ST. Dual-phase CT of autoimmune pancreatitis: a multireader study. AJR Am J Roentgenol. 2008; 190(2):280–286

[27] Arikawa S, Uchida M, Kunou Y, et al. Comparison of sclerosing cholangitis with autoimmune pancreatitis and infiltrative extrahepatic cholangiocarcinoma: multidetector-row computed tomography findings. Jpn J Radiol. 2010; 28(3):205–213

[28] Kamisawa T, Okamoto A. IgG4-related sclerosing disease. World J Gastroenterol. 2008; 14(25):3948–3955

[29] Sarin SK, Bhatia V, Makwane U. Portal biliopathy in extra hepatic portal vein obstruction. Indian J Gastroenterol. 1992; 2:A82

[30] Khuroo MS, Yattoo GN, Zargar SA, et al. Biliary abnormalities associated with extrahepatic portal venous obstruction. Hepatology. 1993; 17(5):807–813

[31] Aguirre DA, Farhadi FA, Rattansingh A, Jhaveri KS. Portal biliopathy: imaging manifestations on multidetector computed tomography and magnetic resonance imaging. Clin Imaging. 2012; 36(2):126–134

[32] Colle I, Van Vlierberghe H, Pattyn P, et al. Cholestasis as presenting symptom of portal cavernoma. Hepatol Res. 2003; 25(1):32–37

[33] Agarwal AK, Sharma D, Singh S, Agarwal S, Girish SP. Portal biliopathy: a study of 39 surgically treated patients. HPB (Oxford). 2011; 13(1):33–39

[34] Kehr H. Die in meiner Klinik geübte Technik der Gallensteinoperationen mit einem Hinweis auf die Indikationen und die Dauererfolge. Auf Grund eigener, bei 1000 Laparotomien gesammelter Erfahrungen. München, Germany: J.F. Lehmann's Verlag; 1905

[35] Ruge E. Beitraege zur chirurgischen anatomie der grossen gallenwege (ductus hepaticus, cysticus, choledochus und pancreaticus. Arch Klin Chir. 1908; 87:47–78

[36] Mirizzi P. Syndrome del conducto hepatico. J Int Chir. 1948; 8:731–777

[37] Erben Y, Benavente-Chenhalls LA, Donohue JM, et al. Diagnosis and treatment of Mirizzi syndrome: 23-year Mayo Clinic experience. J Am Coll Surg. 2011; 213(1):114–119, discussion 120–121

[38] Benhamou Y, Caumes E, Gerosa Y, et al. AIDS-related cholangiopathy. Critical analysis of a prospective series of 26 patients. Dig Dis Sci. 1993; 38(6):1113–1118

[39] Dolmatch BL, Laing FC, Federle MP, Jeffrey RB, Cello J. AIDS-related cholangitis: radiographic findings in nine patients. Radiology. 1987; 163(2):313–316

[40] Romano AJ, vanSonnenberg E, Casola G, et al. Gallbladder and bile duct abnormalities in AIDS: sonographic findings in eight patients. AJR Am J Roentgenol. 1988; 150(1):123–127

[41] Lim JH. Oriental cholangiohepatitis: pathologic, clinical, and radiologic features. AJR Am J Roentgenol. 1991; 157(1):1–8

[42] Reichman TW, Sandroussi C, Grant DR, et al. Surgical revision of biliary strictures following adult live donor liver transplantation: patient selection, morbidity, and outcomes. Transpl Int. 2012; 25(1):69–77

[43] Gwon DI, Sung KB, Ko GY, Yoon HK, Lee SG. Dual catheter placement technique for treatment of biliary anastomotic strictures after liver transplantation. Liver Transpl. 2011; 17(2):159–166

[44] Kim J, Ko GY, Sung KB, et al. Percutaneously placed covered retrievable stents for the treatment of biliary anastomotic strictures following living donor liver transplantation. Liver Transpl. 2010; 16(12):1410–1420

[45] Fidelman N. Benign biliary strictures: diagnostic evaluation and approaches to percutaneous treatment. Tech Vasc Interv Radiol. 2015; 18(4):210–217

[46] Köcher M, Cerná M, Havlík R, Král V, Gryga A, Duda M. Percutaneous treatment of benign bile duct strictures. Eur J Radiol. 2007; 62(2):170–174

[47] Cantwell CP, Pena CS, Gervais DA, Hahn PF, Dawson SL, Mueller PR. Thirty years' experience with balloon dilation of benign postoperative biliary strictures: long-term outcomes. Radiology. 2008; 249(3):1050–1057

[48] Janssen JJ, van Delden OM, van Lienden KP, et al. Percutaneous balloon dilatation and long-term drainage as treatment of anastomotic and nonanastomotic benign biliary strictures. Cardiovasc Intervent Radiol. 2014; 37(6):1559–1567

[49] Zajko AB, Sheng R, Zetti GM, Madariaga JR, Bron KM. Transhepatic balloon dilation of biliary strictures in liver transplant patients: a 10-year experience. J Vasc Interv Radiol. 1995; 6(1):79–83

[50] Weber A, Rosca B, Neu B, et al. Long-term follow-up of percutaneous transhepatic biliary drainage (PTBD) in patients with benign bilioenterostomy stricture. Endoscopy. 2009; 41(4):323–328

[51] Ramos-De la Medina A, Misra S, Leroy AJ, Sarr MG. Management of benign biliary strictures by percutaneous interventional radiologic techniques (PIRT). HPB (Oxford). 2008; 10(6):428–432

[52] Ludwig JM, Webber GR, Knechtle SJ, Spivey JR, Xing M, Kim HS. Percutaneous management of benign biliary strictures with large-bore catheters: comparison between patients with and without orthotopic liver transplantation. J Vasc Interv Radiol. 2016; 27(2):219–225.e1

[53] DePietro DM, Shlansky-Goldberg RD, Soulen MC, et al. Long-term outcomes of a benign biliary stricture protocol. J Vasc Interv Radiol. 2015; 26(7):1032–1039

[54] Kim JH, Gwon DI, Ko GY, et al. Temporary placement of retrievable fully covered metallic stents versus percutaneous balloon dilation in the treatment of benign biliary strictures. J Vasc Interv Radiol. 2011; 22(6):893–899

[55] Mauri G, Michelozzi C, Melchiorre F, et al. Benign biliary strictures refractory to standard bilioplasty treated using polydoxanone biodegradable biliary stents: retrospective multicentric data analysis on 107 patients. Eur Radiol. 2016; 26(11):4057–4063

[56] Kapoor BS, Esparaz A, Levitin A, McLennan G, Moon E, Sands M. Nonvascular and portal vein applications of cone-beam computed tomography: current status. Tech Vasc Interv Radiol. 2013; 16(3):150–160

12 Malignant Obstructive Jaundice

Christopher R. Bailey and Kelvin Hong

12.1 Introduction

Malignant tumors cause approximately 70 to 90% of all biliary obstructions. Several types of malignancies can lead to bile outflow obstruction from the liver to the intestinal tract, including pancreatic adenocarcinoma, cholangiocarcinoma, and metastatic disease.[1,2] Although biliary obstruction primarily occurs in advanced disease, it is often the initial presenting sign of malignancy. As such, many of these cancers remain undiagnosed until the later stages of the disease.

Malignant biliary obstruction typically presents as painless jaundice (yellowing of the skin, sclera, and mucous membranes) and dark urine secondary to hyperbilirubinemia.[2,3] Patients with obstructive jaundice also complain of pruritus and are at risk of developing life-threatening biliary infections, including cholangitis, because of persistent biliary stasis. Interventions that restore biliary flow through stenting or external drainage can decrease serum bilirubin levels and improve quality of life through symptomatic relief[2] (▶ Fig. 12.1). In addition, these interventions may allow for further medical and surgical therapies to treat the patient's underlying malignancy.[3]

The management of these complex and debilitating conditions requires a multidisciplinary medical, surgical, and interventional approach. Interventional radiologists and gastroenterologists use diagnostic imaging and image-guided percutaneous and endoscopic methods for both treatment and symptomatic palliation.[4] In the discussion that follows, we review preprocedural imaging and evaluation, indications for percutaneous intervention, specific interventional and endoscopic techniques, and treatments for malignant obstructive jaundice.

12.2 Patient Evaluation and Preprocedural Imaging

It is important to take into account the patient's baseline liver function and overall functional status before any procedure is performed.[2] Although percutaneous and endoscopic interventions are minimally invasive, patients with significant hepatic dysfunction may not have the functional reserve to overcome even minimal complications.[5] Baseline renal function must also

be taken into account as iodinated contrast is often needed to opacify the biliary system and surrounding vascular structures. In addition, patients with gastrointestinal and neuroendocrine cancers affecting biliary drainage often have significant coagulopathies that may also alter the risk/benefit ratio for a particular intervention. Finally, the clinician must also obtain baseline imaging of the biliary system and surrounding extrahepatic structures.

Cross-sectional imaging with multidetector computed tomography (MDCT) and magnetic resonance imaging (MRI) is useful when evaluating a patient with malignant obstructive jaundice before interventions are performed. CT allows for reformatting of images in multiple planes with 3D (three-dimensional) reconstruction to better define metastatic spread, including lymph node and vascular involvement and the type/degree of biliary obstruction.[2,4,6] MRI, specifically MR cholangiopancreatography (MRCP), also allows for multiplanar evaluation of the biliary system and surrounding organs (▶ Fig. 12.2). MRCP has a high sensitivity for the detection and localization of biliary obstruction (96–99%) but lower specificity with respect to differentiating between benign and malignant causes (85%).[7,8] The major disadvantage of MRCP is the length of time required for image acquisition, but this is accompanied by the benefit of greater image resolution and freedom from ionizing radiation. Finally, evaluation with ultrasound (US) allows for point-of-care evaluation of biliary ductal dilation and stone disease and identification of vascular structures. However, patient positioning, body habitus, and the presence of surrounding extrahepatic structures can limit US evaluation; additionally, US imaging is an operator-dependent modality.[6]

12.3 Diagnostic Endoscopic Evaluation

12.3.1 Endoscopic Retrograde Cholangiopancreatography

Patients with biliary obstruction usually undergo initial evaluation with endoscopic retrograde cholangiopancreatography (ERCP). ERCP is an outpatient procedure that combines gastrointestinal

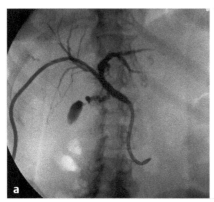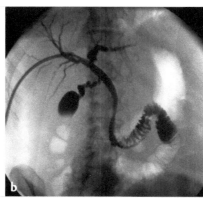

Fig. 12.1 (a) Percutaneous biliary drainage (PBD) in a patient with adenocarcinoma of the pancreas after percutaneous transhepatic cholangiography (PTC). **(b)** PBD with covered self-expanding stent (Viabil, WL Gore Inc., Flagstaff, AZ) in the common bile duct in a patient with adenocarcinoma of the pancreas.

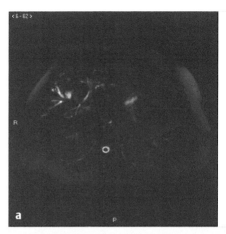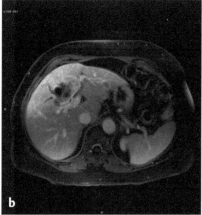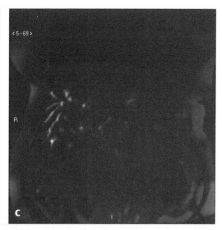

Fig. 12.2 **(a)** Axial magnetic resonance cholangiopancreatography (MRCP) image demonstrating central cholangiocarcinoma (Klatskin tumor). **(b)** Axial MRCP T1 postcontrast image of central cholangiocarcinoma. **(c)** Coronal MRCP image of central cholangiocarcinoma.

endoscopy with fluoroscopy to evaluate the pancreatic and bile ducts. With the patient under procedural sedation or general anesthesia, an endoscope is inserted into the oral pharynx and is advanced into the second part of the duodenum to the level of the ampulla of Vater, an anatomic landmark where the common bile duct (CBD) and pancreatic duct join and enter the duodenum. The ampulla is cannulated and contrast is injected into the confluence to opacify the CBD, pancreatic duct, and proximal bile ducts.[9] After identification of a biliary stricture, ERCP is used to obtain brush cytology or biliary biopsy, if the obstruction is more distal (closer to the ampulla of Vater). The sensitivity of brush cytology is poor for diagnosing a malignant cause of stricture (23–56%); however, the specificity is quite high (95%).[7,9] The sensitivity is improved to 70% when brush cytology is combined with endobiliary biopsy with high specificity (100%).[7] Because ERCP allows for access to the intrahepatic and extrahepatic bile ducts through natural orifices, patients with contraindications to percutaneous methods such as significant coagulopathies, ascites, and polycystic liver disease can be safely evaluated with this technique.[6]

The most common complication is post-ERCP pancreatitis, which can occur in up to 5 to 7% of all procedures and is usually mild and self-limited.[10] Other risks include intestinal perforation from endoscopic insertion and bleeding from the sphincterotomy. The decision to pursue ERCP should be made carefully. If therapeutic interventions are unlikely to be performed, most academic centers opt for noninvasive imaging methods such as MRCP to investigate biliary obstruction and determine whether it is secondary to a benign or malignant process.[8,11] Although cannulation of the ampulla of Vater is successful in approximately 85 to 98% of procedures, this technique is operator dependent and can be quite difficult to perform in patients with surgically altered anatomy.[12]

12.3.2 Endoscopic Ultrasound

Endoscopic US (EUS) employs a technique similar to that of ERCP to evaluate causes of biliary obstruction. First, an endoscope with a US probe and biopsy needle is inserted through the mouth. The scope is advanced through the gastrointestinal tract to the level of the culprit lesion. The needle is deployed from the endoscope into the mass/stricture under US guidance and a fine needle aspirate (FNA) is obtained. For diagnosing

malignancy, EUS has an overall sensitivity of 43 to 86%, with better sensitivity for more distal lesions.[7,13] The complications associated with EUS-FNA are similar to those seen with ERCP. The rates of pancreatitis associated with EUS-FNA through pancreatic tissue have been reported to be approximately 2%.[14] As with any endoscopic procedure, there is a risk of intestinal perforation.[7] Infection and hemorrhage have also been reported after EUS, but the incidence of these complications is low. Finally, there is a theoretical risk of malignant seeding with EUS given that the needle is advanced into malignant tissues and retracted back into the gastrointestinal tract.[7,15]

12.3.3 Intraductal Ultrasound

Intraductal US (IDUS) is a relatively new technology that is used in combination with ERCP. IDUS allows for US evaluation directly within a bile duct. The sensitivity of IDUS for identifying malignant lesions ranges from 80 to 90% with a specificity of 83%.[7] IDUS does not itself provide tissue diagnosis but does allow for limited staging using a set of established imaging criteria for determining whether a lesion is benign or malignant.[16,17] The potential complications of IDUS are similar to those of ERCP and EUS, given the endoscopic approach and required cannulation of the CBD or pancreatic duct.

12.3.4 Peroral Cholangioscopy

Peroral cholangioscopy (POC) allows for direct visualization of the bile ducts and evaluation of stone disease with the use of an optical probe. Cholangioscopy is usually performed after noninvasive imaging and ERCP with diagnostic brushing have failed to provide a diagnosis.[18] A series of diagnostic criteria has been established to determine whether a biliary stricture is malignant or benign. The most sensitive and specific sign for malignancy is the visualization of dilated and tortuous blood vessels.[7] With regard to tissue diagnosis, POC with forceps biopsy has demonstrated a diagnostic accuracy ranging from 49 to 82% when used to evaluate indeterminate biliary lesions.[7,19,20] Cholangitis is the most common complication reported with POC, occurring in up to 14% of procedures.[7] Other complications associated with cannulation of the bile ducts and endoscopy may include pancreatitis and bowel perforation.[18]

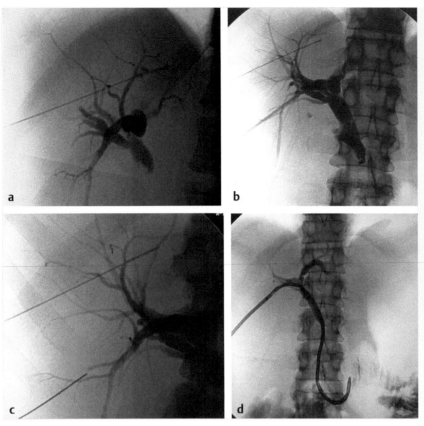

Fig. 12.3 Percutaneous transhepatic cholangiography (PTC)/percutaneous biliary drainage (PBD) procedure. **(a)** Insertion of a Chiba needle into peripheral bile duct under ultrasound guidance. **(b)** Opacification of the biliary system. **(c)** The right posterior biliary duct is accessed and opacified. **(d)** After a wire is advanced into the small bowel, a biliary catheter is advanced over the wire into position. A cholangiogram is performed to confirm positioning.

12.4 Diagnostic Percutaneous Evaluation

12.4.1 Percutaneous Transhepatic Cholangiography

Percutaneous transhepatic cholangiography (PTC) is reserved for situations in which less invasive methods such as MRCP and ERCP are unable to fully opacify the biliary system and identify the area of obstruction. PTC is also helpful in patients with surgically altered anatomy, when cannulation of the bile ducts with ERCP is difficult.[6] PTC allows for delineation of the intrahepatic and extrahepatic biliary tree, characterization of lesions, and identification of any bile leaks. As mentioned earlier, PTC is contraindicated in patients with significant ascites, severe coagulopathies, or polycystic liver disease. In addition to being used to evaluate the biliary system, PTC is performed as the first step before percutaneous biliary drainage (PBD) and percutaneous transhepatic biliary stenting are attempted.

After an appropriate preprocedural evaluation has been carried out (as described earlier), the patient is placed in a supine position and is administered procedural sedation or general anesthesia. After sterile preparation and draping are performed, the skin is anesthetized inferior to the costophrenic angle but superior to the hepatic flexure of the colon.[6,21] Under US guidance, a 22-guage Chiba needle (Cook Inc., Bloomington, IN) is inserted at approximately the mid-axillary line into one of the peripheral ducts. Once the interventional radiologist is satisfied with positioning of the needle, the inner stylet is removed to check for

bile reflux and/or to inject a mixture of 1:1 water-soluble contrast to confirm positioning within a peripheral duct. Once contrast is seen flowing away from the entry point opacifying the biliary system, a cholangiogram can be performed to thoroughly examine the biliary tree and identify obstructions.[6,22] If an obstruction is identified, PBD can be performed for palliation, preoperative staging and decompression, or diversion of bile away from an identified bile leak (▸ Fig. 12.3) and can be utilized for unilateral or bilateral lobe drainage (▸ Fig. 12.4). In addition, endobiliary biopsy can be performed at the time of PTC as a secondary method for obtaining a tissue diagnosis.

12.5 Percutaneous and Endoscopic Interventions

12.5.1 Percutaneous Biliary Drainage

After PTC has been performed, a guidewire can be inserted and advanced into the small bowel. If the original access point is too central or if a guidewire cannot be advanced from the initial access point, a second thin needle can be inserted more peripherally. A coaxial exchange set can then be used to obtain biliary access.[23] Once the guidewire has been passed into the small bowel, the biliary drainage catheter can be advanced over the wire into position. Ideally, a biliary drainage catheter should cross the biliary stricture and be positioned with multiple side holes within the small bowel to restore biliary–enteric bile flow.[6] External drainage may lead to electrolyte disturbances, nutrient malabsorption, and, ultimately, failure to thrive.[6]

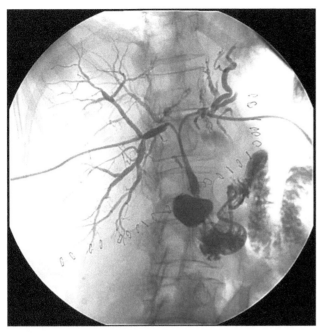

Fig. 12.4 Bilateral percutaneous biliary drainage (PBD) for a Klatskin cholangiocarcinoma tumor.

After PBD is performed, external drainage catheters require ongoing care and maintenance if they are left in place over the long term. Drainage catheters are usually placed to empty into an external drainage bag. The catheter itself must be flushed at least two times daily to maintain adequate patency without aspirating fluid back through the tube.[24] Aspiration may cause seeding of the bile ducts with enteric bacteria. If the catheter is left in place chronically, tubes should be exchanged every 2 to 3 months. This is usually done over a guidewire, using the same tract. Tubes can be upsized if adequate drainage is not being achieved with the current tube size.[6,23]

PTC/PBD is a very well-tolerated procedure with high success rates. Based on the current literature, major complications such as hemobilia, sepsis, hepatic abscesses, bile leak, cholangitis, and peritonitis occur in 4 to 8% of patients.[25,26] Periprocedural fatalities associated with PBD occur in roughly 1 to 6% of patients, with higher fatality rates in patients with malignant strictures, likely because of poorer baseline health and functional status. In addition to major complications, minor delayed complications can occur in up to 20 to 30% of patients and may include catheter occlusion and displacement/dislodgement. Hemobilia results from injury to the hepatic vasculature during PTC/PBD and is estimated to occur in 2 to 8% of procedures. Patients with hemobilia most commonly present with bloody output from their drainage catheter, right upper quadrant pain, or an upper gastrointestinal bleed.[26] Venous bleeding usually occurs from a fistulous connection between a peripheral duct and a branch of the portal vein. These bleeds are usually managed with catheter repositioning or upsizing and rarely require embolization. Arterial bleeds, on the other hand, are brisk and pulsatile and require urgent intervention with coil embolization.[6,26] These bleeds are usually the result of a fistulous connection between the bile duct and the hepatic artery. Arterial bleeds are more likely to lead to massive hemobilia/hemorrhage, given the higher pressure of the arterial system.

Cholangitis is a more common complication after PBD. Cholangitis after PBD often results from a combination of transpapillary reflux of gastrointestinal flora into the biliary system and blockage from either catheter dysfunction or multiple sites of obstruction throughout the liver. The estimated incidence of cholangitis after PTC/PBD ranges from 22 to 54%, with higher incidences in patients with malignancy.[27] In addition, the prevalence of cholangitis appears to increase with the amount of time the drainage catheter is in place. Although the incidence of cholangitis is high, this condition is easily treated with intravenous antibiotics and catheter changes/exchanges and rarely results in fatality.

12.5.2 Internal Biliary Stenting

Patients who have unresectable disease or are poor surgical candidates may undergo endoscopic or percutaneous internal biliary stenting. Biliary stents can be plastic or bare metal (covered or uncovered). Plastic stents are larger in diameter at the time of insertion and often require ERCP with balloon dilation for placement; these stents are usually placed by a gastroenterologist endoscopist. Plastic stents are cheaper than metal stents, but they tend to become occluded within 3 to 4 months.[1,28] A seminal randomized controlled study conducted by Lammer et al[29] in the mid-1990s revealed higher rates of obstruction, higher 30-day mortality, longer length of hospital stay, and decreased patency for plastic stents compared to self-expanding metal stents (SEMs). Thus, plastic stents are often reserved for patients with shorter life expectancies (i.e., < 4 months).

SEMs are more expensive but have been observed to have significantly greater patency times (median: 6–9 months) in multiple randomized controlled studies.[30] Given this longer patency time, metal stents are in fact a more cost-effective choice in patients with expected survival greater than 4 months.[1,30] In addition, these stents can be delivered through either a percutaneous or endoscopic route.[31,32,33]

Percutaneous placement of SEMs begins similarly to the technique used for PTC/PBD. After the target biliary duct is accessed, a guidewire is advanced across the stricture. A large sheath is placed to accommodate the stent, and a sheath cholangiogram is performed to better characterize the area of the stricture and determine the length and caliber of stent that should be placed. Once the stent type is determined, the stent is deployed distal to the obstruction and pulled back into position. The stent will continue to expand to its optimal caliber over time without the need for balloon dilation. A poststenting cholangiogram is then obtained to confirm successful biliary stenting[2] (▶ Fig. 12.5).

SEMs become occluded because of tumor ingrowth into the lumen of an uncovered stent or because of overgrowth of tumor that blocks either end of the stent; this has limited the utility of bare metal SEMs in patients with a life expectancy greater than 6 months. For malignant obstructions involving the CBD, the position of the stent can also affect stent patency rates (▶ Fig. 12.6). A recent study demonstrated that uncovered stent placement above the main duodenal papilla (suprapapillary) results in significantly longer stent patency than stent placement across the duodenal papilla; however, this increased patency associated with suprapapillary stent placement has not been universally demonstrated.[34,35] With regard to complications, suprapapillary stent placement in patients with malignant CBD

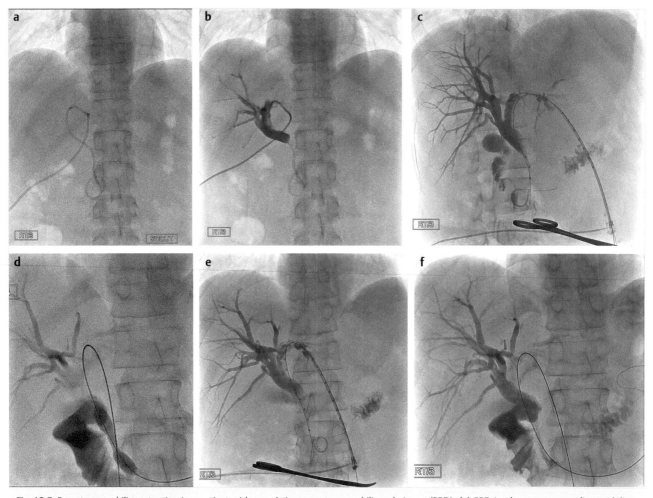

Fig. 12.5 Percutaneous biliary stenting in a patient with an existing percutaneous biliary drainage (PBD). (a) PBD in place across a malignant biliary stricture. (b) Cholangiogram is performed by injecting contrast into the PBD. (c) A guidewire is passed through the existing PBD, and the PBD is removed and replaced with a large sheath. (d) The bile duct is balloon dilated to allow for stent placement. (e) The stent is moved into position and deployment begins. (f) A poststenting cholangiogram is obtained, demonstrating successful stenting of the biliary obstruction.

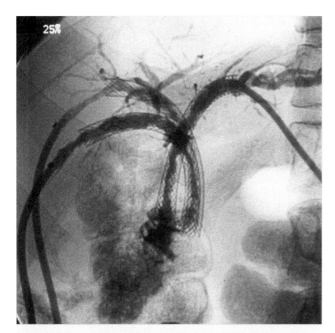

Fig. 12.6 Three uncovered bare metal self-expanding stents in a patient with recurrent cholangiocarcinoma after undergoing a Roux-en-Y hepaticojejunostomy.

obstruction appears to result in decreased rates of infectious complications such as cholangitis and pancreatitis compared to transpapillary placement.[34,35]

To prolong overall stent patency, covered SEMs were developed to prevent occlusion from tumor ingrowth.[36] The current body of evidence suggests that covered stents result in overall better outcomes. Isayama et al[37] conducted a prospective randomized trial investigating covered versus uncovered stents in patients with distal biliary obstruction. Overall, the study demonstrated that covered stents had a lower rate of occlusion and tumor ingrowth and had significantly longer patency than uncovered stents. Similarly, other trials have demonstrated lower rates of stent occlusion and tumor ingrowth and greater lengths of patency with covered stents in cases of cholangiocarcinoma and pancreatic head adenocarcinoma.[38,39] A 2011 meta-analysis comparing the patency of covered versus uncovered stents reported significantly longer patency and survival with covered SEMs in patients with distal biliary obstruction.[40]

Although there is a growing body of evidence to suggest the superiority of covered stents, some conflicting evidence has also been reported.[1,41,42] A recent meta-analysis and several recent studies demonstrated no significant difference between

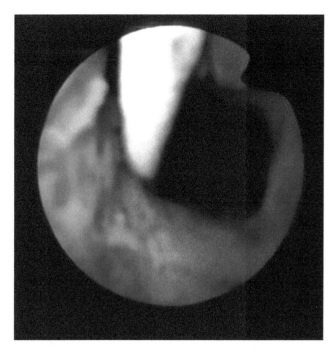

Fig. 12.7 Percutaneous cholangiogram in a patient with cholangiocarcinoma, demonstrating serpiginous neovascularity in a biliary ductal structure.

covered and uncovered stent patency times in patients with distal malignant biliary obstruction.[43,44,45] However, a subgroup analysis of percutaneously placed stents in the meta-analysis by Almadi et al[44] did reveal increased stent patency rates and decreased rates of tumor ingrowth in patients who received covered stents. Overall, there appears to be no significant difference in major complications such as pancreatitis, cholangitis, cholecystitis, and bleeding between covered and uncovered stents.[44] Complications unique to stent placement include ingrowth and overgrowth occlusion (as described earlier), biliary sludge, stent migration, and ulceration.[41,42,43,44,45]

12.5.3 Percutaneous Transhepatic Cholangioscopy

Similar to POC, percutaneous transhepatic cholangioscopy (PTCS), performed by interventional radiologists, also allows for direct visualization of the bile ducts through a percutaneous approach. PTCS has the diagnostic capability to better define malignant versus benign causes of biliary obstruction through a series of visual criteria and direct biopsy (▶ Fig. 12.7). There are several advantages to PTCS. This procedure allows for the evaluation of biliary lesions that cannot be reached with ERCP because of surgically altered anatomy (e.g., as in patients who have undergone gastric bypass or surgical biliary–enteric anastomosis after undergoing a Whipple procedure and Roux-en-Y loop creation). It also allows for the evaluation of intrahepatic and hilar lesions that are traditionally very difficult to reach with ERCP.[46]

Biliary access must be obtained to perform PTCS. Through the methods described earlier, an 8- to 10-Fr biliary drain is placed into the duct of interest. Ductal drainage before cholangioscopy

is critical for tract formation/maturation to prevent hemobilia, peritonitis from biliary spillage, and cholangitis. The drainage tract is left to mature for at least 2 weeks before a cholangioscope is inserted.[47]

For diagnostic visualization with biopsy, PTCS can be performed through a sheath or though the bare tract. After a cholangiogram is performed to confirm the location of the target lesion, a stiff guidewire is placed through the tract into the small bowel, with the sheath placed to allow for the cholangioscope and instruments to be advanced under fluoroscopic guidance toward the target stricture, mass, or stone. The interventional radiologist steers the cholangioscope under scope vision, which has 180° of distal scope tip deflection; by torqueing the entire scope clockwise or counterclockwise, the radiologist can visualize the entire 360° field. Tip deflection and advancement under scope vision allow the scope to be guided/navigated from peripheral PTC access through the central bile ducts, down the CBD, and through to the small bowel. In fact, with the option of 180° deflection, the interventionalist can usually visualize into the first- and second-order bile ducts from the hilum. Once adequate visualization has been obtained, a biopsy can be performed.[46] The sensitivity and specificity of diagnosing biliary malignancy with PTCS visualization and biopsy are greater than 95%.[48] Importantly, PTCS can also be used for treatment, particularly in the setting of symptomatic biliary stones. PTCS access can be used to treat stone disease through retrieval and/or laser lithotripsy under scope visualization.

PTCS is generally very safe; most risks associated with PTCS occur during initial biliary access. Specific complications associated with the insertion of the cholangioscope include cholangitis, bacterial translocation and peritonitis, bacteremia, hemobilia, and ductal perforation.[49] However, complications are minimal when an experienced interventional radiologist performs the procedure.

12.6 Intraductal Treatment

12.6.1 Intraductal Radiofrequency Ablation

Radiofrequency ablation (RFA) uses an alternating current passed through an electrode to generate heat and destroy target tissue, such as a tumor. Recently, intraductal RFA has become available for biliary interventions.[50] With an endobiliary catheter device, RFA can be delivered from either an endoscopic or a percutaneous approach. Multiple studies have demonstrated significantly increased luminal diameters of malignant biliary strictures with the use of intraductal RFA.[50,51,52] Stenting after endoscopic RFA has also been shown to be efficacious. One study reported a median stent patency after endoscopic RFA of 170 days.[53] Endoscopic RFA has also been successfully used to treat SEM occlusions. Percutaneous intraductal RFA with stenting has demonstrated short-term efficacy *for malignant biliary obstructions* in small patient cohorts.[54] In addition, percutaneous RFA has been used to relieve SEM obstructions.[50] Unique to intraductal RFA is the risk of thermal injury to surrounding structures within the hepatic parenchyma. Hemobilia has also been reported after endoscopic RFA; this complication was likely caused by thermal injury to an adjacent portal vein branch.[53]

12.6.2 Photodynamic Therapy

Photodynamic therapy (PDT) is a relatively new treatment modality within the field of interventional oncology. PDT uses a photosensitizer, which is delivered intravenously to the target tumor tissue, and visible or ultraviolet light to generate singlet oxygen molecules. These singlet oxygen molecules cause photo-damage to tumor tissue, resulting in cell death and vascular thrombosis.[55,56] Percutaneous and endoscopic PDT appears to be a well-tolerated palliative treatment option for various biliary malignancies such as cholangiocarcinoma and colorectal liver metastasis.[55,56] Although evidence is scarce, palliative PDT in patients with nonresectable cholangiocarcinoma has been found to result in increased survival time and reduced tumor growth. In addition, this technique appears to be an efficacious treatment option for cholestasis secondary to biliary stenosis, with a favorable side effect profile compared to that of conventional palliative chemotherapy and radiation therapy.[56]

12.7 Conclusion

Malignant causes of biliary obstruction are often difficult-to-treat cancers that present at late stages and are best managed by a multidisciplinary approach. Fortunately, there are many diagnostic and therapeutic interventional and endoscopic technologies available to facilitate rapid and accurate diagnosis and treatment. Diagnostic strategies range from noninvasive imaging to endoscopic fluoroscopy and US to facilitate biopsy, as well as direct visualization through cholangioscopy. Endoscopic diagnostics overall have high sensitivities and specificities for the diagnosis of malignant processes and are generally well tolerated by patients, with few serious complications. Therapeutic options include biliary stricture dilation, stenting, and drainage, both for symptomatic/palliative management and to allow for further medical and surgical management. Regardless of approach, the management of these debilitating cancers requires a multidisciplinary team of interventional radiologists, gastroenterologists, oncologic surgeons, and medical oncologists. As interventional technologies continue to evolve, multidisciplinary collaboration will become increasingly important. In the years ahead, we will see a continued push to develop novel technologies that facilitate accurate diagnosis, reduce procedure-associated complications, and improve overall outcomes and survival.

References

[1] Nam HS, Kang DH. Current status of biliary metal stents. Clin Endosc. 2016; 49(2):124–130

[2] Sutter CM, Ryu RK. Percutaneous management of malignant biliary obstruction. Tech Vasc Interv Radiol. 2015; 18(4):218–226

[3] Levy JL, Sudheendra D, Dagli M, et al. Percutaneous biliary drainage effectively lowers serum bilirubin to permit chemotherapy treatment. Abdom Radiol (NY). 2016; 41(2):317–323

[4] Bowlus CL, Olson KA, Gershwin ME. Evaluation of indeterminate biliary strictures. Nat Rev Gastroenterol Hepatol. 2016; 13(1):28–37

[5] Hayat JO, Loew CJ, Asrress KN, McIntyre AS, Gorard DA. Contrasting liver function test patterns in obstructive jaundice due to biliary strictures [corrected] and stones. QJM. 2005; 98(1):35–40

[6] Venbrux AC, Yadav B, Hossain R, et al. Transhepatic interventions for obstructive jaundice. In: Cameron J, ed. Current Surgical Therapy, 8th ed. St Louis, MO: Elsevier; 2004:448–452

[7] Xu MM, Sethi A. Diagnosing biliary malignancy. Gastrointest Endosc Clin N Am. 2015; 25(4):677–690

[8] Suthar M, Purohit S, Bhargav V, Goyal P. Role of MRCP in differentiation of benign and malignant causes of biliary obstruction. J Clin Diagn Res. 2015; 9 (11):TC08–TC12

[9] Burnett AS, Calvert TJ, Chokshi RJ. Sensitivity of endoscopic retrograde cholangiopancreatography standard cytology: 10-y review of the literature. J Surg Res. 2013; 184(1):304–311

[10] Głuszek S, Matykiewicz J, Kozieł D, Klimer D, Wawrzycka I, Ogonowska A. Risk factors of pancreatitis after endoscopic retrograde cholangio-pancreatography: a retrospective cohort study. Pol Przegl Chir. 2015; 87 (10):499–505

[11] Kim MJ, Mitchell DG, Ito K, Outwater EK. Biliary dilatation: differentiation of benign from malignant causes–value of adding conventional MR imaging to MR cholangiopancreatography. Radiology. 2000; 214(1):173–181

[12] Davee T, Garcia JA, Baron TH. Precut sphincterotomy for selective biliary duct cannulation during endoscopic retrograde cholangiopancreatography. Ann Gastroenterol. 2012; 25(4):291–302

[13] Khashab MA, Valeshabad AK, Afghani E, et al. A comparative evaluation of EUS-guided biliary drainage and percutaneous drainage in patients with distal malignant biliary obstruction and failed ERCP. Dig Dis Sci. 2015; 60(2): 557–565

[14] Wiersema MJ, Vilmann P, Giovannini M, Chang KJ, Wiersema LM. Endosonography-guided fine-needle aspiration biopsy: diagnostic accuracy and complication assessment. Gastroenterology. 1997; 112(4):1087–1095

[15] Heimbach JK, Sanchez W, Rosen CB, Gores GJ. Trans-peritoneal fine needle aspiration biopsy of hilar cholangiocarcinoma is associated with disease dissemination. HPB (Oxford). 2011; 13(5):356–360

[16] Stavropoulos S, Larghi A, Verna E, Battezzati P, Stevens P. Intraductal ultrasound for the evaluation of patients with biliary strictures and no abdominal mass on computed tomography. Endoscopy. 2005; 37(8):715–721

[17] Vazquez-Sequeiros E, Baron TH, Clain JE, et al. Evaluation of indeterminate bile duct strictures by intraductal US. Gastrointest Endosc. 2002; 56(3):372–379

[18] Ghersi S, Fuccio L, Bassi M, Fabbri C, Cennamo V. Current status of peroral cholangioscopy in biliary tract diseases. World J Gastrointest Endosc. 2015; 7(5):510–517

[19] Chen YK, Parsi MA, Binmoeller KF, et al. Single-operator cholangioscopy in patients requiring evaluation of bile duct disease or therapy of biliary stones (with videos). Gastrointest Endosc. 2011; 74(4):805–814

[20] Nishikawa T, Tsuyuguchi T, Sakai Y, Sugiyama H, Miyazaki M, Yokosuka O. Comparison of the diagnostic accuracy of peroral video-cholangioscopic visual findings and cholangioscopy-guided forceps biopsy findings for indeterminate biliary lesions: a prospective study. Gastrointest Endosc. 2013; 77(2):219–226

[21] Covey AM, Brown KT. Percutaneous transhepatic biliary drainage. Tech Vasc Interv Radiol. 2008; 11(1):14–20

[22] Ferrucci JT, Jr, Mueller PR, Harbin WP. Percutaneous transhepatic biliary drainage: technique, results, and applications. Radiology. 1980; 135(1):1–13

[23] Valji K. The Practice of Interventional Radiology. Philadelphia, PA: Saunders Elsevier; 2012

[24] Maher MM, Kealey S, McNamara A, O'Laoide R, Gibney RG, Malone DE. Management of visceral interventional radiology catheters: a troubleshooting guide for interventional radiologists. Radiographics. 2002; 22(2):305–322

[25] Clavien PA, Baillie J, Eds. Diseases of the Gallbladder and Bile Ducts: Diagnosis and Treatment, 2nd ed. Malden, MA: Blackwell Publishing; 2006

[26] Thompson CM, Saad NE, Quazi RR, Darcy MD, Picus DD, Menias CO. Management of iatrogenic bile duct injuries: role of the interventional radiologist. Radiographics. 2013; 33(1):117–134

[27] Nomura T, Shirai Y, Hatakeyama K. Bacteribilia and cholangitis after percutaneous transhepatic biliary drainage for malignant biliary obstruction. Dig Dis Sci. 1999; 44(3):542–546

[28] Kaassis M, Boyer J, Dumas R, et al. Plastic or metal stents for malignant stricture of the common bile duct? Results of a randomized prospective study. Gastrointest Endosc. 2003; 57(2):178–182

[29] Lammer J, Hausegger KA, Flückiger F, et al. Common bile duct obstruction due to malignancy: treatment with plastic versus metal stents. Radiology. 1996; 201(1):167–172

[30] Jaganmohan S, Lee JH. Self-expandable metal stents in malignant biliary obstruction. Expert Rev Gastroenterol Hepatol. 2012; 6(1):105–114

[31] Srinivasan I, Kahaleh M. Biliary stents in the millennium. Adv Ther. 2011; 28 (11):960–972

[32] Moy BT, Birk JW. An update to hepatobiliary stents. J Clin Transl Hepatol. 2015; 3(1):67–77

[33] Dumonceau JM, Tringali A, Blero D, et al. European Society of Gastrointestinal Endoscopy. Biliary stenting: indications, choice of stents and results: European Society of Gastrointestinal Endoscopy (ESGE) clinical guideline. Endoscopy. 2012; 44(3):277–298

[34] Huang X, Shen L, Jin Y, et al. Comparison of uncovered stent placement across versus above the main duodenal papilla for malignant biliary obstruction. J Vasc Interv Radiol. 2015; 26(3):432–437

[35] Jo JH, Park BH. Suprapapillary versus transpapillary stent placement for malignant biliary obstruction: which is better? J Vasc Interv Radiol. 2015; 26(4):573–582

[36] Bakhru M, Ho HC, Gohil V, et al. Fully-covered, self-expandable metal stents (CSEMS) in malignant distal biliary strictures: mid-term evaluation. J Gastroenterol Hepatol. 2011; 26(6):1022–1027

[37] Isayama H, Komatsu Y, Tsujino T, et al. A prospective randomised study of "covered" versus "uncovered" diamond stents for the management of distal malignant biliary obstruction. Gut. 2004; 53(5):729–734

[38] Krokidis M, Fanelli F, Orgera G, Bezzi M, Passariello R, Hatzidakis A. Percutaneous treatment of malignant jaundice due to extrahepatic cholangiocarcinoma: covered Viabil stent versus uncovered Wallstents. Cardiovasc Intervent Radiol. 2010; 33(1):97–106

[39] Krokidis M, Fanelli F, Orgera G, et al. Percutaneous palliation of pancreatic head cancer: randomized comparison of ePTFE/FEP-covered versus uncovered nitinol biliary stents. Cardiovasc Intervent Radiol. 2011; 34(2):352–361

[40] Jeong S, Lee DH. Review of current metal stent. Korean J Gastrointest Endosc.. 2010; 40 Suppl 1:348–353

[41] Kwon CI, Jeong S. Choice of stents for distal biliary obstruction. Clin Endosc. 2013; 46 Suppl:295–302

[42] Saleem A, Leggett CL, Murad MH, Baron TH. Meta-analysis of randomized trials comparing the patency of covered and uncovered self-expandable metal stents for palliation of distal malignant bile duct obstruction. Gastrointest Endosc. 2011; 74(2):321–327.e1, 3

[43] Kullman E, Frozanpor F, Söderlund C, et al. Covered versus uncovered self-expandable nitinol stents in the palliative treatment of malignant distal biliary obstruction: results from a randomized, multicenter study. Gastrointest Endosc. 2010; 72(5):915–923

[44] Almadi MA, Barkun AN, Martel M. No benefit of covered vs uncovered self-expandable metal stents in patients with malignant distal biliary obstruction: a meta-analysis. Clin Gastroenterol Hepatol. 2013; 11(1):27–37.e1

[45] Flores Carmona DY, Alonso Lárraga JO, Hernández Guerrero A, Ramírez Solís ME. Comparison of covered and uncovered self-expandable stents in the treatment of malignant biliary obstruction. Rev Esp Enferm Dig. 2016; 108 (5):246–249

[46] Ahmed S, Schlachter TR, Hong K. Percutaneous transhepatic cholangioscopy. Tech Vasc Interv Radiol. 2015; 18(4):201–209

[47] Bonnel DH, Liguory CE, Cornud FE, Lefebvre JF. Common bile duct and intrahepatic stones: results of transhepatic electrohydraulic lithotripsy in 50 patients. Radiology. 1991; 180(2):345–348

[48] Kim EH, Kim HJ, Oh HC, et al. The usefulness of percutaneous transhepatic cholangioscopy for identifying malignancies in distal common [corrected] bile duct strictures. J Korean Med Sci. 2008; 23(4):579–585

[49] Darcy M, Picus D. Cholangioscopy. Tech Vasc Interv Radiol. 2008; 11(2):133–142

[50] Rustagi T, Jamidar PA. Intraductal radiofrequency ablation for management of malignant biliary obstruction. Dig Dis Sci. 2014; 59(11):2635–2641

[51] Figueroa-Barojas P, Bakhru MR, Habib NA, et al. Safety and efficacy of radiofrequency ablation in the management of unresectable bile duct and pancreatic cancer: a novel palliation technique. J Oncol. 2013; 2013:910897

[52] Alis H, Sengoz C, Gonenc M, Kalayci MU, Kocatas A. Endobiliary radiofrequency ablation for malignant biliary obstruction. Hepatobiliary Pancreat Dis Int. 2013; 12(4):423–427

[53] Dolak W, Schreiber F, Schwaighofer H, et al. Austrian Biliary RFA Study Group. Endoscopic radiofrequency ablation for malignant biliary obstruction: a nationwide retrospective study of 84 consecutive applications. Surg Endosc. 2014; 28(3):854–860

[54] Li TF, Huang GH, Li Z, et al. Percutaneous transhepatic cholangiography and intraductal radiofrequency ablation combined with biliary stent placement for malignant biliary obstruction. J Vasc Interv Radiol. 2015; 26(5):715–721

[55] Vogl TJ, Eichler K, Mack MG, et al. Interstitial photodynamic laser therapy in interventional oncology. Eur Radiol. 2004; 14(6):1063–1073

[56] Ortner MA. Photodynamic therapy for cholangiocarcinoma. Lasers Surg Med. 2011; 43(7):776–780

13 Acute Cholecystitis, Cholelithiasis, and Choledocholithiasis

Daniel B. Gans, Jon C. Davidson, and Indravadan J. Patel

13.1 Introduction

Cholelithiasis, a common condition seen in approximately 10% of the Western population, is symptomatic in only approximately 20% of afflicted patients.[1] When gallstones do become pathologic, the associated conditions are potentially fatal, including acute cholecystitis, ascending cholangitis, pancreatitis, Mirizzi's syndrome, and gallstone ileus. The advent of minimally invasive image-guided procedures has allowed for safer and, at times, more effective treatment for acute cholecystitis, cholelithiasis, and choledocholithiasis. Often, patients present to interventional radiology for treatment when their condition is too unstable for surgery or when their anatomy is too complex for endoscopic therapy. In such cases, radiologists have a unique opportunity to independently treat the patient or work in concert with the gastroenterology and/or surgical teams. This chapter aims to discuss the different treatment options for acute cholecystitis, cholelithiasis, and choledocholithiasis, including a historical perspective and the indications, contraindications, and techniques involved in treating such pathology.

13.2 Acute Cholecystitis

Acute calculous cholecystitis carries a low risk of mortality in patients younger than 80 years, approximately 0.5%; however, the mortality risk can be as high as 11.6% in patients older than 80 years.[2] The pathogenesis involves a gallstone or biliary sludge obstructing the cystic duct, resulting in increased intraluminal pressure. This pressure, in combination with cholesterol supersaturated bile, triggers an inflammatory response. Superimposed infection occurs in approximately 20% of cases, usually from enteric organisms such as *Escherichia coli*, *Klebsiella* species, and *Streptococcus faecalis*. If left untreated, potential sequelae include gangrenous cholecystitis, gallbladder perforation, cholecystoenteric fistulas, and/or gallstone ileus.[1]

In comparison, acute acalculous cholecystitis, which accounts for 10% of all cases, is a much more fatal condition, with a mortality rate of 41% irrespective of age. The majority of these cases occur in critically ill patients or in patients recovering from trauma or nonbiliary tract operations.[3] Acalculous cholecystitis is thought to be the result of biliary stasis and gallbladder ischemia, commonly seen with fasting states or in patients receiving total parenteral nutrition.[4]

13.2.1 Treatment

The first documented surgical percutaneous cholecystostomy (PC) was performed in 1867 by Bobbs,[5,6] and Langebuch performed the first open cholecystectomy (OC) in 1882.[7] For a century, these were the only treatment options for acute cholecystitis until Radder performed the first image-guided PC in 1980. In this case, Radder described an ultrasound (US) guided catheter drainage of a gallbladder empyema.[8] The first laparoscopic cholecystectomy (LC) was performed a few years later in 1985 by Mühe.[7]

The treatment of choice for acute cholecystitis differs based on the severity of the cholecystitis and the presence of comorbidities. The Tokyo Guidelines offer a severity grading system that can be used to determine the optimal treatment strategy (▶ Table 13.1).[9] Using this grading system, Miura et al[10] created a flowchart for the treatment of acute cholecystitis (▶ Fig. 13.1).

In most cases, the treatment of choice for acute cholecystitis is LC. The choice between whether to perform an "early" cholecystectomy (during first presenting admission) or a "delayed" cholecystectomy (6–12 weeks after initial nonoperative management) remains under debate. Although multiple studies have demonstrated that early cholecystectomy is associated with less morbidity,[11,12] studies in which patients underwent PC followed by delayed cholecystectomy found that these patients had shorter mean postoperative hospital stays, a lower frequency of surgical complications, and a lower frequency of conversion to open surgery.[13]

Although LC and PC are currently the most common treatment options, newer techniques are also being used. These include natural orifice transluminal endoscopic surgery (NOTES) and peroral endoscopic transpapillary/transmural drainage. NOTES cholecystectomy involves removal of the gallbladder through a natural orifice, via a transgastric, transrectal, or transvaginal approach. Peroral endoscopic transpapillary drainage entails placement of a double pigtail stent extending from the duodenum through the papilla and cystic duct into the gallbladder.[14] Transmural drainage is performed under

Table 13.1 Tokyo Guidelines for grading acute cholecystitis

Grade	Description
Grade I (mild)	Disease that does not meet the criteria of grade III or II acute cholecystitis. Grade I disease can also be defined as acute cholecystitis in a healthy patient with no organ dysfunction and mild inflammatory changes in the gallbladder, making cholecystectomy a safe and low-risk operative procedure
Grade II (moderate)	Associated with any one of the following conditions: • Elevated white blood cell count (>18,000/mm³) • Palpable tender mass in the right upper abdominal quadrant • Duration of complaints > 72 h • Marked local inflammation (gangrenous cholecystitis, pericholecystic abscess, hepatic abscess, biliary peritonitis, emphysematous cholecystitis)
Grade III (severe)	Associated with dysfunction of any one of the following organs/systems: • Cardiovascular (hypotension requiring treatment with dopamine ≥ 5 μg/kg/min or any dose of norepinephrine) • Neurological (decreased level of consciousness) • Respiratory (ratio of partial pressure arterial oxygen to fraction of inspired oxygen [PaO_2/FiO_2 ratio] < 300) • Renal (oliguria, creatinine > 2.0 mg/dL) • Hepatic (prothrombin time/international normalized ratio > 1.5) • Hematological (platelet count < 100,000/mm³)

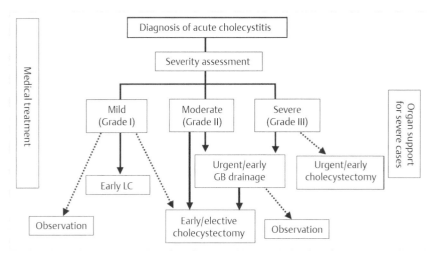

Fig. 13.1 Management strategy for biliary inflammation/infection. (Reproduced *with permission of Miura et al 2007.*[10])

endoscopic ultrasound (EUS), in which there is a direct puncture into the gallbladder through the small bowel wall.[15]

Percutaneous Cholecystostomy

Indications and Contraindications

Although cholecystectomy is considered a safe procedure with a mortality risk of 0.8%, the mortality risk increases significantly in the presence of comorbidities, reaching upward of 30%.[16] In such cases, medical management is typically initiated first. If there is no clinical improvement after 72 hours of medical management, PC is considered to be a reasonable alternative to surgery. In a study of 82 critically ill patients with unexplained sepsis who underwent PC, Boland et al[17] observed substantial clinical improvement within 48 hours in 48 (59%) of these patients. Similarly, Boggi et al[18] found that 10 of 11 critically ill patients (91%) with acute cholecystitis who underwent PC had subsequent resolution of their sepsis. In a retrospective study of 57 patients with acute acalculous cholecystitis, a condition most commonly seen in the intensive care unit, Chung et al[19] observed resolution of symptoms in 53 (93%) patients after 4 days of PC tube placement.

Other conditions associated with acute cholecystitis that expose patients to higher perioperative risk include pregnancy[20] and diabetes mellitus. Cholelithiasis has long been associated with pregnancy, with acute cholecystitis occurring in approximately 1/1,000 pregnancies.[21] PC may be performed as a definitive treatment or a temporizing measure in such cases. Diabetes mellitus is a risk factor for acute acalculous cholecystitis,[22] a poor prognostic factor for acute cholecystitis, and is associated with complications of cholecystectomy such as biliary sepsis, gangrenous changes, and gallbladder wall perforation.[23] Therefore, PC should be considered in such cases.

Contraindications to PC are shown in ▶ Table 13.2.[20,24,25]

Preprocedural Considerations

All cross-sectional imaging results should be reviewed before the procedure. Laboratory studies, including prothrombin time/international normalized ratio and a complete blood count, should be obtained. According to the Society of Interventional Radiology consensus guidelines, PC is considered a category II procedure (moderate risk of bleeding); therefore, an international normalized ratio ≤ 1.5 and a platelet count ≥ 50,000/µL are recommended.[26] Fresh frozen plasma, vitamin K, and/or platelets should be administered to meet these thresholds. The patient's medication list should be reviewed, and pertinent anticoagulants should be withheld. The patient take nothing by mouth the night before the procedure to maximally distend the gallbladder and decompress the bowel.[27] If the patient has not received antibiotics before the procedure, a prophylactic antibiotic should be administered. Although there is no consensus on which medication to use, commonly used antibiotics include ceftriaxone, ampicillin/sulbactam, or vancomycin if the patient is allergic to penicillin.[28]

Technique

Two approaches have been described: transhepatic and transperitoneal. With a transhepatic approach, a catheter is passed through the hepatic parenchyma into the gallbladder via the bare area of the liver (▶ Fig. 13.2a,b). In contradistinction, a transperitoneal approach involves cannulating the gallbladder directly through the fundus without traversing the hepatic parenchyma (▶ Fig. 13.2c,d).

Although the transhepatic route is generally the preferred method, several factors must be considered. The transhepatic route is associated with earlier tract maturation[29] but is considered riskier in the setting of bleeding diathesis. Additional potential risks include pneumothorax, hemobiliary fistula formation, and an increased theoretical risk of bile leak, although this remains controversial.[20,27] The transperitoneal approach is advantageous if this access will be used as a portal for future intervention, such as stone extraction or cystic duct cannulation.[27]

Table 13.2 Contraindications to percutaneous cholecystostomy

Bleeding diathesis
Interposing bowel
Bile peritonitis
Ascites
Decompressed gallbladder due to decompression
Gallbladder completely packed with calculi
Gallbladder cancer (risk of seeding the track)

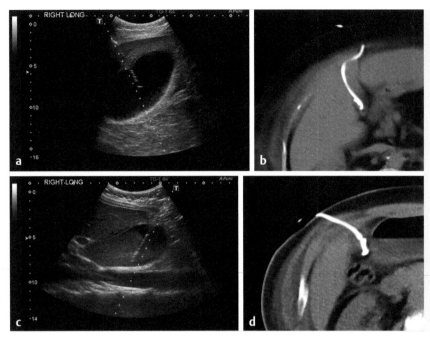

Fig. 13.2 Transhepatic and transperitoneal gallbladder puncture techniques.
(a) Transhepatic gallbladder puncture under ultrasound (US) guidance. **(b)** Axial computed tomography (CT) image in a patient who underwent transhepatic percutaneous cholecystostomy (PC) tube placement.
(c) Transperitoneal gallbladder puncture under US guidance. **(d)** Axial CT image in a patient who underwent transperitoneal PC tube placement.

Loberant et al[30] compared 59 patients who underwent transhepatic PC with 73 patients who underwent transperitoneal PC. There were no significant differences in short-term complications between the two groups, although a tendency toward the transhepatic approach was noted with CT guidance, while a transperitoneal approach was performed more commonly under US guidance.

For this procedure, the patient is typically placed in a supine position, with the right side elevated slightly (if possible). The cutaneous tissues should be prepared and draped before subcutaneous local anesthesia is administered. Two general techniques for PC have been described in the literature: the modified Seldinger technique and the trocar technique.[4,15,16,20,31,32,33,34,35,36,37] In the modified Seldinger technique, a small-diameter needle such as an 18- to 22-gauge Chiba needle is used to perform a micropuncture through the gallbladder wall under US or CT guidance. Confirmation of the needle's location is achieved through aspiration of bile. A 0.018-inch guidewire is then advanced through the needle, and the needle is exchanged over the wire for a coaxial dilator. The coaxial dilator is then used to maintain access within the gallbladder for exchange of the 0.018-inch guidewire for a 0.035-inch guidewire. The coaxial dilator can then be exchanged over the wire for serial dilators and eventually a 6- to 12-Fr Cope Loop drain.[16,38] The trocar technique involves a combination drainage catheter, inner metal stiffener, and a sharp stylet. Under US or CT guidance, a single stick puncture is made into the gallbladder. The drain is advanced over the metal stiffener and sharp stylet into the gallbladder.[25,39] With both techniques, a Cope Loop catheter is preferred to prevent dislodgement from the gallbladder.

Each technique has advantages and disadvantages. The modified Seldinger technique allows for confirmation of access into the gallbladder before the formation of a large-bore cholecystostomy. Additionally, there are less severe consequences if nontarget puncture occurs. However, the multiple steps involved in the modified Seldinger technique make this technique less appealing when urgent drainage is required, when only one operator is present, or when the procedure is being performed at the bedside. Another disadvantage of the Seldinger technique is the risk of fluid leak while exchanging dilators. Therefore, the trocar technique can be advantageous under time constraints and when attempting to limit bile leak. However, when using this technique, nontarget puncture can result in more severe consequences due to the large size of the trocar.[38]

There is very limited research comparing the outcomes of these two techniques for PC, although one study comparing the techniques for peritoneal dialysis catheter placement demonstrated a significantly lower risk of leak and longer catheter survival when placed via the modified Seldinger technique.[40]

The final step of the procedure with either technique is to secure the catheter to the skin with sutures and sterile dressing and connect the catheter to a drainage container. Vital signs should be monitored for 4 to 6 hours after the procedure. A sample of bile may be sent for Gram stain and culture.

Outcomes

With technical success rates ranging from 90 to 100%, PC is an efficient and safe procedure.[29,35,41,42,43] Causes for unsuccessful PC drain placement include loss of wire access,[41] gallbladder full of calculi,[44] bile too thick for aspiration,[44] suboptimal patient cooperation,[29] lack of operator experience,[29] and porcelain gallbladder/thickened gallbladder wall.[45] Clinical response rates in studies have ranged from 59 to 94%, likely in part because of variations in patient populations and clinical response definitions.[17,18,19,33,34,35,41,42,44,46,47,48] The most common indicators of a clinical response included reduction in white blood cell count, defervescence, and reduction of abdominal pain. Most clinical responses were noted in the first 48 hours.

Although PC is considered a safe procedure, complications can occur either immediately after the procedure or slightly later. Potential complications are shown in ▶ Table 13.3.[31,34,35,44] In a study of 127 patients who underwent PC, the total complication rate was 13%, with vagal hypotension and bradycardia most

Table 13.3 Potential complications of percutaneous cholecystostomy

Immediate complications	Delayed complications
Biliary leak and peritonitis	Tube dislodgement
Hematoma	Tube obstruction
Vagal reaction	Abscess formation
Hypotension	Biliary fistula
Pneumothorax	
Respiratory distress	
Severe pain	
Intestinal perforation	

commonly reported (combination occurring in total of 5 patients [4%]).[49] Vagal reactions can be treated with intravenous fluids and atropine. The most lethal complication observed was biliary peritonitis requiring surgical intervention, seen in 3 patients (2%). The 30-day mortality rate was 3.1%, although in each case the cause of death was sepsis and was not directly related to the procedure itself. More recent studies have reported 30-day mortality rates as high as 25%, although only 4% of deaths were attributed to gallbladder-related disease; most were due to preexisting comorbidities.[50]

Follow-Up

While the drain is in place, flushing once or twice daily with 10 mL of saline is recommended to prevent obstruction. Based on the results of the bacterial culture, proper antibiotic therapy should be continued. If an obstructing calculus was present, percutaneous cholecystolithotomy can be considered (discussed later in this chapter).

"Delayed" or "interval" cholecystectomy can be performed 6 to 12 weeks after PC, particularly if the patient is too unstable for surgery at presentation. There is debate about whether this procedure is necessary; the percentage of patients undergoing delayed LC ranges from 3 to 87%.[51] In a retrospective study of 55 patients who had PC for acute cholecystitis, 28 patients (51%) underwent delayed LC. Conversion to OC occurred in only 4 (14%) of these patients, significantly fewer than in the emergent setting. Additionally, no bile duct injuries or major surgical complications occurred.[36] In another study, 11 patients with acute cholecystitis who underwent PC with delayed LC were followed, and conversion to OC was needed in only 1 patient (9%).[52] Although PC with delayed LC is associated with less risk and a lower rate of conversion to OC, one study demonstrated a significantly higher risk of conversion to OC and complications when delayed LC was compared with elective cholecystectomy.[51] One disadvantage of not performing delayed LC is the risk for recurrence. In one study of patients who received a PC drain but did not have delayed cholecystectomy, recurrence of gallbladder-related disease was found to be as high as 41%.[42] However, Chung et al[19] reported a lower risk of recurrence (7%) when a PC drain was placed for acute acalculous cholecystitis. Therefore, PC and eventual drain removal can be considered as definitive treatment in cases of acute acalculous cholecystitis, although interval LC may be necessary in cases of calculous cholecystitis due to the high risk of recurrence.

Cholecystostomy tube removal can only be performed when the tract has matured, which typically occurs approximately 3 to 6 weeks after initial placement. Tract maturity can be assessed beginning at 14 days after tube placement via "tractography." The process involves placing a guidewire

through the existing catheter and exchanging the catheter for a 6- to 8-Fr sheath with its tip at the skin site. Undiluted contrast is then injected through the sheath. The tract is considered mature if there is no leakage of contrast into the peritoneal cavity, subhepatic, subcapsular, or subdiaphragmatic spaces. In the presence of leakage, a new catheter of equal or greater size should be placed over the wire back into the gallbladder.[16] One study comparing time to maturation based on approach demonstrated that 93% of transhepatic PC tracts were mature at 14 days, with the remaining mature at 3 weeks. In comparison, only 13% of transperitoneal PC tracts were mature at 14 days, with maturation rates of 87% at 3 weeks and 100% at 4 weeks.[29]

13.3 Cholelithiasis and Choledocholithiasis

Gallstone disease is an increasingly common entity, with > 20% more cases since the 1980s.[53] The estimated annual combined direct and indirect cost of gallbladder disease in the United States is $6.2 billion.[54] Risk factors for cholelithiasis can be classified into modifiable and nonmodifiable categories (▶ Table 13.4).[53,55]

There are two major types of gallbladder calculi: cholesterol and pigment stones. Cholesterol stones, which are more common in the Western hemisphere, are caused by overproduction of cholesterol by the liver, with associated gallbladder hypomobility. Pigmented stones, which are subclassified into black pigment and brown pigment stones, occur more often in the Eastern hemisphere. Black pigment stones are formed by extremely hard bilirubin polymers, whereas brown pigment stones are polymers of calcium bilirubinate and are often associated with biliary infections.[56]

An impacted gallstone in the gallbladder neck or cystic duct can result in acute calculous cholecystitis or can extrinsically compress the common hepatic duct in a condition known as Mirizzi's syndrome. Choledocholithiasis has long been known to be a risk factor for acute biliary pancreatitis and ascending cholangitis. The simple presence of gallstones is a risk factor for infected bile.[57] The detection of choledocholithiasis can be difficult, both clinically and radiologically. Several studies have been performed to analyze risk factors and predictors for choledocholithiasis,[58,59,60,61] and the American Society for Gastrointestinal Endoscopy has used this information to stratify cases into low-, intermediate-, and high-risk categories based on laboratory, sonographic, and clinical findings (▶ Table 13.5).

Table 13.4 Risk factors for cholelithiasis

Modifiable risk factors	Nonmodifiable risk factors
Diet (low fiber, high calorie)	Familial/genetic
Female sex hormone use (oral contraceptive pills)	Ethnicity (greatest risk in North American Indians)
Obesity/metabolic syndrome	Female sex
Rapid weight loss	Increased age
Low physical activity	
Underlying disease (Crohn's disease, cirrhosis, cystic fibrosis)	
Use of certain drugs (octreotide, ceftriaxone, statins)	
Use of total parenteral nutrition (leads to gallbladder stasis)	
Pregnancy and parity	

Table 13.5 Predictors of choledocholithiasis

Very strong predictors	Strong predictors	Moderate predictors
• CBD stone seen on US • Clinical ascending cholangitis • Bilirubin level > 4 mg/dL	• Dilated CBD > 6 mm (with gallbladder in situ) • Bilirubin level 1.8–4.0 mg/dL	• Abnormal liver biochemical test other than bilirubin level • Age > 55 y • Clinical gallstone pancreatitis

Assigning a likelihood of choledocholithiasis based on clinical predictors

Presence of predictor	Likelihood of choledocholithiasis
Presence of any very strong predictor	High
Presence of both strong predictors	High
No predictors present	Low
All other patients	Intermediate

Abbreviation: CBD, common bile duct.

13.3.1 Cholelithiasis: Treatment

Current treatment options for cholelithiasis include oral dissolution therapy with bile acids such as ursodeoxycholic acid (UDCA), extracorporeal shock wave lithotripsy, LC, and percutaneous therapies. Uncomplicated gallstone pain can be controlled with nonsteroidal anti-inflammatory drugs and/or narcotic analgesics. Decisions regarding when and how to treat are not always clear-cut, as most patients with cholecystitis are asymptomatic. Factors that influence this decision include the presence of symptoms and complications and whether the patient is a surgical candidate. Portincasa et al[62] has developed a flowchart to assist in this decision-making (▶ Fig. 13.3).

UDCA was first shown to be an effective oral dissolution agent in a prospective clinical trial in 1977.[63] Although UDCA is a convenient once-daily medication, its efficacy is limited to the treatment of small, nonpigmented, noncalcified gallstones. Additionally, complete dissolution of the gallstone can take up to 3 years or longer, and sometimes complete dissolution does not occur.[64] Extracorporeal shock wave lithotripsy was first performed in 1986[65] and is an effective noninvasive therapy for gallstones. Disadvantages include the need for adjuvant therapy such as UDCA and high recurrence rates (10% at 6 months after therapy).[66] LC is a safe and definitive treatment for cholecystolithiasis, although this procedure is limited to patients who are poor surgical candidates. Additionally, 5 to 47% of postcholecystectomy patients experience continued or recurrent dyspepsia and upper abdominal pain, a condition known as "postcholecystectomy syndrome."[67,68]

Percutaneous Treatment

Patients with symptomatic cholelithiasis who are poor surgical candidates may require percutaneous gallstone therapy. Patients with Mirizzi's syndrome can benefit from percutaneous therapy

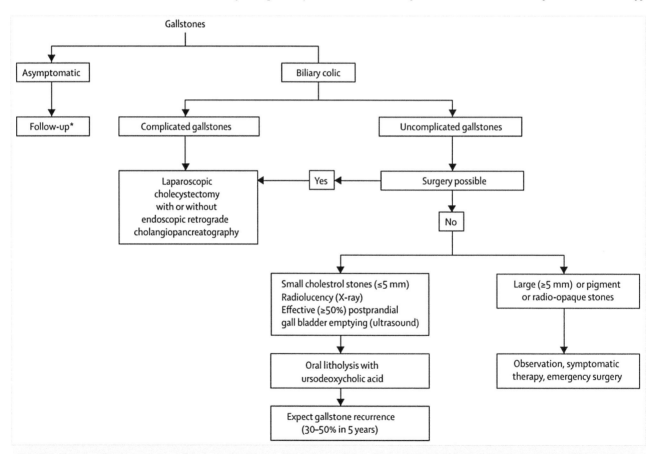

Fig. 13.3 Flowchart for the treatment of cholesterol gallstones. *Exceptions include patients at high risk of becoming symptomatic (i.e., children, morbidly obese) and patients at high risk for gallbladder cancer (i.e., large gallstones, porcelain gallbladder).* (Reproduced with permission of Portincasa et al 2006.[62])

if surgery is not an option.[69] Contact dissolution of cholesterol gallstones using methyl tert-butyl ether was performed throughout the 1980s and 1990s,[2,70,71,72] although this technique fell out of favor because of concerns about toxicity.[73] In 1982, LiPuma et al[74] performed the first percutaneous cholecystolithotomy using a stone basket through an existing PC drain in a patient with acute cholecystitis.

Contraindications to percutaneous cholecystolithotripsy are not as well documented but are generally the same as those reported for PC (▶ Table 13.2).

There are three steps to performing percutaneous cholecystolithotomy: transperitoneal PC drain placement, tract dilation/stone removal, and tract evaluation/tube removal. In the setting of acute cholecystitis with subsequent PC drain placement, tract dilation/stone removal should be performed only after the acute symptoms have resolved. In chronic cholecystitis, tract dilation/stone removal can be performed the day after PC. In this procedure, a 0.035-inch guidewire is placed through the PC drain into the gallbladder. The drain is then exchanged over the wire for subsequent dilators to at least an 18-Fr sheath. Alternatively, the tract can be dilated with a high-pressure noncompliant balloon. Sheaths up to 28 Fr have also been reported.[75,76] A large sheath is then required for the removal of calculi and for the possible passage of a 15-Fr flexible choledochoscope. Some reports suggest using a second PC for passage of the choledochoscope.[77] Occasionally, dilatation of the gallbladder can be technically difficult because of wall thickening. In such cases, T-fasteners can be used to anchor the wall. Then, under fluoroscopic and endoscopic guidance, calculi can be removed with graspers or baskets. Larger stones may require electrohydraulic lithotripsy (EHL) before removal. An 8- to 16-Fr pigtail drain is left in place in the gallbladder to allow for external drainage. Approximately 1 to 2 weeks after the procedure, the drain can be capped to allow for internal drainage. The patient can then return in an additional 1 to 2 weeks for tractography (see above). If the tract has matured, the drain can be removed.[75,76,78,79,80,81,82]

Some limitations to this method include the potential for significant pain during tract dilation and prolonged time for tract maturity. Kim et al[83] suggested a new methodology using a 12-Fr sheath under only fluoroscopic guidance. Two to 3 days following placement of a transhepatic PC drain, the drain can be exchanged for a 12-Fr sheath in a Wittich nitinol stone basket without dilating the tract. A 0.035-inch guidewire can then be advanced through the sheath into the lumen of the gallbladder for stone removal using the Wittich nitinol stone basket under fluoroscopic guidance. Larger stones may require initial fragmentation with a snare technique or by passing a bent Amplatz Extra-Stiff wire through the sheath. Complete stone retrieval was successful in 94% of patients. Causes of incomplete stone retrieval included the inability to grasp large stones and loss of the tract due to a decompressed gallbladder.

The technical success rate for this procedure ranges from 88 to 100%.[75,76,78,79,84] Common factors that preclude success include unsuccessful PC and inability to dilate the tract. The most common major complications are bile leak and bile peritonitis. Other potential complications include transient cholangitis, skin site infection, chest infection, and deep vein thrombosis. Occasionally, multiple removal sessions are required.[76,78,85] Recurrence of gallstones at 14 months occurs in approximately 40% of patients,

although recurrent symptomatic cholelithiasis after 33 months occurs in only 12% of patients.[85]

13.3.2 Choledocholithiasis: Treatment

Current first-line therapies for choledocholithiasis include endoscopic retrograde cholangiopancreatography (ERCP) and surgical common bile duct (CBD) exploration. Because it is presumed that the gallstones originated in the gallbladder, LC should be performed in patients who are surgical candidates. As mentioned earlier, the mere presence of CBD gallstones is not always clear. Therefore, timing of ERCP should be related to the index of suspicion for choledocholithiasis. Tse et al[86] used the aforementioned American Society for Gastrointestinal Endoscopy risk stratification (▶ Table 13.5) to propose a treatment algorithm for patients with planned LC (▶ Fig. 13.4). According to this algorithm, only the intermediate-risk group should have further evaluation, including preoperative ERCP (both diagnostic and therapeutic), EUS, magnetic resonance cholangiopancreatography (MRCP), or intraoperative cholangiogram. All patients in the high-risk category should undergo preoperative ERCP. In the presence of choledocholithiasis, postoperative ERCP or CBD exploration should be performed.

Although ERCP is a minimally invasive procedure, a large Cochrane meta-analysis demonstrated similar rates of successful stone clearance, morbidity, and mortality with ERCP and laparoscopic choledochotomy.[87] Furthermore, ERCP was associated with more repeat procedures and longer hospital stays. Additional risks of ERCP include pancreatitis, hemorrhage, perforation, and cholangitis.[88]

Percutaneous Treatment

Although ERCP and CBD exploration are the mainstay therapies for choledocholithiasis, there are occasional instances in which percutaneous therapy may be indicated. ERCP is successful at CBD clearance in 88% of cases,[87] leaving 12% of cases in which additional therapy is required. Access to the papilla with ERCP can be technically challenging in the setting of a periampullary duodenal diverticulum,[89] after Roux-en-Y gastrojejunostomy, or after gastrectomy with Billroth II reconstruction.[90,91] Retained or overlooked CBD calculi after CBD exploration and T-tube placement range from 1.6 to 7%.[92] Percutaneous options for such patients include basket retrieval, balloon dilation/stone expulsion, and lithotripsy.

Basket Extraction

Burhenne et al[93,94] first described biliary tract stone extraction in 1972. The authors used an existing T-tube and a Dormia ureteral basket. If biliary tract calculi were present on a 7-day postoperative cholangiogram, the patient would return to the radiology department as an outpatient 5 weeks later. At this point, T-tube tract maturation would have occurred. The authors recommended the use of basket extraction only for T-tubes that were 14 Fr or larger. With this technique, a safety guidewire is placed through the existing T-tube before tube removal. A steerable catheter is then advanced through the tract alongside the safety guidewire with the tip beyond the calculus. A basket is advanced through the catheter, and the basket is retracted to engage the stone. For larger calculi, closure of

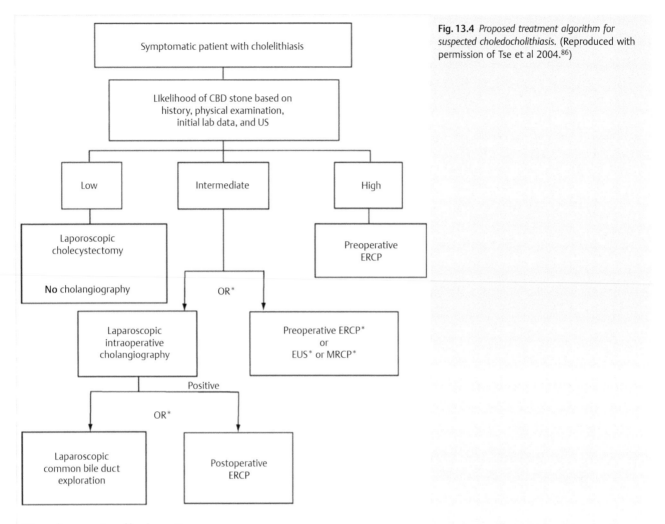

Fig. 13.4 *Proposed treatment algorithm for suspected choledocholithiasis.* (Reproduced with permission of Tse et al 2004.[86])

*Depending on costs and local expertise

the basket is used to break up the stones. Once the stone and/or its fragments are engaged, the catheter/basket combination is retracted through the sinus tract, leaving the safety guidewire in place. When all of the visualized calculi are removed, the guidewire is removed, and a straight catheter is left in the ductal system for drainage.

In a study of 661 patients who underwent this procedure, 95% of cases were technically successful, although approximately one-third of the patients required more than one session.[95] Complications occurred in 4.1% of cases and included (from most to least common) fever, sinus tract leak, peritoneal spill, bile collections, sepsis, pancreatitis, and vasovagal reaction.

In the absence of a T-tube, transcystic and transhepatic modifications to the Burhenne technique have been reported. Transcystic basket retrieval of a CBD calculus was reported by Amberg et al[96] in 1981. Transhepatic retrieval of CBD calculi is not recommended because of the risk of damaging intrahepatic bile ducts. However, successful basket expulsion of CBD calculi into the duodenum via a percutaneous transhepatic approach has been reported.[97,98]

Antegrade Papillary Balloon Dilation and Stone Clearance

Another percutaneous option for patients with endoscopically inaccessible CBD calculi involves using a Fogarty balloon to dilate the papilla and push the calculi through the papilla into the duodenum (▶ Fig. 13.5). Papillary balloon dilation and balloon-push stone clearance can be performed through an existing T-tube, transhepatic tube, or transcystic tube.

In this procedure, a 0.035-inch hydrophilic guidewire is advanced through the existing tube. The tube is then exchanged over the wire for a steerable catheter (Multipurpose or Cobra catheters). Through wire/catheter manipulation, the guidewire is advanced past the papilla into the duodenum. The hydrophilic wire can then be exchanged for an Amplatz Super Stiff Guidewire, and the steerable catheter is exchanged for a peripheral balloon angioplasty catheter. The balloon is placed across the papilla and inflated until the waste of the sphincter disappears; inflation should then be maintained for 30 to 60 seconds. The size of the balloon should be equal to or slightly larger than the largest stone. Multiple balloons of increasing sizes may be used to achieve this effect while preventing laceration of the CBD or papilla. The balloon should then be deflated

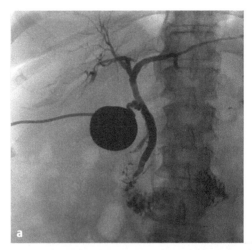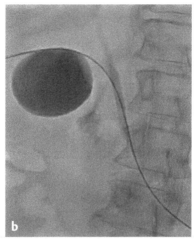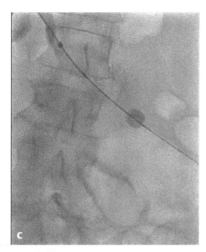

Fig. 13.5 Balloon push technique for choledocholithiasis. **(a)** Choledocholithiasis with PC (percutaneous cholecystostomy) drain in place. **(b)** Wire advanced past calculi into the duodenum. **(c)** Fogarty balloon push.

and reflated to a low pressure proximal to the calculi. Alternatively, the stones can be pushed using a steerable catheter and guidewire. The calculi can then be pushed into the duodenum.

Technical success rates for this procedure range from 95% to 100%. Causes for technical failure include tortuous access tracts and loss of access. Major complications occur in up to 7% of cases (▶ Table 13.6).[99,100,101,102]

Intracorporeal Lithotripsy

Mechanical, ultrasonic, electrohydraulic, and laser lithotripsy procedures have all been used in the percutaneous treatment of biliary calculi.[90,103,104,105] For the purposes of this chapter, only electrohydraulic and laser lithotripsy will be discussed, as these are the most common percutaneous methods.

In EHL, two isolated electrodes are used at the tip of a fiber to create electric high-voltage shock pulses. These shock pulses immediately expand the plasma (liquid), creating spherical shock waves that oscillate, leading to pressure waves that fragment the stone.[106] Laser lithotripsy involves the photothermal destruction of a calculus using a holmium:YAG laser.[107]

EHL is typically performed via transhepatic biliary access, although this procedure can be performed via T-tube or transcystic access. To pass a choledochoscope, a tract of at least 18 Fr is required; the tract should be dilated over the course of a few days to weeks. When the tract is mature, the choledochoscope can be advanced through an 18-Fr sheath or directly into the skin tract. When the electrode is in contact with a stone, EHL can be performed. Passing the stone fragments usually requires either endoscopic or transhepatic sphincterotomy. The stone fragments can then be passed into the duodenum with aggressive

Table 13.6 Major complications from percutaneous papillary balloon dilation and stone clearance

Cholangitis
Subcapsular biloma
Subcapsular hematoma
Subcapsular abscess
Bile peritonitis
Duodenal or common bile duct perforation
Vascular pseudoaneurysm or transection
Biliary pleural effusion

irrigation. Technical success rates for EHL range from 97 to 100%. Major complication rates range from 0 to 22%; complications include hemobilia, CBD perforation, cholangitis, bile peritonitis, biloma, gallbladder necrosis, and empyema/hemothorax.[104,108,109]

Laser lithotripsy requires percutaneous transhepatic access as well as direct visualization with a choledochoscope. Therefore, this procedure is often performed with the assistance of experts in interventional radiology and endourology.[105,110] An 8- to 10-Fr percutaneous transhepatic biliary catheter is first placed. Over the course of several weeks, this catheter should be upsized, usually to between 12 and 16 Fr, to allow passage of a 7-Fr choledochoscope. Lithotripsy can then be performed through this access. Only small population studies have been reported for this procedure, as this technique is typically performed endoscopically. The few studies available have reported technical success rates ranging from 92 to 100%, with total stone clearance usually achieved in one to two sessions. No major complications were noted in these studies, although theoretical complications mirror those seen with EHL.[105,111,112]

13.4 Conclusion

Although more commonly asymptomatic, cholelithiasis occasionally requires treatment, as in the setting of acute cholecystitis, choledocholithiasis, Mirizzi's syndrome, gallstone pancreatitis, ascending cholangitis, etc. While first-line therapy for such conditions includes surgery or endoscopy, interventional radiology plays a large therapeutic role in many circumstances. In the setting of acute cholecystitis, PC tube placement may be considered for patients too unstable for surgery, either as a temporizing measure until more stable or, potentially, as a definitive therapy. Endoscopic therapy for choledocholithiasis can be much more technically challenging in patients with altered gastrointestinal anatomy. Therefore, percutaneous procedures, such as antegrade papillary dilation with stone clearance or extraction of stones with a basket, may prove beneficial. Interventional radiology may even collaborate with other specialists to perform intracorporeal lithotripsy. The above procedures have been proven to be effective and practical with little risk of complication, and should be considered as first-line therapy or alternative therapy when appropriate.

References

[1] Indar AA, Beckingham IJ. Acute cholecystitis. BMJ. 2002; 325(7365):639–643

[2] Gouma DJ, Obertop H. Acute calculous cholecystitis. What is new in diagnosis and therapy? HPB Surg. 1992; 6(2):69–78

[3] Kalliafas S, Ziegler DW, Flancbaum L, Choban PS. Acute acalculous cholecystitis: incidence, risk factors, diagnosis, and outcome. Am Surg. 1998; 64(5):471–475

[4] Barie PS, Eachempati SR. Acute acalculous cholecystitis. Gastroenterol Clin North Am. 2010; 39(2):343–357, x

[5] Sparkman RS. Bobbs centennial: the first cholecystotomy. Surgery. 1967; 61(6):965–971

[6] Sparkman RS. Dr. John S. Bobbs of Indiana. The first cholecystotomist. J Indiana State Med Assoc. 1967; 60(5):541–548

[7] Reynolds W, Jr. The first laparoscopic cholecystectomy. JSLS. 2001; 5(1):89–94

[8] Radder RW. Ultrasonically guided percutaneous catheter drainage for gallbladder empyema. Diagn Imaging. 1980; 49(6):330–333

[9] Yokoe M, Takada T, Strasberg SM, et al. Tokyo Guidelines Revision Committee. TG13 diagnostic criteria and severity grading of acute cholecystitis (with videos). J Hepatobiliary Pancreat Sci. 2013; 20(1):35–46

[10] Miura F, Takada T, Kawarada Y, et al. Flowcharts for the diagnosis and treatment of acute cholangitis and cholecystitis: Tokyo Guidelines. J Hepatobiliary Pancreat Surg. 2007; 14(1):27–34

[11] de Mestral C, Rotstein OD, Laupacis A, et al. Comparative operative outcomes of early and delayed cholecystectomy for acute cholecystitis: a population-based propensity score analysis. Ann Surg. 2014; 259(1):10–15

[12] Gutt CN, Encke J, Köninger J, et al. Acute cholecystitis: early versus delayed cholecystectomy, a multicenter randomized trial (ACDC study, NCT00447304). Ann Surg. 2013; 258(3):385–393

[13] Karakayali FY, Akdur A, Kirnap M, Harman A, Ekici Y, Moray G. Emergency cholecystectomy vs percutaneous cholecystostomy plus delayed cholecystectomy for patients with acute cholecystitis. Hepatobiliary Pancreat Dis Int. 2014; 13(3):316–322

[14] Pannala R, Petersen BT, Gostout CJ, Topazian MD, Levy MJ, Baron TH. Endoscopic transpapillary gallbladder drainage: 10-year single center experience. Minerva Gastroenterol Dietol. 2008; 54(2):107–113

[15] Baron TH, Grimm IS, Swanstrom LL, Swanstrom LL. Interventional approaches to gallbladder disease. N Engl J Med. 2015; 373(4):357–365

[16] Akhan O, Akinci D, Özmen MN. Percutaneous cholecystostomy. Eur J Radiol. 2002; 43(3):229–236

[17] Boland GW, Lee MJ, Leung J, Mueller PR. Percutaneous cholecystostomy in critically ill patients: early response and final outcome in 82 patients. AJR Am J Roentgenol. 1994; 163(2):339–342

[18] Boggi U, Di Candio G, Campatelli A, et al. Percutaneous cholecystostomy for acute cholecystitis in critically ill patients. Hepatogastroenterology. 1999; 46(25):121–125

[19] Chung YH, Choi ER, Kim KM, et al. Can percutaneous cholecystostomy be a definitive management for acute acalculous cholecystitis? J Clin Gastroenterol. 2012; 46(3):216–219

[20] Little MW, Briggs JH, Tapping CR, et al. Percutaneous cholecystostomy: the radiologist's role in treating acute cholecystitis. Clin Radiol. 2013; 68(7):654–660

[21] Casey BM, Cox SM. Cholecystitis in pregnancy. Infect Dis Obstet Gynecol. 1996; 4(5):303–309

[22] Huffman JL, Schenker S. Acute acalculous cholecystitis: a review. Clin Gastroenterol Hepatol. 2010; 8(1):15–22

[23] Landau O, Deutsch AA, Kott I, Rivlin E, Reiss R. The risk of cholecystectomy for acute cholecystitis in diabetic patients. Hepatogastroenterology. 1992; 39(5):437–438

[24] Saad WE, Wallace MJ, Wojak JC, Kundu S, Cardella JF. Quality improvement guidelines for percutaneous transhepatic cholangiography, biliary drainage, and percutaneous cholecystostomy. J Vasc Interv Radiol. 2010; 21(6):789–795

[25] Venara A, Carretier V, Lebigot J, Lermite E. Technique and indications of percutaneous cholecystostomy in the management of cholecystitis in 2014. J Visc Surg. 2014; 151(6):435–439

[26] Patel IJ, Davidson JC, Nikolic B, et al. Standards of Practice Committee, with Cardiovascular and Interventional Radiological Society of Europe (CIRSE) Endorsement, Standards of Practice Committee of the Society of Interventional Radiology. Addendum of newer anticoagulants to the SIR consensus guideline. J Vasc Interv Radiol. 2013; 24(5):641–645

[27] Ginat D, Saad WE. Cholecystostomy and transcholecystic biliary access. Tech Vasc Interv Radiol. 2008; 11(1):2–13

[28] Venkatesan AM, Kundu S, Sacks D, et al. Society of Interventional Radiology Standards of Practice Committee. Practice guidelines for adult antibiotic prophylaxis during vascular and interventional radiology procedures. J Vasc Interv Radiol. 2010; 21(11):1611–1630, quiz 1631

[29] Hatjidakis AA, Karampekios S, Prassopoulos P, et al. Maturation of the tract after percutaneous cholecystostomy with regard to the access route. Cardiovasc Intervent Radiol. 1998; 21(1):36–40

[30] Loberant N, Notes Y, Eitan A, Yakir O, Bickel A. Comparison of early outcome from transperitoneal versus transhepatic percutaneous cholecystostomy. Hepatogastroenterology. 2010; 57(97):12–17

[31] Kiviniemi H, Mäkelä JT, Autio R, et al. Percutaneous cholecystostomy in acute cholecystitis in high-risk patients: an analysis of 69 patients. Int Surg. 1998; 83(4):299–302

[32] Sosna J, Kruskal JB, Copel L, Goldberg SN, Kane RA. US-guided percutaneous cholecystostomy: features predicting culture-positive bile and clinical outcome. Radiology. 2004; 230(3):785–791

[33] van Overhagen H, Meyers H, Tilanus HW, Jeekel J, Laméris JS. Percutaneous cholecystectomy for patients with acute cholecystitis and an increased surgical risk. Cardiovasc Intervent Radiol. 1996; 19(2):72–76

[34] Browning PD, McGahan JP, Gerscovich EO. Percutaneous cholecystostomy for suspected acute cholecystitis in the hospitalized patient. J Vasc Interv Radiol. 1993; 4(4):531–537, discussion 537–538

[35] Hatzidakis AA, Prassopoulos P, Petinarakis I, et al. Acute cholecystitis in high-risk patients: percutaneous cholecystostomy vs conservative treatment. Eur Radiol. 2002; 12(7):1778–1784

[36] Spira RM, Nissan A, Zamir O, Cohen T, Fields SI, Freund HR. Percutaneous transhepatic cholecystostomy and delayed laparoscopic cholecystectomy in critically ill patients with acute calculus cholecystitis. Am J Surg. 2002; 183(1):62–66

[37] Abi-Haidar Y, Sanchez V, Williams SA, Itani KM. Revisiting percutaneous cholecystostomy for acute cholecystitis based on a 10-year experience. Arch Surg. 2012; 147(5):416–422

[38] Lorenz J, Thomas JL. Complications of percutaneous fluid drainage. Semin Intervent Radiol. 2006; 23(2):194–204

[39] García-García L, Lanciego C. Percutaneous treatment of biliary stones: sphincteroplasty and occlusion balloon for the clearance of bile duct calculi. AJR Am J Roentgenol. 2004; 182(3):663–670

[40] Ponce D, Banin VB, Bueloni TN, Barretti P, Caramori J, Balbi AL. Different outcomes of peritoneal catheter percutaneous placement by nephrologists using a trocar versus the Seldinger technique: the experience of two Brazilian centers. Int Urol Nephrol. 2014; 46(10):2029–2034

[41] Teoh WM, Cade RJ, Banting SW, Mackay S, Hassen AS. Percutaneous cholecystostomy in the management of acute cholecystitis. ANZ J Surg. 2005; 75(6):396–398

[42] McKay A, Abulfaraj M, Lipschitz J. Short- and long-term outcomes following percutaneous cholecystostomy for acute cholecystitis in high-risk patients. Surg Endosc. 2012; 26(5):1343–1351

[43] Akyürek N, Salman B, Yüksel O, et al. Management of acute calculous cholecystitis in high-risk patients: percutaneous cholecystotomy followed by early laparoscopic cholecystectomy. Surg Laparosc Endosc Percutan Tech. 2005; 15(6):315–320

[44] Chopra S, Dodd GD, III, Mumbower AL, et al. Treatment of acute cholecystitis in non-critically ill patients at high surgical risk: comparison of clinical outcomes after gallbladder aspiration and after percutaneous cholecystostomy. AJR Am J Roentgenol. 2001; 176(4):1025–1031

[45] England RE, McDermott VG, Smith TP, Suhocki PV, Payne CS, Newman GE. Percutaneous cholecystostomy: who responds? AJR Am J Roentgenol. 1997; 168(5):1247–1251

[46] Atar E, Bachar GN, Berlin S, et al. Percutaneous cholecystostomy in critically ill patients with acute cholecystitis: complications and late outcome. Clin Radiol. 2014; 69(6):e247–e252

[47] Ghahreman A, McCall JL, Windsor JA. Cholecystostomy: a review of recent experience. Aust N Z J Surg. 1999; 69(12):837–840

[48] Davis CA, Landercasper J, Gundersen LH, Lambert PJ. Effective use of percutaneous cholecystostomy in high-risk surgical patients: techniques, tube management, and results. Arch Surg. 1999; 134(7):727–731, discussion 731–732

[49] vanSonnenberg E, D'Agostino HB, Goodacre BW, Sanchez RB, Casola G. Percutaneous gallbladder puncture and cholecystostomy: results, complications, and caveats for safety. Radiology. 1992; 183(1):167–170

[50] Chang L, Moonka R, Stelzner M. Percutaneous cholecystostomy for acute cholecystitis in veteran patients. Am J Surg. 2000; 180(3):198–202

[51] Suzuki K, Bower M, Cassaro S, Patel RI, Karpeh MS, Leitman IM. Tube cholecystostomy before cholecystectomy for the treatment of acute cholecystitis. JSLS. 2015; 19(1):00200

[52] Berber E, Engle KL, String A, et al. Selective use of tube cholecystostomy with interval laparoscopic cholecystectomy in acute cholecystitis. Arch Surg. 2000; 135(3):341–346

[53] Stinton LM, Myers RP, Shaffer EA. Epidemiology of gallstones. Gastroenterol Clin North Am. 2010; 39(2):157–169, vii

[54] Everhart JE, Ruhl CE. Burden of digestive diseases in the United States part I: overall and upper gastrointestinal diseases. Gastroenterology. 2009; 136(2): 376–386

[55] Attasaranya S, Fogel EL, Lehman GA. Choledocholithiasis, ascending cholangitis, and gallstone pancreatitis. Med Clin North Am. 2008; 92(4):925–960

[56] Bouchier IA. The formation of gallstones. Keio J Med. 1992; 41(1):1–5

[57] Csendes A, Becerra M, Burdiles P, Demian I, Bancalari K, Csendes P. Bacteriological studies of bile from the gallbladder in patients with carcinoma of the gallbladder, cholelithiasis, common bile duct stones and no gallstones disease. Eur J Surg. 1994; 160(6–7):363–367

[58] Alponat A, Kum CK, Rajnakova A, Koh BC, Goh PM. Predictive factors for synchronous common bile duct stones in patients with cholelithiasis. Surg Endosc. 1997; 11(9):928–932

[59] Abboud PA, Malet PF, Berlin JA, et al. Predictors of common bile duct stones prior to cholecystectomy: a meta-analysis. Gastrointest Endosc. 1996; 44(4): 450–455

[60] Prat F, Meduri B, Ducot B, Chiche R, Salimbeni-Bartolini R, Pelletier G. Prediction of common bile duct stones by noninvasive tests. Ann Surg. 1999; 229(3):362–368

[61] Onken JE, Brazer SR, Eisen GM, et al. Predicting the presence of choledocholithiasis in patients with symptomatic cholelithiasis. Am J Gastroenterol. 1996; 91(4):762–767

[62] Portincasa P, Moschetta A, Palasciano G. Cholesterol gallstone disease. Lancet. 2006; 368(9531):230–239

[63] Nakagawa S, Makino I, Ishizaki T, Dohi I. Dissolution of cholesterol gallstones by ursodeoxycholic acid. Lancet. 1977; 2(8034):367–369

[64] Thistle JL. Ursodeoxycholic acid treatment of gallstones. Semin Liver Dis. 1983; 3(2):146–156

[65] Sauerbruch T, Delius M, Paumgartner G, et al. Fragmentation of gallstones by extracorporeal shock waves. N Engl J Med. 1986; 314(13):818–822

[66] Vergunst H, Terpstra OT, Brakel K, Laméris JS, van Blankenstein M, Schröder FH. Extracorporeal shockwave lithotripsy of gallstones. Possibilities and limitations. Ann Surg. 1989; 210(5):565–575

[67] Schofer JM. Biliary causes of postcholecystectomy syndrome. J Emerg Med. 2010; 39(4):406–410

[68] Girometti R, Brondani G, Cereser L, et al. Post-cholecystectomy syndrome: spectrum of biliary findings at magnetic resonance cholangiopancreatography. Br J Radiol. 2010; 83(988):351–361

[69] Oxtoby JW, Yeong CC, West DJ. Mirizzi syndrome treated by percutaneous stone removal. Cardiovasc Intervent Radiol. 1994; 17(4):207–209

[70] Thistle JL, May GR, Bender CE, et al. Dissolution of cholesterol gallbladder stones by methyl tert-butyl ether administered by percutaneous transhepatic catheter. N Engl J Med. 1989; 320(10):633–639

[71] Pauletzki J, Holl J, Sackmann M, et al. Gallstone recurrence after direct contact dissolution with methyl tert-butyl ether. Dig Dis Sci. 1995; 40(8): 1775–1781

[72] Allen MJ, Borody TJ, Bugliosi TF, May GR, LaRusso NF, Thistle JL. Rapid dissolution of gallstones by methyl tert-butyl ether. Preliminary observations. N Engl J Med. 1985; 312(4):217–220

[73] Akimoto R, Rieger E, Moossa AR, Hofmann AF, Wahlstrom HE. Systemic and local toxicity in the rat of methyl tert-butyl ether: a gallstone dissolution agent. J Surg Res. 1992; 53(6):572–577

[74] LiPuma JP, Haaga JR, Haranath BS. Gall stone removal via a postoperative cholecystotomy catheter tract. Cardiovasc Intervent Radiol. 1982; 5(2):85–86

[75] Kellett MJ, Wickham JE, Russell RC. Percutaneous cholecystolithotomy. Br Med J (Clin Res Ed). 1988; 296(6620):453–455

[76] Gillams A, Curtis SC, Donald J, Russell C, Lees W. Technical considerations in 113 percutaneous cholecystolithotomies. Radiology. 1992; 183(1):163–166

[77] Wang T, Chen T, Zou S, et al. Ultrasound-guided double-tract percutaneous cholecystostomy combined with a choledochoscope for performing cholecystolithotomies in high-risk surgical patients. Surg Endosc. 2014; 28 (7):2236–2242

[78] Picus D, Hicks ME, Darcy MD, et al. Percutaneous cholecystolithotomy: analysis of results and complications in 58 consecutive patients. Radiology. 1992; 183(3):779–784

[79] Chiverton SG, Inglis JA, Hudd C, Kellett MJ, Russell RC, Wickham JE. Percutaneous cholecystolithotomy: the first 60 patients. BMJ. 1990; 300 (6735):1310–1312

[80] Akiyama H, Nagusa Y, Fujita T, et al. A new method for nonsurgical cholecystolithotomy. Surg Gynecol Obstet. 1985; 161(1):72–74

[81] Kerlan RK, Jr, LaBerge JM, Ring EJ. Percutaneous cholecystolithotomy: preliminary experience. Radiology. 1985; 157(3):653–656

[82] Cope C, Burke DR, Meranze SG. Percutaneous extraction of gallstones in 20 patients. Radiology. 1990; 176(1):19–24

[83] Kim YH, Kim YJ, Shin TB. Fluoroscopy-guided percutaneous gallstone removal using a 12-Fr sheath in high-risk surgical patients with acute cholecystitis. Korean J Radiol. 2011; 12(2):210–215

[84] Picus D, Marx MV, Hicks ME, Lang EV, Edmundowicz SA. Percutaneous cholecystolithotomy: preliminary experience and technical considerations. Radiology. 1989; 173(2):487–491

[85] Courtois CS, Picus DD, Hicks ME, et al. Percutaneous gallstone removal: long-term follow-up. J Vasc Interv Radiol. 1996; 7(2):229–234

[86] Tse F, Barkun JS, Barkun AN. The elective evaluation of patients with suspected choledocholithiasis undergoing laparoscopic cholecystectomy. Gastrointest Endosc. 2004; 60(3):437–448

[87] Martin DJ, Vernon DR, Toouli J. Surgical versus endoscopic treatment of bile duct stones. Cochrane Database Syst Rev. 2006(2):CD003327

[88] Anderson MA, Fisher L, Jain R, et al. ASGE Standards of Practice Committee. Complications of ERCP. Gastrointest Endosc. 2012; 75(3):467–473

[89] Lobo DN, Balfour TW, Iftikhar SY. Periampullary diverticula: consequences of failed ERCP. Ann R Coll Surg Engl. 1998; 80(5):326–331

[90] Hoang JK, Little AF, Clarke A. Percutaneous intracorporeal lithotripsy of biliary calculi. Australas Radiol. 2007; 51 Suppl:B324–B327

[91] Itoi T, Shinohara Y, Takeda K, et al. A novel technique for endoscopic sphincterotomy when using a percutaneous transhepatic cholangioscope in patients with an endoscopically inaccessible papilla. Gastrointest Endosc. 2004; 59(6):708–711

[92] Glenn F. Retained calculi within the biliary ductal system. Ann Surg. 1974; 179(5):528–539

[93] Burhenne HJ. Non-operative retained biliary tract stone extraction. Calif Med. 1972; 117(6):57

[94] Burhenne HJ. The technique of biliary duct stone extraction. Experience with 126 cases. Radiology. 1974; 113(3):567–572

[95] Burhenne HJ. Garland lecture. Percutaneous extraction of retained biliary tract stones: 661 patients. AJR Am J Roentgenol. 1980; 134(5):889–898

[96] Amberg JR, Chun G. Transcystic duct treatment of common bile duct stones. Gastrointest Radiol. 1981; 6(4):361–362

[97] Dotter CT, Bilbao MK, Katon RM. Percutaneous transhepatic gallstone removal by needle tract. Radiology. 1979; 133(1):242–243

[98] Clouse ME. Dormia basket modification for percutaneous transhepatic common bile duct stone removal. AJR Am J Roentgenol. 1983; 140(2):395–397

[99] Szulman C, Giménez M, Sierre S. Antegrade papillary balloon dilation for extrahepatic bile duct stone clearance: lessons learned from treating 300 patients. J Vasc Interv Radiol. 2011; 22(3):346–353

[100] Gil S, de la Iglesia P, Verdú JF, de España F, Arenas J, Irurzun J. Effectiveness and safety of balloon dilation of the papilla and the use of an occlusion balloon for clearance of bile duct calculi. AJR Am J Roentgenol. 2000; 174(5): 1455–1460

[101] Ozcan N, Kahriman G, Mavili E. Percutaneous transhepatic removal of bile duct stones: results of 261 patients. Cardiovasc Intervent Radiol. 2012; 35 (4):890–897

[102] Muchart J, Perendreu J, Casas JD, Díaz-Ruíz MJ. Balloon catheter sphincteroplasty and biliary stone expulsion into the duodenum in patients with an indwelling T tube. Abdom Imaging. 1999; 24(1):69–71

[103] Ho CS, Yee AC, McLoughlin MJ. Biliary lithotripsy with a mechanical lithotripter. Radiology. 1987; 165(3):791–793

[104] Bonnel DH, Liguory CE, Cornud FE, Lefebvre JF. Common bile duct and intrahepatic stones: results of transhepatic electrohydraulic lithotripsy in 50 patients. Radiology. 1991; 180(2):345–348

[105] Hazey JW, McCreary M, Guy G, Melvin WS. Efficacy of percutaneous treatment of biliary tract calculi using the holmium:YAG laser. Surg Endosc. 2007; 21(7):1180–1183

[106] Raijman I. Intracorporeal lithotripsy in the management of biliary stone disease. Semin Laparosc Surg. 2000; 7(4):295–301

[107] Chan KF, Vassar GJ, Pfefer TJ, et al. Holmium:YAG laser lithotripsy: a dominant photothermal ablative mechanism with chemical decomposition of urinary calculi. Lasers Surg Med. 1999; 25(1):22–37

[108] Burton KE, Picus D, Hicks ME, et al. Fragmentation of biliary calculi in 71 patients by use of intracorporeal electrohydraulic lithotripsy. J Vasc Interv Radiol. 1993; 4(2):251–256

[109] Picus D, Weyman PJ, Marx MV. Role of percutaneous intracorporeal electrohydraulic lithotripsy in the treatment of biliary tract calculi. Work in progress. Radiology. 1989; 170(3, Pt 2):989–993

[110] Copelan A, Kapoor BS. Choledocholithiasis: Diagnosis and Management. Tech Vasc Interv Radiol. 2015; 18(4):244–255

[111] Ray AA, Davies ET, Duvdevani M, Razvi H, Denstedt JD. The management of treatment-resistant biliary calculi using percutaneous endourologic techniques. Can J Surg. 2009; 52(5):407–412

[112] Das AK, Chiura A, Conlin MJ, Eschelman D, Bagley DH. Treatment of biliary calculi using holmium: yttrium aluminum garnet laser. Gastrointest Endosc. 1998; 48(2):207–209

14 Imaging of Liver Tumors

Christopher P. Coppa

14.1 Introduction

This review will discuss the imaging features of commonly encountered malignant hepatic neoplasms. The computed tomography (CT) and magnetic resonance (MR) imaging appearances of hepatic metastases and primary hepatic neoplasms, including hepatocellular carcinoma (HCC) and cholangiocarcinoma (CCA), are summarized, with a focus on techniques for detection and patterns of enhancement using dynamic contrast-enhanced imaging. Further, CT and MR findings after locoregional therapy are reviewed, as is the application of these findings to different anatomic and functional-based treatment response models.

14.2 Technical Considerations

Multiphase dynamic contrast-enhanced imaging is the primary method used to characterize liver lesions on CT, and this technique also plays an important but not exclusive role in characterizing hepatic lesions on MR imaging. The patterns of enhancement observed in various hepatic lesions are the same on CT and MR imaging when extracellular contrast agents are administered. However, MR imaging can also use additional pulse sequences (e.g., T1-weighted, T2-weighted, and diffusion-weighted images) in conjunction with postcontrast images to better characterize lesions. As such, MR imaging is the imaging modality of choice for initial lesion characterization, whereas CT is generally reserved for patients who cannot undergo MR imaging.[1]

Regardless of the modality used, dynamic contrast-enhanced liver imaging typically involves late arterial, portal venous, and delayed phases. While portal venous and delayed-phase images are typically acquired at fixed time points after the injection of contrast, the timing of the late arterial phase acquisition is usually tailored to the individual patient. Achieving satisfactory late arterial phase images requires optimization of the time delay between the administration of intravenous contrast material and the initiation of image acquisition. Fixed time-delay techniques are generally considered less reliable given variability in patient factors (such as cardiac output); therefore, bolus tracking or timing-bolus techniques are generally recommended.[2,3,4] High temporal resolution MR imaging performed with multiple arterial acquisitions may also be used to increase the likelihood of obtaining diagnostic arterial phase images.[5]

Meticulous timing of the arterial phase acquisition is crucial, as hypervascular tumors, including HCC and hypervascular metastases, demonstrate maximum enhancement during the late arterial phase. Radiographically, this phase is achieved when there is uniform contrast opacification of arteries and some early portal venous filling but an absence of hepatic vein opacification. Improper timing of the arterial phase may reduce the conspicuity of HCC and hypervascular metastases. Improper timing may involve imaging too early (i.e., the early arterial or angiographic phase, during which there is opacification of arteries but no portal or hepatic venous filling; ▸ Fig. 14.1) or imaging too late (i.e., when there is portal and hepatic venous opacification; ▸ Fig. 14.2).[6]

The importance of well-timed dynamic contrast-enhanced imaging cannot be overstated. The Organ Procurement and Transplantation Network (OPTN) developed a policy in 2011 recommending that transplantation centers across the United States adopt certain technical specifications for dynamic contrast-enhanced imaging to optimize the diagnosis of HCC.[6] This stems from the fact that patients diagnosed with HCC are eligible for Model for End-Stage Liver Disease (MELD) exception points and may therefore gain higher priority on the liver transplant waiting list.[7] If the radiologic criteria for diagnosing HCC cannot be applied because of a technically insufficient study, the results of the study cannot be used to assign automatic exception points for transplant.[6] These OPTN technical specifications set minimum levels of functionality for CT and MR scanners and emphasize the importance of correct timing of image acquisition, especially for the late arterial phase.

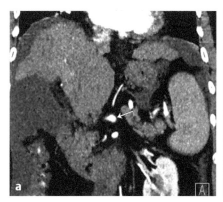 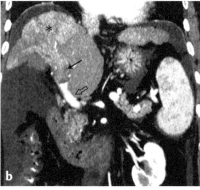

Fig. 14.1 Importance of late arterial phase versus early arterial phase in the detection of HCC (hepatocellular carcinoma). **(a)** There is contrast opacification of arteries (*arrow*) on early arterial phase coronal computed tomography (CT) but no opacification of the portal vein. The liver has a cirrhotic morphology, but a hepatic mass is not identified after contrast administration. **(b)** CT of the same region performed during the late arterial phase shows a large infiltrative hypervascular mass (*) in the right hepatic dome contiguous with enhancing portal venous tumor thrombus (*arrow*). There is contrast opacification of both arterial branches and the main portal vein (*open arrow*) in the late arterial phase but no contrast opacification of the hepatic veins (not shown) as these veins usually do not fill with contrast until the portal venous phase.

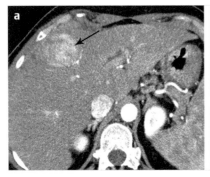 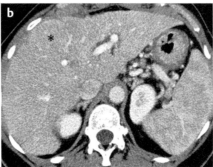

Fig. 14.2 Importance of arterial phase imaging for detection of HCC (hepatocellular carcinoma). **(a)** Hypervascular mass (*arrow*) in a patient with cirrhosis is compatible with HCC and is quite obvious on the arterial phase of the contrast-enhanced CT (computed tomography). **(b)** The same mass (*) is essentially isodense to the background liver on the portal venous phase and could potentially be overlooked if this scan was reviewed in isolation.

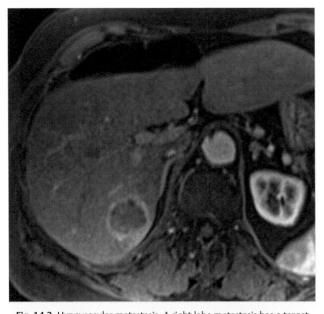

Fig. 14.3 Hypovascular metastasis. A right lobe metastasis has a target appearance created by an early complete ring of peripheral enhancement and a hypoenhancing center in a patient with metastatic lung cancer.

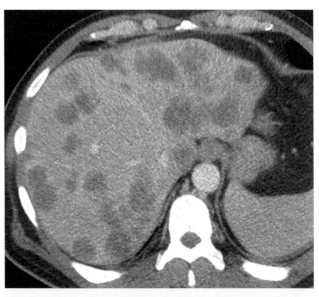

Fig. 14.4 Hypovascular metastases. Multiple masses with ill-defined margins have attenuation greater than cysts and enhance to a lesser degree than the background liver on a CT (computed tomography) scan acquired during the portal venous phase in a patient with metastatic colorectal cancer.

14.3 Metastases

Metastases are the most common hepatic malignancies, occurring significantly more frequently than primary liver tumors. As such, most liver imaging is performed to evaluate metastases.[8]

14.3.1 Enhancement Patterns

Liver metastases have different appearances depending on the histology of the primary tumor and can be broadly classified as hypovascular and hypervascular based on their enhancement patterns.[8] Contrast-enhanced CT and MR examinations can be tailored to assess these differences in enhancement. Although multiphasic contrast-enhanced imaging is routinely performed during every MR scan of the liver, multiphasic contrast-enhanced CT is not always performed because of the ionizing radiation associated with additional phases. Multiphasic CT imaging is indicated for the initial evaluation of an unknown liver mass (in a patient not eligible for MR imaging) and potentially for the surveillance of hypervascular malignancies, but this technique is generally not warranted in cases of hypovascular metastases, which can usually be assessed with a single-phase (i.e., portal venous phase) approach. Ultimately, the use of multiphasic CT imaging depends on the clinical scenario, and protocols for use vary among institutions.

Most metastases are hypovascular and are best visualized during the portal venous phase of enhancement, when enhancement is less than that of the background liver. Colorectal, lung, and gastric cancers classically produce hypovascular liver metastases.[8] These lesions have a "target" appearance created by an early complete ring of peripheral enhancement and a hypoenhancing center (▶ Fig. 14.3), followed by incomplete central progression on the delayed phase.[9]

On CT, hypovascular metastases usually have attenuation greater than that of cysts (> 20 Hounsfield units) but less than that of the surrounding liver (▶ Fig. 14.4). One caveat is that the center of necrotic or mucin-containing metastases can mimic cysts on both CT and MR imaging. The presence of irregular margins or peripheral enhancement helps discriminate such lesions from benign hepatic cysts, which have no associated enhancement.[10,11]

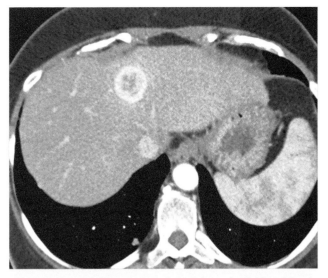

Fig. 14.5 Hypervascular metastasis. Rounded mass has brisk peripheral enhancement greater than that of the normal liver on a CT (computed tomography) scan acquired during the arterial phase in a patient with metastatic renal cell carcinoma. Note the pronounced enhancement of the aorta and the paucity of contrast in the hepatic veins, features indicating an arterial acquisition.

Hypervascular metastases (i.e., metastases predominantly with arterial blood supply) show enhancement greater than that of the background liver during the arterial phase (▶ Fig. 14.5). Hypervascular metastases usually originate from primary tumors such as neuroendocrine tumor, renal cell carcinoma, and melanoma. Breast cancer metastases are usually hypovascular but are sometimes hypervascular.[9]

Diffuse hypervascularity is often present in smaller lesions, whereas peripheral ring enhancement is more characteristic of larger lesions. Some hypervascular metastases, especially lesions of neuroendocrine origin, demonstrate peripheral hypoenhancement or washout compared to the enhancement of the center of the lesion on the delayed phase. This finding is insensitive but highly specific for metastases. When present, it is a feature that can be used to distinguish small hypervascular metastases from hepatic hemangiomas, which retain contrast material on the venous phase.[9,10]

14.3.2 Hepatocyte-Specific Contrast Agents

Thus far, the discussion has applied to enhancement patterns seen after the intravenous administration of extracellular CT and MR contrast agents, which lack hepatocyte uptake. Another type of MR contrast agent, referred to as a hepatocyte-specific agent, has dual pharmacokinetic behavior. Shortly after contrast injection, this agent behaves similarly to extracellular agents, diffusing from the vascular space into the interstitial space. However, unlike extracellular agents, it subsequently accumulates in hepatocytes and is partially excreted by the biliary system. The hepatobiliary phase succeeds the dynamic phase, and the timing of acquisition depends on the agent administered: 20 minutes for gadoxate disodium (gadolinium ethoxybenzyl diethylenetriamine pentaacetic acid [Gd-EOB-DTPA]) and 45 to 120 minutes for gadobenate dimeglumine (Gd-BOPTA).[1]

Images generated during the hepatobiliary phase can be used to discriminate between normal liver (and lesions with functioning hepatocytes) and lesions lacking hepatocytes, thereby providing excellent lesion detection and liver-to-tumor contrast. Lesions with hepatocytes (such as focal nodular hyperplasia) have some degree of contrast accumulation on the hepatobiliary phase, and lesions without hepatocytes (such as metastases, cysts, and hemangiomas) lack uptake. Although the absence of contrast accumulation within a lesion on the hepatobiliary phase is a nonspecific finding in isolation, lesion characterization can be achieved when hepatobiliary phase findings are reviewed in conjunction with the other conventional MR sequences, including the dynamic contrast-enhanced portion of the study.[12]

Gd-EOB-DTPA is particularly useful for detecting very small metastases (< 1 cm) and differentiating these lesions from focal nodular hyperplasia and hepatic cysts. Several studies have shown that MR imaging performed with hepatocyte-specific contrast depicts more liver metastases and improves lesion characterization when compared with CT.[13] For example, MR imaging with Gd-EOB-DTPA is superior to CT in detecting liver metastases from colorectal cancer; some consider this technique the preoperative imaging modality of choice in patients being considered for surgical treatment of such metastases.[14] Further, MR imaging with Gd-EOB-DTPA is more sensitive than positron emission tomography (PET)/CT for detecting liver metastases (▶ Fig. 14.6), especially lesions smaller than 1 cm.[15]

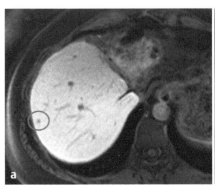
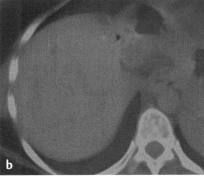

Fig. 14.6 Metastasis evaluation with hepatocyte-specific contrast agent. **(a)** Subcentimeter colorectal metastasis (*circled*) in the periphery of the right lobe is hypointense to the surrounding liver on the hepatobiliary phase acquired 20 minutes after the administration of a hepatocyte-specific contrast agent. **(b)** There is no associated fluorodeoxyglucose (FDG) uptake in the lesion on the PET (positron emission tomography)/CT (computed tomography) performed the previous day, illustrating the benefit of hepatobiliary imaging for lesion detection.

14.3.3 Additional Magnetic Resonance Sequences

Although liver lesions can often be characterized as metastases based on CT or MR enhancement patterns alone, absolute characterization and quantification of metastases is most commonly performed with MR imaging because of the higher specificity gained by adding complementary pulse sequences, including T2-, T1-, and diffusion-weighted sequences.[1] This is especially important in the evaluation of small lesions that are often indeterminate on CT.

T2-Weighted Imaging

Most liver metastases have increased signal on T2-weighted images, with intensity similar to that of the normal splenic parenchyma (▶ Fig. 14.7) but less than the marked signal

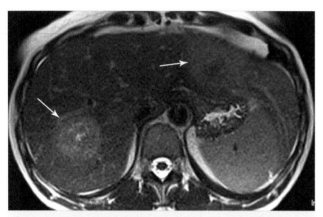

Fig. 14.7 T2-weighted appearance of metastases. Two mildly to moderately hyperintense masses (*arrows*) have signal intensity similar to that of the spleen on a T2-weighted sequence, a rough indicator of malignancy.

hyperintensity generated by hepatic cysts and hemangiomas. This degree of signal intensity is often observed in solid lesions and is not entirely specific for metastases but often indicates malignancy. One exception is mucinous metastases, which may have T2 signal intensity similar to that of a hemangioma because of their high water content.[16] Further, some less common metastases (e.g., lesions containing blood products, smooth muscle, calcification, or fibrotic components) may demonstrate low T2 signal.[17]

T1-Weighted Imaging

Although most metastases are hypointense or isointense to the background liver on T1-weighted images, some metastases have T1 signal hyperintensity because of the presence of paramagnetic substances within the lesion. For example, some melanoma metastases have high T1 signal (▶ Fig. 14.8) because of the presence of melanin and extracellular methemoglobin.[8]

Diffusion-Weighted Imaging

Diffusion-weighted imaging (DWI) is a functional MR technique that is useful for the identification and sometimes characterization of liver lesions based on lesion cellularity. Image contrast is dependent on differences in the mobility of water protons within various tissues, measured as the apparent diffusion coefficient (ADC). This technique is superior to T2-weighted sequences for the detection of liver metastases and is especially useful when gadolinium is contraindicated because of renal insufficiency or allergy.[18,19]

Classically, highly cellular lesions (e.g., tumors) restrict the diffusion of water, which translates into high signal on high b-value DWI and low signal on the corresponding ADC map (▶ Fig. 14.9). In comparison, benign lesions typically permit greater diffusion of water molecules, resulting in decreased signal on high b-value images and high signal on the associated ADC map.

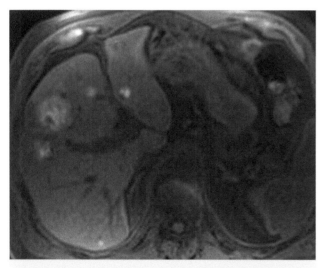

Fig. 14.8 T1 hyperintense liver metastases. Several hyperintense lesions on a noncontrast T1-weighted MR (magnetic resonance) image in a patient with metastatic melanoma have this appearance due to the T1-shortening effect of melanin. Other metastases composed of paramagnetic substances could have a similar appearance. Overall, these metastases are less common than their T1 hypointense counterparts.

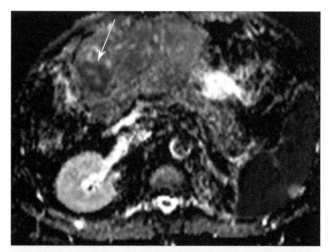

Fig. 14.9 Restricted diffusion in metastatic disease. A patient who previously underwent right hepatectomy for metastatic rectal cancer has a mass with a thick rim of low signal (*arrow*) on the ADC (apparent diffusion coefficient) map, indicative of restricted diffusion in a recurrent metastasis.

Applying these principles, DWI has a role in characterizing liver lesions as benign or malignant. However, it is important to remember that cystic, mucinous, and necrotic metastases may demonstrate high ADC values because of a lack of cellularity (less restriction of water), and some benign lesions (e.g., abscesses and focal nodular hyperplasia) may have low ADC values. As such, there is an overlap in the appearance (and corresponding ADC values) of benign and malignant lesions on DWI, and ultimate characterization often relies on findings from conventional MR sequences.[18,19]

14.4 Hepatocellular Carcinoma

HCC accounts for nearly 90% of all primary liver malignancies. Most cases (70–90%) occur in patients with cirrhosis. HCC can also be seen in noncirrhotic patients who have chronic hepatitis B virus or other chronic liver diseases such as hemochromatosis.[20]

As such, the major international liver societies, including the American Association for the Study of Liver Disease (AASLD), recommend that patients at risk of developing HCC enter surveillance programs. Although the limitations of ultrasound for HCC surveillance are recognized, especially because of the liver heterogeneity often present in cirrhosis, all of the major liver societies recommend ultrasound for HCC surveillance in some capacity because of its affordability and availability. CT and MR imaging are reserved for diagnosis, as the utility of these modalities for surveillance has not been validated.[21]

Current clinical guidelines recommend the use of multiphasic contrast-enhanced CT and MR imaging for the diagnosis and staging of HCC. These examinations should include image acquisition in the late hepatic arterial, portal venous, and delayed phases, as the diagnosis of HCC is based mainly on enhancement criteria.[22] As described earlier, the OPTN has issued minimum technical requirements for performing contrast-enhanced CT and MR imaging of the liver. Included in these specifications is the recommendation that bolus tracking be performed to optimize late arterial phase imaging.[6] As previously mentioned, a hypervascular lesion may be less conspicuous if arterial phase images are not properly timed (▶ Fig. 14.1; ▶ Fig. 14.2).

14.4.1 Enhancement Patterns

The hallmark imaging feature of HCC is hypervascularity (or arterial phase enhancement). This finding is highly sensitive for HCC but not sufficient for diagnosis in isolation. Specificity for the diagnosis of HCC is increased (to approximately 96%) when hypervascularity is followed by washout on portal venous phase or delayed-phase imaging (▶ Fig. 14.10), defined as enhancement less than that of the surrounding parenchyma.[21,23]

Another imaging feature characteristic of HCC is a capsule, which appears as a rim of smooth hyperenhancement on portal venous or delayed-phase imaging (▶ Fig. 14.11). The combination of lesion hypervascularity and a capsule strongly suggests a diagnosis of HCC even when washout is not present.[22]

The OPTN's criteria for the radiographic diagnosis of HCC (i.e., OPTN class 5 lesion) in the setting of chronic liver disease are based on these characteristic enhancement patterns during multiphasic contrast-enhanced CT and MR imaging. Rapid growth (at least 50% growth in a 6-month period) is also incorporated into the classification system. The criteria were created with the intention of optimizing specificity (not sensitivity) such that an unequivocal diagnosis of HCC could be made

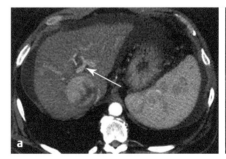
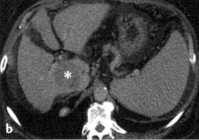

Fig. 14.10 CT (computed tomography) of HCC (hepatocellular carcinoma) with washout. **(a)** A 5-cm mass in the right posterior hepatic lobe hyperenhances on the late arterial phase. There is some contrast opacification of the portal vein (*arrow*), indicative of a satisfactory late arterial phase study. **(b)** The same mass (*) enhances to a lesser degree than the surrounding liver on the delayed phase (performed 180 seconds after contrast injection), compatible with washout. At this size, the lesion is an OPTN (Organ Procurement and Transplantation Network) class 5X.

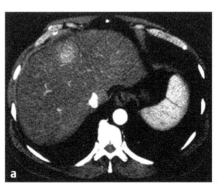
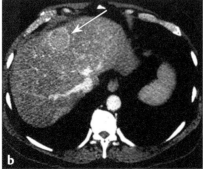

Fig. 14.11 CT (computed tomography) of hepatocellular carcinoma (HCC) with pseudocapsule. **(a)** A 3-cm mass at the junction of hepatic segments IVa and VIII is hypervascular during the late arterial phase. Note the absence of hepatic vein opacification during the arterial phase (and incidental reflux of contrast into the inferior vena cava). **(b)** The mass has an enhancing capsule (*arrow*) in the delayed phase compatible with HCC/OPTN (Organ Procurement and Transplantation Network) class 5B lesion.

before awarding exception points for transplant.[6] The OPTN criteria for radiologic diagnosis of HCC are as follows:

- OPTN 5A: lesions measuring ≥ 1 and < 2 cm are defined as HCC if they are hypervascular AND have washout AND a capsule. Alternatively, lesions of this size are HCC if they are hypervascular AND demonstrate rapid interval growth (OPTN 5A-g).
- OPTN 5B: lesions measuring ≥ 2 and < 5 cm are defined as HCC if they are hypervascular AND have either washout OR a capsule OR rapid growth (▶ Fig. 14.11).
- OPTN 5X: lesions ≥ 5 cm are defined as HCC if they are hypervascular AND have either washout OR a capsule (▶ Fig. 14.10).

Compared to the hypervascular enhancement classically described in HCC, more infiltrative types of HCC usually have minimal arterial enhancement and may be difficult to differentiate from the background liver (▶ Fig. 14.12). Such tumors may be more visible on diffusion-, T1-, and T2-weighted MR images than on contrast-enhanced images. Tumor thrombus, which is often associated with an infiltrative pattern of HCC, may be the most conspicuous indicator that such a pattern of disease is present.[24]

14.4.2 Hepatocyte-Specific Contrast Agents

The use of hepatocyte-specific agents for lesion characterization in the setting of cirrhosis is somewhat controversial.[21] Images obtained during hepatobiliary phase MR imaging can help differentiate premalignant lesions (i.e., high-grade dysplastic nodules) and early HCC from low-grade dysplastic and regenerative nodules. Specifically, hepatobiliary phase signal hypointensity is more typical of premalignant or early HCC and may precede neoarterialization and formation of overt HCC. Comparatively,

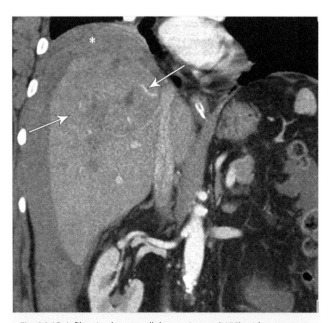

Fig. 14.12 Infiltrative hepatocellular carcinoma (HCC) with rupture. A heterogeneous mass (*arrows*) along the capsule of the right hepatic dome has minimal arterial phase enhancement, a finding described in larger and infiltrative types of HCC. Soft-tissue attenuation material (*) is present within the perihepatic region, consistent with hemoperitoneum from spontaneous HCC rupture.

signal isointensity is generally seen in low-risk nodules.[25] In the absence of hypervascular lesions, identification of such hypointense nodules may help identify patients who require more frequent surveillance.

However, several challenges have prevented the widespread use of hepatocyte-specific agents in patients with cirrhosis. For instance, arterial phase acquisition is compromised by the transient arterial phase motion and subjective dyspnea experienced by some patients after the injection of Gd-EOB-DTPA. Further, administration of lower doses of hepatocyte-specific agents compared with the doses of extracellular agents used may result in less brisk arterial phase enhancement. Finally, the equilibrium phase (usually performed at 3–5 minutes after contrast injection) is replaced by a mixed transitional phase, which has properties of both the equilibrium and the hepatobiliary phases and may compromise the reader's assessment of lesion washout, often crucial in the diagnosis of HCC.[21]

Although all of the major HCC diagnostic and surveillance systems permit the use of extracellular or hepatocyte-specific contrast agents, the diagnosis of HCC is still dependent on the dynamic contrast-enhanced features.[21] The Liver Imaging Reporting and Data System (LI-RADS), an algorithm created by the American College of Radiology to standardize CT and MR image interpretation in patients at risk for HCC, recognizes hepatobiliary phase hypointensity as an ancillary feature of HCC, but the AASLD and OPTN have yet to include this finding as a feature of HCC.[21,26]

14.4.3 Additional Magnetic Resonance Features

Additional imaging features such as the presence of intracellular lipid, iron sparing, T2 signal hyperintensity, and restricted diffusion are findings that support the diagnosis of HCC but are not entirely specific. Some diagnostic guidelines, such as LI-RADS (the details of which are beyond the scope of this discussion[26]), place greater emphasis on these ancillary features than other guidelines do. As suggested earlier, ancillary features are not incorporated into the stricter OPTN guidelines, and the presence of such features cannot be used to grant transplant exception points in the absence of specific HCC enhancement and growth characteristics.

Intracellular Lipid

Signal loss within a mass on out-of-phase compared to in-phase T1-weighted gradient echo images is indicative of intralesional fat. In patients with cirrhosis, a steatotic nodule is likely to be a dysplastic nodule or an early HCC (but not CCA). The lipid usually regresses with progression to overt HCC, but some progressed HCCs may also contain fat (i.e., the steatohepatitic variant of HCC).[22,25]

Iron Sparing

Iron sparing within a mass relative to an otherwise iron-overloaded liver is not entirely specific but favors a diagnosis of premalignancy (e.g., high-grade dysplastic nodule) or malignancy (e.g., HCC, CCA).[22] Sparing is present on T1-weighted gradient echo images when the mass appears hyperintense compared to the hypointense (i.e., siderotic) liver parenchyma on the second/longer echo of the dual-echo sequence.

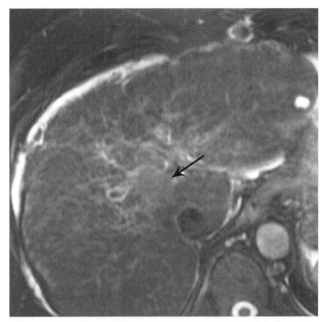

Fig. 14.13 T2-weighted signal hyperintensity associated with hepatocellular carcinoma (HCC). There is mild signal hyperintensity associated with a nodule (*arrow*) in the center of a cirrhotic liver. These results, when reviewed in conjunction with the findings of hypervascularity and washout on the dynamic contrast-enhanced portion of the study (not shown), indicate that the lesion is compatible with HCC; the finding of T2 signal hyperintensity is not entirely specific in isolation.

T2-Signal Hyperintensity

Mild to moderate T2 signal hyperintensity (▶ Fig. 14.13) is suggestive of malignancy (as described earlier) but is not specific for HCC because intrahepatic CCA and metastases can have similar signal intensity (the latter being relatively rare in the cirrhotic population).[27] This finding also lacks sensitivity, as many well-differentiated and moderately differentiated HCCs have T2 signal similar to that of the background liver. Ultimately, the diagnostic value of this finding is limited, as most T2 hyperintense HCCs are progressed lesions readily diagnosed on the dynamic contrast-enhanced portion of the study.[21,22]

Restricted Diffusion

Although contrast-enhanced MR studies outperform DWI for the detection of HCC, some studies have shown that adding DWI to contrast-enhanced T1-weighted images slightly increases the detection rate of HCC.[28] Restricted diffusion is characterized by signal intensity greater than that of background on DWI acquired with at least moderate b-values. The lesion will have a signal similar or lower than that of the surrounding liver on the corresponding ADC map. Unfortunately, the overall sensitivity of DWI for detecting HCC is low, as more well-differentiated lesions do not significantly restrict diffusion.[22] Nonetheless, DWI may play a role in detecting HCC in patients not eligible for contrast-enhanced studies (▶ Fig. 14.14).

All of these additional MR imaging features (from the presence of intracellular lipid to restricted diffusion) are integrated to varying degrees into the currently accepted HCC staging systems and can sometimes be used as a substitute for biopsy. However, biopsy may be warranted if a lesion does not demonstrate typical features of HCC.

14.4.4 Staging

Once the number and size of HCC nodules and the presence of vascular invasion or distant metastases are defined radiographically, a patient's eligibility for liver transplant or other treatment strategies can be determined.[22] Patients with cirrhosis who have a tumor burden within the Milan criteria (single lesion no larger than 5 cm; or up to three separate lesions, none larger than 3 cm) are eligible for transplant and may receive priority on the transplant waiting list in the form of MELD exception points. Patients with tumor burden outside the Milan criteria are not transplant candidates unless they are effectively down staged with locoregional therapies.[7]

Venous invasion is a feature of progressed HCC and helps distinguish HCC from liver metastases, which rarely invade vessels. Although invasion first occurs at the microvascular level (detected microscopically), it is the macrovascular form that is identified by gross pathologic inspection and with imaging. The presence of venous invasion or malignant thrombosis is associated with a worse prognosis and is a contraindication to transplant. As such, differentiating malignant thrombus from bland thrombus, which can develop concomitantly in patients with cirrhosis, has management and prognostic implications. Imaging features of malignant thrombus include contiguity with an HCC, enhancement of the thrombus, and expansion of the vein containing the thrombus (▶ Fig. 14.1b). Although hepatic venous invasion can occur, portal venous involvement is more common.[21,25]

Patients with distant metastases are not eligible for transplant. As such, a chest CT scan and bone scan are performed in

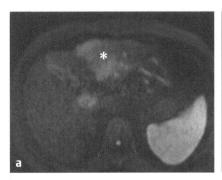
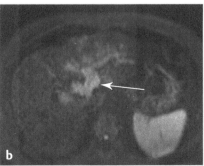

Fig. 14.14 Hepatocellular carcinoma (HCC) detection with diffusion-weighted imaging (DWI). **(a)** A poorly marginated lesion in hepatic segment III (*) has signal intensity greater than that of the surrounding liver on high B-value DWI, compatible with restricted diffusion. **(b)** The adjacent left portal vein is expanded and has similarly high signal intensity (*arrow*). Despite the inability to administer intravenous contrast in this patient with advanced chronic renal disease, these findings were indicative of HCC and tumor in the vein.

patients with HCC being considered for liver transplant to exclude extrahepatic spread.[7]

14.5 Intrahepatic Cholangiocarcinoma

Intrahepatic CCA is the second most common primary hepatic malignancy after HCC. The prevalence of CCA varies in different parts of the world based largely on region-specific risk factors. For instance, infection with liver flukes and hepatolithiasis predispose patients to CCA in Eastern Asia, whereas primary sclerosing cholangitis, liver cirrhosis, chronic hepatitis C virus infection, and heavy alcohol consumption are more common risk factors in Western countries.[29]

Intrahepatic CCA is classified into three types based on morphologic and growth features: mass-forming, periductal infiltrating, and intraductal variants.[30]

14.5.1 Mass-Forming Cholangiocarcinoma

Mass-forming (or peripheral) CCA, the most common variant, usually presents as a large hypoenhancing mass that has irregular peripheral enhancement during the arterial phase of CT or MR examinations. On subsequent phases, there is gradual centripetal enhancement. These masses also commonly enhance more than the background liver during the delayed phases, a reflection of the fibrous stroma that is often present.[29] These masses can cause upstream bile duct dilation and are associated with retraction of the overlying liver capsule (▶ Fig. 14.15).[30] Satellite nodules and vascular encasement without visible tumor thrombus are other imaging features.[29]

On MR imaging, mass-forming CCA may have mild to moderate T2 signal hyperintensity (▶ Fig. 14.16a). However, this is not a feature specific to CCA, as other solid malignancies including HCC and metastases can have a similar appearance. Further, when CCA is small, it may have uniform hypervascular enhancement, similar to HCC. Although differentiating between these lesion types can be difficult, particularly in the cirrhotic population, the presence of delayed enhancement (as opposed to washout) is characteristic of CCA (▶ Fig. 14.16b,c).[21]

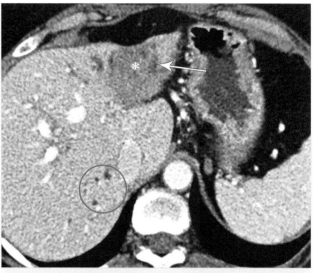

Fig. 14.15 Mass-forming cholangiocarcinoma (CCA). Portal venous phase CT (computed tomography) demonstrates a hypoenhancing mass (*) in the lateral segment of the liver causing overlying capsular retraction and peripheral biliary ductal dilation (*arrow*). Of note, there is also mild biliary ductal dilation scattered throughout the rest of the liver (*circle*) in this patient with a history of primary sclerosing cholangitis, but the degree of dilation is less pronounced than upstream to the mass.

14.5.2 Periductal Infiltrating Cholangiocarcinoma

The periductal infiltrating subtype of CCA is characterized by branchlike growth of the tumor along the biliary tree, resulting in irregular ductal narrowing (▶ Fig. 14.17).[30] On CT and MR imaging, there is periductal thickening and hyperenhancement from tumor infiltration without mass formation. Eventually, ductal narrowing and obliteration will result in obstruction, as evidenced by biliary ductal dilation peripheral to the mass.[29] Although the commonly observed infiltrating hilar CCA has an identical pattern of growth, a purely intrahepatic periductal infiltrating carcinoma is relatively rare because it is by definition exclusively located upstream to the secondary biliary confluence.[31]

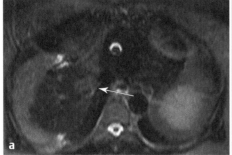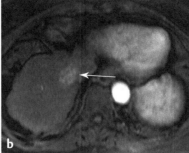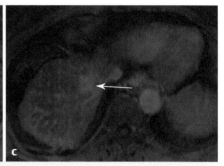

Fig. 14.16 Hypervascular cholangiocarcinoma (CCA). **(a)** A small mass in a cirrhotic liver is mildly T2 hyperintense (*arrow*), a feature suggestive of malignancy but not specific. **(b)** The mass is hyperenhancing on the arterial phase (*arrow*) and **(c)** has persistent enhancement (*arrow*) on the delayed phase, a feature used to distinguish CCA from hepatocellular carcinoma (HCC). Compared to the washout observed in HCC, CCAs classically demonstrate delayed enhancement because of their fibrotic components.

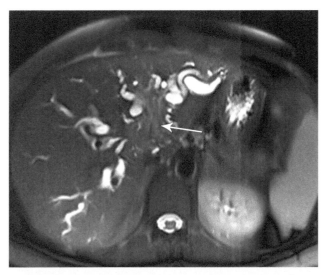

Fig. 14.17 Periductal infiltrating cholangiocarcinoma (CCA). An ill-defined mildly T2 hyperintense infiltrative lesion (*arrow*) tracks from the biliary confluence along the left bile duct system. The mass causes severe upstream biliary ductal dilation and encases the left portal vein.

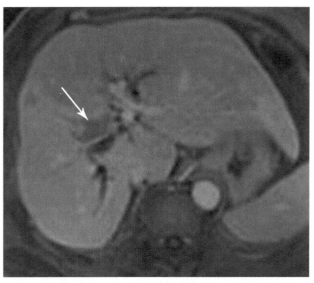

Fig. 14.18 Intraductal cholangiocarcinoma (CCA). An enhancing tubular filling defect (*arrow*) within a dilated right lobe bile duct on venous phase MR (magnetic resonance) imaging is a biopsy-proven CCA.

14.5.3 Intraductal Cholangiocarcinoma

Intraductal CCA is the malignant subtype of intraductal papillary mucinous neoplasm (IPMN) of the bile duct, which is the biliary counterpart to pancreatic IPMN. Its pattern of growth makes it more amenable to resection, and this subtype of CCA has a better prognosis than the mass-forming and periductal infiltrating variants.[32] The appearance that is most often diagnostic of this subtype is an enhancing plaquelike mass or filling defect within a markedly dilated bile duct.[29] Despite the potential for intraductal mucosal spread, the tumor is contained within the bile duct, and the outer margin of the bile duct wall is smooth (▶ Fig. 14.18).[30] The extent of biliary ductal dilation is variable; sometimes there is ductal dilation downstream to the mass due to mucin secretion, in addition to upstream ductal dilation. Enhancement within the intraductal mass is an important feature that distinguishes this tumor from other filling defects, namely, hepatoliths, but these two entities can occur concurrently.[29]

Although hilar CCA (Klatskin's tumor) is sometimes erroneously included in the intrahepatic classification, this tumor type should be classified as an extrahepatic CCA[29] and is beyond the scope of this discussion.

14.6 Other Hepatic Malignancies

Additional rare primary hepatic malignancies, including angiosarcoma, epithelioid hemangioendothelioma, primary hepatic lymphoma, and fibrolamellar HCC, are beyond the scope of this chapter.

14.7 Assessing Response to Treatment

Locoregional therapies, including intra-arterial and ablative therapies, provide an alternative to systemic chemotherapy for the treatment of HCC and hepatic metastases. The traditional anatomic or size-based models for assessing treatment response (e.g., World Health Organization [WHO] and Response Evaluation Criteria in Solid Tumors [RECIST] criteria) may underestimate the efficacy of these therapies.[33] Locoregional therapies induce tumor necrosis, creating nonviable cavities that are similar in size or even larger than the tumor before treatment, so size reduction may not be apparent in the short term. Therefore, functional models, which take into account the amount of tumor necrosis and residual enhancement within lesions after locoregional therapy, are used in conjunction with size-based models to better assess treatment response.[33] This is akin to assessing reduction in lesion attenuation after molecular-targeted therapies (e.g., tyrosine inhibitors for the treatment of metastatic gastrointestinal stromal tumors) as a measure of treatment response, instead of using size measurements, which may be static immediately after treatment.[34] Size-based models alone may be more appropriate for patients receiving classic systemic cytotoxic therapies because these agents significantly reduce the size of lesions and optimally result in their disappearance.[33,34]

The European Association for the Study of the Liver (EASL) and modified RECIST (mRECIST) guidelines are functional treatment response models that take into account treatment-induced tumor necrosis in patients with HCC. They were created as an alternative to conventional response models to better reflect clinical benefits provided by locoregional therapies.[35] Not unexpectedly, research suggests that enhancement-based response criteria outperform size-based guidelines for predicting survival in patients with HCC who are treated with chemoembolization.[36]

Compared to the two-dimensional measurement approach used in the EASL guidelines, the less labor-intensive mRECIST assessment measures only the longest diameter of the remaining hypervascular mass after treatment.[34,37] By mRECIST guidelines, the absence of any residual hypervascular mass indicates a complete response (▶ Fig. 14.19), a greater than 30% decrease in the longest diameter of the viable (i.e., hyperenhancing)

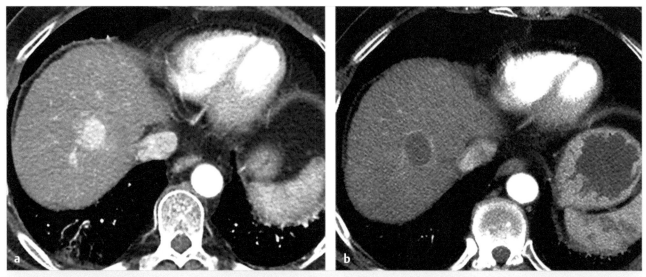

Fig. 14.19 Monitoring treatment response after locoregional therapy. **(a)** Arterial phase computed tomography (CT) performed before transarterial chemoembolization shows a 2.2-cm hypervascular mass compatible with HCC (hepatocellular carcinoma). **(b)** On arterial phase CT performed after transarterial chemoembolization, the lesion is marginally larger with a thin rim of peripheral enhancement but has no residual internal hypervascularity. This is considered a complete treatment response when using enhancement-based response criteria such as modified Response Evaluation Criteria in Solid Tumors (mRECIST) and EASL (European Association for the Study of Liver) but is considered stable disease when using size-based criteria such as RECIST.

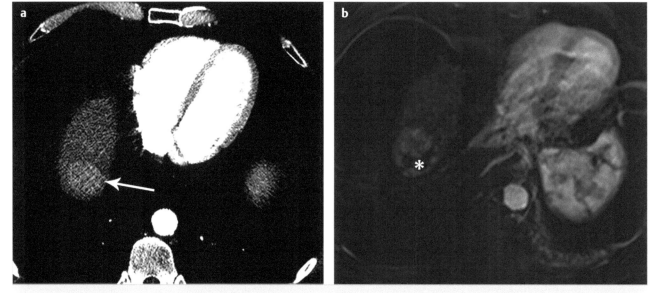

Fig. 14.20 Monitoring treatment response after locoregional therapy. **(a)** Arterial phase CT (computed tomography) performed before transarterial chemoembolization shows a 3-cm hypervascular mass (*arrow*) in the right hepatic dome compatible with HCC (hepatocellular carcinoma). **(b)** On the arterial phase, subtraction images created from magnetic resonance (MR) imaging performed after transarterial chemoembolization, there is still a hypervascular nodule along the anterior margin of the treated lesion that is only slightly smaller than the original lesion when measured in both axes. There is also a small dark crescent along the posterior margin of the treated lesion (*) that is devoid of signal on the subtraction MR image, compatible with treatment necrosis. However, there is an insufficient amount of necrosis to constitute a partial response by mRECIST (modified Response Evaluation Criteria in Solid Tumors) and EASL (European Association for the Study of Liver) criteria (calculations not shown), and so this is considered stable disease. This is also considered stable disease according to the RECIST criteria. Repeat transarterial chemoembolization was subsequently performed.

lesion indicates a partial response, and a greater than 20% increase in the longest diameter of the viable lesion indicates progressive disease. If the changes in diameter fall between the partial response and progressive disease categories, the disease is considered stable (► Fig. 14.20).[35,36]

Enhancement is usually assessed by comparing CT density or MR signal intensity before and after contrast administration. Compared to hypovascular malignancies (e.g., colorectal metasta-ses), hypervascular lesions such as HCC and hypervascular metastases are easier to assess after locoregional treatment because the absence of hypervascularity is more conspicuous. Perceiving decreased or absent enhancement in hypoenhancing tumors is more difficult. In either case, subtraction images obtained during MR imaging have the potential to improve detec-tion of residual enhancement (► Fig. 14.20b). This is especially true when the treated lesion displays T1 signal hyperintensity from hemorrhage (commonly present after locoregional therapy) that can prohibit the interpreter from perceiving enhancement.[33]

A thin (<5 mm thickness) rim of enhancement is often seen around treated lesions after intra-arterial therapy; this rim may persist for several months. This pattern of enhancement is usually considered a benign finding from posttreatment inflammation and is usually not indicative of residual tumor (▶ Fig. 14.19b).[33] Additionally, transient hepatic attenuation/intensity differences are commonly encountered in the early postembolization period because of altered perfusion. These patterns appear as wedge-shaped or geographic areas of hyperenhancement in the liver parenchyma surrounding the treated lesion and usually resolve within 6 to 12 months. They are usually of little clinical significance, but radiologists should be cognizant of their appearance as they could be misinterpreted as residual or recurrent tumor.[33,38]

Assessing response in patients after radioembolization differs from assessing response after other types of transarterial embolization (e.g., transarterial chemoembolization and bland embolization) because the radiation-induced necrosis takes longer and tumoral enhancement may persist for months after radioembolization. Comparatively, any intralesional enhancement on surveillance imaging after transarterial chemoembolization or bland embolization is suggestive of residual tumor, as the embolic effects of these therapies induce necrosis more rapidly.[33]

As mentioned earlier, the cavities that are created after locoregional therapy are similar in size or larger than the pretreatment tumor, the latter being especially true after ablative therapy. An ablation zone larger than the treated tumor is desirable to ensure a sufficient margin around the tumor. The ablation zones typically involute over time;[33] enlargement or change in the morphology of the zone is an indicator of disease recurrence.

DWI is an additional technique that can be used to assess treatment response, as decrease in restriction (i.e., increased ADC value) after therapy is an indicator of necrosis. Because DWI can potentially differentiate between the viable and necrotic portions of a mass after locoregional therapy, it may play a role in assessing treatment response in patients not eligible for contrast administration or may serve as an adjunct to contrast-enhanced images.[19,33]

References

[1] Liu PS. Liver mass evaluation in patients without cirrhosis: a technique-based method. Radiol Clin North Am. 2015; 53(5):903–918

[2] Itoh S, Ikeda M, Achiwa M, Satake H, Iwano S, Ishigaki T. Late-arterial and portal-venous phase imaging of the liver with a multislice CT scanner in patients without circulatory disturbances: automatic bolus tracking or empirical scan delay? Eur Radiol. 2004; 14(9):1665–1673

[3] Hussain HK, Londy FJ, Francis IR, et al. Hepatic arterial phase MR imaging with automated bolus-detection three-dimensional fast gradient-recalled-echo sequence: comparison with test-bolus method. Radiology. 2003; 226(2):558–566

[4] Earls JP, Rofsky NM, DeCorato DR, Krinsky GA, Weinreb JC. Hepatic arterial-phase dynamic gadolinium-enhanced MR imaging: optimization with a test examination and a power injector. Radiology. 1997; 202(1):268–273

[5] Hong HS, Kim HS, Kim MJ, De Becker J, Mitchell DG, Kanematsu M. Single breath-hold multiarterial dynamic MRI of the liver at 3T using a 3D fat-suppressed keyhole technique. J Magn Reson Imaging. 2008; 28(2):396–402

[6] Wald C, Russo MW, Heimbach JK, Hussain HK, Pomfret EA, Bruix J. New OPTN/UNOS policy for liver transplant allocation: standardization of liver imaging, diagnosis, classification, and reporting of hepatocellular carcinoma. Radiology. 2013; 266(2):376–382

[7] Rude MK, Crippin JS. Liver transplantation for hepatocellular carcinoma. Curr Gastroenterol Rep. 2015; 17(3):11

[8] Namasivayam S, Martin DR, Saini S. Imaging of liver metastases: MRI. Cancer Imaging. 2007; 7:2–9

[9] Danet IM, Semelka RC, Leonardou P, et al. Spectrum of MRI appearances of untreated metastases of the liver. AJR Am J Roentgenol. 2003; 181(3):809–817

[10] Gore RM, Thakrar KH, Wenzke DR, Newmark GM, Mehta UK, Berlin JW. That liver lesion on MDCT in the oncology patient: is it important? Cancer Imaging. 2012; 12:373–384

[11] Sica GT, Ji H, Ros PR. CT and MR imaging of hepatic metastases. AJR Am J Roentgenol. 2000; 174(3):691–698

[12] Vogl TJ, Kümmel S, Hammerstingl R, et al. Liver tumors: comparison of MR imaging with Gd-EOB-DTPA and Gd-DTPA. Radiology. 1996; 200(1):59–67

[13] Ringe KI, Husarik DB, Sirlin CB, Merkle EM. Gadoxetate disodium-enhanced MRI of the liver: part 1, protocol optimization and lesion appearance in the noncirrhotic liver. AJR Am J Roentgenol. 2010; 195(1):13–28

[14] Patel S, Cheek S, Osman H, Jeyarajah DR. MRI with gadoxetate disodium for colorectal liver metastasis: is it the new "imaging modality of choice"? J Gastrointest Surg. 2014; 18(12):2130–2135

[15] Donati OF, Hany TF, Reiner CS, et al. Value of retrospective fusion of PET and MR images in detection of hepatic metastases: comparison with 18F-FDG PET/CT and Gd-EOB-DTPA-enhanced MRI. J Nucl Med. 2010; 51(5):692–699

[16] Siegelman ES, Chauhan A. MR characterization of focal liver lesions: pearls and pitfalls. Magn Reson Imaging Clin N Am. 2014; 22(3):295–313

[17] Curvo-Semedo L, Brito JB, Seco MF, Marques CB, Caseiro-Alves F. The hypointense liver lesion on T2-weighted MR images and what it means. Radiographics. 2010; 30(1):e38

[18] Moore WA, Khatri G, Madhuranthakam AJ, Sims RD, Pedrosa I. Added value of diffusion-weighted acquisitions in MRI of the abdomen and pelvis. AJR Am J Roentgenol. 2014; 202(5):995–1006

[19] Taouli B, Koh DM. Diffusion-weighted MR imaging of the liver. Radiology. 2010; 254(1):47–66

[20] Khatri G, Merrick L, Miller FH. MR imaging of hepatocellular carcinoma. Magn Reson Imaging Clin N Am. 2010; 18(3):421–450, x

[21] Bashir MR, Hussain HK. Imaging in patients with cirrhosis: current evidence. Radiol Clin North Am. 2015; 53(5):919–931

[22] Choi JY, Lee JM, Sirlin CBCT. CT and MR imaging diagnosis and staging of hepatocellular carcinoma: part II. Extracellular agents, hepatobiliary agents, and ancillary imaging features. Radiology. 2014; 273(1):30–50

[23] Marrero JA, Hussain HK, Nghiem HV, Umar R, Fontana RJ, Lok AS. Improving the prediction of hepatocellular carcinoma in cirrhotic patients with an arterially-enhancing liver mass. Liver Transpl. 2005; 11(3):281–289

[24] Reynolds AR, Furlan A, Fetzer DT, et al. Infiltrative hepatocellular carcinoma: what radiologists need to know. Radiographics. 2015; 35(2):371–386

[25] Choi JY, Lee JM, Sirlin CBCT. CT and MR imaging diagnosis and staging of hepatocellular carcinoma: part I. Development, growth, and spread: key pathologic and imaging aspects. Radiology. 2014; 272(3):635–654

[26] American College of Radiology. Liver Imaging and Reporting Data System. www.acr.org/quality-safety/resources/LIRADS. Published 2014. Accessed February 2, 2016

[27] Ruebner BH, Green R, Miyai K, Caranasos G, Abbey H. The rarity of intrahepatic metastasis in cirrhosis of the liver. A statistical explanation with some comments on the interpretation of necropsy data. Am J Pathol. 1961; 39:739–746

[28] Park MS, Kim S, Patel J, et al. Hepatocellular carcinoma: detection with diffusion-weighted versus contrast-enhanced magnetic resonance imaging in pretransplant patients. Hepatology. 2012; 56(1):140–148

[29] Chung YE, Kim MJ, Park YN, et al. Varying appearances of cholangiocar-cinoma: radiologic-pathologic correlation. Radiographics. 2009; 29(3):683–700

[30] Lim JH. Cholangiocarcinoma: morphologic classification according to growth pattern and imaging findings. AJR Am J Roentgenol. 2003; 181(3):819–827

[31] Han JK, Choi BI, Kim AY, et al. Cholangiocarcinoma: pictorial essay of CT and cholangiographic findings. Radiographics. 2002; 22(1):173–187

[32] Takanami K, Yamada T, Tsuda M, et al. Intraductal papillary mucininous neoplasm of the bile ducts: multimodality assessment with pathologic correlation. Abdom Imaging. 2011; 36(4):447–456

[33] Adam SZ, Miller FH. Imaging of the liver following interventional therapy for hepatic neoplasms. Radiol Clin North Am. 2015; 53(5):1061–1076

[34] Gonzalez-Guindalini FD, Botelho MP, Harmath CB, et al. Assessment of liver tumor response to therapy: role of quantitative imaging. Radiographics. 2013; 33(6):1781–1800

[35] Minocha J, Lewandowski RJ. Assessing imaging response to therapy. Radiol Clin North Am. 2015; 53(5):1077–1088

[36] Shim JH, Lee HC, Kim SO, et al. Which response criteria best help predict survival of patients with hepatocellular carcinoma following chemoembolization? A validation study of old and new models. Radiology. 2012; 262(2):708–718

[37] Lencioni R, Llovet JM. Modified RECIST (mRECIST) assessment for hepatocellular carcinoma. Semin Liver Dis. 2010; 30(1):52–60

[38] Hwang SH, Yu JS, Chung J, Chung JJ, Kim JH, Kim KW. Transient hepatic attenuation difference (THAD) following transcatheter arterial chemoembolization for hepatic malignancy: changes on serial CT examinations. Eur Radiol. 2008; 18(8):1596–1603

15 Hepatocellular Carcinoma: Staging and Clinical Management

K. V. Narayanan Menon, Arvind R. Murali, Baljendra S. Kapoor, and Federico N. Aucejo

15.1 Introduction: Definition and Epidemiology

Hepatocellular carcinoma (HCC) is the most common primary malignancy of the liver and is the fifth most common cancer in men and the seventh most common cancer in women worldwide.[1] Men are more commonly affected than women. The male-to-female ratio has been reported to vary regionally from 2:1 to 4:1,[2] with an overall male-to-female ratio of 2.4:1. In the United States, the incidence rates of liver cancer per 100,000 person-years are 2.0 for women and 3.7 for men, with a male-to-female ratio of 2.83:1.

High-incidence areas of HCC include Sub-Saharan Africa and eastern Asia, whereas Canada and the United States are low-incidence areas for HCC; this is because of the increased prevalence of hepatitis B in Sub-Saharan Africa and eastern Asia. The presence of hepatitis B and C increases the risk for cirrhosis, which is seen in 80 to 90% of patients with HCC. However, recent data have shown a downward trend of HCC in eastern Asia, whereas the incidence is increasing in North America.[3]

Viral hepatitis is the main risk factor for the development of cirrhosis and HCC, although other risk factors such as alcohol abuse, diabetes mellitus, and obesity can also lead to the development of HCC. Diabetes mellitus can predispose patients to the development of nonalcoholic steatohepatitis, which can subsequently progress to cirrhosis, thus increasing the risk for HCC. It has been reported that obese individuals (body mass index > 30 kg/m^2) have higher HCC-related mortality rates than leaner individuals.[4] With the increasing incidence of obesity, the mortality rates associated with HCC could very well increase, as well.

Other etiologies that predispose patients to the development of HCC include hereditary hemochromatosis, alpha-1-antitrypsin deficiency, primary biliary cirrhosis, autoimmune hepatitis, glycogen storage disease, and other hereditary metabolic conditions.

15.2 Surveillance and Staging of Hepatocellular Carcinoma

Surveillance should be performed in patients at high risk for developing liver cancer (▶ Table 15.1). Decision analysis models have demonstrated that surveillance for HCC in patients with cirrhosis is cost effective and improves survival if the incidence of HCC exceeds 1.5% per year.[5] Based on this model, all patients with cirrhosis irrespective of the etiology should be screened biannually. This includes patients with cirrhosis secondary to hepatitis C, hepatitis B, hemochromatosis, primary biliary cirrhosis, primary sclerosing cholangitis, nonalcoholic steatohepatitis, alpha-1-antitrypsin deficiency, and autoimmune hepatitis. Surveillance is also indicated in select hepatitis B carriers (▶ Table 15.1); in these patients, a history of HCC in a first-degree relative is an independent risk factor for the development of HCC.[6] Also, Africans with hepatitis B have been shown

to develop HCC early in life.[7] Although initiation of HCC surveillance at a younger age has been recommended for these patients,[8] the exact age at which surveillance should begin has not been clearly established. In addition, it is not clear whether Black patients born outside of Africa are at an increased risk for HCC.

HCC surveillance has been shown to decrease mortality. In a randomized controlled trial in China, patients with hepatitis B were either not screened or were screened with abdominal ultrasound and analysis of alpha-fetoprotein (AFP) levels; screening was associated with a 37% decrease in mortality.[9] Studies have also established that patients with early-stage HCC have better survival than those with more advanced disease,[10,11] which is largely explained by the availability of effective treatment, including liver transplant, for patients with early-stage cancer. Therefore, asymptomatic patients with early-stage disease who are identified by a surveillance program should have improved survival compared with symptomatic patients.

The most commonly used surveillance methods for HCC are analysis of serum AFP levels and liver ultrasound. Analysis of serum AFP alone has not been shown to be useful, whereas the combination of AFP plus ultrasound has been shown to reduce mortality when used for HCC surveillance.[9] A recent study reported that the combination of AFP and ultrasound had a higher sensitivity (90%) when compared to ultrasound alone (58%) but at the expense of a lower specificity.[12] Studies have also shown that AFP alone has a low sensitivity (54%) for diagnosing HCC.[13] Tumor size has been described as one of the factors limiting the sensitivity of AFP,[13] suggesting that evaluation of AFP might not be useful in the detection of early-stage HCC. Ongoing studies suggest that analysis of AFP-L3, an isoform of AFP, may be helpful in patients with AFP levels in the intermediate range.[14]

The current American Association for the Study of Liver Diseases (AASLD) guidelines recommend that ultrasound alone be performed once every 6 months for HCC surveillance. However, it may be premature to conclude that AFP analysis is no longer required for surveillance of HCC, as liver ultrasound is operator dependent, and its efficacy may be negatively affected in overweight or obese individuals.

Patients at high risk for the development of HCC should enter surveillance programs.[8] Patients on the waiting list for a liver transplant are also screened for HCC, as priority, or exclusion

Table 15.1 Indications for surveillance for hepatocellular carcinoma (HCC)

Cirrhosis from any etiology
Asian male hepatitis B carriers aged > 40 y
Asian female hepatitis B carriers aged > 50 y
Hepatitis B carriers with a family history of HCC
African/North American Black patients with hepatitis B
Source: Data from Bruix et al.[27]

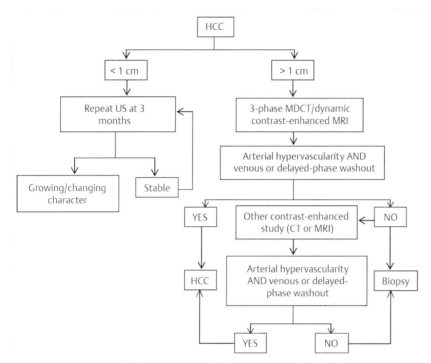

Fig. 15.1 Algorithm for investigation of small nodules found on screening in patients at risk for HCC. HCC, hepatocellular carcinoma; MDCT, multidetector computed tomography scan. (Reproduced with permission from Bruix J, Sherman M. Management of hepatocellular carcinoma: an update. Hepatology 2011;53:1020-1022.)

from the list is dictated by the extent of HCC as defined by the Milan criteria.[6]

Contrast-enhanced multiphase computed tomography (CT) or magnetic resonance imaging (MRI) can be used as an alternative screening modality for individuals in whom ultrasound is suboptimal or nondiagnostic (e.g., patients with extremely fatty or nodular livers).

Any abnormality (e.g., a new or enlarging nodule) detected by screening requires additional investigation and/or follow-up to confirm the presence of HCC as follows (▶ Fig. 15.1):

- Nodules measuring < 1 cm by ultrasound surveillance should be reassessed with ultrasound in 3 to 6 months. If the nodule is stable for 2 years, routine 6-month surveillance is resumed.
- Nodules measuring > 1 cm should be investigated with multiphase contrast-enhanced CT or MRI using the technical specifications outlined by Organ Procurement and Transplantation Network (OPTN)/United Network for Organ Sharing (UNOS; ▶ Table 15.2).[15]
- Although MRI provides better contrast resolution than CT, MRI is contraindicated in patients with certain metallic implants (e.g., pacemakers) and is more time consuming than CT. MR image quality is degraded by respiratory artifacts, some metallic objects (e.g., surgical clips), and perihepatic ascites, and MRI is not well tolerated by patients with claustrophobia. All of these factors should be taken into consideration when choosing the appropriate imaging modality for the patient.
- The risk of nephrogenic systemic fibrosis and radiocontrast-induced nephropathy in individuals undergoing contrast-enhanced MRI and CT, respectively, is a special concern in the subset of patients with severe renal insufficiency (glomerular filtration rate < 30 mL/min/1.73 m^2). The relative risks and benefits of using intravenous contrast in this patient population must be considered by the referring physician, the radiologist, and a nephrologist. Contrast-enhanced

examinations that are determined to be critical to clinical management take precedence over cautionary measures and can be performed using prophylactic techniques after the radiologist obtains an informed consent from the patient.[16] In some instances, noncontrast MRI of the liver may be of value.

- If the imaging appearance is typical of HCC, the lesion should be treated as HCC.
- Radiologic criteria typical of HCC include late arterial phase enhancement and delayed phase washout or hypervascularity with short-term growth as outlined by the OPTN classification system for nodules identified in the setting of cirrhosis (▶ Table 15.2). If features are atypical for HCC, a second contrast-enhanced study can be performed or the lesion can be biopsied. If the biopsy is negative, the lesion should be reassessed every 3 to 6 months until the nodule resolves, grows, or exhibits imaging characteristics typical of HCC.

15.2.1 Staging

Multiple staging systems are available for the management of HCC. However, no single staging system has been found to reliably predict outcomes of HCC. This is largely because the prognosis of HCC depends not only on the stage of the cancer but also on the degree of the underlying liver dysfunction. Various staging systems in use take into account the size of the tumors, severity of underlying liver disease, extension of the tumor into adjacent structures, and presence or absence of metastases. The most common staging systems used are the TNM staging system, the Okuda staging system, the Barcelona Clinic Liver Cancer (BCLC) system, the Chinese University Prognostic Index (CUPI), the Cancer of the Liver Italian Program (CLIP) score, and the biomarker-combined Japanese Integrated Staging (JIS) system (▶ Table 15.3). The BCLC has been externally validated in Western populations, whereas the JIS has been externally

Table 15.2 OPTN HCC classification for patients undergoing evaluation for liver transplant

Class and description	Comment
OPTN class 0: incomplete or technically inadequate study	Repeat study required for adequate assessment; automatic priority model for end-stage liver disease points cannot be assigned on basis of an imaging study categorized as class 0
OPTN class 5: meets radiologic criteria for HCC	May qualify for automatic exception, depending on stage
Class 5A: ≥ 1 and < 2 cm measured on late arterial or portal venous phase images	Increased contrast enhancement in late hepatic arterial phase AND washout during later phases of contrast enhancement AND peripheral rim enhancement (capsule or pseudocapsule)
Class 5A-g: same size as class 5A	Increased contrast enhancement in late hepatic arterial phase AND growth by ≥ 50% documented on serial CT or MR images obtained ≤ 6 mo apart
Class 5B: maximum diameter ≥ 2 and ≤ 5 cm	Increased contrast enhancement in late hepatic arterial phase AND either washout during later contrast phases OR peripheral rim enhancement (capsule or pseudocapsule) OR growth by ≥ 50% documented on serial CT or MR images obtained ≤ 6 mo apart (OPTN class 5B-g)
Class 5T: previous regional treatment for HCC	Any residual lesion or perfusion defect at site of previous UNOS class 5 lesion
Class 5X: maximum diameter ≥ 5 cm	Increased contrast enhancement in late hepatic arterial phase AND either washout during later contrast phases OR peripheral rim enhancement (capsule or pseudocapsule)

Abbreviations: CT, computed tomography; HCC, hepatocellular carcinoma; MR, magnetic resonance; OPTN, Organ Procurement and Transplantation Network; UNOS, United Network for Organ Sharing.

Notes: OPTN class number denotes whether an imaging examination is nondiagnostic (OPTN class 0) or whether the study includes an image that contains at least one treated or untreated HCC lesion (OPTN class 5). OPTN class 5 is further subdivided by adding a capital letter to denote UNOS stage 1 disease (OPTN class 5A), UNOS stage 2 disease (OPTN class 5B), a treated HCC (OPTN class 5T), or HCC beyond acceptable size for transplant (OPTN class 5X). The "g" in OPTN class 5A-g and OPTN class 5B-g is used to indicate that evidence of lesion growth was used to arrive at the HCC diagnosis.

validated in Eastern populations. Because of regional differences in the risk factors for HCC and other comorbidities, a common global classification system has not yet been established.[17]

The TNM staging system is commonly used for all solid malignancies. It involves assessment of the primary tumor size (T), regional lymph node involvement (N), and metastases beyond the regional lymph nodes (M). TNM staging for HCC is performed clinically by means of imaging studies, but the presence of a cirrhotic nodular liver and benign enlargement of lymph nodes that are commonly seen in patients with advanced cirrhosis make clinical TNM staging in these patients challenging. Pathological TNM staging is performed in patients who have undergone resection of HCC. Pathological TNM staging has been shown to be superior to the Okuda, CLIP, and CUPI systems among patients who have undergone curative

resection of HCC.[19] The main drawback of pathological TNM staging is that it can be used in only a minority of patients, as very few patients with HCC undergo surgical resection. In addition, TNM staging does not take into account the severity of liver dysfunction and hence may not be accurate in patients with advanced cirrhosis.

The Okuda staging system is based on both tumor characteristics and the degree of liver dysfunction. This classification involves four factors: tumor size (involving > 50 or < 50% of the liver), serum albumin level, serum bilirubin level, and presence or absence of ascites. Patients with tumor involving < 50% of the liver, albumin level > 3 g/dL, bilirubin level < 3 mg/dL, and no ascites are considered to have Okuda stage I disease; these patients have higher survival rates than those with Okuda stage 2 (one to two factors) or stage 3 (three to four factors) disease.[20] The major drawback of this classification system is that a number of cases are identified as Okuda stage 1 through HCC screening, and this system lacks discrimination among Okuda stage 1 cases.

The BCLC staging system for HCC is the most commonly used staging system. It is endorsed by the European Association for the Study of the Liver (EASL) and the AASLD. The BCLC system incorporates tumor characteristics (tumor size, tumor extent, portal venous invasion, and presence or absence of metastasis), severity of liver dysfunction (Child–Pugh score, portal hypertension), performance status of the individual, and constitutional symptoms from HCC into the disease score.[21] Based on these factors, cases are divided into four categories (BCLC class A, early disease; class B, intermediate disease; class C, advanced disease; and class D, end-stage disease). Treatment recommendations have been provided for each BCLC class. The BCLC classification system has been externally validated in Western populations and has been identified as the best independent prognostic predictive indicator versus six other staging systems in the United States.[22]

The CLIP system uses four factors (Child–Pugh score, tumor morphology, AFP level, and presence/absence of portal vein thrombosis) to determine HCC disease stage.[23] Each factor is assigned a score of 0, 1, or 2, with the total score ranging from 0 to 6. This scoring system has been validated prospectively in an Italian cohort, but in the Japanese population, the median survival for each CLIP score was higher than that in the Western population.[17,24] In addition, the group with the best prognosis in the CLIP staging system is considered to have advanced HCC; therefore, the ability of this system to identify patients who would benefit from curative therapy has been questioned.[25]

The JIS system was developed and proposed by the Liver Cancer Study Group of Japan.[25] This system incorporates tumor characteristics (Japanese TNM staging system) and the degree of liver dysfunction (Child–Pugh class). The JIS system has been validated in the Japanese population, with excellent discrimination demonstrated among patients with early-stage HCC. The JIS system has been further modified by adding biomarkers (AFP, lecithin reactive AFP, and des-gamma-carboxy prothrombin) to the model, and this modified system was shown to have a better prognostic value than the original JIS model.[26] However, the JIS and modified JIS systems have not been validated in Western populations.

The multitude of factors affecting prognosis in patients with HCC has made it challenging to develop a universally accepted

Table 15.3 Proposed staging classifications for HCC

Staging classification	Tumor staging	Variables measured		
		Liver function	Performance status	Serum tumor markers
CLIP	Tumor morphology (uninodular and extension ≤ 50%, multinodular and extension ≤ 50%, massive or extension > 50%), portal vein thrombosis	Child–Pugh	No	AFP
BCLC	Tumor size, number of nodules, portal vein thrombosis	Child–Pugh, bilirubin, portal hypertension	PST	No
GRETCH	Portal vein thrombosis	Bilirubin, alkaline phosphatase	Karnofsky	AFP
U.S. nomogram	Resection margins status, tumor size > 5 cm, satellite lesions, vascular invasion	No	Age, operative blood loss	AFP
Okuda	Tumor size (< 50 or > 50% of liver)	Ascites, albumin, bilirubin	No	No
CUPI	TNM fifth edition	Ascites, bilirubin, alkaline phosphatase	Presence of symptoms	AFP
JIS	Japanese TNM fourth edition	Child–Pugh	No	No
bm-JIS	Japanese TNM fourth edition	Child–Pugh	No	AFP, AFP-L3, DCP
SLiDe	Stage and liver damage categories from the Japanese TNM fourth edition	No	No	DCP
Tokyo	Size and number of tumors	Albumin, bilirubin	No	No
BALAD	No	Albumin, bilirubin	No	AFP, AFP-L3, DCP
ALCPS	Tumor size, portal vein thrombosis, lung metastases	Ascites, Child–Pugh, alkaline phosphatase, bilirubin, urea	Abdominal pain, weight loss	AFP

Abbreviations: AFP, alpha-fetoprotein; AFP-L3, lens culinaris agglutinin-reactive AFP; ALCPS, Advanced Liver Cancer Prognostic System; BALAD, bilirubin, albumin, AFP-L3, AFP, DCP; BCLC, Barcelona Clinic Liver Cancer; bm-JIS, biomarker-combined JIS; CLIP, Cancer of the Liver Italian Program; CUPI, Chinese University Prognostic Index; DCP, des-gamma-carboxy prothrombin; GRETCH, Groupe d'Etude et de Traitement du Carcinome Hépatocellulaire; HCC, hepatocellular carcinoma; JIS, Japanese Integrated Staging; PST, performance status test; SLiDe, Stage, Liver damage, DCP; TNM, tumor–node–metastasis.

Source: Data from Meier V, Ramadori G. Clinical staging of hepatocellular carcinoma. Dig Dis 2009; 27:131–141.[18]

staging system. In addition to tumor morphological characteristics and the severity of liver dysfunction, tumor biology and the etiology of liver disease (such as nonalcoholic fatty liver disease) may influence prognosis. Further research is clearly needed to better define staging systems for HCC and to determine appropriate treatment strategies for each stage of HCC.

15.3 Management of Hepatocellular Carcinoma

Multiple therapeutic modalities are currently available for the management of HCC (▶ Table 15.4). These can be divided into two main categories: curative and palliative treatments. Curative treatment includes surgical resection, liver transplant, and radiofrequency ablation. All other treatment modalities are palliative, including transarterial chemoembolization, stereotactic body radiation therapy, and medical therapy with sorafenib. The decision to choose a particular treatment modality depends on tumor characteristics, the degree of liver dysfunction, and patient performance. The BCLC system is widely used for treatment decisions, as this system incorporates both clinical features and tumor stage.[27] We have provided a simplified management algorithm in ▶ Fig. 15.2.

Table 15.4 Treatment modalities for the management of hepatocellular carcinoma (HCC)

Treatment modality	Procedure
Surgical resection[a]	Orthotopic liver transplant[a]
Locoregional therapies:	
• Ablative therapies	Radiofrequency ablation Percutaneous ethanol injection Microwave ablation Cryotherapy Laser ablation Electroporation Light-activated drug therapy Stereotactic body radiation therapy
• Perfusion-based therapies	Transarterial chemoembolization Drug-eluting bead transarterial chemoembolization Bland embolization Radioembolization
Systemic therapies	Sorafenib Cytotoxic chemotherapy

[a]Indicates curative treatment for HCC.

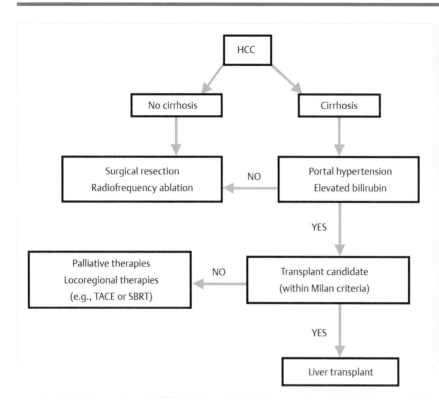

Fig. 15.2 Management algorithm for HCC. HCC, hepatocellular carcinoma; TACE, transarterial chemoembolization; SBRT, stereotactic body radiation therapy.

15.3.1 Surgical Management

Surgical management is the mainstay of treatment for HCC.[28] Although only approximately one-third of patients are candidates for either liver resection or transplant (advanced tumor stage and/or liver dysfunction with portal hypertension often precludes surgery), surgical therapy can be curative.[29]

Liver Resection

Liver resection is the treatment of choice for patients presenting with or without minimal portal hypertension as a consequence of cirrhosis.[30] In general, patients with chronic liver disease with well-compensated liver function and a transhepatic venous pressure gradient less than 10 mm Hg are able to tolerate liver resection.[31] The patient's ability to tolerate liver resection can also be measured through analysis of indocyanine green clearance and retention at 15 minutes; this is a sensitive tool to evaluate liver function and predict tolerability of liver resection.[32,33]

Surgery-related mortality and morbidity rates depend on multiple factors such as Child–Pugh class, pretransplant renal insufficiency, malnutrition, and complexity of the surgical procedure. Reported surgery-related mortality and morbidity rates range from 1 to 2% and 20 to 30%, respectively.[34,35,36]

Complete tumor resection (R0 resection) is associated with a postsurgical 5-year overall survival rate of more than 50%.[37] However, the risk of disease recurrence is high because of metastasis from the primary tumor or de novo tumor formation as a consequence of a defective pro-oncogenic field.[38] Anatomic liver resection is associated with better oncologic results than nonanatomic liver resection, as HCC disseminates mainly via the portal venous system.[39]

When a major liver resection is required, volumetric calculations of the future liver remnant (FLR) should be performed. If the calculated FLR is less than 30% of the whole liver volume, the risk of liver failure is significant. In these cases, portal vein embolization of the lobe that will be removed is indicated to induce hypertrophy of the FLR.[40] Hypertrophy takes approximately 4 to 6 weeks, with a growth rate of approximately 2% per week.[41]

A minimally invasive approach to HCC liver resection via laparoscopy or robotic technology has been practiced for a number of years. Published data suggest that clinical and oncologic outcomes are not inferior when these techniques are compared with open surgery.[42] However, proper patient selection is important; these techniques are most successful in patients with peripherally located unifocal tumors that are sized less than 5 cm.[43]

Liver Transplant

Liver transplant remains the most important surgical therapy for patients with HCC and end-stage liver disease and for those in whom liver resection has failed.[28,29] However, a main drawback is the scarcity of liver grafts,[44] with a transplant waitlist dropout rate as high as 20% because of tumor progression and/or evolution of end-stage organ disease.[31]

When the use of liver transplant for HCC was first introduced, the initial results were dismal because of poor selection criteria (aggressive tumor burden and biology, leading to high tumor recurrence rates after transplant).[45] However, a landmark study published by Mazzaferro et al[44] in 1996 demonstrated that patients fulfilling the Milan criteria (single lesion ≤ 5 cm or up to three lesions no larger than 3 cm each and absence of tumor vascular invasion) achieved 4-year post-transplant survival rates higher than 75% and post-transplant tumor recurrence rates of

Table 15.5 Proposed expanded criteria for cadaveric and living donor liver transplant in patients with HCC

Study	Year	Description	Donor category
Mazzaferro et al[44]	1996	1 lesion ≤ 5 cm, or 2–3 lesions ≤ 3 cm each	Cadaveric
Yao et al[47]	2001	1 lesion ≤ 6.5 cm, or 2–3 lesions ≤ 4.5 cm each; total tumor diameter ≤ 8 cm	Cadaveric
Herrero et al[48]	2001	1 lesion ≤ 6 cm, or 2–3 lesions ≤ 5 cm each	Cadaveric
Roayaie et al[49]	2002	Any number of lesions 5–7 cm each	Cadaveric
Kneteman et al[50]	2004	1 lesion < 7.5 cm, or multiple lesions < 5 cm each	Cadaveric
Onaca et al[51]	2007	1 lesion ≤ 6 cm, or 2–4 lesions ≤ 5 cm each (according to pathological examination)	Cadaveric
Silva et al[52]	2008	1–3 lesions ≤ 5 cm each; total tumor diameter ≤ 10 cm	Cadaveric
Zheng et al[53]	2008	Total tumor diameter ≤ 8 cm; AFP ≤ 400 ng/mL; histopathologic grade I or II if total tumor diameter > 8 cm	Cadaveric
Mazzaferro et al[54]	2009	The sum of the size and number of tumors should not exceed 7	Both
Soejima et al[55]	2007	Any number of lesions ≤ 5 cm each	Living
Jonas et al[56]	2007	Any number of lesions ≤ 6 cm each; total tumor diameter ≤ 15 cm	Living
Kwon et al[57]	2007	Any number of lesions ≤ 5 cm each; AFP ≤ 400 ng/mL	Living
Sugawara et al[58]	2007	Up to 5 lesions ≤ 5 cm each	Living
Takada et al[59]	2007	Up to 10 lesions ≤ 5 cm each	Living

Abbreviations: AFP, alpha-fetoprotein; HCC, hepatocellular carcinoma.

Table 15.6 Proposed expanded criteria including biomarkers for HCC liver transplant

Study	Year	Radiologic criteria	Biomarker criteria
Kwon et al[57]	2007	Any number of lesions ≤ 5 cm each	AFP ≤ 400 ng/mL
Zheng et al[53]	2008	Total tumor diameter > 8 cm	AFP ≤ 400 ng/mL
Fujiki et al[60]	2009	Up to 10 lesions ≤ 5 cm each	DCP ≤ 400 mAU/mL
Lai et al[61]	2012	Total tumor diameter ≤ 8 cm	AFP ≤ 400 ng/mL
Grąt et al[62]	2014	UCSF or up to seven criteria	AFP < 100 ng/mL
Toso et al[63]	2015	Total tumor volume ≤ 115 cm³	AFP ≤ 400 ng/mL
Lee et al[64]	2015	Total tumor diameter ≤ 10 cm	PET/CT negative uptake

Abbreviations: AFP, alpha-fetoprotein; CT, computed tomography; DCP, des-gamma-carboxy prothrombin; HCC, hepatocellular carcinoma; PET, positron emission tomography; UCSF, University of California at San Francisco.

absence of tumor progression during a 3-month observation period were associated with good post-transplant outcomes.[67] Similarly, research has demonstrated good post-transplant outcomes in patients with significantly elevated AFP levels that decreased in response to locoregional therapy.[68] This suggests that morphometric variables along with biomarkers should be assessed when considering transplant appropriateness.

HCC molecular signatures have been described but have not yet been incorporated into clinical practice or scoring systems.[69]

In this era of severe organ shortage and increasing incidence of HCC, researchers should continue to identify predictive biomarkers that can be incorporated into selection criteria, thus improving organ allocation.

15.3.2 Systemic Therapies

Systemic therapies are indicated for the treatment of metastatic HCC and advanced liver-confined HCC not amenable to locoregional therapy. Systemic chemotherapy and targeted agents are not indicated for use in conjunction with locoregional therapies such as radioembolization or chemoembolization unless those therapies were indicated for palliation during the course of systemic treatment for metastatic disease.

With the exception of clinical trials, systemic therapies are not indicated for use as adjuvant therapy after complete resection, ablation, or orthotopic liver transplant regardless of risk stratification. Systemic therapies are also generally not indicated for the treatment of advanced liver disease due to cirrhosis (e.g., Child–Pugh class B or C disease or BCLC stage D disease). Systemic therapies should be avoided in the presence of grade 3 or greater hematologic, renal, or hepatic toxicities.

Systemic therapy should also be avoided in patients with a poor performance status (Eastern Cooperative Oncology Group performance status ≥ 3; Karnofsky Performance Status [KPS] ≤ 50).

Patients who are candidates for systemic therapy should be encouraged to enroll in clinical trials where available.

approximately 8%. As this survival rate was comparable to survival among patients without HCC undergoing liver transplant, the Milan criteria were further validated worldwide and adopted by transplant centers as standard transplant criteria.[47]

A shortcoming of the Milan criteria is the exclusion of tumor biomarkers; because of this exclusion, strict adherence to these criteria can lead to over-selectivity. As numerous single-center studies have demonstrated, a significant number of patients with HCC beyond the Milan criteria can achieve post-transplant outcomes comparable to those achieved in patients with HCC within the Milan criteria.[48] Proposed expanded HCC criteria for cadaveric and live-donor liver transplant are described in ▶ Table 15.5[46,49,50,51,52,53,54,55,56,57,58,59,60,61]; examples of criteria that include biomarkers are shown in ▶ Table 15.6.[55,59,62,63,64,65,66]

One rudimentary but effective method for determining tumor biology is the assessment of response to locoregional therapy in patients with HCC beyond the Milan criteria ("treat and wait approach"). In one study, successful downstaging and

Table 15.7 Randomized control trials of sorafenib versus placebo in survival of patients with hepatocellular carcinoma (HCC)

Trial	Patients	Arm	Median time to progression (mo)	Median overall survival (mo)	p-value for overall survival
SHARP	600	Placebo	2.8	7.9	<0.01
		Sorafenib	5.5	10.7	
Asia-Pacific	270	Placebo	1.4	4.2	<0.01
		Sorafenib	2.8	6.5	

Sorafenib is the only Food and Drug Administration (FDA) approved systemic therapy available for the treatment of advanced HCC. Although other systemic cytotoxic chemotherapies have been studied (mainly in phase II studies), the routine use of these agents is discouraged except in patients with very good performance status. There is no evidence that systemic cytotoxic chemotherapy improves survival.

Sorafenib

The benefits of sorafenib were demonstrated in 2 large randomized clinical trials comparing sorafenib to placebo in patients with advanced or metastatic HCC and normal liver function or Child–Pugh class A cirrhosis (▶ Table 15.7).[70,71]

Sorafenib is supplied as a 200-mg tablet and is usually dispensed by a specialty pharmacy. Patients should be encouraged to complete an application for the drug assistance program through Bayer/onyx, given the potential for suboptimal insurance coverage for this medication.

All patients treated with sorafenib should undergo a thorough physical examination, with clinicians paying careful attention to symptoms, vital signs, and the presence or absence of hepatic encephalopathy and ascites. Hypertension should be controlled before the initiation of sorafenib. Baseline laboratory values should be obtained, including complete blood count with differential, liver function tests, basic metabolic profile, thyroid function test, and AFP level when appropriate. A baseline electrocardiogram is also recommended to check for QT prolongation.

Patients should be seen within 2 weeks of beginning sorafenib treatment to assess for acute toxicity (▶ Table 15.8). Patients should also undergo a physical examination at least monthly

Table 15.8 Notable toxicities of sorafenib and suggested management

Toxicity	Management
Fatigue	Energy conservation, encourage exercise
Hypertension	Aggressive management before sorafenib initiation Aggressive management with antihypertensive agents Dose reduction or cessation might be indicated
Mouth sores	Use of salt and soda mouthwashes Use of Benadryl–Maalox–lidocaine (BMX) solution
Diarrhea	Use of over-the-counter antidiarrheal agent Use of prescription antidiarrheal agent Dose reduction might be indicated
Hand–foot syndrome (palmar–plantar erythema)	Prophylaxis with daily moisturizing of the hands and feet; urea-based ointment may be advantageous Avoidance of repeated traumatic pressure on hands and feet Dose reduction or cessation might be indicated

while taking this agent. Routine blood work (including complete blood count, comprehensive metabolic profile, and AFP level, if previously elevated) should be performed 2 weeks after patients begin sorafenib therapy and then monthly thereafter. Thyroid function tests and electrocardiogram should be ordered when clinically indicated.

Optimal dosing of sorafenib is 400 mg by mouth twice daily. The drug should be administered on an empty stomach. Patients with early Child–Pugh class B cirrhosis should be started on 50% of the dose, given the decreased tolerance to sorafenib seen with impaired liver function. Dose reductions should be based on clinical judgment and evaluation of side effects and hematological and biochemical toxicities:

- Dose level 1: 200 mg twice daily (or 400 mg once daily).
- Dose level 2: 400 mg every other day (or 200 mg once daily).
- Dose level 3: not applicable; sorafenib therapy should be discontinued.

Second-Line Treatments

Patients with advanced HCC that is resistant to sorafenib should be considered for clinical trials when appropriate. Cytotoxic chemotherapy such as oxaliplatin, gemcitabine, doxorubicin, 5-Fluorouracil, or cisplatin has been used in advanced HCC. However, these agents are not considered standard of care and should be used only on a case-by-case basis. Many patients will not be able to tolerate cytotoxic chemotherapies because of underlying liver dysfunction and performance status.

Patients who are not eligible for second-line treatments or clinical trials should be offered palliative and supportive care and should have a discussion with their health care providers regarding hospice referral.

Regorafenib

Regorafenib, an oral multikinase inhibitor blocking VEGFR 1-3, TIE-2, RAF-1, BRAF, BRAFV600, KIT, RET, PDGFR and FGFR, has been recently approved by the FDA as a second line therapy for patients with HCC progressing on sorafenib.

Through the phase III RESORCE trial, 573 HCC patients who previously failed to respond to sorafenib were randomized to regorafenib or placebo.[72] Rogorafenib was associated with improved overall survival compared to placebo (10.6 months vs. 7.8 months, respectively). In addition, progression free survival was 3.1 months with regorafenib vs. 1.5 months with placebo.

Immunotherapy

Nivolumab is a PD-L1 blocker, impeding interaction between PD-L1 (expressed in cancer cells) and PD-1 (expressed in T cells). By blocking PDL1/PD1 interaction, immune suppression induced by cancer cells is precluded.

Nivolumab has been recently approved by FDA for HCC patients previously treated with sorafenib. The approval was based on the phase I/II CheckMate-040 trial that enrolled 154 patients and exhibited 18.2% overall response and 3.2% complete response per m-RECIST criteria.[73]

References

[1] Ferlay J, Shin HR, Bray F, Forman D, Mathers C, Parkin DM. Estimates of worldwide burden of cancer in 2008: GLOBOCAN 2008. Int J Cancer. 2010; 127(12):2893–2917

[2] El-Serag HB, Rudolph KL. Hepatocellular carcinoma: epidemiology and molecular carcinogenesis. Gastroenterology. 2007; 132(7):2557–2576

[3] El-Serag HB. Epidemiology of viral hepatitis and hepatocellular carcinoma. Gastroenterology. 2012; 142(6):1264–1273.e1

[4] Calle EE, Rodriguez C, Walker-Thurmond K, Thun MJ. Overweight, obesity, and mortality from cancer in a prospectively studied cohort of U.S. adults. N Engl J Med. 2003; 348(17):1625–1638

[5] Zhang BH, Yang BH, Tang ZY. Randomized controlled trial of screening for hepatocellular carcinoma. J Cancer Res Clin Oncol. 2004; 130(7):417–422

[6] Bruix J, Llovet JM. Major achievements in hepatocellular carcinoma. Lancet. 2009; 373(9664):614–616

[7] Gómez-Rodríguez R, Romero-Gutiérrez M, Artaza-Varasa T, et al. The value of the Barcelona Clinic Liver Cancer and alpha-fetoprotein in the prognosis of hepatocellular carcinoma. Rev Esp Enferm Dig. 2012; 104 (6):298–304

[8] Sarasin FP, Giostra E, Hadengue A. Cost-effectiveness of screening for detection of small hepatocellular carcinoma in western patients with Child-Pugh class A cirrhosis. Am J Med. 1996; 101(4):422–434

[9] Giannini EG, Erroi V, Trevisani F. Effectiveness of α-fetoprotein for hepatocellular carcinoma surveillance: the return of the living-dead? Expert Rev Gastroenterol Hepatol. 2012; 6(4):441–444

[10] Farinati F, Marino D, De Giorgio M, et al. Diagnostic and prognostic role of alpha-fetoprotein in hepatocellular carcinoma: both or neither? Am J Gastroenterol. 2006; 101(3):524–532

[11] Lang K, Danchenko N, Gondek K, Shah S, Thompson D. The burden of illness associated with hepatocellular carcinoma in the United States. J Hepatol. 2009; 50(1):89–99

[12] Garcia M, Jemal A, Ward EM, et al. Global Cancer Facts and Figures 2007. Atlanta, GA: American Cancer Society; 2007

[13] Wald C, Russo MW, Heimbach JK, Hussain HK, Pomfret EA, Bruix J. New OPTN/UNOS policy for liver transplant allocation: standardization of liver imaging, diagnosis, classification, and reporting of hepatocellular carcinoma. Radiology. 2013; 266(2):376–382

[14] Leerapun A, Suravarapu SV, Bida JP, et al. The utility of Lens culinaris agglutinin-reactive alpha-fetoprotein in the diagnosis of hepatocellular carcinoma: evaluation in a United States referral population. Clin Gastroenterol Hepatol. 2007; 5(3):394–402, quiz 267

[15] Turner JM, Perazella MA. Imaging patients with kidney disease: weighing the risks and benefits. US Nephrology.. 2011; 6:131–137

[16] Santambrogio R, Kluger MD, Costa M, et al. Hepatic resection for hepatocellular carcinoma in patients with Child-Pugh's A cirrhosis: is clinical evidence of portal hypertension a contraindication? HPB (Oxford). 2013; 15 (1):78–84

[17] Marrero JA, Kudo M, Bronowicki JP. The challenge of prognosis and staging for hepatocellular carcinoma. Oncologist. 2010; 15 Suppl 4:23–33

[18] Meier V, Ramadori G. Clinical staging of hepatocellular carcinoma. Dig Dis. 2009; 27:131–141

[19] Lu W, Dong J, Huang Z, Guo D, Liu Y, Shi S. Comparison of four current staging systems for Chinese patients with hepatocellular carcinoma undergoing curative resection: Okuda, CLIP, TNM and CUPI. J Gastroenterol Hepatol. 2008; 23(12):1874–1878

[20] Okuda K, Ohtsuki T, Obata H, et al. Natural history of hepatocellular carcinoma and prognosis in relation to treatment. Study of 850 patients. Cancer. 1985; 56(4):918–928

[21] Llovet JM, Brú C, Bruix J. Prognosis of hepatocellular carcinoma: the BCLC staging classification. Semin Liver Dis. 1999; 19(3):329–338

[22] Guglielmi A, Ruzzenente A, Pachera S, et al. Comparison of seven staging systems in cirrhotic patients with hepatocellular carcinoma in a cohort of patients who underwent radiofrequency ablation with complete response. Am J Gastroenterol. 2008; 103(3):597–604

[23] A new prognostic system for hepatocellular carcinoma: a retrospective study of 435 patients: the Cancer of the Liver Italian Program (CLIP) investigators. Hepatology. 1998; 28(3):751–755

[24] Ueno S, Tanabe G, Sako K, et al. Discrimination value of the new western prognostic system (CLIP score) for hepatocellular carcinoma in 662 Japanese patients. Cancer of the Liver Italian Program. Hepatology. 2001; 34(3):529–534

[25] Kudo M, Chung H, Osaki Y. Prognostic staging system for hepatocellular carcinoma (CLIP score): its value and limitations, and a proposal for a new staging system, the Japan Integrated Staging Score (JIS score). J Gastroenterol. 2003; 38(3):207–215

[26] Kitai S, Kudo M, Minami Y, et al. A new prognostic staging system for hepatocellular carcinoma: value of the biomarker combined Japan integrated staging score. Intervirology. 2008; 51 Suppl 1:86–94

[27] Bruix J, Sherman M, American Association for the Study of Liver Diseases. Management of hepatocellular carcinoma: an update. Hepatology. 2011; 53 (3):1020–1022

[28] Fonseca AL, Cha CH. Hepatocellular carcinoma: a comprehensive overview of surgical therapy. J Surg Oncol. 2014; 110(6):712–719

[29] Llovet JM, Fuster J, Bruix J. Intention-to-treat analysis of surgical treatment for early hepatocellular carcinoma: resection versus transplantation. Hepatology. 1999; 30(6):1434–1440

[30] Lau H, Man K, Fan ST, Yu WC, Lo CM, Wong J. Evaluation of preoperative hepatic function in patients with hepatocellular carcinoma undergoing hepatectomy. Br J Surg. 1997; 84(9):1255–1259

[31] Hemming AW, Scudamore CH, Shackleton CR, Pudek M, Erb SR. Indocyanine green clearance as a predictor of successful hepatic resection in cirrhotic patients. Am J Surg. 1992; 163(5):515–518

[32] Jarnagin WR, Gonen M, Fong Y, et al. Improvement in perioperative outcome after hepatic resection: analysis of 1,803 consecutive cases over the past decade. Ann Surg. 2002; 236(4):397–406, discussion 406–407

[33] Kingham TP, Correa-Gallego C, D'Angelica MI, et al. Hepatic parenchymal preservation surgery: decreasing morbidity and mortality rates in 4,152 resections for malignancy. J Am Coll Surg. 2015; 220(4):471–479

[34] Kneuertz PJ, Pitt HA, Bilimoria KY, et al. Risk of morbidity and mortality following hepato-pancreato-biliary surgery. J Gastrointest Surg. 2012; 16(9): 1727–1735

[35] Bruix J, Sherman M, Practice Guidelines Committee, American Association for the Study of Liver Diseases. Management of hepatocellular carcinoma. Hepatology. 2005; 42(5):1208–1236

[36] Yamamoto J, Kosuge T, Takayama T, et al. Recurrence of hepatocellular carcinoma after surgery. Br J Surg. 1996; 83(9):1219–1222

[37] Agrawal S, Belghiti J. Oncologic resection for malignant tumors of the liver. Ann Surg. 2011; 253(4):656–665

[38] Abulkhir A, Limongelli P, Healey AJ, et al. Preoperative portal vein embolization for major liver resection: a meta-analysis. Ann Surg. 2008; 247 (1):49–57

[39] Shindoh J, Truty MJ, Aloia TA, et al. Kinetic growth rate after portal vein embolization predicts posthepatectomy outcomes: toward zero liver-related mortality in patients with colorectal liver metastases and small future liver remnant. J Am Coll Surg. 2013; 216(2):201–209

[40] Zhou YM, Shao WY, Zhao YF, Xu DH, Li B. Meta-analysis of laparoscopic versus open resection for hepatocellular carcinoma. Dig Dis Sci. 2011; 56(7): 1937–1943

[41] Leong WQ, Ganpathi IS, Kow AW, Madhavan K, Chang SK. Comparative study and systematic review of laparoscopic liver resection for hepatocellular carcinoma. World J Hepatol. 2015; 7(27):2765–2773

[42] Kim WR, Lake JR, Smith JM, et al. OPTN/SRTR 2013 Annual Data Report: liver. Am J Transplant. 2015; 15 Suppl 2:1–28

[43] Iwatsuki S, Gordon RD, Shaw BW, Jr, Starzl TE. Role of liver transplantation in cancer therapy. Ann Surg. 1985; 202(4):401–407

[44] Mazzaferro V, Regalia E, Doci R, et al. Liver transplantation for the treatment of small hepatocellular carcinomas in patients with cirrhosis. N Engl J Med. 1996; 334(11):693–699

[45] Mazzaferro V, Bhoori S, Sposito C, et al. Milan criteria in liver transplantation for hepatocellular carcinoma: an evidence-based analysis of 15 years of experience. Liver Transpl. 2011; 17 Suppl 2:S44–S57

[46] Prasad KR, Young RS, Burra P, et al. Summary of candidate selection and expanded criteria for liver transplantation for hepatocellular carcinoma: a review and consensus statement. Liver Transpl. 2011; 17 Suppl 2:S81–S89

[47] Yao FY, Ferrell L, Bass NM, et al. Liver transplantation for hepatocellular carcinoma: expansion of the tumor size limits does not adversely impact survival. Hepatology. 2001; 33(6):1394–1403

[48] Herrero JI, Sangro B, Quiroga J, et al. Influence of tumor characteristics on the outcome of liver transplantation among patients with liver cirrhosis and hepatocellular carcinoma. Liver Transpl. 2001; 7(7):631–636

[49] Roayaie S, Frischer JS, Emre SH, et al. Long-term results with multimodal adjuvant therapy and liver transplantation for the treatment of hepatocellular carcinomas larger than 5 centimeters. Ann Surg. 2002; 235(4):533–539

[50] Kneteman NM, Oberholzer J, Al Saghier M, et al. Sirolimus-based immunosuppression for liver transplantation in the presence of extended criteria for hepatocellular carcinoma. Liver Transpl. 2004; 10(10):1301–1311

[51] Onaca N, Davis GL, Goldstein RM, Jennings LW, Klintmalm GB. Expanded criteria for liver transplantation in patients with hepatocellular carcinoma: a report from the International Registry of Hepatic Tumors in Liver Transplantation. Liver Transpl. 2007; 13(3):391–399

[52] Silva M, Moya A, Berenguer M, et al. Expanded criteria for liver transplantation in patients with cirrhosis and hepatocellular carcinoma. Liver Transpl. 2008; 14(10):1449–1460

[53] Zheng SS, Xu X, Wu J, et al. Liver transplantation for hepatocellular carcinoma: Hangzhou experiences. Transplantation. 2008; 85(12):1726–1732

[54] Mazzaferro V, Llovet JM, Miceli R, et al. Metroticket Investigator Study Group. Predicting survival after liver transplantation in patients with hepatocellular carcinoma beyond the Milan criteria: a retrospective, exploratory analysis. Lancet Oncol. 2009; 10(1):35–43

[55] Soejima Y, Taketomi A, Yoshizumi T, et al. Extended indication for living donor liver transplantation in patients with hepatocellular carcinoma. Transplantation. 2007; 83(7):893–899

[56] Jonas S, Mittler J, Pascher A, et al. Living donor liver transplantation of the right lobe for hepatocellular carcinoma in cirrhosis in a European center. Liver Transpl. 2007; 13(6):896–903

[57] Kwon CH, Kim DJ, Han YS, et al. HCC in living donor liver transplantation: can we expand the Milan criteria? Dig Dis. 2007; 25(4):313–319

[58] Sugawara Y, Tamura S, Makuuchi M. Living donor liver transplantation for hepatocellular carcinoma: Tokyo University series. Dig Dis. 2007; 25(4):310–312

[59] Takada Y, Ito T, Ueda M, et al. Living donor liver transplantation for patients with HCC exceeding the Milan criteria: a proposal of expanded criteria. Dig Dis. 2007; 25(4):299–302

[60] Fujiki M, Takada Y, Ogura Y, et al. Significance of des-gamma-carboxy prothrombin in selection criteria for living donor liver transplantation for hepatocellular carcinoma. Am J Transplant. 2009; 9(10):2362–2371

[61] Lai Q, Avolio AW, Manzia TM, et al. Combination of biological and morphological parameters for the selection of patients with hepatocellular carcinoma waiting for liver transplantation. Clin Transplant. 2012; 26(2):E125–E131

[62] Grąt M, Kornasiewicz O, Lewandowski Z, et al. Combination of morphologic criteria and α-fetoprotein in selection of patients with hepatocellular carcinoma for liver transplantation minimizes the problem of posttransplant tumor recurrence. World J Surg. 2014; 38(10):2698–2707

[63] Toso C, Meeberg G, Hernandez-Alejandro R, et al. Total tumor volume and alpha-fetoprotein for selection of transplant candidates with hepatocellular carcinoma: a prospective validation. Hepatology. 2015; 62(1):158–165

[64] Lee SD, Kim SH, Kim SK, Kim YK, Park SJ. Clinical impact of 18F-fluorodeoxyglucose positron emission tomography/computed tomography in living donor liver transplantation for advanced hepatocellular carcinoma. Transplantation. 2015; 99(10):2142–2149

[65] Roberts JP, Venook A, Kerlan R, Yao F. Hepatocellular carcinoma: ablate and wait versus rapid transplantation. Liver Transpl. 2010; 16(8):925–929

[66] Lai Q, Avolio AW, Graziadei I, et al. European Hepatocellular Cancer Liver Transplant Study Group. Alpha-fetoprotein and modified response evaluation criteria in solid tumors progression after locoregional therapy as predictors of hepatocellular cancer recurrence and death after transplantation. Liver Transpl. 2013; 19(10):1108–1118

[67] Woo HG, Park ES, Thorgeirsson SS, Kim YJ. Exploring genomic profiles of hepatocellular carcinoma. Mol Carcinog. 2011; 50(4):235–243

[68] Llovet JM, Ricci S, Mazzaferro V, et al. SHARP Investigators Study Group. Sorafenib in advanced hepatocellular carcinoma. N Engl J Med. 2008; 359(4):378–390

[69] Cheng AL, Kang YK, Chen Z, et al. Efficacy and safety of sorafenib in patients in the Asia-Pacific region with advanced hepatocellular carcinoma: a phase III randomised, double-blind, placebo-controlled trial. Lancet Oncol. 2009; 10(1):25–34

[70] Varela M, Real MI, Burrel M, et al. Chemoembolization of hepatocellular carcinoma with drug eluting beads: efficacy and doxorubicin pharmacokinetics. J Hepatol. 2007; 46(3):474–481

[71] Chok KS, Chan SC, Cheung TT, Chan AC, Fan ST, Lo CM. Late recurrence of hepatocellular carcinoma after liver transplantation. World J Surg. 2011; 35(9):2058–2062

[72] Bruix J, Qin S, Merle P, Granito A, Huang YH, Bodoky G, et al. Regorafenib for patients with hepatocellular carcinoma who progressed on sorafenib treatment (RESORCE): a randomized, double-blind, placebo-controlled, phase 3 trial. Lancet. 2017; 389:56–66

[73] Kudo M. Immune checkpoint inhibition in hepatocellular carcinoma: basics and ongoing clinical trials. Oncology. 2017; 92:50–62

16 Management of Locally Advanced Hepatocellular Carcinoma

Olaguoke (Goke) Akinwande and Hyun S. Kim

16.1 Introduction

Hepatocellular carcinoma (HCC) is an aggressive primary liver tumor that typically occurs in the background of chronic liver disease or cirrhosis. The prognosis is related to the patient's treatment options and hepatic reserve. Patients with small volume disease (solitary mass < 5 cm or few masses < 3 cm) with good performance status and preserved hepatic function have more treatment options that include resection, transplantation, and ablation with curative intent. These patients generally have good prognosis. On the other hand, patients with advanced HCC have fewer treatment options. These patients are usually not surgical candidates and some do not qualify for locoregional therapies (LRT) such as chemoembolization and radioembolization. As a result, their prognosis is poor, sometimes dismal.

Advanced HCC comprises those patients with any one or combination of the following characteristics: Eastern Cooperative Oncology Group (ECOG) performance status > 0, presence of vascular invasion, and extrahepatic disease. These patients typically fall in the Barcelona Clinic Liver Cancer (BCLC) stage C category. The BCLC staging system is widely utilized and endorsed by the American Association for the Study of Liver Diseases (AASLD). This staging system, which pairs each stage of the disease with a recommended treatment based on best available evidence, recommends that patients with advanced HCC be treated with systemic therapy (i.e., sorafenib). However, new studies have provided insight into the value of other treatment options such as LRT and radiation therapy (RT) in this patient population. This chapter will give insight into the management approach of treating locally advanced HCC.

16.2 Establishment of Locally Advanced Hepatocellular Carcinoma

As mentioned earlier, advanced HCC includes those with any one or combination of ECOG performance status > 0, macrovascular invasion, and extrahepatic disease. The background liver function can are variable, including those with Child–Pugh (CP) status A and B. CP C patients are in the terminal stage of HCC and may not tolerate any therapy more aggressive than best supportive care. The ECOG score, which highly correlates with the patient's prognosis, is established clinically by taking into account the patient's symptomatology and level of activity. Vascular invasion and the presence of extrahepatic disease require imaging evaluation. The imaging characteristics of typical HCC on contrast computed tomography (CT) or magnetic resonance imaging (MRI) show a hypervascular mass on the arterial phase with enhancement washout on the venous phase of imaging. On contrast-enhanced CT, nonopacification of the portal vein in the portal-venous phase indicates vascular invasion. This is a poor prognostic sign. The corresponding finding on T1 contrast-enhanced MRI is lack of contrast filling in the portal vein. Increased intravascular T2 signal on MRI is also indicative of vascular invasion. The most common sites of metastatic disease from HCC are the lung, abdominal lymph nodes, and bone.[1]

16.2.1 Staging and Treatment Approach

Using tumor stage to determine the appropriate treatment for HCC is difficult because every case is unique, differing in disease state and geographic variability. Another challenge in treating HCC is that differences in patient demographic and background liver disease etiology may affect the efficacy of therapy. For instance, Asian populations tend to involve younger patients with chronic hepatitis B or C and well-compensated cirrhosis. In the western world, patients with HCC are older with alcoholic cirrhosis or nonalcoholic fatty liver disease. These demographic differences can significantly impact the efficacy of treatment; therefore, studies that apply to a specific population cannot be extrapolated to serve another. Constant development of new treatments and new indications for older treatments also affect the ability to formalize rigid criteria regarding HCC treatment.

Nonetheless, the treatment of HCC is still in large part determined by the stage of disease. The stage of disease provides a starting point in deciding how aggressive the treatment approach should be. Many staging systems currently exist, but those that are pathologically based (i.e., Liver Cancer Study Group of Japan [LCSGJ], Chinese University Prognostic Index [CUPI]) are not the most helpful in determining the choice of therapy in advanced stage disease. This is because the diagnosis of HCC can be established in most cases without a pathological specimen. Also, often the goal of this treatment is palliation and rarely curative (for unresectable HCC); therefore, obtaining a pathologic specimen is redundant. Clinical staging systems are more helpful because the diagnosis of HCC is largely imaged based and imaging is assessable and convenient.

Most of the available clinical staging systems are more useful in directing surgical and transplantation decisions (Okuda, Cancer of the Liver Italian Program [CLIP], etc.). The BCLC staging system is of particular interest to oncologists and interventional radiologists because it has been validated as a prognosticator and each stage is paired with a particular treatment based on the best available evidence.[2] This staging system is based on tumor size, number of lesions, vascular invasion, hepatic function (Child–Pugh score), extrahepatic disease, and performance status. In brief, curative surgery (resection/transplant) is recommended for early-stage disease (BCLC A), transarterial chemoembolization (TACE) for intermediate-stage disease (BCLC B), sorafenib for advanced-stage disease (BCLC C), and best supportive care for terminal stage disease (BCLC D; ▶ Table 16.1).

While quite comprehensive, some argue that the BCLC staging system may be too rigid. In other words, it may not reflect novel advances in knowledge, aggressive surgical strategies, new medications, or new technologies. For example, it does not

Table 16.1 Barcelona Clinic Liver Cancer staging classification

Stage	Performance status (ECOG score)	Tumor stage	Child–Pugh status	Liver features	Treatment options
Very early (0)	0	Single lesion < 2 cm	A	No portal hypertension	Surgical resection
Early A1	0	Single lesion < 5 cm	A	No portal hypertension	Surgical resection
Early A2	0	Single lesion < 5 cm	A	Portal hypertension, normal total bilirubin	Liver transplant or ablation
Early A3	0	Single lesion < 5 cm	A	Portal hypertension, abnormal bilirubin	Liver transplant or ablation
Early A4	0	3 lesions < 3 cm	A	N/A	Liver transplant or ablation
Intermediate B	0	Large, multinodular	A–B	N/A	Chemoembolization
Advanced C	1–2	Portal invasion, metastases	A–B	N/A	Sorafenib
Terminal D	3–4	Any size or number	C	N/A	Best supportive care

Abbreviations: ECOG, European Cooperative Oncology Group; N/A, not applicable.

advocate transarterial therapy for patients with advanced HCC who may potentially benefit from it. Further, there are intermediate-stage patients that may benefit from a more aggressive surgical approach.[3] The Hong Kong Liver Cancer staging system is less rigid and may outperform BCLC staging in prognostic significance, but it needs to be validated in non-Asian populations.[4] The Americas Hepato-Pancreato-Biliary Association consensus statement advocated the need to utilize different systems in different patients. They recommended using the TNM system to predict prognosis after surgery (resection or transplant) and the BCLC criteria for nonsurgical HCC patients. To that end, interventional oncologists may find the BCLC criteria the most useful as they plan treatment strategies for patients with advanced HCC.[3]

16.3 Response Assessment

In patients with elevated alpha-fetoprotein (AFP) levels, AFP trends can screen for disease progression after treatment. When the AFP level decreases by 20% from baseline after treatment, the median survival has been found to be greater than nonresponders. Any decrease in AFP should be verified with imaging as the AFP trend should mirror the imaging findings.[5] The limitation of AFP is that a nontrivial fraction of patients with HCC may not have significantly elevated AFP levels to allow biochemical response assessment.

A more effective and practical way of assessing response is using cross-sectional imaging (i.e., CT, MRI). Imaging biomarkers can be used as a surrogate for survival. There are three commonly used imaging criteria used to assess solid liver tumors after treatment: Response Evaluation Criteria in Solid Tumors (RECIST), modified RECIST (mRECIST), and European Association for the Study of the Liver (EASL; ▸ Table 16.2).

The RECIST, which grades response based on variations in tumor size, was established to assess cytotoxic treatment effect on solid tumors. However, size-based criteria are not optimal in this patient population[6,7] because HCC behaves differently when treated with LRT or biologic agents (which are cytostatic not cytotoxic). Specifically, sometimes the post-treatment target lesion may remain stable in size or even increase in size compared to baseline. To circumvent these limitations,

Table 16.2 Radiographic response criteria

Response category	Response criteria		
	RECIST 1.0	mRECIST	EASL
Complete response	Disappearance of target lesions	Disappearance of viable lesions (2 total)	Disappearance of all viable lesions
Partial response	≥ 30% decrease in sum of one-dimensional diameter	≥ 30% decrease in the sum of one-dimensional diameter of viable portion	≥ 50% decrease in the sum of the product of two-dimensional diameter of viable portion
Progressive disease	≥ 20% increase in the sum of one-dimensional diameter	≥ 20% increase in the sum of one-dimensional diameter of viable portion	≥ 25% increase in the sum of the product of two-dimensional diameter of viable portion
Stable disease	Neither partial response nor progressive disease	Neither partial response nor progressive disease	Neither partial response nor progressive disease

Abbreviations: RECIST, response evaluation criteria in solid tumors; mRECIST, modified response evaluation criteria in solid tumors; EASL, European Association for the Study of the Liver.

viability-based criteria were developed. The EASL and mRECIST were both developed to take advantage of the exuberant enhancement of HCC. Rather than evaluating treatment response using differences in size, changes in the amount or pattern of enhancement are prioritized. These enhancement (viability) based imaging criteria are superior to anatomic imaging biomarkers in evaluating patients with HCC treated with LRT.[8,9,10,11] The main difference between EASL and mRECIST is that the former is two-dimensional and the latter is unidimensional. With these imaging criteria, one can assign the following categories based on the strict guidelines: complete response (CR), partial response (PR), stable disease (SD), and progressive disease (PD). Each of these categories correlates with the prognosis of the patient after treatment.

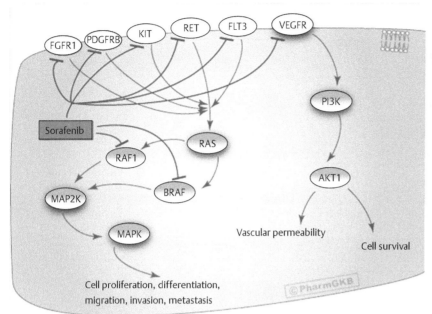

Fig. 16.1 Sorafenib mechanism of action. Sorafenib slows tumor progression by inhibiting intracellular and cell surface kinases involved in the regulation of cancer phenotypes including several members of the RAF/MEK/extracellular signal–regulated kinase (ERK) signaling cascade (RAF1, BRAF). In addition, sorafenib exerts its anticancer properties by inhibiting multiple proangiogenic receptor tyrosine kinases (VEGFR [vascular endothelial growth factor receptor], PDGFRB [platelet-derived growth factor receptor], KIT, RET). (Reproduced with permission of Whirl-Carrillo M, McDonagh EM, Hebert JM, et al. Pharmacogenomics knowledge for personalized medicine. Clin Pharmacol Ther 2012;92:414–417.)

16.4 Therapeutic Options for Advanced Hepatocellular Carcinoma

The decisions regarding the management of patients with advanced HCC must be performed in a multidisciplinary setting, as the treatment spans many specialties and expertise. According to the BCLC criteria, the management of advanced HCC is systemic therapy; however, there is growing evidence supporting the use of other modalities such as LRT. Therefore, treatment decisions should not be made in isolation. The treatment options for advanced HCC are discussed below.

16.4.1 Systemic Therapy

Cytotoxic chemotherapy has limited utility in the treatment of advanced HCC because HCC is a relatively chemorefractory tumor. On the other hand, molecular systemic therapy shows more promise in this setting because of HCC tumor biology. Fortunately, HCC tumors are very vascular tumors that markedly express vascular endothelial growth factors (VEGF) and the RAF/mitogen-activated protein kinase (MAPK)/extracellular signal–regulated kinase (ERK) pathway is important for HCC tumorigenesis. These elements provide useful targets for systemic treatment. Sorafenib, a biologic agent, has been proven to provide some efficacy as monotherapy in treating advanced HCC. Other biologic agents have been studied, but none so far has been proven in this patient population. Detailed description of these biologic agents is outside the scope of this chapter.

Sorafenib

The generally accepted standard of care for patients with advanced HCC is systemic administration of sorafenib. Sorafenib is currently the only molecularly targeted therapy approved by the U.S. Food and Drug Administration (FDA) for the treatment of HCC. Sorafenib is a multitargeted tyrosine kinase inhibitor (TKI) that acts by inhibiting the VEGF receptor pathway and Raf kinases (▶ Fig. 16.1).

Its effect mechanism induces autophagy, thereby leading to suppression of cancer cell growth. The pivotal trial that led to its widespread use was the Study of Heart and Renal Protection (SHARP) trial, which was a multicenter study comprising 602 patients. This European study randomized patients to sorafenib and placebo groups. The result of this trial was an overall survival (OS) that favored the treatment group (treatment group 10.7 months; control group 7.9 months; *p* < 0.001).[12] This study established sorafenib monotherapy as the treatment of choice for advanced HCC in a western population. However, most HCC cases are found in hepatitis B virus (HBV)/hepatitis C virus (HCV) endemic areas (Asia-Pacific, Africa); therefore, the etiology is very different from the Western HCC population. Therefore, the SHARP trial population did not address the HBV/HCV endemic populations. To address this problem, another phase III randomized control trial from the Asia-Pacific region was performed on 226 patients. OS was again noted to favor the treatment group (6.5 vs. 4.2 months, *p* = 0.014), thereby validating the SHARP trial in an HBV/HCV endemic population. Positive results in both trials demonstrate that sorafenib is effective regardless of the HCC sample population.

Treatment of advanced HCC patients should be limited to those with CP A and B cirrhosis. Patients with CP C cirrhosis have a short prognosis due to severe hepatic disease; therefore, they are unlikely to benefit from sorafenib.[13] Of note, there is a higher risk of serious adverse effects in CP B patients compared with CP A (60 vs. 33%).[14] Common side effects associated with sorafenib usage include hand–foot syndrome, diarrhea, alopecia, liver dysfunction, nausea, fatigue, and anorexia.

Sorafenib should be considered for any patient with advanced HCC. There are ongoing trials evaluating sorafenib-based combination therapies to enhance the efficacy of this treatment.

16.4.2 Locoregional Therapy: Chemoembolization and Bland Embolization

As mentioned earlier, HCC is an extremely vascular tumor that derives the majority of its blood supply from the hepatic artery rather than the portal vein. On the contrary, the liver derives most of its blood supply from the portal vein. This differential perfusion provides a convenient target for LRT. Bland embolization involves the use of particles (beads, etc.) to embolize the target hepatic artery without the addition of chemotherapy. TACE involves combining intrahepatic delivery of chemotherapy with embolization of the feeding arteries. TACE can be performed in a conventional fashion (cTACE) using ethiodized oil combined with one or more chemotherapeutic agents (mitomycin C, doxorubicin, cisplatin) to form an emulsion (▶ Fig. 16.2, ▶ Fig. 16.3, ▶ Fig. 16.4).

This is followed by administration of embolic particles. More recently, TACE using drug-eluting beads (DEBTACE) has gained more popularity. DEBTACE involves the use of beads that can be loaded with doxorubicin and injected into the hepatic artery. Once delivered, it provides slow release of the chemotherapeutic agent, thereby optimizing the pharmacokinetics.[15] Bland embolization, cTACE, and DEBTACE have proven to be efficacious for the treatment of unresectable HCC with definitive survival benefit compared with best supportive care.[16,17,18]

Although chemoembolization and bland embolization are well-established treatments for intermediate-stage HCC (BCLC stage B), their roles in treating advanced-stage HCC are not well established despite several studies supporting their benefits.[19,20] In theory, LRT may not be ideal as a treatment device for HCC with associated portal vein thrombosis (PVT) as those livers are more dependent on hepatic artery perfusion. In those cases, embolization in theory may lead to ischemic hepatitis. However, there are several studies that show that LRT is well tolerated in

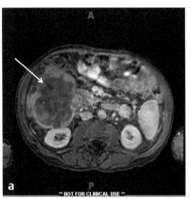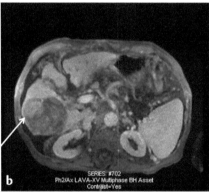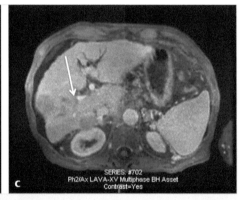

Fig. 16.2 MR (magnetic resonance) image of the abdomen with contrast. **(a)** A large heterogeneous mass (*arrow*) with profound necrosis was seen in this patient with liver cirrhosis. **(b)** There were areas of internal enhancement (*arrow*) along with subjacent areas of necrosis. **(c)** Associated portal vein thrombosis was also seen (*arrow*).

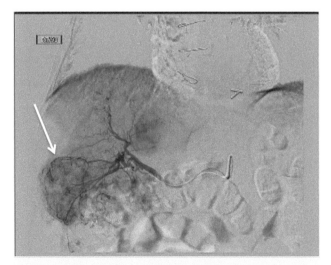

Fig. 16.3 Right hepatic angiogram. Image shows robust hepatic arterial phase perfusion of a known right hepatic mass (*arrow*). This mass was treated in a conventional fashion with a doxorubicin–ethiodized oil emulsion. The infusion was followed by embolization with 100- to 300-μm beads.

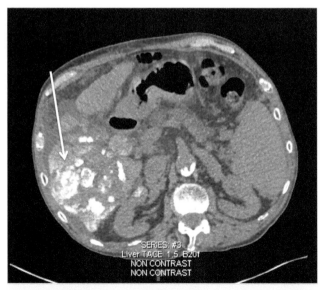

Fig. 16.4 Computed tomography (CT) image of the abdomen without contrast after embolization. Image shows deposition of the high-attenuating ethiodized oil within the tumor substance (*arrow*). Patient underwent another CT scan 3 months later (not shown), which demonstrated stable disease.

those patients.[21] A potential explanation is that there are enough portal vein collaterals to mitigate hepatic parenchymal reliance on the hepatic artery supply. An argument can be made that there is no need for LRT if there is extrahepatic disease; however, the prognosis of most of these patients are linked to liver tumoral disease (especially those with otherwise good liver function and performance status). Therefore, it is reasonable to expect that LRT may potentially prolong survival.

Contraindications of chemoembolization include decompensated liver disease (CP C), poor performance status (~ECOG > 2), uncontrollable coagulopathy, active infection, and encephalopathy. Relative contraindications include extensive extrahepatic disease (TACE is only useful for patients with hepatic-dominant disease or for those whose prognosis is tied to hepatic tumor burden), nondecompressed biliary obstruction, and bilirubin > 2. The most common adverse effect of TACE is postembolization syndrome (nausea, fever, and abdominal pain). Possible complications of TACE include liver failure, nontarget embolization, liver abscess (especially in patients with a compromised sphincter of Oddi), and renal insufficiency (from contrast media). The risk of liver abscess can be minimized with preprocedural antibiotics.

Bland Embolization versus Chemoembolization

The AASLD guidelines recommend chemoembolization—not bland embolization—for the treatment of HCC. Moreover, an expert consensus group from the Americas Hepato-Pancreato-Biliary Association also supports the use of chemoembolization.[22] On the contrary, the National Comprehensive Cancer Network (NCCN) guidelines recommend both. One meta-analysis showed improvement of 2-year survival with chemoembolization compared with the control, which was not seen with bland embolization.[16] Another meta-analysis failed to show any survival advantage for TACE over bland embolization.[23] Of note, these studies were performed on heterogeneous groups with unresectable HCC and not specifically on the advanced HCC subset. Therefore, a conclusion about the superiority of one mode of therapy over the other in that population cannot be derived. Chemoembolization has been more widely studied, and therefore more widely adopted; however, some institutions still favor the use of bland embolization.[24] Further studies are indeed needed to evaluate the difference between bland embolization and chemoembolization specifically in the setting of advanced HCC. The authors favor the use of chemoembolization in this population when indicated.

Conventional TACE versus Drug-Eluting Beads TACE

There is no consensus regarding the optimal technique for chemoembolization because no study has proven one to be better than the other. A seven-study meta-analysis comparing cTACE with DEBTACE ($n = 693$) concluded that tumor response was not different for either treatment.[25] The PRECISION V study, a randomized control study comparing cTACE (doxorubicin) with DEBTACE (loaded with doxorubicin) in 212 patients, showed no advantage in objective response between both modalities.

However, DEBTACE may be favored in the setting of advanced tumoral and background liver disease as the study reported increased objective response with DEBTACE in those subsets. Further studies are required to show any superiority specifically in patients with advanced HCC. Of note, DEBTACE has been shown to be safer with reduction of serious liver toxicity and lower rate of doxorubicin-related side effects.[26,27] Therefore, while both treatments are probably interchangeable, DEBTACE is more widely adopted in this patient population.

16.4.3 Locoregional Therapy: Radioembolization

Radioembolization is another treatment device that takes advantage of differential perfusion for tumor targeting. [90]Y is delivered to liver tumors via the hepatic artery, causing preferential necrosis to the tumor while sparing the adjacent liver parenchyma. With ^{90}Y, the embolic effect is not as prominent as with chemoembolization. Rather, the treatment relies on the penetration of radioactive particles (^{90}Y) into the tumor substance and the subjacent vascular bed.

[90]Y particles decay and release beta particles that form a dose cloud with a range of 2.5 mm. The dose cloud in turn leads to tumor necrosis. The half-life of ^{90}Y is 64 hours with a decay energy of 2.28 MeV.

There are two types of radioactive microspheres: glass (TheraSphere, BTG International) and resin (SIR-Sphere, Sirtex Medical). TheraSphere microspheres have a mean diameter of 25±10 μm with a specific gravity of 2,467 Bq/microspheres, while SIR-Sphere microspheres have a median diameter of 32.5 μm (20 and 60 μm) with a specific gravity of 40 Bq/microspheres. Glass microspheres were approved by the FDA for the treatment of HCC. On the other hand, resin microspheres were approved by the FDA for the treatment of colorectal metastases to the liver. The utilization of resin microspheres for the treatment of HCC is considered off-label.

Expert groups offer different recommendations regarding its place in the HCC treatment population. The AASLD does not recommend radioembolization outside of clinical trials. The Americas Hepato-Pancreato-Biliary Association advocates its use in the setting of PVT, advanced disease, or to bridge/down-stage patients to transplantation or resection. The NCCN guidelines recommend radioembolization for patients with liver-only HCC who are not candidates for definitive treatment (i.e., surgery, ablation). Currently, there are no large randomized trials comparing ^{90}Y to other more established treatments (i.e., chemoembolization or sorafenib), but there is at least one ongoing study (NCT identifiers 01482442, 01556490, 01887717 on ClinicalTrials.gov). Comparative studies suggest ^{90}Y has similar efficacy to chemoembolization in intermediate-stage HCC,[28,29,30,31,32] but how these studies apply to advanced HCC is up for debate. Some experienced practitioners favor radioembolization over chemoembolization in patients with advanced HCC with PVT because its therapeutic effect is not reliant on embolization. Profound embolization is thought to be detrimental in patients with PVT (especially patients without developed portal collaterals); however, this theory has not been proven.

Contraindications to ^{90}Y treatment include acute renal failure, uncontrollable coagulopathy, profound hepatopulmonary shunting that delivers 30 Gy (single treatment) or 50 Gy (aggregate treatment) to the lung, lung shunt fraction > 20% (SIR-Spheres) and extrahepatic flow that is uncorrectable by optimizing catheter placement or coil embolization. Relative contraindications include severe hepatic dysfunction (i.e., CP C or total bilirubin > 2–2.5), poor performance status (ECOG > 2), and non-decompressed biliary obstruction (may lead to biliary necrosis). Hepatopulmonary shunting and extrahepatic flow are evaluated on the initial ^{90}Y shunt mapping study prior to treatment. Side effects of ^{90}Y tend to be milder than those seen with chemoembolization and include fatigue, nausea, abdominal pain, and sometimes fevers. Common complications include abscess formation, nontarget embolization, and radiation cystitis. As with chemoembolization, patients with compromised sphincter of Oddi have a higher propensity to develop liver abscesses.

16.4.4 Other Treatment Strategies

Percutaneous Ablation

Percutaneous ablative therapy can be considered for patients with early-stage HCC who are not amenable to surgery. The advantage of ablation is to provide definitive treatment of HCC in a hepatocyte sparing fashion. In patients with locally advanced HCC, ablation is not currently recommended. In those patients, the prognosis is relatively poor and the disease is not curable (due to large tumor size, extrahepatic disease, etc.); therefore, it is of little utility in using curative techniques that carry inherent risk. In a very few selected cases, ablation may be of benefit for palliative purposes (i.e., painful lesions).

Radiation Therapy

HCC is known to be a radiosensitive tumor; however, the liver parenchyma is even more sensitive to radiation and therefore prone to radiation-induced liver disease. A mean radiation dose of 30 Gy or less is considered safe, but radiation tolerance could be considerably lower in patients with background liver disease as seen in most patients with HCC.[33] Therefore, external beam radiation is challenging to perform without significant collateral damage. On the other hand, stereotactic body radiation therapy (SBRT) may have utility in this setting. SBRT involves precise delivery of a single or limited number of high-dose radiation fractions to a small defined target using focused radiation beams. There is growing evidence that SBRT may be beneficial for small HCC lesions in patients who are not surgical candidates;[34,35] however, its utility specifically in the setting of advanced HCC has not been well established. Usage of RT for HCC should be limited to clinical trials until more evidence emerges.

16.4.5 Combination Therapies

TACE with Sorafenib

As mentioned earlier, sorafenib monotherapy has been shown to prolong survival in patients with advanced HCC, but the survival benefit is only modest. This sparked interest in establishing combinations with sorafenib that can further enhance efficacy. Experts argue that aggressive tumor control in the liver may lead to increased survival since liver tumoral disease dictates the prognosis of most patients. A not so recent large retrospective study (n = 372) comparing TACE with sorafenib in patients with advanced HCC reported longer overall survival in the TACE treatment group compared to the sorafenib group; however, the difference did not reach statistical significance.[36] Given the lethargy of evidence supporting TACE as a superior treatment to the more-studied sorafenib, most centers will rather administer sorafenib. Instead, an argument can be made for combining TACE with sorafenib—a combination that may be synergistic. The premise behind combining the two treatments is that arterial embolization results in the upregulation of angiogenic factors, and some of these factors are inhibited by sorafenib.

Contrary to well-placed scientific logic, combination therapy has not been shown to provide any survival advantage over sorafenib monotherapy in intermediate-stage HCC.[37] On the contrary, there may be additional benefit in treating advanced HCC. Studies have demonstrated the combined TACE–sorafenib therapy to be safe and efficacious[38,39] and may outperform sorafenib monotherapy in advanced-stage disease.[40,41] A recent meta-analysis reported improved OS, thrombotic thrombocytopenic purpura (TTP), and response with combination therapy compared to sorafenib monotherapy.[42] Of note, the analysis also reported an increased rate of grade 3/4 adverse events in the combination therapy group that included diarrhea, rash, foot skin reaction, and hypertension. Therefore, the selection of patients for this aggressive treatment strategy should be exercised with caution and discussed in a multidisciplinary setting.

TACE–sorafenib combination therapy is well tolerated and efficacious, but its additional benefit when compared with sorafenib monotherapy needs to be established with high-quality controlled trials. The increased adverse events should be weighed against the potential benefits of combination therapy on a patient-to-patient basis.

Sorafenib with Radiation

There is convincing preclinical evidence that suggests that sorafenib sensitizes HCC cells to RT.[43] However, this finding has not been sufficiently studied in a clinical setting. A recent phase I study evaluating the combination of sorafenib and SBRT for the treatment of locally advanced HCC reported significant dose-related toxicity and toxicity-related patient dropout. Despite the reported toxicity, they did report a respectable response rate of 50 and 36% for small- and large-volume diseases, respectively.[44] As a result, we suggest (as did the authors) that this combination should not be performed outside of clinical trials. There is at least one ongoing phase III study evaluating the use of SBRT with subsequent sorafenib compared with sorafenib monotherapy.[45]

Sorafenib with Cytotoxic Chemotherapy

A randomized phase II study evaluated the combination of sorafenib and doxorubicin compared with doxorubicin monotherapy in patients with advanced HCC. The authors reported improved TTP (6.4 vs. 2.8 months; p = 0.02), progression-free survival (6 vs. 2.7 months; p = 0.006), and OS (13.7 vs. 6.5 months; p = 0.006) in the combination group. In addition, the toxicity profile was similar in both groups. Unfortunately, doxorubicin is not standard of care for the treatment of advanced HCC; therefore, the control group was not ideal. In other words, the degree of synergy between sorafenib and doxorubicin compared to standard of care sorafenib monotherapy cannot be derived from that study. An ongoing trial is currently studying the effects of the sorafenib–doxorubicin combination treatment compared with sorafenib monotherapy.[46] When completed, this study will give insight into any additional efficacy the combination treatment provides over standard of care.

16.5 Conclusion

Advanced HCC comes with a grave prognosis and is very challenging to treat. Sorafenib is the treatment of choice in this patient population with improved survival compared with best supportive care. Unfortunately, the survival benefit derived from sorafenib is modest at best. Chemoembolization may provide additional survival benefit, but this should be weighed against the potential increase in adverse effects. Radioembolization is probably interchangeable with chemoembolization, but comparative evidence is scant. A potential utility for radioembolization could be for patients with advanced HCC who are not candidates for chemoembolization or failed chemoembolization treatment. SBRT is a promising treatment, but more studies are needed to establish its place in the treatment algorithm. In general, patients with advanced HCC should be discussed in a multidisciplinary setting including surgical oncologists, medical oncologists, radiation oncologists, and interventional radiologists. The final treatment option would come down to local expertise and multidisciplinary consensus.

References

[1] Katyal S, Oliver JH, III, Peterson MS, Ferris JV, Carr BS, Baron RL. Extrahepatic metastases of hepatocellular carcinoma. Radiology. 2000; 216(3):698–703

[2] Bruix J, Sherman M, American Association for the Study of Liver Diseases. Management of hepatocellular carcinoma: an update. Hepatology. 2011; 53 (3):1020–1022

[3] Vauthey JN, Dixon E, Abdalla EK, et al. American Hepato-Pancreato-Biliary Association, Society of Surgical Oncology, Society for Surgery of the Alimentary Tract. Pretreatment assessment of hepatocellular carcinoma: expert consensus statement. HPB (Oxford). 2010; 12(5):289–299

[4] Yau T, Tang VY, Yao TJ, Fan ST, Lo CM, Poon RT. Development of Hong Kong Liver Cancer staging system with treatment stratification for patients with hepatocellular carcinoma. Gastroenterology. 2014; 146(7):1691–700.e3

[5] Chan SL, Mo FK, Johnson PJ, et al. New utility of an old marker: serial alpha-fetoprotein measurement in predicting radiologic response and survival of patients with hepatocellular carcinoma undergoing systemic chemotherapy. J Clin Oncol. 2009; 27(3):446–452

[6] Sharma MR, Maitland ML, Ratain MJ. RECIST: no longer the sharpest tool in the oncology clinical trials toolbox—point. Cancer Res. 2012; 72(20):5145–5149, discussion 5150

[7] Sharma MR, Maitland ML, Ratain MJ. Why RECIST works and why it should stay-reply to counterpoint. Cancer Res. 2012; 72(20):5158

[8] Prajapati HJ, Spivey JR, Hanish SI, et al. mRECIST and EASL responses at early time point by contrast-enhanced dynamic MRI predict survival in patients with unresectable hepatocellular carcinoma (HCC) treated by doxorubicin drug-eluting beads transarterial chemoembolization (DEB TACE). Ann Oncol. 2013; 24(4):965–973

[9] Jung ES, Kim JH, Yoon EL, et al. Comparison of the methods for tumor response assessment in patients with hepatocellular carcinoma undergoing transarterial chemoembolization. J Hepatol. 2013; 58(6):1181–1187

[10] Shim JH, Lee HC, Kim SO, et al. Which response criteria best help predict survival of patients with hepatocellular carcinoma following chemoembolization? A validation study of old and new models. Radiology. 2012; 262(2): 708–718

[11] Memon K, Kulik L, Lewandowski RJ, et al. Radiographic response to locoregional therapy in hepatocellular carcinoma predicts patient survival times. Gastroenterology. 2011; 141(2):526–535, 535.e1–535.e2

[12] Llovet JM, Ricci S, Mazzaferro V, et al. SHARP Investigators Study Group. Sorafenib in advanced hepatocellular carcinoma. N Engl J Med. 2008; 359(4):378–390

[13] Pinter M, Sieghart W, Graziadei I, et al. Sorafenib in unresectable hepatocellular carcinoma from mild to advanced stage liver cirrhosis. Oncologist. 2009; 14(1):70–76

[14] Lencioni R, Kudo M, Ye SL, et al. First interim analysis of the GIDEON (Global Investigation of therapeutic decisions in hepatocellular carcinoma and of its treatment with sorafeNib) non-interventional study. Int J Clin Pract. 2012; 66 (7):675–683

[15] Varela M, Real MI, Burrel M, et al. Chemoembolization of hepatocellular carcinoma with drug eluting beads: efficacy and doxorubicin pharmacokinetics. J Hepatol. 2007; 46(3):474–481

[16] Llovet JM, Bruix J. Systematic review of randomized trials for unresectable hepatocellular carcinoma: chemoembolization improves survival. Hepatology. 2003; 37(2):429–442

[17] Llovet JM, Real MI, Montaña X, et al. Barcelona Liver Cancer Group. Arterial embolisation or chemoembolisation versus symptomatic treatment in patients with unresectable hepatocellular carcinoma: a randomised controlled trial. Lancet. 2002; 359(9319):1734–1739

[18] Lo CM, Ngan H, Tso WK, et al. Randomized controlled trial of transarterial lipiodol chemoembolization for unresectable hepatocellular carcinoma. Hepatology. 2002; 35(5):1164–1171

[19] Vetter D, Wenger JJ, Bergier JM, Doffoel M, Bockel R. Transcatheter oily chemoembolization in the management of advanced hepatocellular carcinoma in cirrhosis: results of a Western comparative study in 60 patients. Hepatology. 1991; 13(3):427–433

[20] Carr BI. Hepatic artery chemoembolization for advanced stage HCC: experience of 650 patients. Hepatogastroenterology. 2002; 49(43):79–86

[21] Xue TC, Xie XY, Zhang L, Yin X, Zhang BH, Ren ZG. Transarterial chemoembolization for hepatocellular carcinoma with portal vein tumor thrombus: a meta-analysis. BMC Gastroenterol. 2013; 13:60

[22] Schwarz RE, Abou-Alfa GK, Geschwind JF, Krishnan S, Salem R, Venook AP, American Hepato-Pancreato-Biliary Association, Society of Surgical Oncology, Society for Surgery of the Alimentary Tract. Nonoperative therapies for combined modality treatment of hepatocellular cancer: expert consensus statement. HPB (Oxford). 2010; 12(5):313–320

[23] Marelli L, Stigliano R, Triantos C, et al. Transarterial therapy for hepatocellular carcinoma: which technique is more effective? A systematic review of cohort and randomized studies. Cardiovasc Intervent Radiol. 2007; 30(1):6–25

[24] Maluccio MA, Covey AM, Porat LB, et al. Transcatheter arterial embolization with only particles for the treatment of unresectable hepatocellular carcinoma. J Vasc Interv Radiol. 2008; 19(6):862–869

[25] Gao S, Yang Z, Zheng Z, et al. Doxorubicin-eluting bead versus conventional TACE for unresectable hepatocellular carcinoma: a meta-analysis. Hepatogastroenterology. 2013; 60(124):813–820

[26] Lammer J, Malagari K, Vogl T, et al. PRECISION V Investigators. Prospective randomized study of doxorubicin-eluting-bead embolization in the treatment of hepatocellular carcinoma: results of the PRECISION V study. Cardiovasc Intervent Radiol. 2010; 33(1):41–52

[27] Vogl TJ, Lammer J, Lencioni R, et al. Liver, gastrointestinal, and cardiac toxicity in intermediate hepatocellular carcinoma treated with PRECISION TACE with drug-eluting beads: results from the PRECISION V randomized trial. AJR Am J Roentgenol. 2011; 197(4):W562–W570

[28] Lewandowski RJ, Kulik LM, Riaz A, et al. A comparative analysis of transarterial downstaging for hepatocellular carcinoma: chemoembolization versus radioembolization. Am J Transplant. 2009; 9(8):1920–1928

[29] Kooby DA, Egnatashvili V, Srinivasan S, et al. Comparison of yttrium-90 radioembolization and transcatheter arterial chemoembolization for the treatment of unresectable hepatocellular carcinoma. J Vasc Interv Radiol. 2010; 21(2):224–230

[30] Moreno-Luna LE, Yang JD, Sanchez W, et al. Efficacy and safety of transarterial radioembolization versus chemoembolization in patients with hepatocellular carcinoma. Cardiovasc Intervent Radiol. 2013; 36(3):714–723

[31] El Fouly A, Ertle J, El Dorry A, et al. In intermediate stage hepatocellular carcinoma: radioembolization with yttrium 90 or chemoembolization? Liver Int. 2015; 35(2):627–635

[32] Lance C, McLennan G, Obuchowski N, et al. Comparative analysis of the safety and efficacy of transcatheter arterial chemoembolization and yttrium-90 radioembolization in patients with unresectable hepatocellular carcinoma. J Vasc Interv Radiol. 2011; 22(12):1697–1705

[33] Dawson LA, Normolle D, Balter JM, McGinn CJ, Lawrence TS, Ten Haken RK. Analysis of radiation-induced liver disease using the Lyman NTCP model. Int J Radiat Oncol Biol Phys. 2002; 53(4):810–821

[34] Yoon SM, Lim YS, Park MJ, et al. Stereotactic body radiation therapy as an alternative treatment for small hepatocellular carcinoma. PLoS One. 2013; 8 (11):e79854

[35] Bujold A, Massey CA, Kim JJ, et al. Sequential phase I and II trials of stereotactic body radiotherapy for locally advanced hepatocellular carcinoma. J Clin Oncol. 2013; 31(13):1631–1639

[36] Pinter M, Hucke F, Graziadei I, et al. Advanced-stage hepatocellular carcinoma: transarterial chemoembolization versus sorafenib. Radiology. 2012; 263(2):590–599

[37] Sansonno D, Lauletta G, Russi S, Conteduca V, Sansonno L, Dammacco F. Transarterial chemoembolization plus sorafenib: a sequential therapeutic scheme for HCV-related intermediate-stage hepatocellular carcinoma: a randomized clinical trial. Oncologist. 2012; 17(3):359–366

[38] Pawlik TM, Reyes DK, Cosgrove D, Kamel IR, Bhagat N, Geschwind JF. Phase II trial of sorafenib combined with concurrent transarterial chemoembolization with drug-eluting beads for hepatocellular carcinoma. J Clin Oncol. 2011; 29 (30):3960–3967

[39] Zhao Y, Wang WJ, Guan S, et al. Sorafenib combined with transarterial chemoembolization for the treatment of advanced hepatocellular carcinoma: a large-scale multicenter study of 222 patients. Ann Oncol. 2013; 24(7): 1786–1792

[40] Abdel-Rahman O, Elsayed ZA. Combination trans arterial chemoembolization (TACE) plus sorafenib for the management of unresectable hepatocellular carcinoma: a systematic review of the literature. Dig Dis Sci. 2013; 58(12): 3389–3396

[41] Choi GH, Shim JH, Kim MJ, et al. Sorafenib alone versus sorafenib combined with transarterial chemoembolization for advanced-stage hepatocellular carcinoma: results of propensity score analyses. Radiology. 2013; 269(2): 603–611

[42] Zhang L, Hu P, Chen X, Bie P. Transarterial chemoembolization (TACE) plus sorafenib versus TACE for intermediate or advanced stage hepatocellular carcinoma: a meta-analysis. PLoS One. 2014; 9(6):e100305

[43] Huang CY, Lin CS, Tai WT, et al. Sorafenib enhances radiation-induced apoptosis in hepatocellular carcinoma by inhibiting STAT3. Int J Radiat Oncol Biol Phys. 2013; 86(3):456–462

[44] Dawson L.. Phase I. Study of sorafenib and SBRT for advanced hepatocellular carcinoma. Int J Radiat Oncol Biol Phys. 2012; 84(3):s10–s11

[45] Dawson L. Sorafenib tosylate with or without stereotactic body radiation therapy in treating patients with liver cancer [clinical trial]. Available at: https://clinicaltrials.gov/ct2/show/NCT017309372015 [updated November]

[46] NCI. Sorafenib tosylate with or without doxorubicin hydrochloride in treating patients with locally advanced or metastatic liver cancer. Available at: http://clinicaltrials.gov/ct2/show/NCT01015833?term=sorafenib + and + doxorubicin + and + hepatocellular + cancer&rank=3.2015

17 Management of Liver Metastases

Terence P. F. Gade and Gregory J. Nadolski

17.1 Introduction

The liver is a frequent site of metastatic disease. Although extra-abdominal malignancies can spread to the liver, these tend to be late manifestations of the disease process. On the other hand, intra-abdominal malignancies frequently metastasize to the liver at an early time in the disease course and may be present at the time of diagnosis. This chapter will focus on the management of liver metastases with a focus on two malignancies commonly encountered in the interventional oncology practice: colorectal cancer (CRC) and neuroendocrine tumors (NETs). Other types of metastatic disease to the liver will be briefly discussed at the end of the chapter. A more detailed review of the treatment of cholangiocarcinoma and pancreatic adenocarcinoma metastases can be found in Chapters 18 and 21, respectively, of this book.

17.2 Colorectal Cancer

17.2.1 Incidence, Demographics, and Epidemiology

Among all cancers, CRC has the fourth highest incidence in the United States, with approximately 130,000 new cases diagnosed annually and over 1 million people living with the disease. Worldwide, it is the third most commonly diagnosed cancer and the fourth leading cause of cancer death. Of newly diagnosed patients, nearly 25% will present with distant metastases (stage IV disease, as defined by the American Joint Committee on Cancer).[1] Additionally, up to 50% of patients will develop liver metastases in their lifetime.[1,2] The median 5-year survival for metastatic CRC is less than 15%.

CRC incidence varies with geographical location; more than half of all cases occur in more developed nations, with the highest incidence rates occurring in Australia/New Zealand, Europe, and North America. The increased incidence in these regions is partially related to higher rates of physical inactivity, unhealthy diet, smoking, and obesity.[3] Incidence of CRC is higher among people of lower socioeconomic background and educational level in the United States, even when controlling for other known risk factors of the disease, reflecting differences in screening rates among these groups. Racial and sex differences also exist in the United States, with lower rates of CRC among Caucasians and women. Similarly, men worldwide are significantly more likely to develop CRC than women. These differences in incidence are believed to be the result of complex interactions among etiological factors and differences in screening rates.[4] Regardless of race, sex, and socioeconomic status, the incidence of CRC increases with age beginning in the fifth decade of life.

Approximately 90% of CRCs are sporadic, whereas 10% occur in association with one of several genetic conditions predisposing one to CRC. Of these genetic predispositions, the two most common and well understood are familial adenomatous polyposis (FAP) and hereditary nonpolyposis colorectal cancer (HNPCC), formerly referred to as Lynch's syndrome. In FAP, carcinogenesis is driven by chromosomal instability involving chromosomes 5q, 17p, and 18q.[5] Alterations of these chromosomes lead to deletions and loss of function of the tumor suppressor genes adenomatous polyposis coli (*APC*), tumor protein P53 (*p53*), and deleted in colorectal carcinoma (*DCC*) with subsequent mutational activation of the oncogene *KRAS*. HNPCC is characterized by microsatellite instability with alterations in mismatch repair genes, leading to accumulation of mutations and carcinogenesis. Both of these patterns of carcinogenesis are observed in sporadic cancers as well, although microsatellite instability in sporadic cancer is an epigenetic phenomenon regulated by methylation of mismatch repair genes as opposed to mutational loss of function of the genes encoding the proteins involved in this deoxyribonucleic acid (DNA) repair mechanism.

17.2.2 Diagnosis and Prognosis

CRC may be suspected when a patient presents with a gradual change in bowel habits, gastrointestinal bleeding, or bowel obstruction. For symptomatic CRC, colonoscopy is usually performed first, as this procedure allows tissue sampling for diagnostic purposes and tissue staging. Alternatively, CRC may be discovered by routine screening. The American College of Gastroenterologists recommends performing screening colonoscopy every 10 years beginning at age 50 (45 years of age for African Americans) in patients at average risk for CRC. Alternative strategies for individuals at average risk include flexible sigmoidoscopy every 5 years, computed tomography (CT) colonography every 5 years, or a fecal immunochemical test for blood annually. Screening strategies for patients with above-average risk because of family history, prior adenomatous polyp, or genetic predisposition to CRC are beyond the scope of this chapter but may be reviewed elsewhere.[6,7]

Once a diagnosis of CRC has been established based on histological evaluation of the endoscopic biopsy, clinical staging is performed with cross-sectional imaging to evaluate for distant metastases. The National Comprehensive Cancer Network (NCCN) supports the use of CT of the chest, abdomen, and pelvis for all patients with CRC before resection of the primary tumor. Alternatively, contrast-enhanced magnetic resonance imaging (MRI) of the abdomen and pelvis combined with unenhanced CT of the chest can be performed for clinical staging. MRI is more sensitive to detecting liver metastases in treatment-naïve patients and may be particularly advantageous when steatosis of the liver makes the detection of hypoattenuating metastases difficult on CT. The NCCN recommends the use of positron emission tomography (PET)/CT only in the setting of equivocal findings on CT or MRI. In a study comparing preoperative PET/CT with CT, PET/CT was similar to conventional CT in regard to tumor detection rate (100% with PET/CT vs. 95% with CT) and nodal accuracy (59% with PET/CT vs. 62% with CT). Furthermore, findings on PET/CT resulted in treatment changes in only one patient (2%).[8]

Overall, the 1- and 5-year survival rates for patients with CRC are 83 and 65%, respectively. A modest decrease in survival is observed at 10 years after diagnosis (~58%). For stage I and IIa CRCs, the 5-year survival rate can exceed 90%. Unfortunately, less than 40% of tumors are diagnosed at these stages, likely because of underuse of screening. For more advanced stage cancers with involvement of regional lymph nodes, the 5-year survival rate decreases to approximately 70%, and this rate further decreases to 13% when the disease has metastasized to distant organs.[9,10]

Although the colon and rectum will be treated as a single entity in this chapter for simplicity, several factors distinguishing the two entities are worth noting. First, the molecular pathways leading from adenoma to carcinoma differ between the two entities. Colon cancer carcinogenesis is characterized by the two mechanisms mentioned earlier. However, rectal cancer rarely exhibits microsatellite instability, is less *KRAS* dependent for carcinogenesis, and overall develops more genetic mutations than colon cancer.[11] Second, the pattern of metastatic spread is different with rectal cancer; disease more commonly spreads to the lungs without metastatic involvement of the liver, presumably because of the rectum's drainage to the systemic venous circulation through the inferior rectal veins.[12,13] Additionally, rectal cancers tend to present earlier with a change in bowel habits or visible blood in the stool and can be more readily detected with flexible sigmoidoscopy or digital rectal examination. The combination of these factors culminates in diagnosis at an early stage of the disease compared to colon cancer; this ultimately results in slightly better overall survival. Lastly, treatment for these two entities is different, as treatment for rectal cancer involves neoadjuvant and/or adjuvant radiation to the primary site of disease, whereas treatment for colon cancer does not.

17.3 Therapy for Metastatic Colorectal Cancer

17.3.1 Systemic Chemotherapy

Systemic chemotherapy for metastatic CRC (mCRC) has rapidly evolved over the past 25 years and resulted in a near doubling of the median survival from approximately 12 months to nearly 24 months in some clinical trials.[14] For mCRC, chemotherapy regimens are based on the antimetabolite 5-fluoruracil (5-FU), which directly inhibits thymidylate synthase, in combination with the adjuvant folinic acid, also known as leucovorin (L), which augments 5-FU inhibition of thymidylate synthase. In the late 1990s, several trials demonstrated that the addition of the cytotoxic agent oxaliplatin (XELOX) improved progression-free survival in patients with mCRC compared to 5-FU/L alone (from 6.2 to 9 months).[15] Further studies demonstrated the addition of XELOX with 5-FU/L, known commonly as FOLFOX, significantly improved the disease-free survival rate for patients with stage II or III CRC compared to 5-FU/L alone (from 73 to 78%; hazard ratio [HR]: 0.77; confidence interval [CI]: 0.65–0.91, $p = 0.002$).[16,17]

Noninferiority studies of the 5-FU prodrug capecitabine (Xeloda) established its efficacy in intermediate-stage CRC. Subsequently, the use of capecitabine plus XELOX compared to

FOLFOX validated the use of this combination for mCRC.[18] In this noninferiority study, XELOX had a similar overall response rate (42%) to FOLFOX (46%). Additionally, progression-free and median overall survivals in the XELOX arm were similar (8.8 and 19.9 months, respectively) to FOLFOX (9.3 and 20.5 months, respectively) with significantly less neutropenia and neuropathy.

Further refinements to the medical treatment of mCRC have involved the addition of the topoisomerase inhibitor irinotecan to 5-FU/L. Initial studies of irinotecan plus 5-FU/L, a combination known as FOLFIRI, demonstrated improved survival with this regimen versus 5-FU/L alone.[19,20] FOLFIRI gained widespread acceptance for treating mCRC after a crossover design trial demonstrated that the outcomes with this regimen were equivalent to the outcomes seen with six cycles of FOLFOX.[21] In this study, patients assigned to FOLFIRI first had a median survival of 21.5 months compared to 20.6 months for those allocated to FOLFOX6 before FOLFIRI. Importantly, the response rate to either regimen as the first-line agent was similar (56% with FOLFIRI and 54% with FOLFOX). The only differences in outcomes noted by the investigators were the types of toxicity observed, with more mucositis and nausea/vomiting occurring with irinotecan and more neutropenia and neuropathy occurring with XELOX.[21] The success of FOLFIRI has led some investigators to consider treating mCRC with FOLFIRI plus XELOX, a triplet regimen termed FOLFOXIRI.

Monoclonal antibodies to vascular endothelial growth factor (VEGF) and epidermal growth factor receptor (EGFR) have been used in combination with FOLFOX or FOLFIRI to treat mCRC, particularly in patients who do not carry mutations in *KRAS*.[22,23,24] In one trial, patients with mCRC were randomized to FOLFIRI plus the EGFR antagonist cetuximab or to FOLFIRI plus bevacizumab, a monoclonal antibody to VEGF. The objective response rate was similar for the two groups (62% for cetuximab and 58% for bevacizumab). The median overall survival was nearly 29 months in the cetuximab group, about 3 months longer than overall survival in the bevacizumab group, suggesting the potential superiority of cetuximab as a first-line biologic in combination with FOLFIRI.[22]

Within the past 15 years, chemotherapy regimens for mCRC have been repeatedly refined increasing overall survival from the time of diagnosis. As a result, surgical and minimally invasive therapies to enhance survival have become more common in the care of these patients. Therefore, knowledge of the toxicities of mCRC chemotherapies that may alter or preclude the use of invasive procedures is mandatory. One well-recognized phenomenon that can occur after treatment with XELOX is hepatic sinusoidal dilation and congestion, which may be seen in up to 19% of patients undergoing liver resection after receiving this agent; however, this effect is not associated with a significant increase in mortality after surgery.[25] 5-FU and its prodrug capecitabine are known to cause fatty liver disease, found in nearly half of patients on CT follow-up of hepatic metastases. Unfortunately, the exact relationships among the cumulative dose of 5-FU, changes in liver function tests, and progression to steatohepatitis remain unclear. Although steatosis has been linked to increased complication rates after hepatic resection of colon cancer metastases, mortality is not affected by this condition.[26,27] Steatohepatitis is most commonly observed in patients treated with irinotecan (~8%). Unlike steatosis, steatohepatitis is associated with increased 90-day mortality after liver resection

(14.7 vs. 1.6% 90-day mortality in patients without steatohepatitis).[25] Lastly, bevacizumab has been found to impair wound healing. Although recommendations regarding bevacizumab treatment differ based on the type of intervention used and other health parameters, in general, the drug must be held both before and after interventions to prevent an increased risk of wound complications. Generally, incisions should be fully healed before bevacizumab therapy is reinitiated.[28]

17.3.2 Surgical Management

For patients with liver-only mCRC, surgical resection and/or ablation is the only potentially curative therapy. Many studies have demonstrated a survival benefit with resection including 5-year overall survival of 30 to 60% and 10-year survival of approximately 20%.[29,30] However, this treatment strategy has two major limitations. First, the number of patients whose distribution of hepatic metastases is considered resectable at the time of diagnosis is limited, constituting approximately 15% of all patients with mCRC. Second, the eventual failure rate of hepatic resection alone is high, with up to 75% of patients relapsing in some studies and approximately half of all recurrences occurring in the liver.[31] Thus, treatment of mCRC becomes truly multidisciplinary, as the use of neoadjuvant or adjuvant chemotherapy can mitigate both limitations and potentially prolong survival after resection.

Just as the medical management of chemotherapy has evolved over the past three decades, so has the selection of patients for treatment with surgery and neoadjuvant and adjuvant chemotherapy. Although once patients with greater than three hepatic metastases were excluded from resection because of an increased risk of recurrence, current data suggest that although the absolute number of metastases may reflect the likelihood of recurrence, the absolute number of metastases is no longer a contraindication to resection.[32,33] Additionally, the presence of bilobar metastases is no longer an absolute contraindication to resection.[34] In both scenarios, the most critical factor is whether all tumors can be completely resected or ablated while preserving adequate liver function. Complete resection (R0 resection) has been shown to be one of the most powerful predictors of overall survival. For example, John et al observed a 5-year survival rate of 46.7% with R0 resection of liver metastases from CRC compared with a 14.6% rate in patients with incomplete resection.[35] To obtain adequate volume of the future liver remnant, portal vein embolization may need to be performed before resection or after ablation in preparation for two-stage hepatectomy.[36,37] The details of portal vein embolization indications, techniques, and outcomes are covered in Chapter 19.

The use of postoperative chemotherapy after curative resection improves overall survival compared to surgery alone. However, the optimal timing of chemotherapy relative to resection still remains unclear. There is a strong rationale for preoperative neoadjuvant chemotherapy. First, neoadjuvant therapy can be used to treat micrometastases, preventing further spread to other organs. Second, response assessment to chemotherapy before surgery may allow optimization of therapy after surgery or prevent the need for surgery in patients with early-stage disease. However, it should be noted that several clinical trials and retrospective studies have shown that response before resection is not predictive of overall survival.[38,39,40] Lastly, neoadjuvant chemotherapy offers the potential to convert unresectable cases to resection candidates. The rate of conversion varies based on the chemotherapy regimen used but has ranged from 20 to 30% in most trials.[41] One potential risk of neoadjuvant therapy is liver injury precluding resection. The primary concern is steatohepatitis secondary to irinotecan or 5-FU treatment. Sinusoidal injury from XELOX is more common, but this occurrence has not been shown to be predictive of postoperative liver failure.[42]

17.3.3 Hepatic Artery Infusional Chemotherapy

Like other forms of locoregional therapy, hepatic artery infusional (HAI) chemotherapy is based on the premise that hepatic metastases derive the majority of their blood supply and nutrients from the hepatic artery, whereas hepatocytes rely more on portal venous blood flow. Therefore, the tumoricidal effects of direct infusion of chemotherapy can be maximized while minimizing the systemic toxicity from intravenous administration.

To deliver this therapy, a fully implanted pump is typically placed during a usually open abdominal surgery with the infusion catheter placed into the gastroduodenal artery.[43] 5-fluoro 2-deoxyuridine (FUDR), a deoxyribonucleoside derivative of 5-FU, is the typical chemotherapeutic agent infused through HAI pumps. This agent is administered as a continuous infusion in cycles of 2 weeks on and 2 weeks off therapy. FUDR is considered ideal for HAI because it has high first-pass extraction by the liver and, when administered intra-arterially, can reach concentrations in hepatic tumors 400 times greater than the concentrations seen with systemic delivery.[44,45]

Multiple clinical trials have demonstrated the efficacy of HAI in treating mCRC within the liver. A multicenter German study demonstrated similar overall survival for patients treated with HAI 5-FU/L, systemic 5-FU/L, and HAI FUDR.[46] A study by Kemeny et al[47] assessed HAI FUDR versus systemic 5-FU/L and found that overall survival was significantly longer for the HAI therapy group (median: 24 months) than for the systemic therapy group (median: 20 months; $p = 0.0034$). This trial was the first to show a survival benefit for HAI chemotherapy despite not allowing crossover between arms. Despite the limited data showing superiority of HAI over systemic therapy, proponents of HAI point to the high rate of conversion from unresectable disease to resectable or ablatable hepatic metastases as a rationale for using HAI in patients with liver-only mCRC. Overall, the rate of conversion is slightly higher with HAI than with systemic therapy, ranging from 25 to 45% in most studies.[48] The rate of conversion may be further increased by combining HAI with systemic chemotherapy. Phase I studies have demonstrated the safety of combining FUDR HAI with irinotecan, XELOX, and FOLFOX as first- and second-line therapy, with observed response rates near 90% and median overall survival ranging from 17 to 36 months.[49,50]

The most common toxicity observed with HAI therapy is biliary toxicity from FUDR infusion. Mild hyperbilirubinemia is often self-limited and may resolve when the dose is reduced or the infusion is held. Severe or progressive hyperbilirubinemia is often a sign of irreversible biliary toxicity with stricture formation that may require biliary stenting. The addition of dexamethasone to FUDR infusion decreases the rate of biliary toxicity from 30 to less than 10%.[51] Technical complications related to the HAI pump or catheter have been reported to occur in 12 to 41% of patients.[52]

17.3.4 Percutaneous Ablation

Ablation may be performed in conjunction with open resection or may be performed laparoscopically or percutaneously. This technique may be offered in many clinical scenarios, but the most commonly encountered scenarios involve patients with limited hepatic disease (typically defined as < 3 lesions), those who are not surgical candidates, those with unresectable mCRC (in an attempt to treat lesions in the remnant liver after resection), and those with recurrent hepatic metastases. Multiple ablation modalities are available for treating tumors within the liver, including radiofrequency ablation (RFA), cryoablation, microwave ablation (MWA), and irreversible electroporation (IRE). Of these modalities, RFA has been the most extensively discussed in the literature.

RFA works by delivering thermal energy into the tissue using high-frequency alternating current, causing thermal coagulation. Cellular death occurs instantaneously at temperatures in excess of 60 °C. Most retrospective studies in the surgical literature comparing resection to RFA alone found RFA to be inferior to resection.[53] For example, RFA alone was found to have a recurrence rate of 84% and a 4-year survival rate of 22% compared to 52 and 65%, respectively, for resection.[54] Studies from the radiology literature have also reported poorer survival outcomes with RFA than with resection.[55] The median survival after RFA was found to be approximately 3 years, with a 5-year overall survival rate of approximately 25%.[53,56] In a comparison of RFA versus resection of solitary metastases, the two techniques demonstrated similar 3-year overall survival rates (approximately 55%).[57] As technique and patient selection have improved such that patients undergoing RFA have become similar to those undergoing resection, 5- and 10-year overall survival rates with RFA have begun to approach the rates seen with surgery.[58]

RFA remains the second best option after surgical resection in terms of recurrence and overall survival (▶ Fig. 17.1). However, given the high incidence of recurrence after resection,

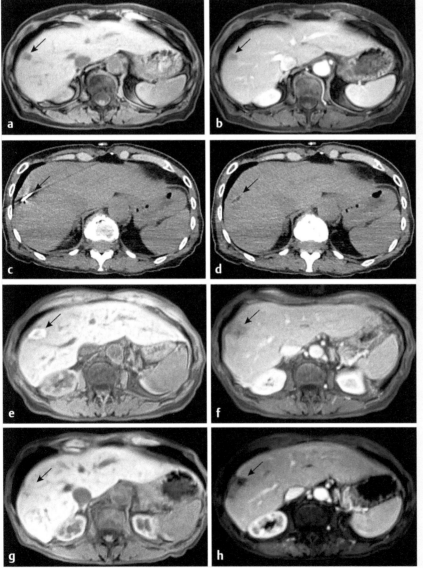

Fig. 17.1 A 61-year-old woman with a history of metastatic colorectal cancer. **(a)** Pre- and **(b)** postcontrast T1-weighted magnetic resonance (MR) images demonstrate a hypointense and nonenhancing metastasis within segment 4 of the liver (*arrows*). **(c)** A preablation noncontrast computed tomography (CT) image demonstrates positioning of a single microwave ablation probe within the target lesion (*arrow*). **(d)** A postablation noncontrast CT image demonstrates gas within the distribution of the target lesion (*arrow*). One month following ablation, **(e)** pre- and **(f)** postcontrast T1-weighted MR images demonstrate hyperintensity within the treatment zone (*arrows*) in keeping with blood products without enhancement. One and a half years following ablation, **(g)** pre- and **(h)** postcontrast T1-weighted MR images demonstrate resolution of blood products within the treatment zone (*arrows*) without contrast enhancement in keeping with a completely treated metastasis.

many clinicians support the use of ablation for oligometastatic disease because patients are spared unnecessary surgery. For example, Livraghi et al[59] found that 98% of patients with oligometastatic mCRC to the liver could be spared surgical resection by undergoing percutaneous ablation; 2% went on to surgery because of incomplete ablation. In this study, approximately half of the patients were disease free at follow-up, whereas the other half had disease that recurred within the liver or elsewhere. The authors suggested that the patients who had disease recurrence would have experienced this recurrence regardless of whether resection or ablation was used and that these individuals therefore benefited by avoiding the morbidity of hepatic resection.

Rather than considering RFA a competitor of resection, many use RFA as a complementary tool for patients with unresectable mCRC. For example, in one trial, RFA was used in combination with resection in patients with unresectable mCRC to potentially cure all metastatic disease. The 5-year overall survival rate for treated patients was 43%, which is similar to the survival achieved with resection alone.[60] Similar results have been seen in the treatment of bilateral unresectable mCRC with ablation. RFA has also been used in combination with chemotherapy for the treatment of unresectable mCRC. Ruers et al[61] found improved progression-free survival in patients randomized to receive RFA in conjunction with systemic chemotherapy (17 months) compared to those treated with systemic chemotherapy alone (10 months).

Despite the success of RFA in some studies and in different applications, this technique remains limited by the size of individual metastases. In general, tumors greater than 3 cm are more difficult to completely ablate with a single probe, and lesions greater than 4 cm almost always require the use of overlapping ablations. These size limitations affect the outcomes of RFA. For example, Livraghi et al[59] observed that the median survival for patients with hepatic mCRC lesions was 38 months for tumors less than 3 cm, 34 months for tumors between 3 and 5 cm, and only 21 months for tumors less than 5 cm. Similarly, the recurrence rate for tumors greater than 4 cm can exceed 70%.[62] An additional limitation of RFA is the potential for incomplete ablation of tumors adjacent to large blood vessels that dissipate heat from the area, the so-called heat sink effect. Also, as tissue desiccates and becomes charred, radiofrequency energy becomes less effective in heating tissue at the periphery, which may result in incomplete ablation. Furthermore, ablation near large central biliary structures is not recommended because of the potential for fistula or biliary stricture. Overall, the major complication rates for RFA are low, with complications occurring in approximately 6% of cases and death occurring in 1%.[63] The most frequently reported major complication is abscess formation in the ablation cavity. Other less common major complications include portal vein thrombosis, pleural effusion, and injury to adjacent bowel. Tract seeding from RFA is extremely rare, occurring in less than 0.2% of ablated tumors.[56,63]

MWA uses a needle-based probe with a microwave antenna near the tip, which is inserted through a tumor under imaging guidance. When microwave energy is applied to the tissue, rapid oscillation of water molecules raises the temperature of the tissue, resulting in coagulative necrosis. This transfer of energy is more rapid and varies less with tissue composition and density compared with RFA because of the shorter wavelength used with MWA.[64] In animal models of ablation, these properties of MWA allow it to be less susceptible to heat sink and to incomplete ablation secondary to charring.[65,66,67] Although this suggests that MWA would be effective in treating larger tumors, several studies have shown that recurrence rates with MWA are higher for lesions greater than 3 cm.[68]

Ablation is not limited to patients with newly diagnosed mCRC or those with liver-only disease (▶ Fig. 17.2). When disease recurs after resection or ablation, survival decreases to approximately 36 months regardless of whether the recurrence is local tumor progression or new metastatic disease.[58] Treatment of these recurrences, particularly local progression, improves survival to approximately 46 months, which is still poorer than the 63-month median survival seen in those without local tumor progression.[58] Although extrahepatic disease is a poor prognostic factor, ablation should still be considered in these patients if the bulk of mCRC is within the liver. Gillams et al[56] demonstrated a median survival of approximately 2 years in patients with extrahepatic mCRC who underwent RFA of liver metastases. Although this is a year less than those without extrahepatic disease, these outcomes may still justify ablation in select cases.

17.3.5 Transarterial Embolotherapy

Multiple transarterial therapies are currently being used to treat mCRC. These interventions were initially reserved for cases of unresectable multifocal disease that had become refractory to systemic chemotherapy. However, the use of transarterial embolotherapy to treat mCRC has progressed over the past two decades.

Conventional lipiodol-based transarterial chemoembolization (cTACE) was the initial embolotherapy used to treat chemorefractory mCRC. This embolization approach uses a variety of chemotherapy agents, typically mitomycin-C, cisplatin, doxorubicin, or irinotecan, in an emulsion with ethiodized oil. Gelfoam- or starch-based embolization material may be mixed with or delivered immediately after the emulsion.[69] One randomized trial suggested that differences in the infused therapy had little effect on response.[70,71] Early experiences with this technique in chemorefractory disease demonstrated a positive effect, with radiologic response in 63% of cases, a median survival of approximately 8 months, and acceptable rates of mild and moderate toxicity.[72] Attempts at using cTACE as a first-line therapy for patients with mCRC with liver-only metastases have been less successful. In an early phase trial of patients with liver-only mCRC, chemoembolization before systemic 5-FU therapy was associated with an overall response rate of only 29%. Furthermore, time to progression was approximately 8 months, and median survival was only 14 months.[73] Subsequent studies of cTACE as a second-line therapy have demonstrated that cTACE leads to results that are similar to those seen with other second-line systemic therapies, although trials directly comparing systemic chemotherapy to cTACE have **not** been performed.[71,74]

The evolution of TACE has brought about the development of drug-eluting beads (DEBs). DEBs contain sulfonate binding sites on polyvinyl alcohol beads, which can be loaded with doxorubicin or irinotecan via an ion-exchange mechanism.[75] The rationale behind DEB-TACE is that more controlled chemotherapy

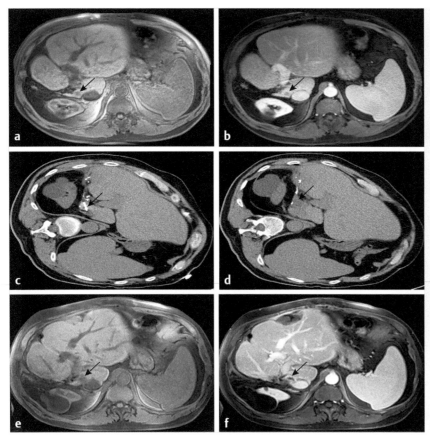

Fig. 17.2 A 67-year-old man with a history of metastatic colorectal cancer. **(a)** Pre- and **(b)** postcontrast T1-weighted magnetic resonance (MR) images demonstrate a hypointense and nonenhancing metastasis within the caudate lobe of the liver (*arrows*). **(c)** Preablation noncontrast computed tomography (CT) demonstrates positioning of one of the two microwave ablation probes within the target lesion (*arrow*). **(d)** Postablation noncontrast CT demonstrates hypoattenuation within the distribution of the target lesion (*arrow*). One year and three months following ablation, **(e)** pre- and **(f)** postcontrast T1-weighted MR images demonstrate hypointensity and hypoenhancement within the treatment zone in keeping with a completely treated lesion (*arrow*).

release can be achieved with this technique, resulting in a more reproducible therapy. DEBs bound with irinotecan (commonly called DEBIRI) were introduced in 2006 for the treatment of mCRC. Preclinical testing of this device in a porcine model demonstrated sustained release of irinotecan into the hepatic parenchyma with systemic plasma levels reduced by 75% when compared with bolus infusion of intra-arterial irinotecan.[75]

DEBIRI has been compared to systemic therapy either alone or in conjunction with systemic chemotherapy. In a randomized trial comparing DEBIRI to FOLFIRI, the DEBIRI group had improved survival and imaging response rate (22 months and 69%, respectively) versus the FOLFIRI group (15 months and 20%, respectively).[76] A recent phase II study evaluating DEBIRI with capecitabine demonstrated the safety of this combination.[77] More recently, a trial comparing FOLFOX plus bevacizumab to FOLFOX plus bevacizumab plus DEBIRI for the treatment of mCRC demonstrated that the overall response rate was significantly higher (by 15–30%) in the DEBIRI arm at 2, 4, and 6 months (**$p = 0.02$, 0.03, and 0.05, respectively**).[78] The frequency of patients being converted to resectability more than doubled in the DEBIRI arm (to 35%) despite 56% of patients in the DEBIRI arm having extrahepatic disease compared to 32% of patients in the chemotherapy arm. Progression-free survival also doubled to 15.3 months in the DEBIRI arm. The rate of toxicity was similar between the two groups (~50%).[78]

The most common side effects and adverse events associated with DEBIRI are similar to those seen with cTACE and seem to be related to postembolization syndrome. These adverse events include nausea/vomiting and abdominal pain, occurring in up to 55 and 60% of patients, respectively. Fatigue is also common.

However, liver dysfunction or failure is rare, occurring in less than 5% of cases.[78,79] Factors associated with adverse events are embolization to complete stasis, treatment with greater than 100 mg of irinotecan in a single session, repeated embolization, degree of liver involvement by tumor, and pre-embolization bilirubin level greater than 2.0 g/dL.[79]

An alternative form of transarterial embolotherapy is intra-arterial injection of nondegradable glass or resin microspheres loaded with the nearly pure beta-emitter yttrium-90 (Y-90). This technique was first introduced in the early 1980s and has evolved from being used in a single whole liver treatment session to being used in multisession lobar or segmental treatments. Y-90 has a half-life of 2.67 days, has an energy level of 0.94 MeV, and demonstrates mean and maximum soft-tissue penetration of 2.5 and 11 mm, respectively.[80] No clinically significant leaching of the Y-90 from either type of microsphere has been observed. Although a greater median radiation dose is delivered with glass microspheres, largely because the ratio of radioactivity per bead is higher for glass spheres (3–10 GBq on 4 million glass spheres) than for resin microspheres (0.75–3.03 GBq on 50 million resin spheres), no difference in response between the two bead types has been reported.[81]

Radioembolization of mCRC was originally almost exclusively performed for chemorefractory disease or in patients who had developed severe toxicity to systemic therapy. Compared to patients treated with best supportive care for chemorefractory disease, which provides an overall survival of less than 6 months, patients treated with radioembolization typically experience an overall survival of 10.5 months and a 2-year survival rate of approximately 20%.[82] Prospective phase II studies of chemorefractory mCRC have demonstrated a median overall survival of approximately 12 months even though most patients in these studies had received ≥ 4 lines of chemotherapy before radioembolization. In this heavily treated cohort, liver failure after embolization was rare, occurring in only a single patient.[83] Factors associated with improved outcomes after radioembolization of chemorefractory mCRC are smaller tumor volume, liver-only disease, and response to radioembolization.[84,85] In this population, patients who demonstrate an imaging response to radioembolization can have an overall survival that is twice as long as those who have progression or no response after therapy.[83]

Researchers have also begun to explore the combination of radioembolization and systemic therapy. A phase I trial of radioembolization plus second-line systemic therapy with irinotecan failed to reach the maximum tolerated dose.[86] Although approximately 50% of patients had grade 3 (G3) toxicities or greater, these toxicities were similar to those previously reported for irinotecan-based therapies. The outcomes of this early phase trial were promising, with progression-free and overall survival of 6 and 12 months, respectively.[86] Radioembolization has also been studied in combination with first-line systemic therapy.[87,88] Based on the promise of early phase studies using radioembolization with 5-FU/L or FOLFOX, two large phase III trials were planned: the SIRFLOX trial, which examined progression-free survival, and the FOXFIRE trial, which aims to examine overall survival and has just completed enrollment.[89] Although the addition of radioembolization to FOLFOX first-line chemotherapy did not improve progression-free survival overall (~10 months) in the SIRFLOX trial, a significant delay in tumor progression within the liver was seen with the addition of radioembolization (20.5 months) compared to chemotherapy only (12.6 months) in patients with mCRC that was either liver-only (60%) or liver-dominant (40%) disease (HR: 0.69; 95% CI: 0.55–0.90; $p = 0.002$).[89]

As with cTACE and DEBIRI, the toxicity and complications of radioembolization are caused by the treatment itself, destruction of normal hepatocytes, and improper delivery to extrahepatic viscera. Postradioembolization syndrome is similar to postembolization syndrome but consists of fatigue and cachexia more commonly than nausea/vomiting or abdominal pain. Reported rates of toxicity range from 20 to 70%. Despite this frequency, toxicity from radioembolization is only rarely severe enough to necessitate hospitalization.[90,91] The most feared complication of radioembolization is liver failure from destruction of normal hepatocytes, termed radioembolization-induced liver disease.[92] Severe radioembolization-induced liver disease, which is most often fatal or at the least will cause severe enough toxicity to prevent additional systemic therapy, occurs in 2 to 13% of cases. The factor most commonly associated with radioembolization-induced liver disease in noncirrhotic patients is prior systemic chemotherapy in the 2 months preceding radioembolization.[92]

17.4 Neuroendocrine Tumors

Once considered an exceedingly rare malignancy, the incidence of NET has increased by fivefold in the United States in the past four decades and is second only to colon cancer in terms of the prevalence of gastrointestinal tract malignancies. This increasing prevalence has spurred the development of new therapies for this disease. As with CRC, metastatic NET requires a multidisciplinary approach involving oncology, gastroenterology, endocrinology, surgery, and interventional oncology. To better care for patients with metastatic NET, interventional oncologists must be familiar with the management of NET by other specialists to fully understand when to apply locoregional therapies and how to guide patients in integration of care.

17.5 Defining Neuroendocrine Disease

17.5.1 Terminology

NET is defined as a spectrum of epithelial neoplasms originating in cells that synthesize and release peptide hormones in response to specific neuronal stimuli. Neuroendocrine neoplasms may arise sporadically or as part of familial syndromes including multiple endocrine neoplasia, von Hippel–Lindau syndrome, and neurofibromatosis. Originally identified in the small intestine, NETs were first thought to be benign based on histology and an indolent growth pattern, and thus were termed carcinoid or carcinoma-like. Since then, NETs have been found to originate primarily from the gastrointestinal tract, pancreas, or epithelium of the airways but may arise from any organ given the widespread distribution of neuroendocrine cells within the body. More importantly, these tumors are not benign; they have the potential to metastasize and develop an aggressive phenotype.

This heterogeneity of origin and invasiveness has created difficulty in nomenclature. Recently, the World Health Organization Classification of Tumors of the Digestive System of 2010 was published with the intent of addressing this issue.[93] This system focuses on criteria that determine malignant potential, incorporating histological features such as tumor differentiation and grade along with site of primary tumor, tumor size, and disease stage. Tumor differentiation is the extent to which the neoplasm resembles nonneoplastic neuroendocrine cells in the primary site of disease. Tumor grade, which is based on proliferative activity, is classified by the number of mitoses per unit area of tumor (mitoses per 10 high-power microscopic fields or per 2 mm^2) or by the proliferative index (the percentage of cells staining for Ki-67). G1 and G2 represent well-differentiated neoplasms based on the proliferative index. The term "neuroendocrine carcinoma" is reserved for G3 neoplasms, which include high-grade, poorly differentiated large cell or small cell neuroendocrine carcinomas.[93]

17.5.2 Incidence, Demographics, and Epidemiology

The Surveillance, Epidemiology, and End Results database of the National Cancer Institute shows a significant increase in the incidence of NET in the United States, from 1.09 per 100,000 in 1973 to 5.25 per 100,000 in 2004.[94] Despite the relatively low incidence of this disease, NET has a relatively high prevalence, estimated to be 35/100,000. This prevalence surpasses other malignancies of the upper gastrointestinal tract, pancreas, and liver, highlighting the indolent course of neuroendocrine neoplasms relative to other epithelial malignancies.[94]

NET has a slight female predominance (52–55%).[94,95] The median age at diagnosis is 63 years; the age at diagnosis of appendiceal and rectal NETs is lower. In a recent analysis of the Surveillance, Epidemiology, and End Results registry, Yao et al[94] found that the gastrointestinal tract remains the primary site of NETs (~50% of all cases). Tracheobronchopulmonary NETs represent the largest group of extragastrointestinal NETs, comprising 27% of all neuroendocrine neoplasms.

17.5.3 Diagnosis and Prognosis

Despite the ability of NETs to secrete peptide hormones, thus causing a wide variety of paraneoplastic syndromes, most NETs are asymptomatic. Thus, at early stages, these neoplasms may be incidentally discovered during surgery or on imaging performed for an unrelated condition. More commonly, this condition is not diagnosed before metastasis occurs. The predilection for advanced disease at the time of diagnosis is emphasized by the fact that most patients develop symptoms such as mass effect, tumor-induced fibrosis, mechanical bowel obstruction, weight loss/abdominal pain, and rectal bleeding.

When NETs are hormonally active, symptoms vary based on the tumor cell of origin and the specific secreted hormone. Potential hormones include serotonin, catecholamine, dopamine, histamine, gastrin, glucagon, and prostaglandins. Although classical carcinoid syndrome resulting in cutaneous flushing, diarrhea, bronchoconstriction, and right-sided heart failure is the most well-known reaction, it is relatively uncommon, occurring in approximately 20% of small bowel neuroendocrine neoplasms and in less than 5% of extraenteric disease cases.[96] The onset of symptoms related to the secretion of these bioactive amines usually coincides with the development of liver metastases. Once the disease has metastasized to the liver, these hormones are no longer metabolized as efficiently, and the frequency of carcinoid syndrome increases to 60%.[97] Carcinoid syndrome in the absence of liver metastases may be encountered when the primary site drains to the systemic circulation, as occurs in thoracic and ovarian primary NETs. When carcinoid syndrome is suspected, the serotonin breakdown product 5-hydroxyindole-3-acetic acid can be measured within urine; this technique has a specificity of 88% for identifying serotonin-producing NETs within the small intestine. Alternatively, the diagnosis of a hormonally active neuroendocrine neoplasm can be confirmed through serum measurements of the relevant peptides and amines. Among these biomarkers, chromogranin A is the most sensitive for NET (99%). Chromogranin A level also correlates with tumor volume. However, this marker is nonspecific and may also be seen in patients with small cell lung cancer, prostate cancer, atrophic gastritis, or renal insufficiency.[96]

Because most NETs are hormonally inactive, imaging plays a pivotal role in the diagnosis and management of this condition. Although some studies suggest that MRI is more effective than CT in the detection of liver metastases, both imaging modalities are recommended for initial evaluation, as these techniques may provide complementary information regarding tumor distribution relative to vascular anatomy and may facilitate post-treatment comparisons.[98] Nuclear medicine studies offer greater sensitivity and specificity than CT or MRI. Approximately 70 to 90% of NETs express multiple somatostatin receptor subtypes, allowing imaging with radiolabeled somatostatin analogues such as ^{111}In-octreotide and ^{111}In-lantreotide (reported sensitivities of 93 and 87%, respectively).[99] ^{111}In-octreotide imaging demonstrates significantly higher sensitivity than imaging with other somatostatin analogues and has therefore become the standard method of imaging NETs; this technique also provides predictive information regarding susceptibility of the tumor to therapy with somatostatin analogues. Recently, PET approaches have shown promise for imaging NETs with even greater sensitivity than nuclear imaging with somatostatin analogues.[100,101,102,103] Although highly differentiated tumors do not demonstrate increased uptake of [18]Flouro-deoxyglucose (FDG), FDG-PET may be as sensitive as ^{111}In-octreotide for imaging neuroendocrine neoplasms with a high Ki-67 proliferative index.[104]

NETs generally evolve with a progressive and indolent growth, with symptoms developing in the late stages of the disease once the tumor has metastasized to the lymph nodes, liver, and/or bones. The frequency of distant metastases at the time of diagnosis differs depending on the primary tumor site, ranging from 5% for rectal NETs to 39% for small bowel NETs to 64% for pancreatic neuroendocrine neoplasms.[94] Tumor grade is correlated with the frequency of metastatic disease at presentation, ranging from 21% for well-differentiated (G1), 30% for moderately differentiated (G2), and 50% for poorly differentiated (G3) tumors. Overtime, hepatic metastases develop in an estimated 46 to 93% of patients with NETs.[105,106,107,108]

Overall survival for patients with neuroendocrine neoplasms is approximately 75 months.[94] Survival varies with tumor grade, from a median survival of 124 months for patients with G1 disease, 64 months for patients with G2 disease, and 10 months for patients with higher grade disease.[94] Likewise, stage of disease is a predictor of survival; patients with low-grade NETs with localized, regional, or distant metastatic disease have median survivals of 223, 111, and 33 months, respectively.

17.6 Therapy for Metastatic Neuroendocrine Tumors

Surgery remains the only potentially curative therapy for patients with NET; however, curative resection is possible in less than 10% of patients.[105] No consensus exists regarding the optimal management of metastatic NET. A variety of approaches, including medical therapy, surgical resection/cytoreduction, and minimally invasive locoregional therapies, may be employed, underscoring the importance of a multidisciplinary approach to metastatic NET.

17.6.1 Medical Therapy

Systemic therapy for metastatic NET has evolved tremendously over the past 30 years; the most important advance may have been the discovery of the antiproliferative effects of somatostatin analogues. The antiproliferative effects of octreotide were established in a study that examined the effect of octreotide long-acting repeatable (LAR) on tumor growth in patients with metastatic small bowel NET.[109,110] This study demonstrated a time to progression of 14.3 months in the octreotide LAR arm versus 6 months in the placebo arm, an effect that was independent of hormonal symptoms or chromogranin A levels. This positive response, along with the low toxicity of treatment, clearly established the role of somatostatin analogue therapy for metastatic NET.

In 2011, two new agents were approved by the U.S. Food and Drug Administration for the treatment of metastatic pancreatic NET. Everolimus (Afinitor) is an inhibitor of the serine/threonine kinase mammalian target of rapamycin (mTOR). In one trial, everolimus improved progression-free survival by 5 months when used in combination with octreotide LAR compared to octreotide LAR alone in patients with well-differentiated or moderately differentiated metastatic NET with carcinoid symptoms.[111] In another trial assessing the efficacy of everolimus for the treatment of progressive metastatic pancreatic NET, everolimus alone improved progression-free survival by 7 months versus placebo.[112] More recent research has demonstrated the effectiveness of everolimus for the treatment of pancreatic, small bowel, and lung NETs.[113]

Tyrosine kinases have also been targeted in the treatment of metastatic NET. Sunitinib (Sutent), a multiple tyrosine kinase receptor inhibitor, was found to increase progression-free survival in patients with metastatic pancreatic NET in a double-blind, placebo-controlled, phase III trial.[114] A phase II clinical trial investigating the combination of the tyrosine kinase receptor inhibitor sorafenib plus bevacizumab for the treatment of metastatic intestinal NET of the gut demonstrated a median progression-free survival of 12.4 months with this therapy; however, this combination was associated with unfavorable side effects, including the hand–foot syndrome.[115]

Cytotoxic chemotherapy has also been used for metastatic NET, particularly for tumors of pancreatic origin. In a phase II clinical trial combining temozolomide with capecitabine, 70% of patients achieved an objective radiographic response, with a median progression-free survival of 18 months. The 2-year survival rate was 92%, with minimal toxicity occurring in only 12% of patients.[116]

17.6.2 Surgical Management

Surgical resection remains the only potentially curative therapy for metastatic NET and should be considered for all patients despite the absence of clinical trials comparing surgery with other therapies. Surgery confers a 5-year survival rate of 50 to 85% in this patient population.[117] This remarkable survival benefit exists in spite of an astonishingly high rate of hepatic recurrence—up to 90% at 5 years in some series.[118,119]

Although complete surgical resection is uncommon (performed in approximately 10% of patients), resection of the primary tumor and subtotal resection (debulking) of liver metastases play an important role in the treatment of metastatic neuroendocrine disease. Resection of small bowel primary NET in the metastatic setting improves survival largely by relieving symptoms from local or regional lymphadenopathy such as bowel obstruction; resection of pancreatic primary NET offers less clear benefits.[120,121] Similarly, research has suggested a role for cytoreduction of unresectable metastases in select patients. Liver transplant has also been performed in select cases of metastatic NET, but in general, the role of transplant in these patients remains unclear. Transplant in such cases should generally be limited to select centers with expertise in case selection and management.[122]

17.6.3 Ablation

Ablation therapy has been developed for both percutaneous and surgical approaches and may be used as an adjunct to liver resection or as an alternative to resection for patients who are not candidates for surgery.[123,124] Although no head-to-head clinical trials examining the superiority of the percutaneous or surgical approach exist, each technique has its advantages and disadvantages. Percutaneous ablation is less invasive and less expensive and is associated with lower morbidity than surgery, whereas open or laparoscopic ablation permits direct visualization of the extent of disease, provides access to sites not conducive to percutaneous ablation, and permits simultaneous resection of the primary NET if indicated. All of these factors should be considered when choosing the ablation approach for a given patient.

Percutaneous ablation of metastatic NET is primarily used to palliate carcinoid symptoms and manage recurrent disease after resection or prior ablation in patients with less than five metastatic lesions each ideally measuring less than 3 cm in diameter.[125,126] As with mCRC, RFA is the most well-studied ablation technique in this patient population. One unique consideration when applying ablation to NET is the potential for release of vasoactive hormones during tumor necrosis. Thus, patients should be premedicated with somatostatin analogs before ablation to minimize the risk of carcinoid crisis.[127] Additionally, as many patients may have undergone prior resection of the pancreas or proximal small bowel with a bilioenteric anastomosis, there is an increased risk of liver abscess with ablation.[128]

The outcomes of RFA treatment of neuroendocrine metastases to the liver are encouraging. Local recurrence rates can be as low as 3%.[123] Symptom relief after RFA is well established and has been effective in cases unresponsive to hepatic artery embolization. The median duration of symptom relief is approximately 2 years, with new metastatic disease in the liver commonly occurring by this time. The 5-year overall survival rate after RFA ranges from 40 to 65%.[123] Morbidity with percutaneous ablation can be less than that seen with transarterial therapies or surgery.[129] As with mCRC, other ablation modalities have been applied to the treatment of neuroendocrine liver metastases. MWA seems to perform similarly to RFA, with local recurrence of approximately 3%, recurrence-free survival of 2 to 3 years, and 5-year overall survival higher than 50%.[68]

17.6.4 Transarterial Embolotherapy

Intra-arterial embolotherapy is primarily a palliative treatment that can be used for patients with unresectable disease that is not amenable to ablation (▶ Fig. 17.3). The two primary indications for liver embolization of NET metastases are palliation of hormone-related symptoms uncontrolled by somatostatin analogues and progression of unresectable hepatic metastases threatening liver function.[130] Given the potential for indolent growth of NET metastases within the liver, the optimal timing of embolization with respect to quantity of metastatic disease in the liver remains undefined, and approaches differ considerably among centers. In general, if the tumor occupies less than 25% of liver volume, documented progression on two consecutive imaging studies is an indication for embolization at some

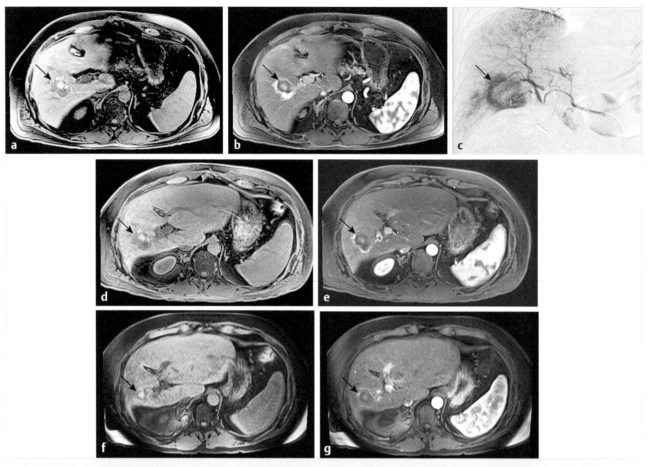

Fig. 17.3 A 44-year-old man with a history of metastatic pancreatic neuroendocrine tumor. **(a)** Pre- and **(b)** postcontrast T1-weighted magnetic resonance (MR) images demonstrate a hypointense and predominantly nonenhancing metastasis (*arrows*) within the inferior right hepatic lobe. **(c)** Right hepatic arteriography demonstrates tumor staining prior to radioembolization of the right hepatic lobe (*arrow*). **(d)** Pre- and **(e)** postcontrast T1-weighted MR images 3 months following radioembolization demonstrate a stable appearance of the targeted metastasis (*arrows*). **(f)** Pre- and **(g)** postcontrast T1-weighted MR images 3 years following radioembolization demonstrate a decrease in size of the treatment zone (*arrows*) without enhancement as well as atrophy of the right hepatic lobe and hypertrophy of the left hepatic lobe.

centers. On the other hand, some institutions would not initiate liver-directed therapy in asymptomatic patients with normal liver function until the tumor burden surpasses 25% of the liver volume, with the rationale that even progressive disease may take years to threaten liver function and embolization therapies can only be used a finite number of times in a patient's lifetime. Extensive tumor replacing approximately half of the liver volume at the time of diagnosis is an indication for prompt embolization, as this degree of tumor invasion limits the likelihood of success and increases the risk of complications from embolotherapy. Embolotherapy is considered the first-line therapy for unresectable liver-dominant low-grade NETs.[131] Extrahepatic disease to the lungs, bones, or lymph nodes is not a contraindication to embolization if the tumor distribution is liver dominant by volume, as the progression of liver involvement will be the primary determinant of life expectancy.

Although intra-arterial infusion of chemotherapy has been tried for metastatic NET, the efficacy of this technique is relatively poor; thus, this option has been supplanted by embolization with or without concurrent infusion of chemotherapy or radioembolization.[132]

First employed in the 1970s, bland embolization of NET can involve a variety of embolic agents including Gelfoam slurry with or without lipiodol, Gelfoam powder, poly vinyl alcohol particles, and tris-acryl particles.[133,134,135,136] Chemoembolization combining intra-arterial chemotherapy with embolics began to be used for NET in the 1980s. A variety of chemotherapeutic agents have been used for chemoembolization in either aqueous or lipid-based preparations without a significant difference in response rates.[137,138] The two most common regimens are doxorubicin (Adriamycin) alone (50 mg/m^2) or a combination of cisplatin (100 mg), Adriamycin (50 mg), and mitomycin-C (10 mg) typically infused as an emulsion with ethiodized oil followed by embolization until near stasis.[139] The addition of ethiodized oil increases chemotherapy dwell time within the tumor as a result of the vascular relaxation induced by the oil's viscosity and permeation of the abnormal tumor vasculature.[140,141] The use of streptozotocin, which has some efficacy as a systemic agent for the treatment of metastatic NET, has not been shown to be as effective as the above agents when used in chemoembolization and is associated with a poorer side effect profile.[142]

More recently, doxorubicin DEBs have been used for metastatic NET, with the rationale that the release of chemotherapy into the ischemic tissue is even greater than with conventional TACE.[143,144,145] The systemic pharmacokinetic profile of DEBs has lower serum levels of doxorubicin compared to conventional TACE, which may translate into fewer systemic side effects.[146] However, two studies have suggested a higher incidence of biliary necrosis and biloma formation after DEB-TACE of NET, with a relative risk ratio of 8:1 compared to conventional TACE.[147,148]

Regardless of the embolization method used, patients with bilioenteric anastomosis are at risk of biloma and abscess formation after embolization.[149] Pre- and postprocedural antibiotic regimens have been shown to decrease the incidence of abscess formation after embolization in this scenario.[150,151] As with ablation, patients should receive somatostatin analogue therapy (octreotide 500 mcg subcutaneously or intravenously) before embolization to minimize the incidence of carcinoid crisis.

Transarterial embolization demonstrates a clear therapeutic benefit regardless of the method used. There are no definitive data demonstrating the relative superiority of chemoembolization over bland embolization or vice versa. Overall, median survival ranges from 23 to 86 months for bland embolization and from 15 to 69 months for chemoembolization. Median survival from first embolization is similar with the two methods, and the median 5-year overall survival rate is approximately 50% for both, with a wide range demonstrated in studies.[121,152,153,154,155,156] The intermediate overall survival of patients receiving bland embolization or chemoembolization is roughly double that of those receiving medical therapy.[106,108] Several studies have demonstrated superior response rates in patients with extrapancreatic NET versus those with pancreatic NET. For example, one study demonstrated significantly higher response rates and longer progression-free survival times for extrapancreatic neuroendocrine neoplasms (66.7% and 22.7 months, respectively) than for islet cell carcinoma (35.2% and 16.1 months, respectively).[157] Several studies have examined predictors of response. In these studies, three patient variables appeared to be associated with a worse outcome: need for urgent embolization to treat symptoms, greater than 50% liver replacement by tumor, and extrahepatic metastasis. Patients with all three risk factors had decreased overall survival (8.5 months) versus those with none (86 months).[152] Recently, higher tumor grade has also been implicated in a poorer response to embolotherapy.[158]

17.6.5 Selective Internal Radiation

For metastatic NET, brachytherapy can be performed using one of two methods for the selective delivery of internal radiation: (1) intra-arterial radioembolization with microspheres loaded with radioactive beta-emitter Y-90 or (2) intravenous administration of a somatostatin analogue labeled with a beta-emitting isotope. As discussed earlier, radioembolization involves selective hepatic arterial injection with nondegradable glass or resin microspheres loaded with the nearly pure beta-emitter Y-90. Studies assessing radioembolization for the treatment of hepatic NET metastases have demonstrated similar benefits to those seen with bland embolization and chemoembolization with regard to local tumor control and symptom relief of

hormonally active NETs.[156] Given the similar clinical outcomes reported in the literature, advocates of radioembolization favor this therapy because of the typically less severe side effect profile, which allows the therapy to be administered on an outpatient basis.[159] A recent multicenter analysis of radioembolization and chemoembolization for metastatic NET suggested that tumor grade may be an important factor in selecting the optimal embolization therapy. The investigators found that radioembolization provided better local tumor control without a survival benefit compared to chemoembolization and bland embolization in low-grade NETs, but radioembolization provided worse local tumor control and survival outcomes compared to the other embolotherapies for G3 NETs.[158] Randomized trials including cost–benefit and quality of life analyses are still needed to determine the optimal transarterial therapy for metastatic NET.

Although a complete discussion of the intravenous injection of somatostatin analogue-based intravenous radiotherapy is beyond the scope of this chapter, interventional oncologists participating in the care of patients with NET should be familiar with the relevant literature to better inform patients of all possible treatment options. Attempts to adapt these systemic radiotherapies for intra-arterial administration have also been reported. McStay et al[160] found that the intra-arterial injection of Y-90-tetraazacyclododecane tetra-acetic acid lanreotide provided a partial response in 16% of patients and stable disease in an additional 63% of patients. Clinical improvement was reported by 61% of the 23 patients treated. Similarly, intra-arterial injection of 131I-labeled methyliodobenzylguanidine, an established nuclear medicine therapy for the treatment of metastatic NET, has been reported, with some studies showing an up to fourfold increase in tumor uptake of the therapeutic radioisotope compared to the uptake with intravenous injection.[161]

17.7 Conclusion

CRC and NET are two of the most common malignancies that present with either liver-only or liver-dominant metastatic disease. Multiple effective systemic and locoregional therapies exist for both conditions, highlighting the need for a multidisciplinary approach in caring for patients with these conditions. This is most evident by the growing number of studies combining multimodality therapy to prolong survival, transforming metastatic cancer into a chronic disease.

References

[1] Pawlik TM, Choti MA. Surgical therapy for colorectal metastases to the liver. J Gastrointest Surg. 2007; 11(8):1057–1077

[2] You YN, Rustin RB, Sullivan JD. Oncotype DX(®) colon cancer assay for prediction of recurrence risk in patients with stage II and III colon cancer: a review of the evidence. Surg Oncol. 2015; 24(2):61–66

[3] Doubeni CA, Major JM, Laiyemo AO, et al. Contribution of behavioral risk factors and obesity to socioeconomic differences in colorectal cancer incidence. J Natl Cancer Inst. 2012; 104(18):1353–1362

[4] Murphy G, Devesa SS, Cross AJ, Inskip PD, McGlynn KA, Cook MB. Sex disparities in colorectal cancer incidence by anatomic subsite, race and age. Int J Cancer. 2011; 128(7):1668–1675

[5] Fearon ER, Vogelstein B. A genetic model for colorectal tumorigenesis. Cell. 1990; 61(5):759–767

[6] Smith RA, Manassaram-Baptiste D, Brooks D, et al. Cancer screening in the United States, 2015: a review of current American cancer society guidelines and current issues in cancer screening. CA Cancer J Clin. 2015; 65(1):30–54

[7] Smith RA, Andrews K, Brooks D, et al. Cancer screening in the United States, 2016: a review of current American Cancer Society guidelines and current issues in cancer screening. CA Cancer J Clin. 2016; 66(2):96–114

[8] Furukawa H, Ikuma H, Seki A, et al. Positron emission tomography scanning is not superior to whole body multidetector helical computed tomography in the preoperative staging of colorectal cancer. Gut. 2006; 55(7):1007–1011

[9] DeSantis CE, Lin CC, Mariotto AB, et al. Cancer treatment and survivorship statistics, 2014. CA Cancer J Clin. 2014; 64(4):252–271

[10] Estimated New Cancer Cases. SEER 1–1. 2015. Available at: http://seer.cancer.gov/archive/csr/1975_2012/results_single/sect_01_table.01.pdf. Accessed April 30, 2016

[11] Frattini M, Balestra D, Suardi S, et al. Different genetic features associated with colon and rectal carcinogenesis. Clin Cancer Res. 2004; 10(12, Pt 1):4015–4021

[12] Tan KK, Lopes GdeL, Jr, Sim R. How uncommon are isolated lung metastases in colorectal cancer? A review from database of 754 patients over 4 years. J Gastrointest Surg. 2009; 13(4):642–648

[13] Kirke R, Rajesh A, Verma R, Bankart MJ. Rectal cancer: incidence of pulmonary metastases on thoracic CT and correlation with T staging. J Comput Assist Tomogr. 2007; 31(4):569–571

[14] Gustavsson B, Carlsson G, Machover D, et al. A review of the evolution of systemic chemotherapy in the management of colorectal cancer. Clin Colorectal Cancer. 2015; 14(1):1–10

[15] de Gramont A, Figer A, Seymour M, et al. Leucovorin and fluorouracil with or without oxaliplatin as first-line treatment in advanced colorectal cancer. J Clin Oncol. 2000; 18(16):2938–2947

[16] André T, Boni C, Navarro M, et al. Improved overall survival with oxaliplatin, fluorouracil, and leucovorin as adjuvant treatment in stage II or III colon cancer in the MOSAIC trial. J Clin Oncol. 2009; 27(19):3109–3116

[17] André T, Boni C, Mounedji-Boudiaf L, et al. Multicenter International Study of Oxaliplatin/5-Fluorouracil/Leucovorin in the Adjuvant Treatment of Colon Cancer (MOSAIC) Investigators. Oxaliplatin, fluorouracil, and leucovorin as adjuvant treatment for colon cancer. N Engl J Med. 2004; 350(23):2343–2351

[18] Ducreux M, Bennouna J, Hebbar M, et al. GI Group of the French Anti-Cancer Centers. Capecitabine plus oxaliplatin (XELOX) versus 5-fluorouracil/leucovorin plus oxaliplatin (FOLFOX-6) as first-line treatment for metastatic colorectal cancer. Int J Cancer. 2011; 128(3):682–690

[19] Douillard JY, Cunningham D, Roth AD, et al. Irinotecan combined with fluorouracil compared with fluorouracil alone as first-line treatment for metastatic colorectal cancer: a multicentre randomised trial. Lancet. 2000; 355(9209):1041–1047

[20] Saltz LB, Cox JV, Blanke C, et al. Irinotecan Study Group. Irinotecan plus fluorouracil and leucovorin for metastatic colorectal cancer. N Engl J Med. 2000; 343(13):905–914

[21] Tournigand C, André T, Achille E, et al. FOLFIRI followed by FOLFOX6 or the reverse sequence in advanced colorectal cancer: a randomized GERCOR study. J Clin Oncol. 2004; 22(2):229–237

[22] Heinemann V, von Weikersthal LF, Decker T, et al. FOLFIRI plus cetuximab versus FOLFIRI plus bevacizumab as first-line treatment for patients with metastatic colorectal cancer (FIRE-3): a randomised, open-label, phase 3 trial. Lancet Oncol. 2014; 15(10):1065–1075

[23] Venook A, et al. O-0019 * CALGB/SWOG 80405: Phase III trial of irinotecan/5-FU/leucovorin (FOLFIRI) or oxaliplatin/5-FU/leucovorin (mFOLFOX6) with bevacizumab (BV) or cetuximab (CET) for patients (PTS) with KRAS wild-type (wt) untreated metastatic adenocarcinoma of the colon. Ann Oncol. 2014; 25:ii112–ii113

[24] Giantonio BJ, Catalano PJ, Meropol NJ, et al. Eastern Cooperative Oncology Group Study E3200. Bevacizumab in combination with oxaliplatin, fluorouracil, and leucovorin (FOLFOX4) for previously treated metastatic colorectal cancer: results from the Eastern Cooperative Oncology Group Study E3200. J Clin Oncol. 2007; 25(12):1539–1544

[25] Vauthey JN, Pawlik TM, Ribero D, et al. Chemotherapy regimen predicts steatohepatitis and an increase in 90-day mortality after surgery for hepatic colorectal metastases. J Clin Oncol. 2006; 24(13):2065–2072

[26] Zorzi D, Laurent A, Pawlik TM, Lauwers GY, Vauthey JN, Abdalla EK. Chemotherapy-associated hepatotoxicity and surgery for colorectal liver metastases. Br J Surg. 2007; 94(3):274–286

[27] Chun YS, Laurent A, Maru D, Vauthey J-N. Management of chemotherapy-associated hepatotoxicity in colorectal liver metastases. Lancet Oncol. 2009; 10(3):278–286

[28] Gordon CR, Rojavin Y, Patel M, et al. A review on bevacizumab and surgical wound healing: an important warning to all surgeons. Ann Plast Surg. 2009; 62(6):707–709

[29] Frankel TL, D'Angelica MI. Hepatic resection for colorectal metastases. J Surg Oncol. 2014; 109(1):2–7

[30] Kanas GP, Taylor A, Primrose JN, et al. Survival after liver resection in metastatic colorectal cancer: review and meta-analysis of prognostic factors. Clin Epidemiol. 2012; 4:283–301

[31] Ciliberto D, Prati U, Roveda L, et al. Role of systemic chemotherapy in the management of resected or resectable colorectal liver metastases: a systematic review and meta-analysis of randomized controlled trials. Oncol Rep. 2012; 27(6):1849–1856

[32] Viganò L, Capussotti L, Majno P, et al. Liver resection in patients with eight or more colorectal liver metastases. Br J Surg. 2015; 102(1):92–101

[33] Smith MD, McCall JL. Systematic review of tumour number and outcome after radical treatment of colorectal liver metastases. Br J Surg. 2009; 96(10):1101–1113

[34] Aloia TA, Vauthey J-N. Management of colorectal liver metastases: past, present, and future. Updates Surg. 2011; 63(1):1–3

[35] John SK, Robinson SM, Rehman S, et al. Prognostic factors and survival after resection of colorectal liver metastasis in the era of preoperative chemotherapy: an 11-year single-centre study. Dig Surg. 2013; 30(4–6):293–301

[36] Jaeck D, Oussoultzoglou E, Rosso E, Greget M, Weber JC, Bachellier P. A two-stage hepatectomy procedure combined with portal vein embolization to achieve curative resection for initially unresectable multiple and bilobar colorectal liver metastases. Ann Surg. 2004; 240(6):1037–1049, discussion 1049–1051

[37] Lam VW, Laurence JM, Johnston E, Hollands MJ, Pleass HC, Richardson AJ. A systematic review of two-stage hepatectomy in patients with initially unresectable colorectal liver metastases. HPB (Oxford). 2013; 15(7):483–491

[38] Nordlinger B, Sorbye H, Glimelius B, et al. EORTC Gastro-Intestinal Tract Cancer Group, Cancer Research UK, Arbeitsgruppe Lebermetastasen und-tumoren in der Chirurgischen Arbeitsgemeinschaft Onkologie (ALM-CAO), Australasian Gastro-Intestinal Trials Group (AGITG), Fédération Francophone de Cancérologie Digestive (FFCD). Perioperative FOLFOX4 chemotherapy and surgery versus surgery alone for resectable liver metastases from colorectal cancer (EORTC 40983): long-term results of a randomised, controlled, phase 3 trial. Lancet Oncol. 2013; 14(12):1208–1215

[39] Gallagher DJ, Zheng J, Capanu M, et al. Response to neoadjuvant chemotherapy does not predict overall survival for patients with synchronous colorectal hepatic metastases. Ann Surg Oncol. 2009; 16(7):1844–1851

[40] Nikfarjam M, Shereef S, Kimchi ET, et al. Survival outcomes of patients with colorectal liver metastases following hepatic resection or ablation in the era of effective chemotherapy. Ann Surg Oncol. 2009; 16(7):1860–1867

[41] Kemeny N. Management of liver metastases from colorectal cancer. Oncol. 2006; 20(10):1161–1176

[42] Kishi Y, Zorzi D, Contreras CM, et al. Extended preoperative chemotherapy does not improve pathologic response and increases postoperative liver insufficiency after hepatic resection for colorectal liver metastases. Ann Surg Oncol. 2010; 17(11):2870–2876

[43] Bacchetti S, Pasqual E, Crozzolo E, Pellarin A, Cagol PP. Intra-arterial hepatic chemotherapy for unresectable colorectal liver metastases: a review of medical devices complications in 3172 patients. Med Devices (Auckl). 2009; 2:31–40

[44] Dizon DS, Schwartz J, Kemeny N. Regional chemotherapy: a focus on hepatic artery infusion for colorectal cancer liver metastases. Surg Oncol Clin N Am. 2008; 17(4):759–771, viii

[45] Ensminger WD, Rosowsky A, Raso V, et al. A clinical-pharmacological evaluation of hepatic arterial infusions of 5-fluoro-2′-deoxyuridine and 5-fluorouracil. Cancer Res. 1978; 38(11, Pt 1):3784–3792

[46] Lorenz M, Hochmuth K, Müller HH. Hepatic arterial infusion of chemotherapy for metastatic colorectal cancer. N Engl J Med. 2000; 342(20):1525–1526, author reply 1526–1527

[47] Kemeny NE, Niedzwiecki D, Hollis DR, et al. Hepatic arterial infusion versus systemic therapy for hepatic metastases from colorectal cancer: a randomized trial of efficacy, quality of life, and molecular markers (CALGB 9481). J Clin Oncol. 2006; 24(9):1395–1403

[48] Ammori JB, Kemeny NE, Fong Y, et al. Conversion to complete resection and/or ablation using hepatic artery infusional chemotherapy in patients with unresectable liver metastases from colorectal cancer: a decade of experience at a single institution. Ann Surg Oncol. 2013; 20(9):2901–2907

[49] Kemeny N, Gonen M, Sullivan D, et al. Phase I study of hepatic arterial infusion of floxuridine and dexamethasone with systemic irinotecan for unresectable hepatic metastases from colorectal cancer. J Clin Oncol. 2001; 19(10):2687–2695

[50] Kemeny N, Jarnagin W, Paty P, et al. Phase I trial of systemic oxaliplatin combination chemotherapy with hepatic arterial infusion in patients with unresectable liver metastases from colorectal cancer. J Clin Oncol. 2005; 23 (22):4888–4896

[51] Kemeny N, Seiter K, Niedzwiecki D, et al. A randomized trial of intrahepatic infusion of fluorodeoxyuridine with dexamethasone versus fluorodeoxy-uridine alone in the treatment of metastatic colorectal cancer. Cancer. 1992; 69(2):327–334

[52] Allen PJ, Nissan A, Picon AI, et al. Technical complications and durability of hepatic artery infusion pumps for unresectable colorectal liver metastases: an institutional experience of 544 consecutive cases. J Am Coll Surg. 2005; 201(1):57–65

[53] Abdalla EK, Bauer TW, Chun YS, D'Angelica M, Kooby DA, Jarnagin WR. Locoregional surgical and interventional therapies for advanced colorectal cancer liver metastases: expert consensus statements. HPB (Oxford). 2013; 15(2):119–130

[54] Abdalla EK, Vauthey JN, Ellis LM, et al. Recurrence and outcomes following hepatic resection, radiofrequency ablation, and combined resection/ablation for colorectal liver metastases. Ann Surg. 2004; 239(6):818–825, discussion 825–827

[55] Lencioni R, Crocetti L, Cioni D, Della Pina C, Bartolozzi C. Percutaneous radiofrequency ablation of hepatic colorectal metastases: technique, indications, results, and new promises. Invest Radiol. 2004; 39(11):689–697

[56] Gillams AR, Lees WR. Five-year survival in 309 patients with colorectal liver metastases treated with radiofrequency ablation. Eur Radiol. 2009; 19(5): 1206–1213

[57] Stang A, Fischbach R, Teichmann W, Bokemeyer C, Braumann D. A systematic review on the clinical benefit and role of radiofrequency ablation as treatment of colorectal liver metastases. Eur J Cancer. 2009; 45(10):1748–1756

[58] Solbiati L, Ahmed M, Cova L, Ierace T, Brioschi M, Goldberg SN. Small liver colorectal metastases treated with percutaneous radiofrequency ablation: local response rate and long-term survival with up to 10-year follow-up. Radiology. 2012; 265(3):958–968

[59] Livraghi T, Solbiati L, Meloni F, Ierace T, Goldberg SN, Gazelle GS. Percutaneous radiofrequency ablation of liver metastases in potential candidates for resection: the "test-of-time approach". Cancer. 2003; 97(12): 3027–3035

[60] Evrard S, Rivoire M, Arnaud J-, et al. Unresectable colorectal cancer liver metastases treated by intraoperative radiofrequency ablation with or without resection. Br J Surg. 2012; 99(4):558–565

[61] Ruers T, Punt C, Van Coevorden F, et al. EORTC Gastro-Intestinal Tract Cancer Group, Arbeitsgruppe Lebermetastasen und—tumoren in der Chirurgischen Arbeitsgemeinschaft Onkologie (ALM-CAO) and the National Cancer Research Institute Colorectal Clinical Study Group (NCRI CCSG). Radiofrequency ablation combined with systemic treatment versus systemic treatment alone in patients with non-resectable colorectal liver metastases: a randomized EORTC Intergroup phase II study (EORTC 40004). Ann Oncol. 2012; 23(10):2619–2626

[62] Solbiati L, Livraghi T, Goldberg SN, et al. Percutaneous radio-frequency ablation of hepatic metastases from colorectal cancer: long-term results in 117 patients. Radiology. 2001; 221(1):159–166

[63] de Baère T, Risse O, Kuoch V, et al. Adverse events during radiofrequency treatment of 582 hepatic tumors. AJR Am J Roentgenol. 2003; 181(3):695–700

[64] Gravante G, Ong SL, Metcalfe MS, Strickland A, Dennison AR, Lloyd DM. Hepatic microwave ablation: a review of the histological changes following thermal damage. Liver Int. 2008; 28(7):911–921

[65] Andreano A, Brace CL. A comparison of direct heating during radiofrequency and microwave ablation in ex vivo liver. Cardiovasc Intervent Radiol. 2013; 36(2):505–511

[66] Bhardwaj N, Dormer J, Ahmad F, et al. Microwave ablation of the liver: a description of lesion evolution over time and an investigation of the heat sink effect. Pathology. 2011; 43(7):725–731

[67] Bhardwaj N, Strickland AD, Ahmad F, Atanesyan L, West K, Lloyd DM. A comparative histological evaluation of the ablations produced by microwave, cryotherapy and radiofrequency in the liver. Pathology. 2009; 41 (2):168–172

[68] Groeschl RT, Pilgrim CH, Hanna EM, et al. Microwave ablation for hepatic malignancies: a multiinstitutional analysis. Ann Surg. 2014; 259(6):1195–1200

[69] Bhutiani N, Martin RC, II. Transarterial therapy for colorectal liver metastases. Surg Clin North Am. 2016; 96(2):369–391

[70] Salman HS, Cynamon J, Jagust M, et al. Randomized phase II trial of embolization therapy versus chemoembolization therapy in previously treated patients with colorectal carcinoma metastatic to the liver. Clin Colorectal Cancer. 2002; 2(3):173–179

[71] Vogl TJ, Gruber T, Balzer JO, Eichler K, Hammerstingl R, Zangos S. Repeated transarterial chemoembolization in the treatment of liver metastases of colorectal cancer: prospective study. Radiology. 2009; 250(1):281–289

[72] Tellez C, Benson AB, III, Lyster MT, et al. Phase II trial of chemoembolization for the treatment of metastatic colorectal carcinoma to the liver and review of the literature. Cancer. 1998; 82(7):1250–1259

[73] Leichman CG, Jacobson JR, Modiano M, et al. Hepatic chemoembolization combined with systemic infusion of 5-fluorouracil and bolus leucovorin for patients with metastatic colorectal carcinoma: a Southwest Oncology Group pilot trial. Cancer. 1999; 86(5):775–781

[74] Gruber-Rouh T, Naguib NN, Eichler K, et al. Transarterial chemoembolization of unresectable systemic chemotherapy-refractory liver metastases from colorectal cancer: long-term results over a 10-year period. Int J Cancer. 2014; 134(5):1225–1231

[75] Taylor RR, Tang Y, Gonzalez MV, Stratford PW, Lewis AL. Irinotecan drug eluting beads for use in chemoembolization: in vitro and in vivo evaluation of drug release properties. Eur J Pharm Sci. 2007; 30(1):7–14

[76] Fiorentini G, Aliberti C, Tilli M, et al. Intra-arterial infusion of irinotecan-loaded drug-eluting beads (DEBIRI) versus intravenous therapy (FOLFIRI) for hepatic metastases from colorectal cancer: final results of a phase III study. Anticancer Res. 2012; 32(4):1387–1395

[77] Iezzi R, Marsico VA, Guerra A, et al. Trans-arterial chemoembolization with irinotecan-loaded drug-eluting beads (DEBIRI) and capecitabine in refractory liver prevalent colorectal metastases: a Phase II single-center study. Cardiovasc Intervent Radiol. 2015; 38(6):1523–1531

[78] Martin RC, II, Scoggins CR, Schreeder M, et al. Randomized controlled trial of irinotecan drug-eluting beads with simultaneous FOLFOX and bevacizumab for patients with unresectable colorectal liver-limited metastasis. Cancer. 2015; 121(20):3649–3658

[79] Martin RC, Howard J, Tomalty D, et al. Toxicity of irinotecan-eluting beads in the treatment of hepatic malignancies: results of a multi-institutional registry. Cardiovasc Intervent Radiol. 2010; 33(5):960–966

[80] Kennedy A, Nag S, Salem R, et al. Recommendations for radioembolization of hepatic malignancies using yttrium-90 microsphere brachytherapy: a consensus panel report from the radioembolization brachytherapy oncology consortium. Int J Radiat Oncol Biol Phys. 2007; 68(1):13–23

[81] Rhee TK, Lewandowski RJ, Liu DM, et al. 90Y Radioembolization for metastatic neuroendocrine liver tumors: preliminary results from a multi-institutional experience. Ann Surg. 2008; 247(6):1029–1035

[82] Saxena A, Meteling B, Kapoor J, Golani S, Morris DL, Bester L. Is yttrium-90 radioembolization a viable treatment option for unresectable, chemorefractory colorectal cancer liver metastases? A large single-center experience of 302 patients. Ann Surg Oncol. 2015; 22(3):794–802

[83] Cosimelli M, Golfieri R, Cagol PP, et al. Italian Society of Locoregional Therapies in Oncology (SITILO). Multi-centre phase II clinical trial of yttrium-90 resin microspheres alone in unresectable, chemotherapy refractory colorectal liver metastases. Br J Cancer. 2010; 103(3):324–331

[84] Lewandowski RJ, Memon K, Mulcahy MF, et al. Twelve-year experience of radioembolization for colorectal hepatic metastases in 214 patients: survival by era and chemotherapy. Eur J Nucl Med Mol Imaging. 2014; 41(10):1861–1869

[85] Kalva SP, et al. Yttrium-90 radioembolization as salvage therapy for liver metastases from colorectal cancer. Am J Clin Oncol. 2017; 40(3):288–293:1

[86] van Hazel GA, Pavlakis N, Goldstein D, et al. Treatment of fluorouracil-refractory patients with liver metastases from colorectal cancer by using yttrium-90 resin microspheres plus concomitant systemic irinotecan chemotherapy. J Clin Oncol. 2009; 27(25):4089–4095

[87] Van Hazel G, Blackwell A, Anderson J, et al. Randomised phase 2 trial of SIR-Spheres plus fluorouracil/leucovorin chemotherapy versus fluorouracil/leucovorin chemotherapy alone in advanced colorectal cancer. J Surg Oncol. 2004; 88(2):78–85

[88] Sharma RA, Van Hazel GA, Morgan B, et al. Radioembolization of liver metastases from colorectal cancer using yttrium-90 microspheres with concomitant systemic oxaliplatin, fluorouracil, and leucovorin chemotherapy. J Clin Oncol. 2007; 25(9):1099–1106

[89] van Hazel GA, Heinemann V, Sharma NK, et al. SIRFLOX: randomized Phase III trial comparing first-line mFOLFOX6 (plus or minus bevacizumab) versus mFOLFOX6 (plus or minus bevacizumab) plus selective internal radiation therapy in patients with metastatic colorectal cancer. J Clin Oncol. 2016; 34 (15):1723–1731

[90] Peterson JL, Vallow LA, Johnson DW, et al. Complications after 90Y microsphere radioembolization for unresectable hepatic tumors: an evaluation of 112 patients. Brachytherapy. 2013; 12(6):573–579

[91] Riaz A, Awais R, Salem R. Side effects of yttrium-90 radioembolization. Front Oncol. 2014; 4:198

[92] Gil-Alzugaray B, Chopitea A, Iñarrairaegui M, et al. Prognostic factors and prevention of radioembolization-induced liver disease. Hepatology. 2013; 57(3):1078–1087

[93] Bosman FT, Carneiro F Hruban RH. WHO Classification of Tumours of the Digestive System. Geneva, Switzerland: World Health Organization; 2010

[94] Yao JC, Hassan M, Phan A, et al. One hundred years after "carcinoid": epidemiology of and prognostic factors for neuroendocrine tumors in 35,825 cases in the United States. J Clin Oncol. 2008; 26(18):3063–3072

[95] Modlin IM, Lye KD, Kidd M. A 5-decade analysis of 13,715 carcinoid tumors. Cancer. 2003; 97(4):934–959

[96] Gustafsson BI, Kidd M, Modlin IM. Neuroendocrine tumors of the diffuse neuroendocrine system. Curr Opin Oncol. 2008; 20(1):1–12

[97] Modlin IM, Kidd M, Latich I, Zikusoka MN, Shapiro MD. Current status of gastrointestinal carcinoids. Gastroenterology. 2005; 128(6):1717–1751

[98] Dromain C, de Baere T, Lumbroso J, et al. Detection of liver metastases from endocrine tumors: a prospective comparison of somatostatin receptor scintigraphy, computed tomography, and magnetic resonance imaging. J Clin Oncol. 2005; 23(1):70–78

[99] Rodrigues M, Traub-Weidinger T, Li S, Ibi B, Virgolini I. Comparison of 111 In-DOTA-DPhe1-Tyr3-octreotide and 111 In-DOTA-lanreotide scintigraphy and dosimetry in patients with neuroendocrine tumours. Eur J Nucl Med Mol Imaging. 2006; 33(5):532–540

[100] Frilling A, Sotiropoulos GC, Radtke A, et al. The impact of 68Ga-DOTATOC positron emission tomography/computed tomography on the multimodal management of patients with neuroendocrine tumors. Ann Surg. 2010; 252 (5):850–856

[101] Hofmann M, Maecke H, Börner R, et al. Biokinetics and imaging with the somatostatin receptor PET radioligand (68)Ga-DOTATOC: preliminary data. Eur J Nucl Med. 2001; 28(12):1751–1757

[102] Carrasquillo JA, Chen CC. Molecular imaging of neuroendocrine tumors. Semin Oncol. 2010; 37(6):662–679

[103] Orlefors H, Sundin A, Garske U, et al. Whole-body (11)C-5-hydroxytryptophan positron emission tomography as a universal imaging technique for neuroendocrine tumors: comparison with somatostatin receptor scintigraphy and computed tomography. J Clin Endocrinol Metab. 2005; 90(6):3392–3400

[104] Abgral R, Leboulleux S, Déandreis D, et al. Performance of (18) fluorodeoxyglucose-positron emission tomography and somatostatin receptor scintigraphy for high Ki67 (≥10%) well-differentiated endocrine carcinoma staging. J Clin Endocrinol Metab. 2011; 96(3):665–671

[105] Frilling A, Li J, Malamutmann E, Schmid KW, Bockisch A, Broelsch CE. Treatment of liver metastases from neuroendocrine tumours in relation to the extent of hepatic disease. Br J Surg. 2009; 96(2):175–184

[106] Chamberlain RS, Canes D, Brown KT, et al. Hepatic neuroendocrine metastases: does intervention alter outcomes? J Am Coll Surg. 2000; 190(4): 432–445

[107] Knox CD, Anderson CD, Lamps LW, Adkins RB, Pinson CW. Long-term survival after resection for primary hepatic carcinoid tumor. Ann Surg Oncol. 2003; 10(10):1171–1175

[108] Touzios JG, Kiely JM, Pitt SC, et al. Neuroendocrine hepatic metastases: does aggressive management improve survival? Ann Surg. 2005; 241(5):776–783, discussion 783–785

[109] Kvols LK, Moertel CG, O'Connell MJ, Schutt AJ, Rubin J, Hahn RG. Treatment of the malignant carcinoid syndrome. Evaluation of a long-acting somatostatin analogue. N Engl J Med. 1986; 315(11):663–666

[110] Rinke A, Müller HH, Schade-Brittinger C, et al. PROMID Study Group. Placebo-controlled, double-blind, prospective, randomized study on the effect of octreotide LAR in the control of tumor growth in patients with metastatic neuroendocrine midgut tumors: a report from the PROMID Study Group. J Clin Oncol. 2009; 27(28):4656–4663

[111] Pavel ME, Hainsworth JD, Baudin E, et al. RADIANT-2 Study Group. Everolimus plus octreotide long-acting repeatable for the treatment of advanced neuroendocrine tumours associated with carcinoid syndrome (RADIANT-2): a randomised, placebo-controlled, phase 3 study. Lancet. 2011; 378(9808):2005–2012

[112] Yao JC, Shah MH, Ito T, et al. RAD001 in Advanced Neuroendocrine Tumors, Third Trial (RADIANT-3) Study Group. Everolimus for advanced pancreatic neuroendocrine tumors. N Engl J Med. 2011; 364(6):514–523

[113] Yao JC, Fazio N, Singh S, et al. RAD001 in Advanced Neuroendocrine Tumours, Fourth Trial (RADIANT-4) Study Group. Everolimus for the treatment of advanced, non-functional neuroendocrine tumours of the lung or gastrointestinal tract (RADIANT-4): a randomised, placebo-controlled, phase 3 study. Lancet. 2016; 387(10022):968–977

[114] Raymond E, Dahan L, Raoul JL, et al. Sunitinib malate for the treatment of pancreatic neuroendocrine tumors. N Engl J Med. 2011; 364(6):501–513

[115] Castellano D, Capdevila J, Sastre J, et al. Sorafenib and bevacizumab combination targeted therapy in advanced neuroendocrine tumour: a phase II study of Spanish Neuroendocrine Tumour Group (GETNE0801). Eur J Cancer. 2013; 49(18):3780–3787

[116] Strosberg JR, Fine RL, Choi J, et al. First-line chemotherapy with capecitabine and temozolomide in patients with metastatic pancreatic endocrine carcinomas. Cancer. 2011; 117(2):268–275

[117] Glazer ES, Tseng JF, Al-Refaie W, et al. Long-term survival after surgical management of neuroendocrine hepatic metastases. HPB (Oxford). 2010; 12 (6):427–433

[118] Mayo SC, de Jong MC, Pawlik TM. Surgical management and emerging therapies to prolong survival in metastatic neuroendocrine cancer. Ann Surg Oncol. 2011; 18 Suppl 3:S220–S221, author reply S222–S223

[119] Mayo SC, de Jong MC, Pulitano C, et al. Surgical management of hepatic neuroendocrine tumor metastasis: results from an international multi-institutional analysis. Ann Surg Oncol. 2010; 17(12):3129–3136

[120] Hellman P, Lundström T, Ohrvall U, et al. Effect of surgery on the outcome of midgut carcinoid disease with lymph node and liver metastases. World J Surg. 2002; 26(8):991–997

[121] Frilling A, Modlin IM, Kidd M, et al. Working Group on Neuroendocrine Liver Metastases. Recommendations for management of patients with neuroendocrine liver metastases. Lancet Oncol. 2014; 15(1):e8–e21

[122] Máthé Z, Tagkalos E, Paul A, et al. Liver transplantation for hepatic metastases of neuroendocrine pancreatic tumors: a survival-based analysis. Transplantation. 2011; 91(5):575–582

[123] Gamblin TC, Christians K, Pappas SG. Radiofrequency ablation of neuroendocrine hepatic metastasis. Surg Oncol Clin N Am. 2011; 20(2):273–279, vii–viii

[124] Taner T, Atwell TD, Zhang L, et al. Adjunctive radiofrequency ablation of metastatic neuroendocrine cancer to the liver complements surgical resection. HPB (Oxford). 2013; 15(3):190–195

[125] Solbiati L, Ierace T, Tonolini M, Osti V, Cova L. Radiofrequency thermal ablation of hepatic metastases. Eur J Ultrasound. 2001; 13(2):149–158

[126] Liu DM, Kennedy A, Turner D, et al. Minimally invasive techniques in management of hepatic neuroendocrine metastatic disease. Am J Clin Oncol. 2009; 32(2):200–215

[127] Wettstein M, Vogt C, Cohnen M, et al. Serotonin release during percutaneous radiofrequency ablation in a patient with symptomatic liver metastases of a neuroendocrine tumor. Hepatogastroenterology. 2004; 51(57):830–832

[128] Elias D, Di Pietroantonio D, Gachot B, Menegon P, Hakime A, De Baere T. Liver abscess after radiofrequency ablation of tumors in patients with a biliary tract procedure. Gastroenterol Clin Biol. 2006; 30(6–7):823–827

[129] Karabulut K, Akyildiz HY, Lance C, et al. Multimodality treatment of neuroendocrine liver metastases. Surgery. 2011; 150(2):316–325

[130] Frilling A, Clift AK. Therapeutic strategies for neuroendocrine liver metastases. Cancer. 2015; 121(8):1172–1186

[131] Roche A, Girish BV, de Baère T, et al. Trans-catheter arterial chemoembolization as first-line treatment for hepatic metastases from endocrine tumors. Eur Radiol. 2003; 13(1):136–140

[132] Engstrom PF, Lavin PT, Moertel CG, Folsch E, Douglass HO, Jr. Streptozocin plus fluorouracil versus doxorubicin therapy for metastatic carcinoid tumor. J Clin Oncol. 1984; 2(11):1255–1259

[133] Schell SR, Camp ER, Caridi JG, Hawkins IF, Jr. Hepatic artery embolization for control of symptoms, octreotide requirements, and tumor progression in metastatic carcinoid tumors. J Gastrointest Surg. 2002; 6(5):664–670

[134] Pueyo I, Jiménez JR, Hernández J, et al. Carcinoid syndrome treated by hepatic embolization. AJR Am J Roentgenol. 1978; 131(3):511–513

[135] Lunderquist A, Ericsson M, Nobin A, Sandén G. Gelfoam powder embolization of the hepatic artery in liver metastases of carcinoid tumors. Radiologe. 1982; 22(2):65–70

[136] Ajani JA, Carrasco CH, Charnsangavej C, Samaan NA, Levin B, Wallace S. Islet cell tumors metastatic to the liver: effective palliation by sequential hepatic artery embolization. Ann Intern Med. 1988; 108(3):340–344

[137] Burns WR, Edil BH. Neuroendocrine pancreatic tumors: guidelines for management and update. Curr Treat Options Oncol. 2012; 13(1):24–34

[138] Madoff DC, Gupta S, Ahrar K, Murthy R, Yao JC. Update on the management of neuroendocrine hepatic metastases. J Vasc Interv Radiol. 2006; 17(8): 1235–1249, quiz 1250

[139] de Baere T, Dufaux J, Roche A, et al. Circulatory alterations induced by intra-arterial injection of iodized oil and emulsions of iodized oil and doxorubicin: experimental study. Radiology. 1995; 194(1):165–170

[140] de Baère T, Denys A, Briquet R, Chevallier P, Dufaux J, Roche A. Modification of arterial and portal hemodynamics after injection of iodized oils and different emulsions of iodized oils in the hepatic artery: an experimental study. J Vasc Interv Radiol. 1998; 9(2):305–310

[141] Imaeda T, Yamawaki Y, Seki M, et al. Lipiodol retention and massive necrosis after lipiodol-chemoembolization of hepatocellular carcinoma: correlation between computed tomography and histopathology. Cardiovasc Intervent Radiol. 1993; 16(4):209–213

[142] Dominguez S, Denys A, Madeira I, et al. Hepatic arterial chemoembolization with streptozotocin in patients with metastatic digestive endocrine tumours. Eur J Gastroenterol Hepatol. 2000; 12(2):151–157

[143] Gaur SK, Friese JL, Sadow CA, et al. Hepatic arterial chemoembolization using drug-eluting beads in gastrointestinal neuroendocrine tumor metastatic to the liver. Cardiovasc Intervent Radiol. 2011; 34(3):566–572

[144] Hong K, Khwaja A, Liapi E, Torbenson MS, Georgiades CS, Geschwind JF. New intra-arterial drug delivery system for the treatment of liver cancer: preclinical assessment in a rabbit model of liver cancer. Clin Cancer Res. 2006; 12(8):2563–2567

[145] Carter S, Martin Ii RCG. Drug-eluting bead therapy in primary and metastatic disease of the liver. HPB (Oxford). 2009; 11(7):541–550

[146] Varela M, Real MI, Burrel M, et al. Chemoembolization of hepatocellular carcinoma with drug eluting beads: efficacy and doxorubicin pharmacokinetics. J Hepatol. 2007; 46(3):474–481

[147] Bhagat N, Reyes DK, Lin M, et al. Phase II study of chemoembolization with drug-eluting beads in patients with hepatic neuroendocrine metastases: high incidence of biliary injury. Cardiovasc Intervent Radiol. 2013; 36(2):449–459

[148] Guiu B, Deschamps F, Aho S, et al. Liver/biliary injuries following chemoembolisation of endocrine tumours and hepatocellular carcinoma: lipiodol vs. drug-eluting beads. J Hepatol. 2012; 56(3):609–617

[149] de Baère T, Roche A, Amenabar JM, et al. Liver abscess formation after local treatment of liver tumors. Hepatology. 1996; 23(6):1436–1440

[150] Khan W, Sullivan KL, McCann JW, et al. Moxifloxacin prophylaxis for chemoembolization or embolization in patients with previous biliary interventions: a pilot study. AJR Am J Roentgenol. 2011; 197(2):W343–5

[151] Patel S, Tuite CM, Mondschein JI, Soulen MC. Effectiveness of an aggressive antibiotic regimen for chemoembolization in patients with previous biliary intervention. J Vasc Interv Radiol. 2006; 17(12):1931–1934

[152] Sofocleous CT, Petre EN, Gonen M, et al. Factors affecting periprocedural morbidity and mortality and long-term patient survival after arterial embolization of hepatic neuroendocrine metastases. J Vasc Interv Radiol. 2014; 25(1):22–30, quiz 31

[153] Memon K, Lewandowski RJ, Riaz A, Salem R. Chemoembolization and radioembolization for metastatic disease to the liver: available data and future studies. Curr Treat Options Oncol. 2012; 13(3):403–415

[154] Vogl TJ, Naguib NN, Zangos S, Eichler K, Hedayati A, Nour-Eldin NE. Liver metastases of neuroendocrine carcinomas: interventional treatment via transarterial embolization, chemoembolization and thermal ablation. Eur J Radiol. 2009; 72(3):517–528

[155] Pitt SC, Knuth J, Keily JM, et al. Hepatic neuroendocrine metastases: chemo- or bland embolization? J Gastrointest Surg. 2008; 12(11):1951–1960

[156] Kennedy AS. Hepatic-directed therapies in patients with neuroendocrine tumors. Hematol Oncol Clin North Am. 2016; 30(1):193–207

[157] Gupta S, Johnson MM, Murthy R, et al. Hepatic arterial embolization and chemoembolization for the treatment of patients with metastatic neuroendocrine tumors: variables affecting response rates and survival. Cancer. 2005; 104(8):1590–1602

[158] Chen J, et al. Embolotherapy for neuroendocrine tumor liver metastases: prognostic factors for hepatic progression-free survival and overall survival. J Vasc Interv Radiol. 2016; 27:S36

[159] Kennedy A, Coldwell D, Sangro B, Wasan H, Salem R. Integrating radioembolization into the treatment paradigm for metastatic neuroendocrine tumors in the liver. Am J Clin Oncol. 2012; 35(4):393–398

[160] McStay MKG, Maudgil D, Williams M, et al. Large-volume liver metastases from neuroendocrine tumors: hepatic intraarterial 90Y-DOTA-lanreotide as effective palliative therapy. Radiology. 2005; 237(2):718–726

[161] Brogsitter C, Pinkert J, Bredow J, Kittner T, Kotzerke J. Enhanced tumor uptake in neuroendocrine tumors after intraarterial application of 131I-MIBG. J Nucl Med. 2005; 46(12):2112–2116

18 Cholangiocarcinoma

Aladin T. Mariano, R. Peter Lokken, and Charles E. Ray Jr.

18.1 Introduction

Cholangiocarcinoma is an aggressive neoplasm of the biliary epithelium associated with significant morbidity and mortality. Diagnosis and treatment of cholangiocarcinoma require a multidisciplinary approach that involves diagnostic and interventional radiologists, gastroenterologists, surgeons, pathologists, and medical oncologists. Interventional radiologists play an increasingly essential role in the diagnosis and management of this devastating disease. The following sections will provide an overview of cholangiocarcinoma, including the epidemiology, pathology, diagnosis, and treatment options for this disease.

18.2 Epidemiology

Cholangiocarcinoma is the second most common primary hepatic malignancy after hepatocellular carcinoma (HCC).[1] On histology, cholangiocarcinoma is most commonly seen as adenocarcinoma with associated fibrous stroma formation (>90%); however, there are rare variants, such as squamous/adenosquamous, clear cell, undifferentiated, mucinous/signet ring, and lymphoproliferative types, among others.[2,3] Numerous risk factors for cholangiocarcinoma have been established, including primary sclerosing cholangitis (PSC), choledochal cysts, chronic viral hepatitis, liver flukes, and hepatolithiasis, although most patients with cholangiocarcinoma have no known risk factors.[4]

The incidence of cholangiocarcinoma varies significantly by geographic region and is highest where hepatobiliary infection with liver flukes is endemic. Thailand has one of the highest annual incidences of cholangiocarcinoma at 96 cases per 100,000; in the United States, the annual incidence is less than 3 cases per 100,000.[5] The disease typically presents in the seventh decade of life, with men at slightly higher risk than women.[6] The most common presenting symptoms include jaundice (84%), weight loss (35%), and abdominal pain (30%).[6]

Cholangiocarcinoma is often categorized anatomically as intrahepatic or extrahepatic. Gallbladder carcinoma, a bile duct epithelial neoplasm, is considered a separate category that has its own management guidelines.[7] Intrahepatic cholangiocarcinoma (ICC) is defined as involving the second-order (or beyond) peripheral bile ducts. Extrahepatic cholangiocarcinoma (ECC) includes perihilar tumors involving the confluence of the left and right hepatic ducts and tumors involving the more inferior common hepatic and common bile ducts.[8] In the United States, the annual incidence of ICC is less than that of ECC, at 0.58 per 100,000 compared to 0.88 per 100,000, although the relative incidence of ICC may be increasing.[9] The Surveillance, Epidemiology, and End Results (SEER) program has reported an increase in the age-adjusted annual incidence of ICC from 0.13 per 100,000 in 1973 to 0.85 per 100,000 in 1995 to 1999 and a concurrent decrease in the incidence of ECC from 1.08 per 100,0000 in 1979 to 0.82 per 100,000 in 1998.[8] Survival is affected by the anatomic distribution at diagnosis. ICC has the best 5-year survival rate of 40%, whereas distal and perihilar ECC have 5-year survival rates of 23 and 10%, respectively.[6]

The prognosis and treatment of cholangiocarcinoma can be further stratified by tumor morphology. The Liver Cancer Study Group of Japan classifies tumors as mass-forming, periductal (infiltrating or sclerosing), intraductal (polypoid or papillary), or mixed mass-forming periductal types.[10] Mass-forming types have a worse prognosis; the intraductal type has a relatively favorable prognosis.[11,12] Because the papillary type does not infiltrate into the submucosal layer, it is associated with improved survival after resection.[13]

Perihilar infiltrating tumors are stratified into four groups by the Bismuth–Corlette system (▶ Fig. 18.1).[14] Type 1 lesions involve

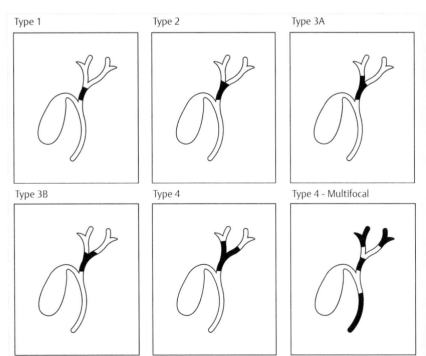

Type 1   Type 2   Type 3A

Type 3B   Type 4   Type 4 - Multifocal

Fig. 18.1 The Bismuth–Corlette classification of perihilar cholangiocarcinoma.

the common hepatic duct more than 2 cm inferior to the confluence. Type 2 lesions involve the common hepatic duct less than 2 cm inferior to the confluence. Type 3 and 4 lesions involve the confluence of the hepatic ducts: type 3 lesions involve the confluence and either the right or left hepatic ducts (type 3a lesions involve the right hepatic duct; type 3b lesions involve the left hepatic duct), and type 4 lesions include tumors involving the biliary confluence and both hepatic ducts and multifocal disease.

Mixed hepatocellular carcinoma–cholangiocarcinoma (HCC-CC) was first recognized in 1949 and has been considered rare, although this disease is being recognized with increasing frequency.[15,16] In one study of patients who received orthotopic liver transplant (OLT) for HCC, HCC-CC, or ICC was present in 10 of 302 explants (3.3%); compared to matched controls with only HCC on explant, patients with HCC-CC had a poorer prognosis with a high rate of tumor recurrence after OLT.[16] On imaging, patients with HCC-CC may demonstrate HCC-predominant, cholangiocarcinoma-predominant, or mixed enhancement characteristics.[17] The HCC component typically enhances during the arterial phase and hypoenhances during the portal venous or delayed phases. Cholangiocarcinoma-predominant mixed disease typically shows gradual enhancement. On magnetic resonance (MR) imaging, combined tumors typically demonstrate moderate hyperintensity on T2-weighted images, and contrast dynamics on enhanced images are similar to those seen on computed tomography (CT).[18,19]

18.3 Diagnosis of Cholangiocarcinoma

The diagnosis of cholangiocarcinoma may be suggested by clinical evidence of cholestasis and hepatic failure, the presence of risk factors, and elevations in the tumor markers carbohydrate antigen 19–9 (CA 19–9) and carcinoembryonic antigen (CEA). However, the clinical presentation is generally nonspecific, and both tumor markers can be elevated by other causes such as other malignancies, nonmalignant biliary obstruction, and liver injury. Imaging and biopsy are therefore often required to establish the diagnosis.[7,20]

18.3.1 Imaging

Ultrasound

Transabdominal ultrasound is frequently performed in patients with cholangiocarcinoma to evaluate biliary obstruction. Periductal or intraductal cholangiocarcinoma may manifest as indirect findings of biliary dilation and parenchymal atrophy if obstruction is long standing. Although the inciting tumor is often not discernible, the site of reduction in biliary caliber may indicate its location. Perihilar infiltrating lesions may appear as a mass disrupting the confluence of the right and left hepatic ducts and possibly involving adjacent vascular structures.[21]

Mass-forming ICC often appears as a solid hypovascular mass with irregular, well-defined margins or as abnormal liver echotexture. The mass may be hypoechoic, hyperechoic, or mixed, without specific features to differentiate it from other solid hepatic lesions.[3,21] Further evaluation with CT, MR imaging, or positron emission tomography (PET) fused with CT (PET/CT) is generally needed to evaluate the extent of intrahepatic and extrahepatic disease.

Computed Tomography

Contrast-enhanced multiphase CT is superior to ultrasound in characterizing the extent of intrahepatic, extrahepatic, and distal metastatic disease in patients with cholangiocarcinoma. Intraductal tumors may present as ductal ectasia with or without discernible plaquelike or papillary intraluminal tissue that enhances mildly on arterial and portal venous phases. Periductal infiltrating tumors tend to manifest as periductal concentric and irregular thickening and enhancement with associated biliary obstruction.[3]

Mass-forming cholangiocarcinoma is typically hypoattenuating on noncontrast phase images with an incomplete, thin rim of enhancement on arterial and portal venous phases and with varying degrees of progressive central enhancement on delayed phase images (▶ Fig. 18.2).[22] Peripheral enhancement correlates to viable neoplasm on pathology, whereas progressive central enhancement represents contrast diffusion into the fibrous

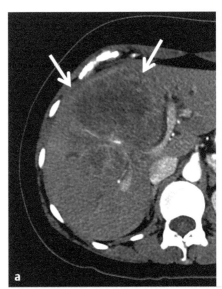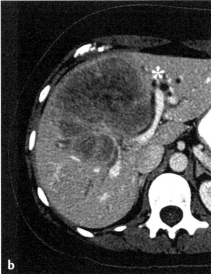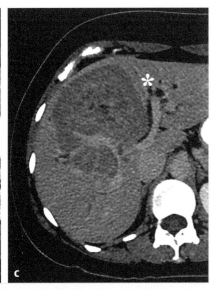

Fig. 18.2 Multiphase CT (computed tomography) in a 43-year-old woman with mass-forming intrahepatic cholangiocarcinoma (ICC; patient A). **(a)** A thin, incomplete rim of enhancement (*arrows*) is seen on the late arterial phase image, with central hypoenhancement. **(b)** The central components gradually enhance on the portal venous phase and **(c)** 5-minute delayed images. Dilated biliary ducts (*asterisk*) are noted peripheral to the mass.

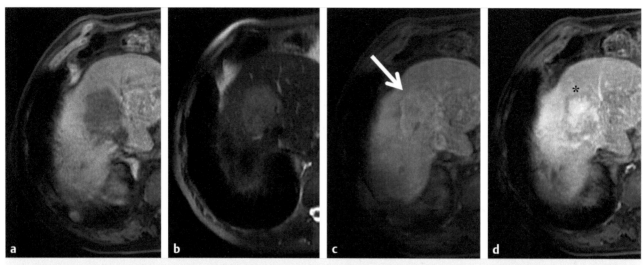

Fig. 18.3 Multiphase 3 T magnetic resonance (MR) images in a 70-year-old man with mass-forming intrahepatic cholangiocarcinoma (ICC; patient B). **(a)** MR images demonstrate T1 prolongation and **(b)** moderate T2 prolongation of the mass relative to liver parenchyma. **(c)** Fat-saturated, postcontrast T1 sequences show a thin peripheral rim (*arrow*) on enhancement with gradual enhancement (**d**; *asterisk*) of the central components on 5-minute delayed images.

interstitial spaces of desmoplastic tissue.[3,23,24] Ancillary features such as capsular retraction secondary to fibrosis, satellite nodules, bile duct dilation, and vascular encasement support the diagnosis of cholangiocarcinoma. Segmental atrophy may also occur secondary to chronic biliary or portal venous obstruction.[25]

Magnetic Resonance Imaging

MR imaging also plays a role in the diagnosis and characterization of cholangiocarcinoma. Mass-forming lesions are typically hypointense or isointense to liver on T1-weighted images and mildly to moderately hyperintense on T2-weighted images peripherally (▶ Fig. 18.3).[26] After administration of gadolinium contrast, mass-forming lesions demonstrate an enhancement pattern similar to that seen on multiphase CT, with early marginal enhancement and progressive enhancement of desmoplastic components. Depending on the degree of necrosis, the central T2 signal can range from low to high in intensity. Central T2 shortening may correlate to severe fibrosis on pathology.[27]

MR imaging with cholangiopancreatography (MRCP) is a valuable adjunct for evaluation of the biliary tree. MRCP is superior to CT in evaluating intraductal tumors and has an efficacy similar to that of CT in delineating extension to the vasculature and lymph nodes.[21,28] MRCP imaging has an efficacy similar to that of percutaneous transhepatic cholangiography in determining the longitudinal extent of hilar cholangiocarcinoma.[29]

Positron Emission Tomography

[18]F-fluorodoxyglucose PET/CT is helpful in determining management strategies and prognosis for patients with cholangiocarcinoma.[30] Identifying the status of the lymph nodes is critical, as this is an important prognostic factor in patients with R0 resection margins.[6] PET/CT has demonstrated higher accuracy than CT in the diagnosis of regional lymph nodes metastases (75.9 vs. 60.9%; $p = 0.004$) and distant metastases (88.3 vs. 78.7%; $p = 0.004$).[31] In one study, approximately 24% of

patients had a change in surgical or medical management after undergoing PET/CT.[32]

18.3.2 Endoscopic Retrograde Cholangiopancreatography

Gastroenterologists perform endoscopic retrograde cholangiopancreatography (ERCP) to access the biliary tree with retrograde cholangiography, allowing access for biopsy and stent placement. The retrograde cholangiogram may identify malignant features of strictures, such as a long segment or shelf-like margin; however, the specificity of this technique is low, as 5 to 25% of these strictures may be benign on histologic analysis.[33,34]

18.3.3 Biopsy

Although imaging is effective in noninvasive characterization of the disease extent, biopsy is often required for diagnostic confirmation of cholangiocarcinoma.[1,7] Common approaches include laparoscopic biopsy, endoscopic fine-needle aspiration (FNA) and cytologic brushings, and percutaneous biopsy.

ERCP enables biliary tree access and visualization and allows for tissue sampling. Endoscopic brush cytology is often performed, although this technique has a relatively low sensitivity of approximately 58%;[35] other studies have reported an accuracy of 9 to 24%.[21] Endoscopic ultrasound (EUS) may be used to visualize hilar lesions and evaluate the involvement of regional lymph nodes and vessels.[1] FNA biopsy with EUS of the distal bile duct lesions has been shown to have a sensitivity of 77 to 89% and a specificity of 100%.[36,37,38] Although tumor seeding after FNA is of concern, particularly in cases of potentially resectable disease, this event appears to be exceedingly rare, occurring at a rate of approximately 1 in 10,000 to 40,000 biopsies.[1]

Percutaneous image-guided biopsy is particularly valuable in cases of mass-forming lesions and can be performed under ultrasound or cross-sectional imaging guidance depending on

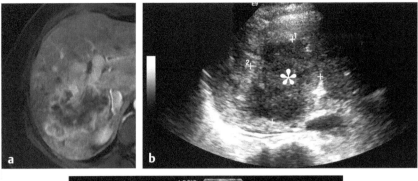

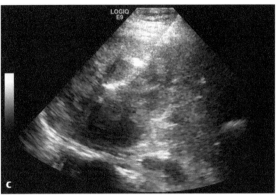

Fig. 18.4 Ultrasound-guided biopsy in a 27-year-old man presenting to the emergency department with abdominal pain (patient C). **(a)** Fat-saturated postcontrast T1-weighted magnetic resonance (MR) image demonstrates a large, heterogeneously enhancing mass in the right hepatic lobe. **(b)** The mass (*asterisk*) is predominantly hypoechoic on sonographic images. **(c)** Under ultrasound guidance, an 18-gauge, 2-cm core biopsy was performed through a 17-gauge introducer needle, demonstrating moderately differentiated ICC (intrahepatic cholangiocarcinoma).

lesion conspicuity and operator preference (▶ Fig. 18.4). In one study, malignant lesions measuring 3 cm or smaller were accurately sampled by core-needle biopsy (18-gauge automated side-cutting needles through a 17-gauge introducer package) in 84.4% of cases and by FNA in 91.7% of cases.[39] Smaller lesions measuring 1.5 cm or less were associated with similar success rates.[40,41]

For intraductal lesions without a targetable mass-forming component, percutaneous brush cytology or forceps biopsy may be used. The sensitivity of transhepatic brush cytologic biopsy in the evaluation of malignant strictures ranges from 30 to 75%.[42,43] Forceps biopsy provides a sample of subepithelial tissue and has been reported to have a higher sensitivity compared to brush biopsy (43–81% or higher).[43,44]

In patients with established transhepatic biliary tracts from prior percutaneous drainage, an endobiliary core biopsy can be performed, although this method is less established. A cohort of 18 patients with suspicious biliary stricture underwent 19-gauge, 2-cm core biopsy through a transhepatic sheath and inner 14-gauge curved metal cannula.[45] Sensitivity and specificity were reported as 76 to 81% and 100%, respectively.

18.4 Management of Cholangiocarcinoma

Management of cholangiocarcinoma often requires a multidisciplinary approach that involves interventional radiologists, radiation oncologists, surgeons, medical oncologists, and gastroenterologists. Interventional radiologists play an important role in providing symptomatic relief with biliary decompression and in controlling the tumor with transcatheter therapies and thermal ablation.

18.4.1 Drainage Procedures

Percutaneous Biliary Drainage

Percutaneous transhepatic biliary drainage (PTBD) to decompress the biliary tree is indicated for cholangitis, hyperbilirubinemia, and hepatic dysfunction related to malignant obstruction that cannot be treated endoscopically with internal biliary stent placement (▶ Fig. 18.5).[46,47] Although ERCP with internal stent placement is generally considered first-line therapy, percutaneous drainage, particularly in perihilar cholangiocarcinoma, has been reported to be as efficacious as endoscopic decompression with a lower risk of complications such as cholangitis.[48,49,50] PTBD may also be considered in cholangiocarcinoma to relieve liver function test derangements precluding systemic chemotherapy or potentially curative resection.[51,52]

Patients undergoing percutaneous cholangiography (PTC) and PTBD placement are at risk for periprocedural sepsis. Patients with a fever, history of prior biliary instrumentation, and bilioenteric anastomoses are at particularly high risk for positive bile cultures. Therefore, the Society of Interventional Radiology (SIR) recommends the use of preprocedural antibiotics.[53] Intravenous antibiotics that cover organisms such as *Enterococcus* should be administered before PTBD, and patients should be closely monitored for at least 6 hours after the procedure for signs of sepsis.[54] Antibiotics may be terminated 24 hours after placement in the absence of clinical signs of infection. Overdistention of the biliary tree with contrast during PTC and PTBD may also increase the risk of bacterial translocation and septicemia and should be avoided.

Placement of an internal/external PTBD that traverses the site of obstruction and terminates within the small bowel is generally preferable to the use of external drainage, as an internal/external PTBD allows physiological drainage and the preservation of bile

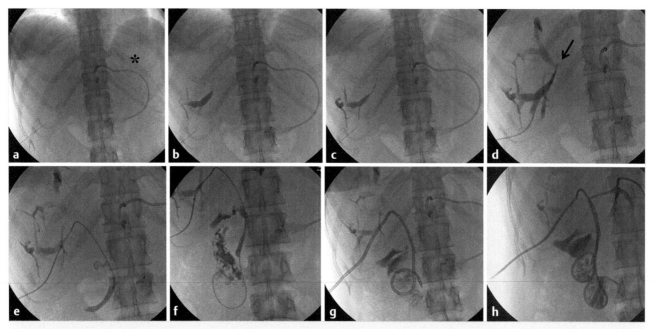

Fig. 18.5 Internal/external biliary drain placement (patient A). **(a)** A left hepatic duct external drain was placed at another institution before admission (*asterisk*). A 21-gauge Chiba needle was advanced under ultrasound guidance (not pictured) into a dilated right hepatic biliary duct peripheral to the obstructing mass. **(b,c)** Contrast was instilled for cholangiography, demonstrating dilated peripheral ducts with abrupt occlusion within the right hepatic lobe. **(d-f)** A 0.018-inch guidewire was advanced through the needle, and the needle was exchanged for a 6-Fr dilator. The guidewire was exchanged for a 0.035-inch guidewire, which was advanced with a 4-Fr catheter past the stricture (*arrow*) and into the duodenum. **(g)** An 8-Fr internal/external biliary drain was placed over the guidewire with opacification of the duodenum to confirm placement. **(h)** The left hepatic duct external biliary drain was then internalized in a similar fashion.

salts. The internal/external drain can be attached to gravity drainage to maximize decompression. Alternatively, the catheter may be capped for internal physiologic biliary drainage, which allows for the preservation of bile salts, prevention of associated electrolyte imbalance, and improved quality of life. If the stricture cannot be traversed, an external PTBD that terminates peripheral to the site of obstruction may be placed and attached to gravity drainage.

The patient should be monitored for signs of catheter dysfunction such as fever, disproportionate abdominal pain, drainage from the skin entry site, and liver function test abnormalities to prompt catheter evaluation and possible exchange. In the absence of clinical symptoms, catheters are generally exchanged every 4 to 6 weeks.

Biliary Stent Placement

After placement of an internal/external PTBD, a stent may be deployed to restore physiological biliary flow, with the main advantage of obviating the need for an indwelling catheter and thereby improving quality of life.[55] Stenting may be performed immediately after PTBD but generally should be preceded by normalization of liver function tests and clearance of infection. Self-expanding bare metal stents or stent grafts may be used. Bare metal stents are permanent and generally less expensive but allow interstitial tumor ingrowth.[56,57] Covered stent grafts may be less susceptible to obstruction from tumor ingrowth and are potentially retrievable but are more susceptible to migration.[58,59] Leaving a capped external biliary drain in place for 1 to 2 weeks after stent placement should be considered as

a precautionary measure to ensure adequate biliary drainage through the stent. Technical success rates for biliary stents range from 75 to 100%.[60,61]

The decision to stent or continue internal/external biliary catheter drainage is based on prognosis and patient preference. The length of patency is of primary concern when placing stents, as occlusion may lead to morbidity with associated hospitalization and intervention. For distal extrahepatic malignant obstruction, it is unclear whether covered or uncovered stents are more effective. In a prospective randomized controlled trial of expanded polytetrafluoroethylene/fluorinated ethylene propylene (ePTFE/FEP) stents versus uncovered self-expanding nitinol stents for inoperable pancreatic head cancer, Krokidis et al[58] reported a mean patency of 166 days for the bare metal stent group and 234 days for the covered stent group ($p = 0.007$), suggesting that a covered stent for distal common bile duct lesions may result in fewer interventions, although survival was not significantly different between the two groups. In contrast, another prospective randomized controlled trial showed improved patency of uncovered stents versus covered stents (413.3 vs. 207.5 days; $p < 0.05$) in patients with distal extrahepatic tumors.[59]

Hilar biliary obstruction involving both hepatic lobes presents unique challenges for stent placement. Although allowing drainage of both lobes is desirable, drainage of approximately 25% of the liver volume may achieve symptomatic palliation and biochemical improvement, and bilobar stent placement may not improve survival when compared with unilobar stent placement.[62,63] With common bile duct strictures, a stent terminating superior to the major duodenal papilla is associated with decreased rates of ascending cholangitis. In a study of 98 patients, Huang et al[64] reported a 23.5% incidence of cholangitis in cases stented across the duodenal major papilla versus an 8.5% incidence in cases with suprapapillary stent termination ($p = 0.44$). In addition, suprapapillary stent termination has been associated with a decreased rate of pancreatitis (25% with transpapillary stent placement vs. 4% with suprapapillary stent placement; $p < 0.001$; $n = 155$).[65]

18.4.2 Primary Tumor Therapies

Surgical Resection

Surgical treatment typically aims for resection with negative margins. In a study of 584 patients at multiple institutions, Spolverato et al[66] found that R1 resections were associated with significantly shorter overall survival (hazard ration [HR] = 1.54; $p = 0.01$) when compared with R0 resections. In addition, thicker R0 resection margins demonstrated improved recurrence-free survival (1–4 mm, HR = 1.32; 5–9 mm, HR = 1.21) and overall survival (1–4 mm, HR = 1.95; 5–9 mm, HR = 1.21) when compared with resection margins thinner than 1 mm. Margin width and status were independent determinants of recurrence-free survival and overall survival on multivariate analysis.[66]

OLT has also been performed to treat cholangiocarcinoma when resection is not possible, although its role in this setting is limited. In a meta-analysis of 14 studies involving 605 patients, survival rates after OLT were 73% at 1 year, 42% at 3 years, and 39% at 5 years.[67] However, there was a high complication rate (65%) that included vascular injury, biliary leakage, and pancreatic leakage. Preoperative adjuvant therapy was associated with improved pooled survival rates of 83% at 1 year, 57% at 3 years, and 65% at 5 years. The Mayo protocol,[68] with OLT after neoadjuvant chemotherapy and radiation of selected early-stage cholangiocarcinoma patients with underlying PSC, has been associated with promising outcomes for selected early-stage cholangiocarcinoma patients with underlying PSC; however, this protocol is highly selective, requiring laparotomy to confirm that the disease is limited to the liver.

Systemic Chemotherapy

Systemic chemotherapy is typically the first-line treatment for unresectable cholangiocarcinoma, demonstrating a survival benefit of 5 to 8 months.[69,70,71,72,73] Per National Comprehensive Cancer Network (NCCN) guidelines, the primary treatment for unresectable ICC involves systemic chemotherapy with gemcitabine and cisplatin. In a phase 3 randomized controlled trial that compared the combination of gemcitabine and cisplatin with gemcitabine alone, the median overall survival in the combination group was 11.7 versus 8.1 months in patients treated with gemcitabine alone (HR = 0.64; confidence interval [CI] = 0.52–0.80; $p < 0.001$).[74] Tumor control based on Response Evaluation Criteria in Solid Tumors (RECIST) was also improved with combination therapy versus single-agent therapy (81.4 vs. 71.8%; $p = 0.49$).[74]

Radiation Therapy

NCCN guidelines recommend the consideration of radiation therapy for unresectable extrahepatic and ICC.[7] In addition,

cases of resectable ICC with R1 margins or positive lymph nodes can be treated with adjuvant chemotherapy and radiation. For cases of resectable ECC, adjuvant radiation and chemotherapy are recommended regardless of margin and nodal status.[7] External beam radiation therapy (EBRT), brachytherapy, and stereotactic body radiation therapy can be used to treat cholangiocarcinoma.

For resectable ECC, adjuvant EBRT has been found to improve survival versus surgery alone (HR = 0.62; 95% CI = 0.48–0.78; $p < 0.001$).[75] Researchers from the Mayo Clinic assessed the use of neoadjuvant chemoradiotherapy before transplant in patients with unresectable perihilar cholangiocarcinoma and PSC.[76] In this small study with strict patient selection criteria ($n = 11$), a combination of EBRT, 5-fluorourocil, and iridium brachytherapy before transplant yielded a median survival of 44 months. A subsequent study in 287 patients at 12 institutions who received chemotherapy, EBRT, and/or brachytherapy before transplant demonstrated that masses larger than 3 cm were associated with a significantly worse 5-year recurrence-free survival rate than smaller masses ($p < 0.001$).[77] No difference was shown between a subgroup of patients who had received brachytherapy versus those who had not (HR = 1.05; 95% CI: 0.60–1.85). For ICC, EBRT is limited secondary to the risk of radiation-induced liver disease. Further investigation of radiation therapy in cholangiocarcinoma is ongoing.

Transarterial Chemoembolization

Transarterial chemoembolization (TACE) involves direct transcatheter instillation of chemotherapy and an embolic agent into the arterial branches that perfuse the targeted tumor (▶ Fig. 18.6; ▶ Fig. 18.7). TACE is a first-line therapy for intermediate-stage HCC and has also been used to treat patients with unresectable cholangiocarcinoma who have liver-dominant disease. However, because of the rarity of cholangiocarcinoma, current evidence supporting this technique is limited to small, uncontrolled, retrospective observational studies. Numerous chemotherapeutic agents (and dosages) have been used in these studies, including doxorubicin, mitomycin C, irinotecan, and cysplatin.[78] Embolic agents studied have included Gelfoam, ethiodized oil, polyvinyl alcohol particles, and drug-eluting beads.[79,80,81,82,83]

A systematic review and meta-analysis of 16 studies that assessed TACE for cholangiocarcinoma included 1,453 procedures in 542 patients with relatively preserved liver function and performance status. No patients had Child–Pugh class C liver disease, and more than 95% of the patients had an Eastern Cooperative Oncology Group (ECOG) score of 0 or 1.[78] In this meta-analysis, which was limited by the heterogeneity in TACE agents used and outcomes reported, the median overall survival was 15.7 months from the date of diagnosis and 13.4 months from the initiation of TACE. In addition, stable disease or tumor response as defined by RECIST or modified RECIST was observed in 77% of patients within 4 months after treatment; 22.8% of patients demonstrated a complete or partial response. Patients treated with TACE survived 2 to 7 months longer than historical controls treated with systemic therapies.[69,70,71,72,73] However, this perceived survival benefit may be attributable to selection bias and confounding variables.[78] TACE was also associated with a low overall 30-day mortality (0.7%), but severe

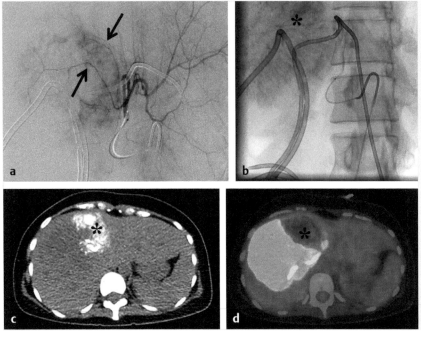

Fig. 18.6 Transarterial chemoembolization (TACE), first treatment (patient A). **(a)** Left hepatic angiogram opacified the medial margin of the mass (*arrows*) that is supplied by the segment 4 hepatic artery. **(b)** An emulsified mixture of cisplatin, doxorubicin, mitomycin c, and ethiodized oil (*asterisk*) was delivered via a segment 4 branch of the left hepatic artery, with associated tumor staining. **(c,d)** At 1 month after TACE, PET (positron emission tomography)/CT (computed tomography) showed photopenia of the portion of the mass with ethiodized oil retention (*asterisk*) and FDG (fluoro-2-deoxy-d-glucose) avidity of the untreated portion of the mass.

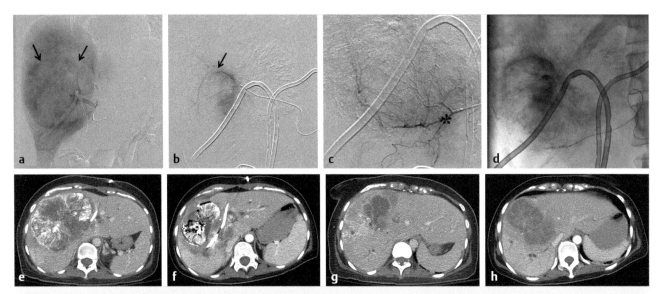

Fig. 18.7 Transarterial chemoembolization (TACE), second treatment (patient A). Patient A underwent further TACE of the untreated areas 1 month after the first TACE procedure. **(a)** Selective angiography of the right hepatic artery demonstrates predominantly peripheral enhancement of the right hepatic lobe tumor (*arrows*). **(b)** Subsegmental branches supplied the tumor (*arrow*), and **(c)** extrahepatic collateral arterial supply via the cystic artery (*asterisk*) was also present. **(d)** TACE was also delivered via the cystic artery after the catheter was guided past branches supplying the gallbladder, with associated ethiodized oil staining of the mass. **(e)** Axial contrast-enhanced computed tomography (CT) image 1 week after TACE demonstrates retained ethiodol within the tumor. **(f)** Contrast-enhanced CT images 3 months later show decrease size of the treated portion of the tumor with associated gas from necrosis or infection, although the patient had no clinical signs of infection. **(g,h)** However, the tumor had increased in size at its superior aspect. The patient opted for home hospice after tumor progression was established.

toxicity (National Cancer Institute/World Health Organization grade 3 or greater) was observed in 18.9% of patients. Although these toxicities were highly variable, numerous studies reported severe complications related to abdominal pain, hepatic toxicity, hepatic abscess, and biliary sepsis.[78]

Hepatic abscess and biliary sepsis have long been known as potential complications of TACE in patients with a history of biliary instrumentation or biliary-enteric anastomosis. For example, a study of TACE for hepatic tumors demonstrated that a history of bilioenteric anastomosis was strongly associated with abscess formation (odds ratio [OR] = 894; $p < 0.0001$); six of seven patients who had undergone a Whipple procedure developed a hepatic abscess after TACE.[84] Similarly, Woo et al[85] demonstrated that 48% of patients with bilioenteric anastomosis developed abscess after TACE for hepatic primary and metastatic tumors. Patients with leukopenia (OR = 17.5; $p = 0.029$) or

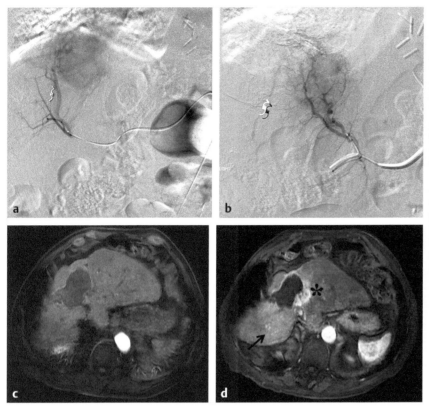

Fig. 18.8 ^{90}Y RE (patient B). [90]Y RE with glass particles was performed in two procedures. **(a)** The anterior segmental branch of the right hepatic artery was selectively catheterized, opacifying the ICC (intrahepatic cholangiocarcinoma); 85 mCi was delivered from this location. **(b)** The second procedure was performed 4 weeks later via a segment 4 branch supplying the medial aspect of the tumor; 50 mCi was delivered from this site. **(c)** MR (magnetic resonance) image obtained 5 weeks after treatment demonstrated tumor response, with a uniformly thin margin of peripheral enhancement and no discernible central enhancement. **(d)** Imaging at 7 months after initial treatment demonstrated a new right hepatic lobe nodule (*arrow*) and increased eccentric nodularity at the superior tumor margin (*asterisk*) that increased in size on further imaging, reflecting disease recurrence.

grade 2 oily portogram (OR = 16.5; p = 0.001) were at particularly high risk. The mechanism of abscess formation is likely related to retrograde contamination of necrotic hepatic tissue after TACE by enteric bacteria. The risk of abscess after TACE may be mitigated by a preprocedural course of moxifloxacin or a bowel preparation regimen, combined with an aggressive periprocedural antibiotic regimen of broad-spectrum intravenous antibiotics.[86,87] However, TACE should be performed with caution in patients with cholangiocarcinoma who have previously undergone procedures for biliary decompression or bilioenteric anastomosis.[88]

Yttrium-90 Radioembolization

Yttrium-90 radioembolization (^{90}Y RE) involves minimally invasive transcatheter delivery of ^{90}Y-labeled particles to hepatic tumors via their arterial supply (▶ Fig. 18.8; ▶ Fig. 18.9).[89] Through β emission, ^{90}Y decays to stable zirconium-90 with a half-life of 64.1 days. The emitted β particles have an average energy of 0.937 MeV volts and tissue penetration of 2.5 mm, with a maximum penetration of 10 mm. Two delivery systems for ^{90}Y are currently available: glass (TheraSphere; MDS Nordion, ON, Canada) and resin (SIR-Sphere; Sirtex Medical, Lane Cove, NSW, Australia) ^{90}Y-embedded particles. [90]Y RE is commonly used to treat HCC and metastatic liver disease and has also been used to treat unresectable ICC. As with TACE for cholangiocarcinoma, the evidence for ^{90}Y RE in this patient population is promising but currently limited to relatively small, uncontrolled observational studies.

Saxena et al[90] prospectively studied ^{90}Y RE with resin in 25 patients with unresectable ICC. All patients had baseline total bilirubin levels of ≤ 2 mg/dL and an ECOG score of 0 to 2; before

[90]Y RE, 68% of the study patients had demonstrated disease progression after systemic chemotherapy, and 40% had demonstrated tumor recurrence after hepatic resection. On follow-up imaging, treatment with ^{90}Y RE was associated with stable disease or partial response in 72% of patients, and the median survival after treatment was 9.3 months. Patients with mass-forming tumors had better median survival than patients with periductal tumors. Treatment was generally well tolerated, although fatigue (64%) and self-limiting abdominal pain (40%) were common.

Mouli et al[91] retrospectively studied ^{90}Y RE with glass for the treatment of unresectable ICC in 46 patients at a single institution over an 8-year period. All patients had total bilirubin levels of ≤ 2 mg/dL and an ECOG score of 0 to 2 before ^{90}Y RE; 39% were treatment naive. Partial or complete response according to the European Association for the Study of Liver Disease criteria was demonstrated in 73% of patients. Survival after the time of first ^{90}Y RE treatment differed by tumor distribution (multifocal, 5.7 months; unifocal, 14.6 months; p < 0.005) and morphology (peripheral, 15.6 months; infiltrative, 6.1 months; p = 0.006). Five patients (11%) were converted to resectable status and underwent R0 resection. The most common adverse events associated with ^{90}Y RE were fatigue (54%) and transient abdominal pain (28%). Grade 3 albumin toxicity occurred in 9% of patients, and grade 3 bilirubin elevations occurred in 7%.[91]

In a systematic review of 12 studies involving 298 patients treated with ^{90}Y RE for unresectable ICC, patients underwent ^{90}Y RE either before, synchronously, or after systemic chemotherapy, with a weighted mean ^{90}Y dose of 1.6 GBq and approximately 1.5 treatments per patient.[92] The weighted median overall survival was 15.5 months. At 3 months after ^{90}Y RE, 28% of patients demonstrated a partial response, and 54% had stable

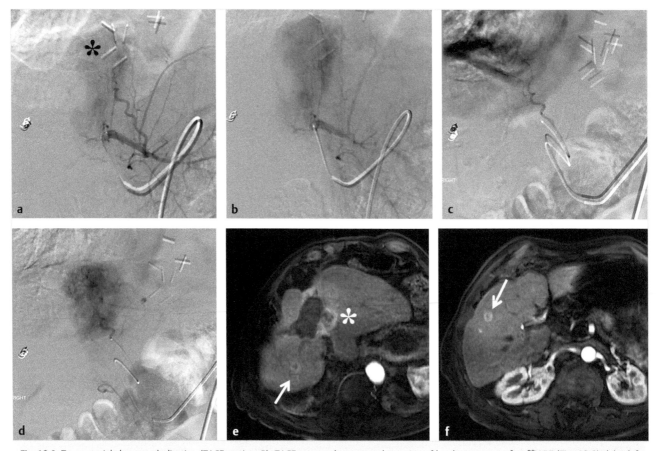

Fig. 18.9 Transarterial chemoembolization (TACE; patient B). TACE was used to target the region of local recurrence after ^{90}Y RE (**Fig. 18.8**). **(a)** A left hepatic artery angiogram shows masslike enhancement corresponding to the area of local recurrence on magnetic resonance (MR) imaging (*black asterisk*). **(b)** A subsegmental branch of the left hepatic artery was selectively catheterized, and **(c,d)** TACE was performed with an emulsified mixture of doxorubicin, mitomycin C, and ethiodized oil, with associated tumor staining. **(e,f)** MR imaging performed 1 month later demonstrated a decrease in the enhancing components of the treated area (*white asterisk*) but an increase in the size of the enhancing hepatic nodules (*arrows*) measuring up to 1.7 cm (previously 1.0 cm), concerning for recurrent disease. These nodules were subsequently treated with percutaneous RFA (radiofrequency ablation).

disease. A total of seven patients from three separate studies were converted to operable disease and underwent surgical resection; the authors therefore suggested that a potential indication for ^{90}Y RE is for the treatment of patients with borderline operable disease at initial presentation. Adverse events were reported in 8 of the 12 studies and most commonly included fever, abdominal pain, or nausea at rates similar to those reported in a systematic review of TACE for unresectable ICC.[78] Several studies reported the development of ascites or hepatitis after ^{90}Y RE, raising the possibility of radiation-induced liver disease.[92] The authors concluded that survival after ^{90}Y RE was comparable to that of historical controls treated with systemic chemotherapy and/or TACE but that randomized controlled trials are needed to determine which therapy is most efficacious.[92]

The risk of postprocedural hepatic abscess formation in patients with a history of biliary instrumentation or bilioenteric anastomosis has not been as thoroughly investigated for ^{90}Y RE as it has been for TACE. Cholapranee et al[93] reported results of 24 ^{90}Y RE procedures in 16 patients with a history of biliary intervention. All patients received a prophylactic regimen of oral levofloxacin and metronidazole and a bowel preparation of oral

neomycin/erythromycin, followed by intravenous levofloxacin and metronidazole on the day of ^{90}Y RE and a 2-week postprocedural course orally. No hepatic abscess was observed on follow-up. In a comparison group of 13 similar patients who underwent TACE, hepatic abscess was observed in 23% of patients.[93] Further research is needed to determine the risk of abscess after ^{90}Y RE in patients with a history of biliary instrumentation and whether the risk is lower compared to the risk with TACE.

Percutaneous Thermal Ablation

Percutaneous thermal ablation with radiofrequency or microwave energy is used extensively to treat HCC and has been investigated for the treatment of primary and recurrent mass-forming ICC (▶ Fig. 18.10). Kim et al[94] retrospectively studied 13 patients with 17 ICC tumors treated with percutaneous radiofrequency ablation (RFA) and reported technical success on 1-month follow-up imaging for all 15 tumors smaller than 5 cm; treatment failure occurred in the 2 tumors larger than 5 cm. The median survival was 38.5 months, with 85% of patients alive at 1 year. One major complication (liver abscess)

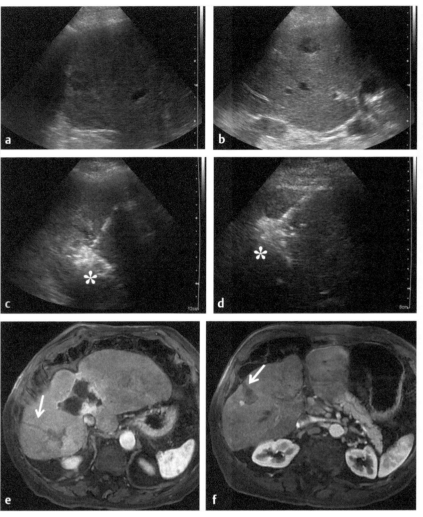

Fig. 18.10 Radiofrequency ablation (RFA; patient B). **(a,b)** The two enlarging nodules in the right hepatic lobe were identified on ultrasound as circumscribed hypoechoic masses. **(c)** A 14-gauge talon RITA applicator (AngioDynamics, Latham, NY) was introduced into the segment 7 mass and the tines were extended to 4 cm, with total ablation time of 10 minutes. **(d)** The anterior inferior right hepatic lobe mass was ablated with a 14-gauge talon RITA applicator with tines deployed at 3 cm for a total of 7 minutes. Echogenicity within the RFA ablation zone during treatment corresponded with expected gas (*asterisk*). **(e,f)** MR (magnetic resonance) imaging performed 1 month later showed the ablation zones (*arrows*) and evidence of technical success; however, the patient ultimately developed multifocal recurrent disease and died 36 months after initial ^{90}Y RE and 25 months after RFA.

occurred; this patient died of sepsis 3.3 months after RFA.[94] Butros et al[95] also studied RFA for primary ICC in seven patients with nine tumors of mean size 2.4 cm (range: 1.3–3.3 cm). Technical success was achieved in eight of the nine tumors. The mean overall survival was 38.5 months, with no major complications observed.

RFA has also been studied for the treatment of recurrent ICC after surgical resection.[96] Although repeat hepatic resection is first-line therapy for recurrent ICC, this is often not feasible because of multifocal recurrence or comorbidities. In one study, 77 patients with 133 recurrent ICC tumors underwent percutaneous RFA; all patients had five or fewer tumors, all measuring 5 cm or smaller, and patients had Child–Pugh class A or B disease without coagulopathy, macrovascular invasion, or extrahepatic disease.[96] TACE was performed before RFA in 45.5% of the study patients. The median overall survival was 21.3 months. Among patients with tumors 3 cm in size or smaller, overall survival was similar in patients who underwent RFA and in a group of 32 similar patients who underwent repeat hepatic resection. In patients with tumors larger than 3 cm, overall survival was slightly improved with hepatic resection. The rate of major complications was significantly lower in the RFA group (3.9%) than in the repeat hepatic resection group (47%); the most common major adverse event in the RFA group was hepatic abscess in two patients.

Further investigation is needed to elucidate the role of percutaneous thermal ablation in ICC. The role of thermal ablation in ECC is likely limited because of the risk of biliary injury.[95]

18.5 Conclusion

Cholangiocarcinoma is a highly aggressive primary hepatic malignancy with an overall poor prognosis. There are many associated risk factors, such as viral hepatitis, PSC, and liver flukes, but most patients with cholangiocarcinoma have no known risk factors. Surgical resection and transplant offer the best opportunity for long-term survival, but most patients are not surgical candidates at the time of diagnosis. Systemic therapy with gemcitabine and cisplatin can lead to improved outcomes, and radiation therapy can play a role in adjuvant therapy. Interventional radiology, in addition to its critical role in providing biliary diversion, also plays a role in controlling tumors through the use of ^{90}Y RE, TACE, and thermal ablation.

References

[1] Khan SA, Davidson BR, Goldin RD, et al. British Society of Gastroenterology. Guidelines for the diagnosis and treatment of cholangiocarcinoma: an update. Gut. 2012; 61(12):1657–1669

[2] Nakanuma Y, Sato Y, Harada K, Sasaki M, Xu J, Ikeda H. Pathological classification of intrahepatic cholangiocarcinoma based on a new concept. World J Hepatol. 2010; 2(12):419–427

[3] Chung YE, Kim MJ, Park YN, et al. Varying appearances of cholangiocarcinoma: radiologic-pathologic correlation. Radiographics. 2009; 29(3):683–700

[4] Ben-Menachem T. Risk factors for cholangiocarcinoma. Eur J Gastroenterol Hepatol. 2007; 19(8):615–617

[5] Shaib Y, El-Serag HB. The epidemiology of cholangiocarcinoma. Semin Liver Dis. 2004; 24(2):115–125

[6] DeOliveira ML, Cunningham SC, Cameron JL, et al. Cholangiocarcinoma: thirty-one-year experience with 564 patients at a single institution. Ann Surg. 2007; 245(5):755–762

[7] National Comprehensive Cancer Network. NCCN Clinical Practice Guidelines in Oncology (NCCN Guidelines): Hepatobiliary Cancers. Version 2. Fort Washington, PA: NCCN; 2013

[8] Lazaridis KN, Gores GJ. Cholangiocarcinoma. Gastroenterology. 2005; 128(6):1655–1667

[9] Tyson GL, El-Serag HB. Risk factors for cholangiocarcinoma. Hepatology. 2011; 54(1):173–184

[10] Lim JH. Cholangiocarcinoma: morphologic classification according to growth pattern and imaging findings. AJR Am J Roentgenol. 2003; 181(3):819–827

[11] Yamasaki S. Intrahepatic cholangiocarcinoma: macroscopic type and stage classification. J Hepatobiliary Pancreat Surg. 2003; 10(4):288–291

[12] Razumilava N, Gores GJ. Classification, diagnosis, and management of cholangiocarcinoma. Clin Gastroenterol Hepatol. 2013; 11(1):13–21.e1, quiz e3–e4

[13] Jarnagin WR, Bowne W, Klimstra DS, et al. Papillary phenotype confers improved survival after resection of hilar cholangiocarcinoma. Ann Surg. 2005; 241(5):703–712, discussion 712–714

[14] Bismuth H, Nakache R, Diamond T. Management strategies in resection for hilar cholangiocarcinoma. Ann Surg. 1992; 215(1):31–38

[15] Allen RA, Lisa JR. Combined liver cell and bile duct carcinoma. Am J Pathol. 1949; 25(4):647–655

[16] Sapisochin G, Fidelman N, Roberts JP, Yao FY. Mixed hepatocellular cholangiocarcinoma and intrahepatic cholangiocarcinoma in patients undergoing transplantation for hepatocellular carcinoma. Liver Transpl. 2011; 17(8):934–942

[17] Nishie A, Yoshimitsu K, Asayama Y, et al. Detection of combined hepatocellular and cholangiocarcinomas on enhanced CT: comparison with histologic findings. AJR Am J Roentgenol. 2005; 184(4):1157–1162

[18] Saboo SS, Krajewski KM, Jagannathan JP, et al. Rapid progression of combined hepatocellular carcinoma and cholangiocarcinoma. Cancer Imaging. 2011; 11:37–41

[19] Shetty AS, Fowler KJ, Brunt EM, Agarwal S, Narra VR, Menias CO. Combined hepatocellular-cholangiocarcinoma: what the radiologist needs to know about biphenotypic liver carcinoma. Abdom Imaging. 2014; 39(2):310–322

[20] Van Beers BE. Diagnosis of cholangiocarcinoma. HPB (Oxford). 2008; 10(2):87–93

[21] Sainani NI, Catalano OA, Holalkere NS, Zhu AX, Hahn PF, Sahani DV. Cholangiocarcinoma: current and novel imaging techniques. Radiographics. 2008; 28(5):1263–1287

[22] Kim TK, Choi BI, Han JK, Jang HJ, Cho SG, Han MC. Peripheral cholangiocarcinoma of the liver: two-phase spiral CT findings. Radiology. 1997; 204(2):539–543

[23] Valls C, Gumà A, Puig I, et al. Intrahepatic peripheral cholangiocarcinoma: CT evaluation. Abdom Imaging. 2000; 25(5):490–496

[24] Honda H, Onitsuka H, Yasumori K, et al. Intrahepatic peripheral cholangiocarcinoma: two-phased dynamic incremental CT and pathologic correlation. J Comput Assist Tomogr. 1993; 17(3):397–402

[25] Hann LE, Getrajdman GI, Brown KT, et al. Hepatic lobar atrophy: association with ipsilateral portal vein obstruction. AJR Am J Roentgenol. 1996; 167(4):1017–1021

[26] Manfredi R, Masselli G, Maresca G, Brizi MG, Vecchioli A, Marano P. MR imaging and MRCP of hilar cholangiocarcinoma. Abdom Imaging. 2003; 28 (3):319–325

[27] Maetani Y, Itoh K, Watanabe C, et al. MR imaging of intrahepatic cholangiocarcinoma with pathologic correlation. AJR Am J Roentgenol. 2001; 176(6):1499–1507

[28] Park HS, Lee JM, Choi JY, et al. Preoperative evaluation of bile duct cancer: MRI combined with MR cholangiopancreatography versus MDCT with direct cholangiography. AJR Am J Roentgenol. 2008; 190(2):396–405

[29] Lee SS, Kim MH, Lee SK, et al. MR cholangiography versus cholangioscopy for evaluation of longitudinal extension of hilar cholangiocarcinoma. Gastrointest Endosc. 2002; 56(1):25–32

[30] Rizvi S, Gores GJ. Pathogenesis, diagnosis, and management of cholangiocarcinoma. Gastroenterology. 2013; 145(6):1215–1229

[31] Kim JY, Kim M-H, Lee TY, et al. Clinical role of 18F-FDG PET-CT in suspected and potentially operable cholangiocarcinoma: a prospective study compared with conventional imaging. Am J Gastroenterol. 2008; 103(5):1145–1151

[32] Corvera CU, Blumgart LH, Akhurst T, et al. 18F-fluorodeoxyglucose positron emission tomography influences management decisions in patients with biliary cancer. J Am Coll Surg. 2008; 206(1):57–65

[33] Adler DG, Baron TH, Davila RE, et al. Standards of Practice Committee of American Society for Gastrointestinal Endoscopy. ASGE guideline: the role of ERCP in diseases of the biliary tract and the pancreas. Gastrointest Endosc. 2005; 62(1):1–8

[34] Wakai T, Shirai Y, Sakata J, et al. Clinicopathological features of benign biliary strictures masquerading as biliary malignancy. Am Surg. 2012; 78(12):1388–1391

[35] Gonda TA, Glick MP, Sethi A, et al. Polysomy and p16 deletion by fluorescence in situ hybridization in the diagnosis of indeterminate biliary strictures. Gastrointest Endosc. 2012; 75(1):74–79

[36] DeWitt J, Misra VL, Leblanc JK, McHenry L, Sherman S. EUS-guided FNA of proximal biliary strictures after negative ERCP brush cytology results. Gastrointest Endosc. 2006; 64(3):325–333

[37] Eloubeidi MA, Chen VK, Jhala NC, et al. Endoscopic ultrasound-guided fine needle aspiration biopsy of suspected cholangiocarcinoma. Clin Gastroenterol Hepatol. 2004; 2(3):209–213

[38] Fritscher-Ravens A, Broering DC, Sriram PV, et al. EUS-guided fine-needle aspiration cytodiagnosis of hilar cholangiocarcinoma: a case series. Gastrointest Endosc. 2000; 52(4):534–540

[39] Ma X, Arellano RS, Gervais DA, Hahn PF, Mueller PR, Sahani DV. Success of image-guided biopsy for small (≤3 cm) focal liver lesions in cirrhotic and noncirrhotic individuals. J Vasc Interv Radiol. 2010; 21(10):1539–1547, quiz 1547

[40] Kim SH, Lim HK, Lee WJ, Cho JM, Jang HJ. Needle-tract implantation in hepatocellular carcinoma: frequency and CT findings after biopsy with a 19.5-gauge automated biopsy gun. Abdom Imaging. 2000; 25(3):246–250

[41] Joyce D, Falk GA, Gandhi N, Hashimoto K. Post liver transplant presentation of needle-track metastasis of hepatocellular carcinoma following percutaneous liver biopsy. BMJ Case Rep. 2014; 2014:bcr2013010076

[42] Xing GS, Geng JC, Han XW, Dai JH, Wu CY. Endobiliary brush cytology during percutaneous transhepatic cholangiodrainage in patients with obstructive jaundice. Hepatobiliary Pancreat Dis Int. 2005; 4(1):98–103

[43] Weber A, Schmid RM, Prinz C. Diagnostic approaches for cholangiocarcinoma. World J Gastroenterol. 2008; 14(26):4131–4136

[44] Tapping CR, Byass OR, Cast JE. Cytological sampling versus forceps biopsy during percutaneous transhepatic biliary drainage and analysis of factors predicting success. Cardiovasc Intervent Radiol. 2012; 35(4):883–889

[45] Andrews JC, Sabater EA, LeRoy AJ, Burgart LJ. Percutaneous transhepatic endoluminal biliary biopsy with use of a 19-gauge gun. J Vasc Interv Radiol. 2001; 12(12):1437–1439

[46] Singhal D, van Gulik TM, Gouma DJ. Palliative management of hilar cholangiocarcinoma. Surg Oncol. 2005; 14(2):59–74

[47] Nagino M, Takada T, Miyazaki M, et al. Japanese Association of Biliary Surgery, Japanese Society of Hepato-Biliary-Pancreatic Surgery, Japan Society of Clinical Oncology. Preoperative biliary drainage for biliary tract and ampullary carcinomas. J Hepatobiliary Pancreat Surg. 2008; 15(1):25–30

[48] Kloek JJ, van der Gaag NA, Aziz Y, et al. Endoscopic and percutaneous preoperative biliary drainage in patients with suspected hilar cholangiocarcinoma. J Gastrointest Surg. 2010; 14(1):119–125

[49] Walter T, Ho CS, Horgan AM, et al. Endoscopic or percutaneous biliary drainage for Klatskin tumors? J Vasc Interv Radiol. 2013; 24(1):113–121

[50] Wiggers JK, Groot Koerkamp B, Coelen RJ, et al. Preoperative biliary drainage in perihilar cholangiocarcinoma: identifying patients who require percutaneous drainage after failed endoscopic drainage. Endoscopy. 2015; 47 (12):1124–1131

[51] Brandi G, Venturi M, Pantaleo MA, Ercolani G. Cholangiocarcinoma: Current opinion on clinical practice diagnostic and therapeutic algorithms: a review of the literature and a long-standing experience of a referral center. Dig Liver Dis. 2015

[52] Fang Y, Gurusamy KS, Wang Q, et al. Pre-operative biliary drainage for obstructive jaundice. Cochrane Database Syst Rev. 2012; 9(9):CD005444

[53] Saad WE, Wallace MJ, Wojak JC, Kundu S, Cardella JF. Quality improvement guidelines for percutaneous transhepatic cholangiography, biliary drainage, and percutaneous cholecystostomy. J Vasc Interv Radiol. 2010; 21(6):789–795

[54] Zarrinpar A, Kerlan RK. A guide to antibiotics for the interventional radiologist. Semin Intervent Radiol. 2005; 22(2):69–79

[55] Abraham NS, Barkun JS, Barkun AN. Palliation of malignant biliary obstruction: a prospective trial examining impact on quality of life. Gastrointest Endosc. 2002; 56(6):835–841

[56] Tsetis D, Krokidis M, Negru D, Prassopoulos P. Malignant biliary obstruction: the current role of interventional radiology. Ann Gastroenterol. 2016; 29(1): 33–36

[57] Krokidis M, Fanelli F, Orgera G, et al. Percutaneous palliation of pancreatic head cancer: randomized comparison of ePTFE/FEP-covered versus uncovered nitinol biliary stents. Cardiovasc Intervent Radiol. 2011; 34(2):352–361

[58] Krokidis M, Fanelli F, Orgera G, Bezzi M, Passariello R, Hatzidakis A. Percutaneous treatment of malignant jaundice due to extrahepatic cholangiocarcinoma: covered Viabil stent versus uncovered Wallstents. Cardiovasc Intervent Radiol. 2010; 33(1):97–106

[59] Lee SJ, Kim MD, Lee MS, et al. Comparison of the efficacy of covered versus uncovered metallic stents in treating inoperable malignant common bile duct obstruction: a randomized trial. J Vasc Interv Radiol. 2014; 25(12):1912–1920

[60] Tesdal IK, Adamus R, Poeckler C, Koepke J, Jaschke W, Georgi M. Therapy for biliary stenoses and occlusions with use of three different metallic stents: single-center experience. J Vasc Interv Radiol. 1997; 8(5):869–879

[61] Rossi P, Bezzi M, Rossi M, et al. Metallic stents in malignant biliary obstruction: results of a multicenter European study of 240 patients. J Vasc Interv Radiol. 1994; 5(2):279–285

[62] Inal M, Akgül E, Aksungur E, Seydaoğlu G. Percutaneous placement of biliary metallic stents in patients with malignant hilar obstruction: unilobar versus bilobar drainage. J Vasc Interv Radiol. 2003; 14(11):1409–1416

[63] van Delden OM, Laméris JS. Percutaneous drainage and stenting for palliation of malignant bile duct obstruction. Eur Radiol. 2008; 18(3):448–456

[64] Huang X, Shen L, Jin Y, et al. Comparison of uncovered stent placement across versus above the main duodenal papilla for malignant biliary obstruction. J Vasc Interv Radiol. 2015; 26(3):432–437

[65] Jo JH, Park BH. Suprapapillary versus transpapillary stent placement for malignant biliary obstruction: which is better? J Vasc Interv Radiol. 2015; 26 (4):573–582

[66] Spolverato G, Yakoob MY, Kim Y, et al. The impact of surgical margin status on long-term outcome after resection for intrahepatic cholangiocarcinoma. Ann Surg Oncol. 2015; 22(12):4020–4028

[67] Gu J, Bai J, Shi X, et al. Efficacy and safety of liver transplantation in patients with cholangiocarcinoma: a systematic review and meta-analysis. Int J Cancer. 2012; 130(9):2155–2163

[68] Rosen CB, Heimbach JK, Gores GJ. Liver transplantation for cholangiocarcinoma. Transpl Int. 2010; 23(7):692–697

[69] Khan SA, Thomas HC, Davidson BR, Taylor-Robinson SD. Cholangiocarcinoma. Lancet. 2005; 366(9493):1303–1314

[70] Alberts SR, Gores GJ, Kim GP, et al. Treatment options for hepatobiliary and pancreatic cancer. Mayo Clin Proc. 2007; 82(5):628–637

[71] Mazhar D, Stebbing J, Bower M. Chemotherapy for advanced cholangiocarcinoma: what is standard treatment? Future Oncol. 2006; 2(4):509–514

[72] Okusaka T, Ishii H, Funakoshi A, et al. Phase II study of single-agent gemcitabine in patients with advanced biliary tract cancer. Cancer Chemother Pharmacol. 2006; 57(5):647–653

[73] Dingle BH, Rumble RB, Brouwers MC, Cancer Care Ontario's Program in Evidence-Based Care's Gastrointestinal Cancer Disease Site Group. The role of gemcitabine in the treatment of cholangiocarcinoma and gallbladder cancer: a systematic review. Can J Gastroenterol. 2005; 19(12):711–716

[74] Valle J, Wasan H, Palmer DH, et al. ABC-02 Trial Investigators. Cisplatin plus gemcitabine versus gemcitabine for biliary tract cancer. N Engl J Med. 2010; 362(14):1273–1281

[75] Bonet Beltrán M, Allal AS, Gich I, Solé JM, Carrió I. Is adjuvant radiotherapy needed after curative resection of extrahepatic biliary tract cancers? A systematic review with a meta-analysis of observational studies. Cancer Treat Rev. 2012; 38(2):111–119

[76] De Vreede I, Steers JL, Burch PA, et al. Prolonged disease-free survival after orthotopic liver transplantation plus adjuvant chemoirradiation for cholangiocarcinoma. Liver Transpl. 2000; 6(3):309–316

[77] Darwish Murad S, Kim WR, Harnois DM, et al. Efficacy of neoadjuvant chemoradiation, followed by liver transplantation, for perihilar cholangiocarcinoma at 12 US centers. Gastroenterology. 2012; 143(1):88–98. e3, quiz e14

[78] Ray CE, Jr, Edwards A, Smith MT, et al. Metaanalysis of survival, complications, and imaging response following chemotherapy-based transarterial therapy in patients with unresectable intrahepatic cholangiocarcinoma. J Vasc Interv Radiol. 2013; 24(8):1218–1226

[79] Aliberti C, Benea G, Tilli M, Fiorentini G. Chemoembolization (TACE) of unresectable intrahepatic cholangiocarcinoma with slow-release doxorubicin-eluting beads: preliminary results. Cardiovasc Intervent Radiol. 2008; 31(5):883–888

[80] Kuhlmann JB, Euringer W, Spangenberg HC, et al. Treatment of unresectable cholangiocarcinoma: conventional transarterial chemoembolization compared with drug eluting bead-transarterial chemoembolization and systemic chemotherapy. Eur J Gastroenterol Hepatol. 2012; 24(4):437–443

[81] Vogl TJ, Naguib NN, Nour-Eldin NE, et al. Transarterial chemoembolization in the treatment of patients with unresectable cholangiocarcinoma: results and prognostic factors governing treatment success. Int J Cancer. 2012; 131(3): 733–740

[82] Schiffman SC, Metzger T, Dubel G, et al. Precision hepatic arterial irinotecan therapy in the treatment of unresectable intrahepatic cholangiocellular carcinoma: optimal tolerance and prolonged overall survival. Ann Surg Oncol. 2011; 18(2):431–438

[83] Poggi G, Amatu A, Montagna B, et al. OEM-TACE: a new therapeutic approach in unresectable intrahepatic cholangiocarcinoma. Cardiovasc Intervent Radiol. 2009; 32(6):1187–1192

[84] Kim W, Clark TW, Baum RA, Soulen MC. Risk factors for liver abscess formation after hepatic chemoembolization. J Vasc Interv Radiol. 2001; 12(8): 965–968

[85] Woo S, Chung JW, Hur S, et al. Liver abscess after transarterial chemoembolization in patients with bilioenteric anastomosis: frequency and risk factors. AJR Am J Roentgenol. 2013; 200(6):1370–1377

[86] Khan W, Sullivan KL, McCann JW, et al. Moxifloxacin prophylaxis for chemoembolization or embolization in patients with previous biliary interventions: a pilot study. AJR Am J Roentgenol. 2011; 197(2):W343–5

[87] Geschwind JF, Kaushik S, Ramsey DE, Choti MA, Fishman EK, Kobeiter H. Influence of a new prophylactic antibiotic therapy on the incidence of liver abscesses after chemoembolization treatment of liver tumors. J Vasc Interv Radiol. 2002; 13(11):1163–1166

[88] Patel S, Tuite CM, Mondschein JI, Soulen MC. Effectiveness of an aggressive antibiotic regimen for chemoembolization in patients with previous biliary intervention. J Vasc Interv Radiol. 2006; 17(12):1931–1934

[89] Salem R, Thurston KG. Radioembolization with 90yttrium microspheres: a state-of-the-art brachytherapy treatment for primary and secondary liver malignancies. Part 2: special topics. J Vasc Interv Radiol. 2006; 17(9):1425–1439

[90] Saxena A, Bester L, Chua TC, Chu FC, Morris DL. Yttrium-90 radiotherapy for unresectable intrahepatic cholangiocarcinoma: a preliminary assessment of this novel treatment option. Ann Surg Oncol. 2010; 17(2):484–491

[91] Mouli S, Memon K, Baker T, et al. Yttrium-90 radioembolization for intrahepatic cholangiocarcinoma: safety, response, and survival analysis. J Vasc Interv Radiol. 2013; 24(8):1227–1234

[92] Al-Adra DP, Gill RS, Axford SJ, Shi X, Kneteman N, Liau SS. Treatment of unresectable intrahepatic cholangiocarcinoma with yttrium-90 radioembolization: a systematic review and pooled analysis. Eur J Surg Oncol. 2015; 41(1):120–127

[93] Cholapranee A, van Houten D, Deitrick G, et al. Risk of liver abscess formation in patients with prior biliary intervention following yttrium-90 radioembolization. Cardiovasc Intervent Radiol. 2015; 38(2):397–400

[94] Kim JH, Won HJ, Shin YM, Kim KA, Kim PN. Radiofrequency ablation for the treatment of primary intrahepatic cholangiocarcinoma. AJR Am J Roentgenol. 2011; 196(2):W205–W209

[95] Butros SR, Shenoy-Bhangle A, Mueller PR, Arellano RS. Radiofrequency ablation of intrahepatic cholangiocarcinoma: feasibility, local tumor control, and long-term outcome. Clin Imaging. 2014; 38(4):490–494

[96] Zhang SJ, Hu P, Wang N, et al. Thermal ablation versus repeated hepatic resection for recurrent intrahepatic cholangiocarcinoma. Ann Surg Oncol. 2013; 20(11):3596–3602

19 Portal Vein Embolization

David Li and David C. Madoff

19.1 Introduction

The anticipated liver remaining after extensive hepatic resection, commonly described as the future liver remnant (FLR), is a critical factor associated with the risk of perioperative liver failure and death.[1,2] Hence, the ability to modulate the FLR has become a key component of modern oncologic hepatobiliary surgery practice.[3] Preoperative portal vein embolization (PVE) serves as a well-established means to improve the safety of extensive hepatic resection by redirecting flow to the FLR in an effort to hypertrophy and ultimately improve the functional reserve of the nonembolized segments.[4,5,6,7]

The liver is unique in its ability to regenerate after injury or resection. In the setting of either liver injury or resection, massive hepatocyte proliferation can occur, resulting in recovery of functional liver mass within 2 weeks after the loss of upward of two-thirds of the liver.[8]

Regeneration of the liver is dependent on both the stimulus of the injury and the condition of the liver parenchyma. Hepatocyte proliferation is proportional to the severity of the liver injury/resection; minor injuries (< 10% parenchymal involvement) induce only localized mitotic reactions, whereas major injuries (> 50% parenchymal involvement) result in multiple mitotic waves throughout the entire liver.[9] Regeneration rates are dependent on the time from injury, with the greatest rate of regeneration after PVE typically occurring within the first 2 weeks (▶ Fig. 19.1).[10] The predominant mechanism of cell death after PVE is cell-mediated apoptosis rather than the necrosis observed after transarterial embolization (TAE).[11] A direct correlation can be observed clinically: unlike TAE, PVE is typically not associated with postembolization syndrome (characterized by nausea, fever, and pain).

In 1990, Makuuchi et al[12] first reported on the utility of PVE in promoting FLR hypertrophy before hepatic resection in 14 patients with hilar cholangiocarcinoma. Since that time, PVE has continued to gain traction as a well-established technique to modulate the FLR. Alternative techniques have recently been proposed to modulate FLR, including transhepatic liver venous deprivation (LVD) and associating liver partition and portal vein ligation (ALPPS).[3,13,14] Transhepatic LVD is in its infancy, and

only limited reports are available to support its clinical adoption. Proponents of ALPPS suggest that greater, more rapid liver hypertrophy occurs with this technique than with PVE.[14] However, recent studies have raised concerns over increased morbidity and mortality associated with ALPPS as compared to PVE; histologically, the regenerative hepatocytes observed with ALPPS are immature compared to those observed with PVE.[15] These findings suggest that although ALPPS is associated with greater absolute size of FLR, the size does not correlate with greater functional increase. Hence, PVE remains the standard of care at many tertiary care centers, with numerous studies validating its clinical utility to modulate the FLR. This chapter reviews the current indications for and technical aspects of PVE before hepatic resection, with an emphasis on strategies to improve outcomes.

19.2 Clinical Considerations

19.2.1 Indications and Contraindications

PVE allows for safe, potentially curative hepatectomy for patients previously considered ineligible for resection based on anticipated small remnant livers.[6,12,16,17,18,19,20,21] Candidates for PVE include hepatic resection candidates with primary or metastatic liver disease who have anticipated FLRs that are too small for adequate function during the perioperative period. If too little liver remains after resection, immediate postresection hepatic failure leads to multisystem organ failure and death. If a marginal volume of liver remains, cirrhotic or not, the lack of reserve often leads to a cascade of complications, prolonged hospital and intensive care unit stays, and slow recovery or slowly progressive liver failure over weeks to months, with eventual death.[1,2,7]

To determine whether a patient will benefit from PVE, several factors must be considered.[5] First, the presence or absence of underlying liver disease will have a major effect on the volume of liver remnant needed for adequate function. A healthy liver has a greater regenerative capacity than a cirrhotic liver, functions more efficiently, and tolerates injury better. Patients can survive resection of up to 90% of the liver in the absence of underlying liver disease, but survival after resection beyond

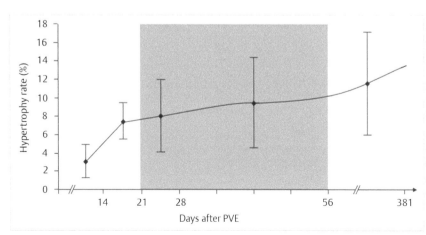

Fig. 19.1 Degree of hypertrophy of the standardized future liver remnant (sFLR) over time after portal vein embolization (PVE) with kinetics of FLR growth, plotted as median degree of hypertrophy after PVE (with interquartile ranges). The shaded zone, days 22 through 56 after PVE, represents the "plateau" period during which the degree of hypertrophy did not change significantly between measurement points. (Reproduced with permission of Ribero et al 2007.[10])

60% of the functional parenchyma in patients with cirrhosis is unlikely.[16] Second, liver volume is directly correlated with a patient's size (larger patients require larger liver remnants); hence, standardizing the anticipated liver volume to a patient's size results in a more accurate assessment of the FLR.[7,22] Third, the extent and complexity of the planned resection and the possibility that associated nonhepatic surgery will be performed at the time of liver resection (e.g., hepatectomy plus pancreaticoduodenectomy) must be considered. These three factors are considered in the setting of the patient's age and comorbidities (e.g., diabetes) that may affect hypertrophy. Thus, once the procedure type and extent of resection necessary to treat the patient have been determined, appropriate liver volumetry is performed so that the standardized FLR (sFLR) volume

expressed as a percentage of the estimated total liver volume (TLV) can be used to determine the need for PVE.

Candidates for PVE include patients with primary or metastatic liver disease who would be hepatic resection candidates but for the following factors:

- Healthy underlying liver and an sFLR less than 20%.[10,16,23]
- Cirrhosis and/or advanced fibrosis and an sFLR less than 40%.[1,24]
- Undergoing extensive chemotherapy and with an sFLR less than 30%.[25]

PVE is an adjunctive procedure to major hepatectomy (▶ Fig. 19.2). Hence, contraindications to PVE mirror those of hepatectomy. Severe portal hypertension precluding surgery is

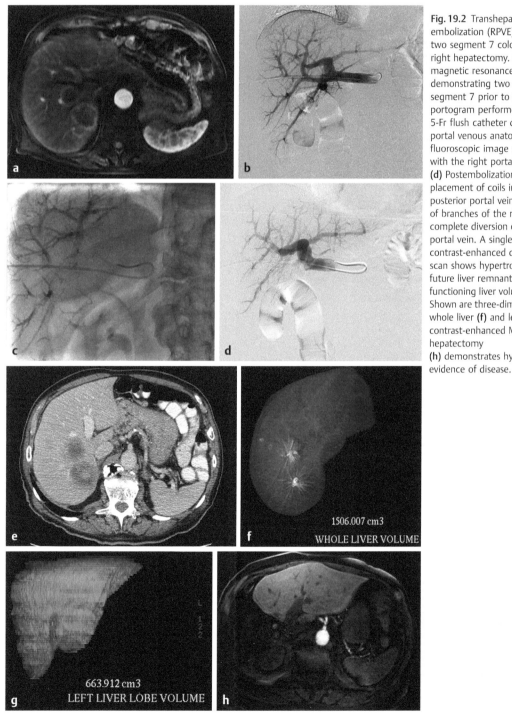

Fig. 19.2 Transhepatic ipsilateral right portal vein embolization (RPVE) in an 87-year-old man with two segment 7 colorectal metastases prior to right hepatectomy. **(a)** Axial contrast-enhanced magnetic resonance imaging (MRI) demonstrating two colorectal metastases in segment 7 prior to RPVE. **(b)** Pre-embolization portogram performed through a 5-Fr flush catheter demonstrates conventional portal venous anatomy. **(c)** Intra-procedural fluoroscopic image showing stasis of contrast with the right portal venous system. **(d)** Postembolization portogram after the placement of coils in the right anterior and right posterior portal veins shows complete occlusion of branches of the right portal vein with complete diversion of blood flow though the left portal vein. A single image **(e)** from post-PVE contrast-enhanced computed tomography (CT) scan shows hypertrophy of the left liver. The future liver remnant (FLR)/total estimated functioning liver volume (TELV) increased to 43%. Shown are three-dimensional reformations of the whole liver **(f)** and left liver **(g)** volumes. Axial contrast-enhanced MRI status post right hepatectomy **(h)** demonstrates hypertrophic left liver with no evidence of disease.

1506.007 cm3
WHOLE LIVER VOLUME

663.912 cm3
LEFT LIVER LOBE VOLUME

the only absolute contraindication to PVE. Also, for cases in which tumor obstructs the portal system in the liver to be resected, PVE is not necessary as portal flow is already redirected to the FLR.[16,26,27] Relative contraindications include uncorrectable coagulopathy, renal failure, and extrahepatic metastasis. The introduction of two-stage hepatectomy has expanded the population of patients with bilobar hepatic disease burden who are eligible for PVE and potential curative resection; however, diffuse hepatic disease burden remains a contraindication to PVE.

19.2.2 Outcomes

PVE is indicated in patients with healthy underlying liver and sFLR less than 20%. Multiple studies have demonstrated that hepatectomy in a setting of sFLR less than 20% is associated with increased postoperative complications.[10,16,23] A study of 112 patients by Ribero et al[10] demonstrated that sFLR less than 20% and degree of sFLR hypertrophy after PVE less than 5% predicted a poor outcome after resection (▶ Fig. 19.3).[10] Kishi et al[23] found that in a series of 301 consecutive patients who underwent extended right hepatectomy, those with a preoperative sFLR less than 20% had significantly higher rates of postoperative liver insufficiency and death from liver failure compared with patients with sFLR greater than 20% ($p < 0.05$). In addition, patients who underwent PVE before surgery to increase their sFLR from less than 20 to greater than 20% had statistically equivalent rates of liver insufficiency as patients with sFLR greater than 20% at baseline (▶ Fig. 19.4).[23] This study confirmed the association between an sFLR threshold less than 20% and increased perioperative complications, as well as the beneficial role of PVE in reducing perioperative complication rates in those patients who undergo liver hypertrophy to an sFLR greater than 20%.

Liver regeneration occurs at a reduced rate and capacity in diseased livers, an observation directly correlated with clinical outcomes. Patients with cirrhosis with marginal liver remnants are not only at high risk for complications but also at increased risk for death from liver failure.[1] As such, the recommended

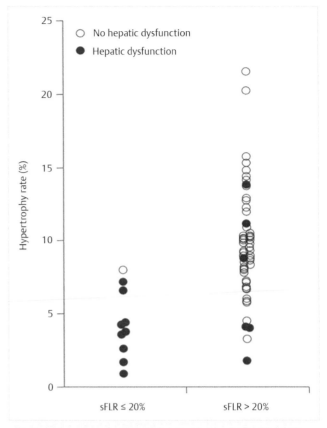

Fig. 19.3 Presence of hepatic dysfunction by standardized future liver remnant (sFLR) volume and degree of hypertrophy. (Reproduced with permission of Ribero et al 2007.[10])

sFLR cutoff in the setting of cirrhosis is 40%, higher than the 20% sFLR cutoff recommended in the setting of healthy underlying liver parenchyma.[6,28,29] In patients with chronic liver disease, hepatectomy outcomes, including the number and severity of complications and the incidence of postoperative liver failure and death, are better with PVE than without.[24,30,31] Azoulay

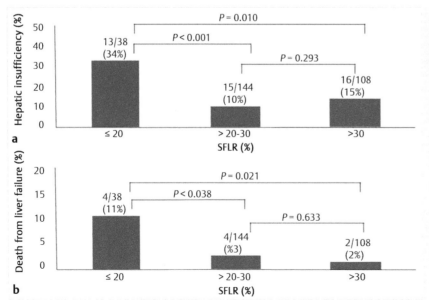

Fig. 19.4 Rates of **(a)** hepatic insufficiency and **(b)** death by preoperative standardized future liver remnant (sFLR) volume. (Adapted from Kishi et al 2009.[23])

et al[30] reported long-term outcomes after resection of ≥ 3 liver segments for hepatocellular carcinoma (HCC) in patients with cirrhosis. PVE was performed when the FLR volume was predicted to be less than 40%, and this procedure led to significant increases in FLR volumes for all embolized patients, correlating with a reduced incidence of liver failure and death without differences in disease-free survival rates. Tanaka et al[31] similarly reported several benefits of PVE in a larger study of patients with HCC and cirrhosis. Disease-free survival rates were similar between patients treated with PVE and those not treated with PVE, but cumulative survival rates were significantly higher in the PVE group than in the non-PVE group. In addition, patients with recurrence after PVE plus resection were more often candidates for further treatments such as TAE, an additional benefit of PVE in the long term. However, the complications of PVE are higher in patients with chronic liver disease than in those with an otherwise healthy liver because of an increased risk of secondary portal vein thrombosis, presumably from slow flow in the portal vein trunk after PVE.[32,33]

In patients with chronic liver disease such as chronic hepatitis, fibrosis, or cirrhosis, the increase in nonembolized liver volumes after PVE varies (range: 28–46%), and hypertrophy after PVE may take greater than 4 weeks because of slower regeneration rates.[34,35] The degree of parenchymal fibrosis is thought to limit regeneration, possibly as a result of reduced portal blood flow.[33] Hence, treatment strategies combining transarterial therapy with PVE are particularly useful in cirrhotic populations to maximize potential liver regeneration and prevent disease progression, as discussed in more detail below.

19.2.3 Role of PVE in Conjunction with Transarterial Therapies

PVE can be combined with other interventional radiology techniques such as TAE (▶ Fig. 19.5) in patients who are not anticipated to have sufficient hypertrophy after PVE alone.[36,37] The mechanism of TAE is complementary, as a component of inflammation and necrosis is added to the apoptosis-mediated cell death induced by PVE to stimulate liver hypertrophy. Nagino et al[37] first described the use of TAE to improve FLR volume in two patients with cholangiocarcinoma who demonstrated inadequate hypertrophy after PVE. In both patients, PVE in the setting of underlying liver disease led to negligible hypertrophy of the FLR. After interval TAE, the FLR volume demonstrated an adequate increase, and both patients underwent successful curative resection. With combination therapies, both arterial and portal venous hepatic supplies are embolized, placing patients at greater risk for liver necrosis. In Nagino et al's original report, only half of the target segments were treated because of the potential risk of hepatic infarction.

TAE is now more commonly performed as a staged procedure before PVE, with an interval of 2 to 3 weeks between the procedures to help prevent hepatic infarction. TAE followed by PVE has been advocated in the setting of cirrhosis complicated by HCC. In this patient population, the rationale for performing TAE before PVE includes preventing tumor progression after PVE, reducing arterioportal shunts that may limit the effectiveness of the subsequent PVE, and boosting the regenerative stimulus in chronically diseased livers.[38,39] Using this regimen, Aoki et al[38] demonstrated increased profound tumor necrosis

without substantial injury to the noncancerous liver in patients with large HCC and chronically injured livers. Similarly, Ogata et al[39] found an increased incidence of complete tumor necrosis (83 vs. 6%; $p < 0.001$) and increased 5-year disease-free survival rate (37 vs. 19%; $p = 0.041$) in patients who underwent transcatheter arterial chemoembolization and PVE versus PVE alone.

With all combination of TAE and PVE regimens, special care must be taken to reduce the risk of hepatic necrosis; this should include staging the procedures at least 2 to 3 weeks apart. Embolization should not be carried out to complete stasis, and the use of nonparticulate embolic agents such as chemoembolization should be favored over particulate agents. After embolization, the interventional radiologist should confirm patency of the hepatic artery supplying the targeted liver segment to avoid occlusion of arterial and portal hepatopetal flow and the potential of parenchymal necrosis.

19.2.4 Role of Concurrent Chemotherapy

PVE has been reported to accelerate tumor growth for both primary and metastatic liver tumors.[40,41,42,43] Progression of disease after PVE may preclude curative intent surgery; in two-stage hepatectomy series, 20% dropout rates due to progression of disease after first-stage resection have been reported.[44,45] Neoadjuvant chemotherapy can be administered to provide tumor control in the interim between PVE and resection; however, concerns have been raised regarding its potential deleterious effects on liver function. Two separate studies have demonstrated an association between chemotherapy agents and sinusoidal dilation and steatohepatitis.[46,47] Given these findings, Shindoh et al[25] performed a retrospective analysis of 194 patients with colorectal liver metastasis to determine the optimal FLR in patients treated with neoadjuvant chemotherapy. The authors found that both long duration of chemotherapy (defined as > 12 weeks) and sFLR ≤ 30% were predictors of hepatic insufficiency (odds ratio [OR] = 5.4; $p = 0.004$; OR = 6.3; $p = 0.019$, respectively; ▶ Fig. 19.6).[25] No cases of postoperative mortality and only two cases of postoperative hepatic insufficiency were reported when the sFLR is greater than 30%, indicating that an sFLR greater than 30% may be a more appropriate cutoff value in patients who have received neoadjuvant chemotherapy, particularly if the duration of treatment is greater than 12 weeks.

The effect of systemic neoadjuvant chemotherapy on liver hypertrophy after PVE has also been addressed by several studies.[48,49,50] Zorzi et al[50] reviewed FLR hypertrophy after PVE in patients with colorectal liver metastases who underwent PVE either with concomitant neoadjuvant chemotherapy ($n = 43$) or without chemotherapy ($n = 22$) before resection. Patients treated with chemotherapy and those not treated with chemotherapy demonstrated similar rates of hypertrophy at 4 weeks after PVE. Covey et al[48] also reported on patients with colorectal liver metastases who underwent PVE either with ($n = 47$) or without ($n = 53$) neoadjuvant chemotherapy and found no significant difference between the groups in the median contralateral liver growth after PVE.

Several studies have examined the effect of chemotherapy on disease progression after PVE performed before hepatectomy.[51,52,53,54] Spelt et al[54] found that the rate of tumor

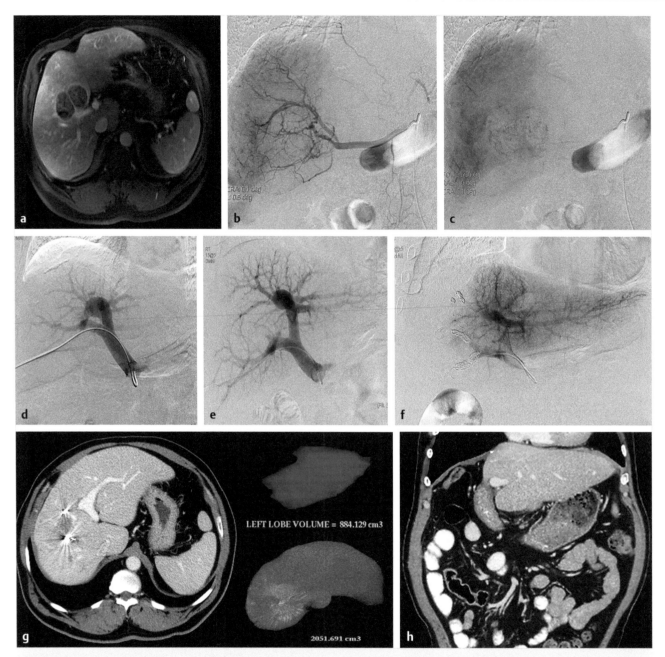

Fig. 19.5 Sequential transcatheter arterial embolization (TAE) followed approximately 1 month later by right portal vein embolization (RPVE) extended to segment 4 prior to extended right hepatectomy in a 69-year-old man with hepatitis C cirrhosis and two adjacent foci of hepatocellular carcinoma spanning up to 7 cm in segments 4, 5, and 8. **(a)** Axial contrast-enhanced magnetic resonance imaging (MRI) demonstrating two foci of hepatocellular carcinoma prior to therapy. **(b)** Early- and **(c)** late-phase hepatic arteriography demonstrating subtle tumor blush corresponding to tumors in segments 4 and 5. Postembolization arteriogram shows successfully the tumor embolized to stasis with 100- to 300-μm tris-acryl microspheres. **(d)** Anteroposterior and **(e)** craniocaudal pre-embolization portography (after TAE) shows conventional portal anatomy. **(f)** Postembolization portogram shows complete occlusion of branches of the right portal vein. The left portal vein remains patent. **(g)** A single image from post-PVE contrast-enhanced computed tomography (CT) scan shows hypertrophy of the left liver. The future liver remnant (FLR)/total estimated functioning liver volume (TELV) increased to 43%. **(h)** Coronal contrast-enhanced CT status post extended right hepatectomy demonstrates hypertrophic left liver.

progression in patients who underwent PVE was low when concomitant chemotherapy was administered; this low rate was seen when the interval between completion of chemotherapy and PVE was short. Fischer et al[51] reported on a series of 64 consecutive patients who underwent PVE, including 25 patients who received chemotherapy and 39 who did not, in preparation for extended right hepatic resection. Although there was no statistical difference between the two groups in the proportion of patients who ultimately underwent hepatic resection, the chemotherapy group had a statistically lower rate of progression by Response Evaluation Criteria in Solid Tumors (RECIST) criteria (18.9 vs. 34.2%; $p = 0.03$). Of greater importance, patients who

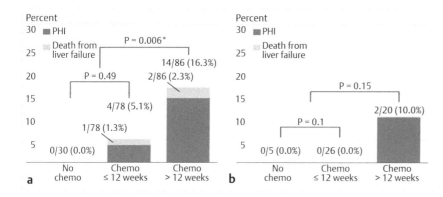

Fig. 19.6 Postoperative liver insufficiency and mortality from liver failure in patients who underwent extended right hepatectomy in the setting of colorectal metastases, stratified by no chemotherapy, chemotherapy, or long-term (>12 week) chemotherapy. **(a)** Image depicts standardized future liver remnant (sFLR) greater than 20% cutoff for resection eligibility. **(b)** Image depicts sFLR > 30% cutoff for resection eligibility. (Reproduced with permission of Shindoh et al 2013.[25])

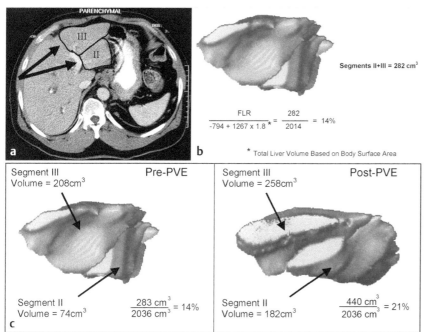

Fig. 19.7 Hypertrophy of the future liver remnant (FLR) after portal vein embolization (PVE) as determined by three-dimensional reconstruction of computed tomography (CT) images. **(a)** Three-dimensional volumetric measurements are determined by outlining the hepatic segmental contours and then calculating the volumes from the surface measurements of each slice. **(b)** The formula for calculating total liver volume is based on the patient's body surface area. **(c)** Before embolization, the volume of segments 2 and 3 was 283 cm³, or 14% of the total liver volume (2,036 cm³). After embolization, the volume of segments 2 and 3 was 440 cm³, or 21% of the total liver volume (an increase of 7%). (Image in **(b)** reproduced with permission of Vauthey et al 2002[20]; image in **(c)** reproduced with permission of Vauthey et al 2000.[7])

received chemotherapy demonstrated a clear survival benefit versus those who did not (5-year survival; 49 vs. 24%; $p = 0.006$) in both the surgical resection and nonsurgical cohorts.

In summary, PVE is likely associated with accelerated tumor growth. Administration of neoadjuvant chemotherapy is helpful in lowering the rate of disease progression and does not interfere with liver regeneration. However, when long-term chemotherapy is administered (>12 weeks), an sFLR cutoff of greater than 30% should be considered, given the potential deleterious effects of chemotherapy on native liver function.

19.3 Technical Considerations

19.3.1 FLR Volumetry and Predicting Liver Function after PVE

PVE is indicated when the anticipated FLR is insufficient to support hepatic function in the postoperative period after hepatectomy. Accurate calculation of the FLR is essential for identifying potential hepatectomy candidates who may benefit from PVE. Liver volume is directly correlated with a patient's size, hence normalizing the anticipated liver volume to a patient's size results in a more accurate assessment of the FLR.[7,22] This

principle led to the proposal and clinical validation of an sFLR by Vauthey et al[7] expressed as a ratio of the FLR over the total estimated functioning liver volume (TELV): sFLR = FLR/TELV.

Computed tomography (CT) volumetry is accurate within ±5% of estimating normal liver parenchymal volumes and is the standard for FLR measurement.[7,55] To measure the TELV, Vauthey et al[20] and Ribero[56] derived the following formula by analyzing liver size and body surface area (BSA) in 292 Western adults: TELV = –794.41 + 1267.28 × BSA. This formula was demonstrated by meta-analysis to be accurate in adult patients as compared to similar formulas (▶ Fig. 19.7).[7,20,56] Other methods that have been used to measure TLV include CT volumetry and assessment of body weight. Determining TLV from CT volumetry can be tedious, as measurements of the tumor volume must be performed and excluded from the overall liver volume. Ribero et al[57] verified that CT volumetry was less accurate than BSA for calculating sFLR by identifying a subset of patients for whom CT volumetry underestimated the risk of hepatic insufficiency. However, a more recent study by Leung et al[58] demonstrated that measured volumetrics using CT volumetry with subtraction methods were more closely correlated with outcomes than estimated volumetrics using the BSA method; however, these results were based on cases from a single tertiary center.

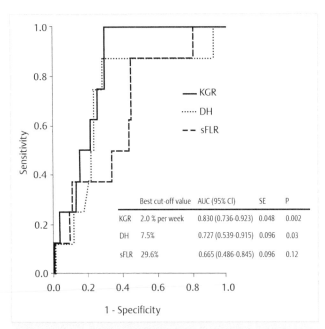

Fig. 19.8 Receiver operating characteristic curves for measured volume parameters in the prediction of postoperative hepatic insufficiency. Area under the curve (AUC) calculated for kinetic growth rate (KGR), degree of hypertrophy (DH), and standardized future liver remnant (sFLR). p-values represent asymptotic significance (null hypothesis; AUC = 0.500). (Adapted from Shindoh et al 2013.[59])

Recent studies have assessed alternative predictors of postoperative liver function in addition to FLR. Through analysis of a series of 107 patients who underwent right PVE and subsequent right hemihepatectomy or extended right hepatectomy, Shindoh et al[59] proposed that the kinetic growth rate (defined as degree of hypertrophy at initial volume assessment divided by number of weeks elapsed after PVE) could be used as a predictor of postoperative complications after hepatectomy. The kinetic growth rate was found to be the most accurate predictor of postoperative hepatic insufficiency and mortality when compared to sFLR or degree of hypertrophy measurements using receiver operating characteristic analysis. Of the three measures, a kinetic growth rate cutoff value of less than 2% per week demonstrated the highest accuracy (81%), with sensitivity of 100% and specificity of 71% in predicting postoperative hepatic insufficiency (▶ Fig. 19.8).[59]

Several groups have begun investigating the effect of PVE on parameters of liver function in addition to liver volumetrics. Malinowski et al[60] evaluated liver function tests (LiMAx) and volumetry before PVE demonstrating an expected correlation with postoperative liver function. Interestingly, a study by Meier et al[61] demonstrated that preoperative PVE positively influenced postoperative liver function independently from changes expected from increased liver volume alone, suggesting that PVE increases not only the postoperative volume but also the functional capacity of the FLR.

19.3.2 Standard Approaches to Portal Vein Embolization

PVE is performed to redirect portal blood flow toward the liver that remains after surgery to promote its hypertrophy before resection of the tumor-bearing liver. To ensure adequate hypertrophy, embolization of the portal branches must be as complete as possible so that recanalization of the occluded portal system is minimized. The entire portal system to be resected must be occluded to avoid the development of intrahepatic portoportal collaterals that may limit regeneration.[62]

PVE is most commonly performed percutaneously using one of two standard approaches: transhepatic portal access is performed via either the FLR (contralateral approach) or the liver to be resected (ipsilateral approach). These approaches are chosen based on operator preference, type of hepatic resection planned, extent of embolization (e.g., right PVE [RPVE] with or without extension to segment 4), and type of embolic agent used.

In the contralateral approach developed by Kinoshita et al,[63] a branch of the left portal system (usually segment 3) is accessed, and the catheter is advanced into the right portal venous system for embolization (▶ Fig. 19.9).[64] The major advantage of this approach is that catheterization of the desired right portal vein branches is more direct via the left system than via the right, making the procedure technically easier. However, the disadvantage of this technique is the risk of injury to the FLR parenchyma and the left portal vein.

In the ipsilateral approach, first described by Nagino et al,[65] a peripheral portal vein branch in the liver to be resected is accessed, and the embolic material is administered through this branch (▶ Fig. 19.10).[66] Because this original ipsilateral approach required the use of specialized catheters, modifications of the technique have been developed to allow for the use of standard angiographic catheters for combined particulate and coil embolization (▶ Fig. 19.11).[26,67,68] When right hepatectomy is planned, RPVE is performed. One advantage of the ipsilateral approach is that the anticipated liver remnant is not instrumented. However, catheterization of the right portal vein branches may be more difficult because of severe angulations between right portal branches, necessitating the use of reverse-curve catheters. Another potential disadvantage of this approach is that some embolic material may be displaced upon catheter removal.

The ipsilateral approach also allows operators to more readily perform segment 4 embolization without the sharp angulations encountered when trying to cannulate segment 4 from a contralateral approach. When two-stage or extended right hepatectomy is planned, RPVE is extended to segment 4 (RPVE + 4; ▶ Fig. 19.12). Ipsilateral RPVE ± 4 is performed after a 5- or 6-Fr sheath is placed into a distal right portal vein branch. When RPVE + 4 is needed, segment 4 embolization is performed first so that the catheters are not manipulated through previously embolized segments. A microcatheter is advanced coaxially through an angled catheter into the portal vein branches in segment 4 so that particulate embolics followed by coils can be delivered. Once segment 4 embolization is completed, a reverse-curve catheter is often needed for RPVE. After complete occlusion of the right portal vein is achieved, embolization of the access tract is performed with coils and/or Gelfoam to reduce the risk of perihepatic hemorrhage at the puncture site.

Published complication rates for the contralateral and ipsilateral approaches are relatively similar. Di Stefano et al[32] reported on 188 patients who underwent contralateral approach PVE and found a 12.8% adverse event rate and only 1 major

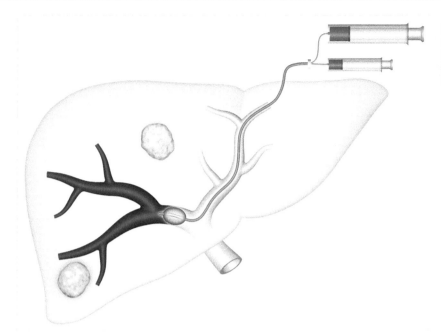

Fig. 19.9 Schematic representation of the contralateral approach. An occlusion balloon catheter is placed from the left lobe into the right portal branch, with delivery of the embolic agent in the antegrade direction.

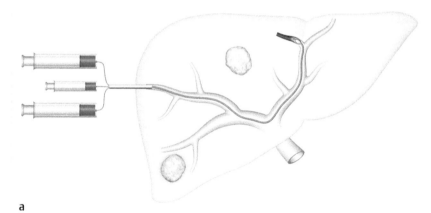

a

Fig. 19.10 Schematic representation of the ipsilateral approach for right portal vein embolization (RPVE) + 4 as described by Nagino et al.[66] Different portions of the balloon catheter are used **(a)** for antegrade embolization of segment 4 veins and **(b)** for retrograde delivery of the embolic agent into the right portal system.

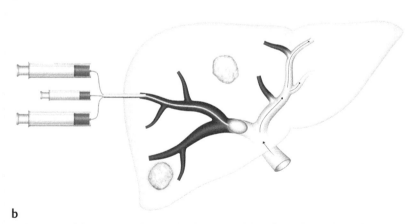

b

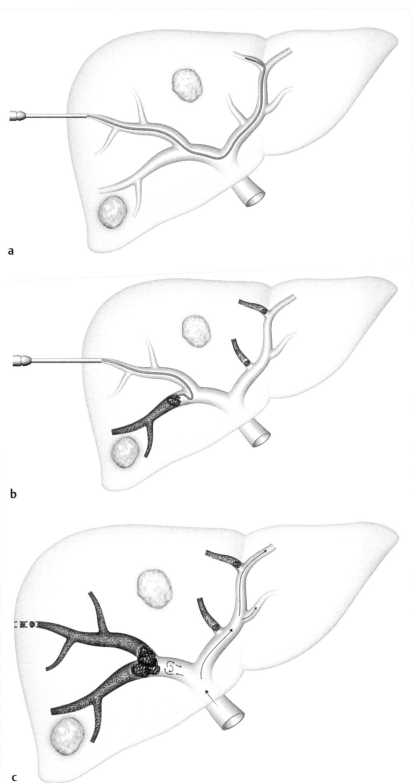

Fig. 19.11 Schematic representation shows modification of the ipsilateral technique for right portal vein embolization (RPVE) + 4. **(a)** Placement of a 6-Fr vascular sheath into the right portal branch. An angled 5-Fr catheter is placed into the left portal system with coaxial placement of a microcatheter into a segment 4 branch. Particulate embolization is performed, followed by placement of coils, until all of the branches are occluded. **(b)** After segment 4 is completely occluded, a 5-Fr reverse-curve catheter is used for RPVE. **(c)** After PVE is complete, the access tract is embolized with coils and/or Gelfoam to prevent subcapsular hemorrhage.

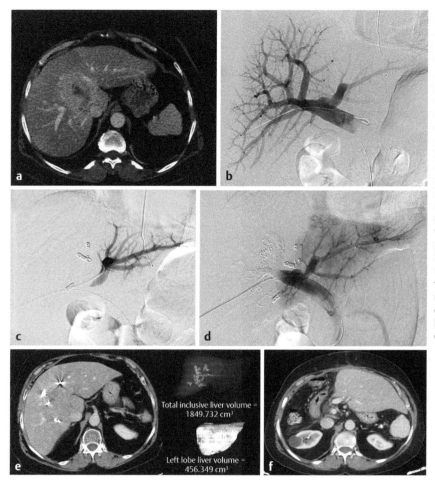

Fig. 19.12 Transhepatic ipsilateral right portal vein embolization (PVE) extended to segment 4 using tris-acryl particles and coils performed in a 74-year-old woman with a 6.2-cm cholangiocarcinoma involving segments 1, 4, 7, and 8. **(a)** Axial contrast-enhanced computed tomography (CT) image of the liver shows the mass with peripheral hyperenhancement. **(b)** Pre-embolization portogram demonstrates patent conventional portal venous anatomy. **(c)** Intraprocedural left portogram after particle and coil embolization of segment 4 branches shows patency of the segment 2 and 3 portal veins. **(d)** Postembolization portogram shows complete occlusion of branches of the right portal vein extended to segment 4. The left lateral portal vein remains patent. **(e)** A single image from post-PVE contrast-enhanced CT scan shows hypertrophy of the left liver. The future liver remnant (FLR)/total estimated functioning liver volume (TELV) increased to 25%. **(f)** Axial magnetic resonance imaging (MRI) status post extended right hepatectomy demonstrates hypertrophic left liver with no evidence of disease.

complication (complete portal vein thrombosis) directly related to the contralateral approach that precluded surgery. Ribero et al[10] reported on 112 patients who underwent ipsilateral approach PVE and found an 8.9% adverse event rate. Accounting for the fact that Di Stefano et al[32] included clinically occult CT findings when calculating the complication rate, the rates are comparable between the two studies. Kodama et al[69] directly compared complication rates for contralateral ($n = 11$) and ipsilateral ($n = 36$) approaches in a series of 47 patients who underwent PVE. Contralateral approach PVE was associated with an 18.1% complication rate versus 13.9% for ipsilateral PVE. Although this difference did not reach statistical significance, the authors recommended the use of the ipsilateral approach because of the potential for injury to the FLR with the contralateral approach.

PVE can also be performed via a transileocolic venous approach during laparotomy by direct cannulation of the ileocolic vein and advancement of a balloon catheter into the portal vein for embolization.[12] This approach is not commonly used in current practice as improvements in experience, imaging equipment, catheter systems, and embolic agents have led to greater use of minimally invasive transhepatic approaches. The transileocolic venous approach necessitates the use of general anesthesia and laparotomy and is typically only performed when an interventional radiology suite is not available, a percutaneous approach is not considered feasible, or additional treatment is needed during the same surgical exploration.[70,71]

19.3.3 Extent of Embolization

Several studies recommend extending RPVE to include segment 4 before performing extended right hepatectomy.[37,72,73,74] In a multicenter survey of surgical preferences for FLR augmentation methods, institutions with the capability to perform RPVE + 4 had significantly higher ratings for both likelihood of technical success and likelihood of subsequent hypertrophy compared to institutions without this capability.[75] Possible benefits include improved hypertrophy of segments 2 and 3, embolization of the entire tumor-bearing liver, and reduction of potentially challenging surgical resections in the setting of segment 4 hypertrophy.[72,73] Kishi et al[73] compared patients who underwent RPVE ($n = 15$) versus those who underwent RPVE + 4 ($n = 58$) and observed significant increases in both the absolute volume and hypertrophy rate of segments 2 and 3 in the RPVE + 4 groups. The complication rates were similar for RPVE and RPVE + 4 groups (7 vs. 10%; $p > 0.99$), and no PVE complications precluded resection. Mise et al[72] reported on the clinical utility of RPVE + 4 performed during two-stage hepatectomy and found that the dynamics of liver regeneration of segments 2 and 3 were impaired with RPVE alone but not with RPVE + 4 after the first stage of resection.

The drawback to performing RPVE + 4 is that catheter manipulation into branches feeding segment 4 is more technically demanding, and inadvertent reflux of embolic material to the FLR has been reported.[76,77] In addition, a study by Capussotti et al[76] evaluated 26 patients who underwent RPVE (n = 13) or RPVE + 4 (n = 13) and found no difference between the groups in volume increase (p = 0.20) or rate of increase (p = 0.40) of segments 2 and 3.

19.3.4 Embolic Material

A wide range of materials and devices have been used for embolization of the portal system, including but not limited to spherical particles, coils, polyvinyl alcohol (PVA) particles, Gelfoam, fibrin glue, N-butyl cyanoacrylate glue (NBCA), sodium tetradecyl sulfate foam, lipiodol, and Amplatzer plugs.[67,78,79,80,81] Ideal agents should be safe, easy to control, well tolerated, and cost effective, and should result in reproducible, sustained, substantial hypertrophy of the FLR.[78] Currently, the two most commonly discussed agents are NBCA and microspheres in combination with coils.

Multiple studies have demonstrated the safety and efficacy of small particle embolization of the liver with both PVA particles and microspheres.[67,82] After catheterization of the portal system, embolization of distal small veins is performed with 100- to 300-µm particles. More proximal veins are embolized with larger particles with a goal of stasis or near stasis. Coils are placed behind the particles to prevent particle dislodgement and recanalization, thus improving hypertrophy of the FLR. Research by Geisel et al[83,84] demonstrated superior FLR hypertrophy with the use of coils and plugs in combination with particles versus the use of particles alone (44 vs. 25.7%; p < 0.001); this improvement in hypertrophy was later shown to be significantly associated with decreased postoperative liver failure rates. In this series, the use of PVA particles plus coils was associated with decreased recanalization rates, suggesting that permanent occlusive agents may be superior to temporary or absorbable occlusive agents in promoting hypertrophy. Relative increased liver hypertrophy with the use of permanent versus absorbable portal venous embolic agents has also been demonstrated in an animal model.[85]

Similarly, the permanent agent NBCA has been shown to produce portal venous occlusion for more than 4 weeks and to induce a larger FLR when compared with coils and gelatin sponge.[64,79,86] NBCA induces an inflammatory reaction resulting in peribiliary fibrosis, with associated rates of liver regeneration believed to be as good as or better than the rates seen with other embolic agents.[64] However, NBCA preparation and administration require advanced knowledge and experience, and the inflammatory reaction sometimes renders surgical resection more difficult.[79,87] NBCA is mixed with lipiodol at a ratio of 1:1–2 and is delivered from second- or third-order portal branches to prevent nontarget embolization. Straight catheters are preferred by some operators to prevent gluing of catheters into the liver. Great care must be taken to prevent embolization of NBCA to nontarget areas; as such, NBCA is routinely administered through a contralateral approach, and embolization is not routinely extended to segment 4 when this agent is used.

19.3.5 Complications

Complications of PVE are similar to those of other image-guided transhepatic procedures and include subscapular hematoma, hemoperitoneum, hemobilia, abscess formation, cholangitis and sepsis, arterioportal shunts, arterioportal fistula, and pneumothorax. In addition, PVE-specific complications include nontarget embolization, recanalization of embolized segments, and extension of portal vein thrombosis to involve the left or main branches.[88] In 2010, the Society of Interventional Radiology established quality improvement guidelines for transcatheter embolization, including a suggested threshold for PVE-related major complications of 6% and a morbidity rate of 11%.[89] Most published complication rates fall well below this range.[87] Abulkhir et al[4] published a meta-analysis of 1,088 PVE cases pooled from 37 studies performed from 1990 to 2005 and reported pooled procedure-related morbidity and mortality rates of 2.2 and 0%, respectively. In this analysis, percutaneous PVE was performed in most cases (72%); the remaining cases were performed via the transileocolic technique.

19.4 Future Prospects

Despite PVE's proven clinical benefits in a large proportion of patients, there are still hepatic resection candidates who undergo PVE but cannot undergo surgery because of either inadequate liver hypertrophy or disease progression during the waiting period after PVE. Augmenting PVE with agents to promote hypertrophy can help overcome these limitations. In keeping with this hypothesis, am Esch et al[90] investigated the co-treatment of patients with PVE and bone marrow–derived stem cells (PVE + SC; n = 11) versus PVE alone (PVE; n = 11) in a series of patients undergoing extended right hepatectomy. The mean hepatic growth of segments 2 and 3 was significantly higher in the PVE + SC group as compared to the PVE group (138.7 ± 66.3 vs. 63.0 mL ± 40.0; p = 0.004) after a waiting period of only 14 days. In this investigation, PVE was performed using a surgical transileocolic approach; a subsequent animal (porcine model) study by Avritscher et al[91] demonstrated the ability to administer mesenchymal SCs using percutaneous endovascular approaches. Using an alternative method of PVE augmentation, Beppu et al[92] prospectively evaluated whether adding branched amino acids to patients' diets would affect functional liver regeneration (as measured by serum albumin scintigraphy) after PVE. Branched chain amino acid diet supplementation was found to improve functional liver regeneration in patients undergoing PVE followed by major resection, as evidenced by ultimately increased liver uptake values 6 months after resection (266.7 vs. 77.6%; p = 0.04). Overall, the augmentation of PVE with these techniques is a promising area of future research and may improve upon the already well-established efficacy of PVE.

19.5 Conclusion

PVE is well established as an invaluable adjunctive procedure to increase candidacy for and the safety of major hepatic resections. Numerous studies have validated PVE's clinical utility in surgical hepatic resection candidates with limited anticipated FLRs. Low associated complication rates in combination with high efficacy in promoting hypertrophy of the FLR have propelled the increased use of PVE and its incorporation into standard of care paradigms. Over the past decade, research has demonstrated the appropriate use of PVE in addition to TAE and chemotherapy in the increasingly complex multidisciplinary clinical scenarios needed to deliver state-of-the-art cancer care. Percutaneous ipsilateral and contralateral approaches using a variety of occlusive embolic agents for PVE are well established. The ipsilateral technique allows for technically easier embolization of segment 4, which is now a well-accepted practice in the setting of either extended or two-stage hepatectomy. An exciting area of future research is the augmentation of the regenerative potential of PVE with SCs or medications. PVE remains an important aspect of oncologic care, in large part because of the substantial foundation of information available demonstrating its clear clinical benefit for hepatic resection candidates with small anticipated FLRs.

References

[1] Shirabe K, Shimada M, Gion T, et al. Postoperative liver failure after major hepatic resection for hepatocellular carcinoma in the modern era with special reference to remnant liver volume. J Am Coll Surg. 1999; 188(3):304–309

[2] Tsao JI, Loftus JP, Nagorney DM, Adson MA, Ilstrup DM. Trends in morbidity and mortality of hepatic resection for malignancy. A matched comparative analysis. Ann Surg. 1994; 220(2):199–205

[3] Aloia TA. Associating liver partition and portal vein ligation for staged hepatectomy: portal vein embolization should remain the gold standard. JAMA Surg. 2015; 150(10):927–928

[4] Abulkhir A, Limongelli P, Healey AJ, et al. Preoperative portal vein embolization for major liver resection: a meta-analysis. Ann Surg. 2008; 247 (1):49–57

[5] Madoff DC, Abdalla EK, Vauthey JN. Portal vein embolization in preparation for major hepatic resection: evolution of a new standard of care. J Vasc Interv Radiol. 2005; 16(6):779–790

[6] May BJ, Talenfeld AD, Madoff DC. Update on portal vein embolization: evidence-based outcomes, controversies, and novel strategies. J Vasc Interv Radiol. 2013; 24(2):241–254

[7] Vauthey JN, Chaoui A, Do KA, et al. Standardized measurement of the future liver remnant prior to extended liver resection: methodology and clinical associations. Surgery. 2000; 127(5):512–519

[8] Black DM, Behrns KE. A scientist revisits the atrophy-hypertrophy complex: hepatic apoptosis and regeneration. Surg Oncol Clin N Am. 2002; 11(4):849–864

[9] Koniaris LG, McKillop IH, Schwartz SI, Zimmers TA. Liver regeneration. J Am Coll Surg. 2003; 197(4):634–659

[10] Ribero D, Abdalla EK, Madoff DC, Donadon M, Loyer EM, Vauthey JN. Portal vein embolization before major hepatectomy and its effects on regeneration, resectability and outcome. Br J Surg. 2007; 94(11):1386–1394

[11] Duncan JR, Hicks ME, Cai SR, Brunt EM, Ponder KP. Embolization of portal vein branches induces hepatocyte replication in swine: a potential step in hepatic gene therapy. Radiology. 1999; 210(2):467–477

[12] Makuuchi M, Thai BL, Takayasu K, et al. Preoperative portal embolization to increase safety of major hepatectomy for hilar bile duct carcinoma: a preliminary report. Surgery. 1990; 107(5):521–527

[13] Guiu B, Chevallier P, Denys A, et al. Simultaneous trans-hepatic portal and hepatic vein embolization before major hepatectomy: the liver venous deprivation technique. Eur Radiol. 2016; 26(12):4259–4267

[14] Pandanaboyana S, Bell R, Hidalgo E, et al. A systematic review and meta-analysis of portal vein ligation versus portal vein embolization for elective liver resection. Surgery. 2015; 157(4):690–698

[15] Matsuo K, Murakami T, Kawaguchi D, et al. Histologic features after surgery associating liver partition and portal vein ligation for staged hepatectomy versus those after hepatectomy with portal vein embolization. Surgery. 2016; 159(5):1289–1298

[16] Abdalla EK, Barnett CC, Doherty D, Curley SA, Vauthey JN. Extended hepatectomy in patients with hepatobiliary malignancies with and without preoperative portal vein embolization. Arch Surg. 2002; 137(6):675–680, discussion 680–681

[17] Azoulay D, Castaing D, Smail A, et al. Resection of nonresectable liver metastases from colorectal cancer after percutaneous portal vein embolization. Ann Surg. 2000; 231(4):480–486

[18] de Baere T, Roche A, Vavasseur D, et al. Portal vein embolization: utility for inducing left hepatic lobe hypertrophy before surgery. Radiology. 1993; 188 (1):73–77

[19] Kubota K, Makuuchi M, Kusaka K, et al. Measurement of liver volume and hepatic functional reserve as a guide to decision-making in resectional surgery for hepatic tumors. Hepatology. 1997; 26(5):1176–1181

[20] Vauthey JN, Abdalla EK, Doherty DA, et al. Body surface area and body weight predict total liver volume in Western adults. Liver Transpl. 2002; 8(3):233–240

[21] Vauthey JN, Pawlik TM, Abdalla EK, et al. Is extended hepatectomy for hepatobiliary malignancy justified? Ann Surg. 2004; 239(5):722–730, discussion 730–732

[22] Johnson TN, Tucker GT, Tanner MS, Rostami-Hodjegan A. Changes in liver volume from birth to adulthood: a meta-analysis. Liver Transpl. 2005; 11 (12):1481–1493

[23] Kishi Y, Abdalla EK, Chun YS, et al. Three hundred and one consecutive extended right hepatectomies: evaluation of outcome based on systematic liver volumetry. Ann Surg. 2009; 250(4):540–548

[24] Farges O, Belghiti J, Kianmanesh R, et al. Portal vein embolization before right hepatectomy: prospective clinical trial. Ann Surg. 2003; 237(2):208–217

[25] Shindoh J, Tzeng CW, Aloia TA, et al. Optimal future liver remnant in patients treated with extensive preoperative chemotherapy for colorectal liver metastases. Ann Surg Oncol. 2013; 20(8):2493–2500

[26] Madoff DC, Hicks ME, Vauthey JN, et al. Transhepatic portal vein embolization: anatomy, indications, and technical considerations. Radiographics. 2002; 22(5):1063–1076

[27] Thakrar PD, Madoff DC. Preoperative portal vein embolization: an approach to improve the safety of major hepatic resection. Semin Roentgenol. 2011; 46 (2):142–153

[28] Benson AB, III, Abrams TA, Ben-Josef E, et al. NCCN clinical practice guidelines in oncology: hepatobiliary cancers. J Natl Compr Canc Netw. 2009; 7(4):350–391

[29] Palavecino M, Chun YS, Madoff DC, et al. Major hepatic resection for hepatocellular carcinoma with or without portal vein embolization: perioperative outcome and survival. Surgery. 2009; 145(4):399–405

[30] Azoulay D, Castaing D, Krissat J, et al. Percutaneous portal vein embolization increases the feasibility and safety of major liver resection for hepatocellular carcinoma in injured liver. Ann Surg. 2000; 232(5):665–672

[31] Tanaka H, Hirohashi K, Kubo S, Shuto T, Higaki I, Kinoshita H. Preoperative portal vein embolization improves prognosis after right hepatectomy for hepatocellular carcinoma in patients with impaired hepatic function. Br J Surg. 2000; 87(7):879–882

[32] Di Stefano DR, de Baere T, Denys A, et al. Preoperative percutaneous portal vein embolization: evaluation of adverse events in 188 patients. Radiology. 2005; 234(2):625–630

[33] Kooby DA, Fong Y, Suriawinata A, et al. Impact of steatosis on perioperative outcome following hepatic resection. J Gastrointest Surg. 2003; 7(8):1034–1044

[34] Nagino M, Nimura Y, Kamiya J, et al. Changes in hepatic lobe volume in biliary tract cancer patients after right portal vein embolization. Hepatology. 1995; 21(2):434–439

[35] Shimamura T, Nakajima Y, Une Y, et al. Efficacy and safety of preoperative percutaneous transhepatic portal embolization with absolute ethanol: a clinical study. Surgery. 1997; 121(2):135–141

[36] Gruttadauria S, Luca A, Mandala' L, Miraglia R, Gridelli B. Sequential preoperative ipsilateral portal and arterial embolization in patients with colorectal liver metastases. World J Surg. 2006; 30(4):576–578

[37] Nagino M, Kanai M, Morioka A, et al. Portal and arterial embolization before extensive liver resection in patients with markedly poor functional reserve. J Vasc Interv Radiol. 2000; 11(8):1063–1068

[38] Aoki T, Imamura H, Hasegawa K, et al. Sequential preoperative arterial and portal venous embolizations in patients with hepatocellular carcinoma. Arch Surg. 2004; 139(7):766–774

[39] Ogata S, Belghiti J, Farges O, Varma D, Sibert A, Vilgrain V. Sequential arterial and portal vein embolizations before right hepatectomy in patients with cirrhosis and hepatocellular carcinoma. Br J Surg. 2006; 93(9):1091–1098

[40] Al-Sharif E, Simoneau E, Hassanain M. Portal vein embolization effect on colorectal cancer liver metastasis progression: lessons learned. World J Clin Oncol. 2015; 6(5):142–146

[41] Elias D, De Baere T, Roche A, Mducreux, Leclere J, Lasser P. During liver regeneration following right portal embolization the growth rate of liver metastases is more rapid than that of the liver parenchyma. Br J Surg. 1999; 86(6):784–788

[42] Kokudo N, Tada K, Seki M, et al. Proliferative activity of intrahepatic colorectal metastases after preoperative hemihepatic portal vein embolization. Hepatology. 2001; 34(2):267–272

[43] Simoneau E, Aljiffry M, Salman A, et al. Portal vein embolization stimulates tumour growth in patients with colorectal cancer liver metastases. HPB (Oxford). 2012; 14(7):461–468

[44] Brouquet A, Abdalla EK, Kopetz S, et al. High survival rate after two-stage resection of advanced colorectal liver metastases: response-based selection and complete resection define outcome. J Clin Oncol. 2011; 29(8):1083–1090

[45] Narita M, Oussoultzoglou E, Jaeck D, et al. Two-stage hepatectomy for multiple bilobar colorectal liver metastases. Br J Surg. 2011; 98(10):1463–1475

[46] Pawlik TM, Olino K, Gleisner AL, Torbenson M, Schulick R, Choti MA. Preoperative chemotherapy for colorectal liver metastases: impact on hepatic histology and postoperative outcome. J Gastrointest Surg. 2007; 11(7):860–868

[47] Vauthey JN, Pawlik TM, Ribero D, et al. Chemotherapy regimen predicts steatohepatitis and an increase in 90-day mortality after surgery for hepatic colorectal metastases. J Clin Oncol. 2006; 24(13):2065–2072

[48] Covey AM, Brown KT, Jarnagin WR, et al. Combined portal vein embolization and neoadjuvant chemotherapy as a treatment strategy for resectable hepatic colorectal metastases. Ann Surg. 2008; 247(3):451–455

[49] Simoneau E, Alanazi R, Alshenaifi J, et al. Neoadjuvant chemotherapy does not impair liver regeneration following hepatectomy or portal vein embolization for colorectal cancer liver metastases. J Surg Oncol. 2016; 113 (4):449–455

[50] Zorzi D, Chun YS, Madoff DC, Abdalla EK, Vauthey JN. Chemotherapy with bevacizumab does not affect liver regeneration after portal vein embolization in the treatment of colorectal liver metastases. Ann Surg Oncol. 2008; 15(10):2765–2772

[51] Fischer C, Melstrom LG, Arnaoutakis D, et al. Chemotherapy after portal vein embolization to protect against tumor growth during liver hypertrophy before hepatectomy. JAMA Surg. 2013; 148(12):1103–1108

[52] Muratore A, Zimmitti G, Ribero D, Mellano A, Viganò L, Capussotti L. Chemotherapy between the first and second stages of a two-stage hepatectomy for colorectal liver metastases: should we routinely recommend it? Ann Surg Oncol. 2012; 19(4):1310–1315

[53] Simoneau E, Hassanain M, Shaheen M, et al. Portal vein embolization and its effect on tumour progression for colorectal cancer liver metastases. Br J Surg. 2015; 102(10):1240–1249

[54] Spelt L, Sparrelid E, Isaksson B, Andersson RG, Sturesson C. Tumour growth after portal vein embolization with pre-procedural chemotherapy for colorectal liver metastases. HPB (Oxford). 2015; 17(6):529–535

[55] Soyer P, Roche A, Elias D, Levesque M. Hepatic metastases from colorectal cancer: influence of hepatic volumetric analysis on surgical decision making. Radiology. 1992; 184(3):695–697

[56] Ribero D, Chun YS, Vauthey JN. Standardized liver volumetry for portal vein embolization. Semin Intervent Radiol. 2008; 25(2):104–109

[57] Ribero D, Amisano M, Bertuzzo F, et al. Measured versus estimated total liver volume to preoperatively assess the adequacy of the future liver remnant: which method should we use? Ann Surg. 2013; 258(5):801–806, discussion 806–807

[58] Leung U, Simpson AL, Araujo RL, et al. Remnant growth rate after portal vein embolization is a good early predictor of post-hepatectomy liver failure. J Am Coll Surg. 2014; 219(4):620–630

[59] Shindoh J, Truty MJ, Aloia TA, et al. Kinetic growth rate after portal vein embolization predicts posthepatectomy outcomes: toward zero liver-related mortality in patients with colorectal liver metastases and small future liver remnant. J Am Coll Surg. 2013; 216(2):201–209

[60] Malinowski M, Lock JF, Seehofer D, et al. Preliminary study on liver function changes after trisectionectomy with versus without prior portal vein embolization. Surg Today. 2016; 46(9):1053–1061

[61] Meier RP, Toso C, Terraz S, et al. Improved liver function after portal vein embolization and an elective right hepatectomy. HPB (Oxford). 2015; 17(11):1009–1018

[62] Denys AL, Abehsera M, Sauvanet A, Sibert A, Belghiti J, Menu Y. Failure of right portal vein ligation to induce left lobe hypertrophy due to intrahepatic portoportal collaterals: successful treatment with portal vein embolization. AJR Am J Roentgenol. 1999; 173(3):633–635

[63] Kinoshita H, Sakai K, Hirohashi K, Igawa S, Yamasaki O, Kubo S. Preoperative portal vein embolization for hepatocellular carcinoma. World J Surg. 1986; 10 (5):803–808

[64] de Baere T, Roche A, Elias D, Lasser P, Lagrange C, Bousson V. Preoperative portal vein embolization for extension of hepatectomy indications. Hepatology. 1996; 24(6):1386–1391

[65] Nagino M, Nimura Y, Kamiya J, Kondo S, Kanai M. Selective percutaneous transhepatic embolization of the portal vein in preparation for extensive liver resection: the ipsilateral approach. Radiology. 1996; 200(2):559–563

[66] Nagino M, Nimura Y, Kamiya J, et al. Right or left trisegment portal vein embolization before hepatic trisegmentectomy for hilar bile duct carcinoma. Surgery. 1995; 117(6):677–681

[67] Madoff DC, Abdalla EK, Gupta S, et al. Transhepatic ipsilateral right portal vein embolization extended to segment IV: improving hypertrophy and resection outcomes with spherical particles and coils. J Vasc Interv Radiol. 2005; 16(2, Pt 1):215–225

[68] Madoff DC, Hicks ME, Abdalla EK, Morris JS, Vauthey JN. Portal vein embolization with polyvinyl alcohol particles and coils in preparation for major liver resection for hepatobiliary malignancy: safety and effectiveness-study in 26 patients. Radiology. 2003; 227(1):251–260

[69] Kodama Y, Shimizu T, Endo H, Miyamoto N, Miyasaka K. Complications of percutaneous transhepatic portal vein embolization. J Vasc Interv Radiol. 2002; 13(12):1233–1237

[70] Azoulay D, Raccuia JS, Castaing D, Bismuth H. Right portal vein embolization in preparation for major hepatic resection. J Am Coll Surg. 1995; 181(3):266–269

[71] Denys A, Madoff DC, Doenz F, et al. Indications for and limitations of portal vein embolization before major hepatic resection for hepatobiliary malignancy. Surg Oncol Clin N Am. 2002; 11(4):955–968

[72] Mise Y, Aloia TA, Conrad C, Huang SY, Wallace MJ, Vauthey JN. Volume regeneration of segments 2 and 3 after right portal vein embolization in patients undergoing two-stage hepatectomy. J Gastrointest Surg. 2015; 19 (1):133–141, discussion 141

[73] Kishi Y, Madoff DC, Abdalla EK, et al. Is embolization of segment 4 portal veins before extended right hepatectomy justified? Surgery. 2008; 144(5):744–751

[74] Mueller L, Hillert C, Möller L, Krupski-Berdien G, Rogiers X, Broering DC. Major hepatectomy for colorectal metastases: is preoperative portal occlusion an oncological risk factor? Ann Surg Oncol. 2008; 15(7):1908–1917

[75] Day RW, Conrad C, Vauthey JN, Aloia TA. Evaluating surgeon attitudes towards the safety and efficacy of portal vein occlusion and associating liver partition and portal vein ligation: a report of the MALINSA survey. HPB (Oxford). 2015; 17(10):936–941

[76] Capussotti L, Muratore A, Ferrero A, Anselmetti GC, Corgnier A, Regge D. Extension of right portal vein embolization to segment IV portal branches. Arch Surg. 2005; 140(11):1100–1103

[77] van Gulik TM, van den Esschert JW, de Graaf W, et al. Controversies in the use of portal vein embolization. Dig Surg. 2008; 25(6):436–444

[78] Madoff DC. Portal vein embolization: the continued search for the ideal embolic agent. J Vasc Interv Radiol. 2014; 25(7):1053–1055

[79] Guiu B, Bize P, Gunthern D, Demartines N, Halkic N, Denys A. Portal vein embolization before right hepatectomy: improved results using n-butyl-cyanoacrylate compared to microparticles plus coils. Cardiovasc Intervent Radiol. 2013; 36(5):1306–1312

[80] Bent CL, Low D, Matson MB, Renfrew I, Fotheringham T. Portal vein embolization using a nitinol plug (Amplatzer vascular plug) in combination with histoacryl glue and iodinized oil: adequate hypertrophy with a reduced risk of nontarget embolization. Cardiovasc Intervent Radiol. 2009; 32(3):471–477

[81] Fischman AM, Ward TJ, Horn JC, et al. Portal vein embolization before right hepatectomy or extended right hepatectomy using sodium tetradecyl sulfate foam: technique and initial results. J Vasc Interv Radiol. 2014; 25(7):1045–1053

[82] Cazejust J, Bessoud B, Le Bail M, Menu Y. Preoperative portal vein embolization with a combination of trisacryl microspheres, gelfoam and coils. Diagn Interv Imaging. 2015; 96(1):57–64

[83] Geisel D, Malinowski M, Powerski MJ, et al. Improved hypertrophy of future remnant liver after portal vein embolization with plugs, coils and particles. Cardiovasc Intervent Radiol. 2013; 96(1):57–64

[84] Malinowski M, Geisel D, Stary V, et al. Portal vein embolization with plug/coils improves hepatectomy outcome. J Surg Res. 2015; 194(1):202–211

[85] van den Esschert JW, van Lienden KP, Alles LK, et al. Liver regeneration after portal vein embolization using absorbable and permanent embolization materials in a rabbit model. Ann Surg. 2012; 255(2):311–318

[86] Matsuoka T, Nakatsuka H, Nakamura K, et al. Long-term embolization of the portal vein with isobutyl-2-cyanoacrylate in hepatoma. Nippon Igaku Hoshasen Gakkai Zasshi. 1986; 46(1):72–74

[87] Denys A, Bize P, Demartines N, Deschamps F, De Baere T, Cardiovascular and Interventional Radiological Society of Europe. Quality improvement for portal vein embolization. Cardiovasc Intervent Radiol. 2010; 33(3):452–456

[88] Yeom YK, Shin JH. Complications of portal vein embolization: evaluation on cross-sectional imaging. Korean J Radiol. 2015; 16(5):1079–1085

[89] Angle JF, Siddiqi NH, Wallace MJ, et al. Society of Interventional Radiology Standards of Practice Committee. Quality improvement guidelines for percutaneous transcatheter embolization: Society of Interventional Radiology Standards of Practice Committee. J Vasc Interv Radiol. 2010; 21 (10):1479–1486

[90] am Esch JS, Schmelzle M, Fürst G, et al. Infusion of CD133 + bone marrow-derived stem cells after selective portal vein embolization enhances functional hepatic reserves after extended right hepatectomy: a retrospective single-center study. Ann Surg. 2012; 255(1):79–85

[91] Avritscher R, Abdelsalam ME, Javadi S, et al. Percutaneous intraportal application of adipose tissue-derived mesenchymal stem cells using a balloon occlusion catheter in a porcine model of liver fibrosis. J Vasc Interv Radiol. 2013; 24(12):1871–1878

[92] Beppu T, Nitta H, Hayashi H, et al. Effect of branched-chain amino acid supplementation on functional liver regeneration in patients undergoing portal vein embolization and sequential hepatectomy: a randomized controlled trial. J Gastroenterol. 2015; 50(12):1197–1205

20 Ablation of Malignant Liver Tumors

Ronald S. Arellano

20.1 Introduction

Over the past 15 years, image-guided tumor ablation has evolved to become a well-established therapeutic option for the treatment of liver tumors.[1,2,3,4,5,6] Thermal ablation offers several distinct advantages over surgical resection including decreased morbidity and mortality, the ability to perform ablations as an outpatient procedure with lower costs, and the potential to offer treatment to patients who might otherwise be poor surgical candidates. Currently available ablation techniques include radiofrequency ablation (RFA), microwave ablation (MWA), cryoablation, and irreversible electroporation (IRE; ▶ Table 20.1). Although each modality has its own unique properties, they all share the common goal of generating necrotic tissue through the use of minimally invasive techniques.[7,8,9] This chapter will describe the currently available ablation techniques and their role in the treatment of liver tumors.

20.2 Ablation Types

20.2.1 Radiofrequency Ablation

RFA is probably the most studied of the thermal ablation techniques. RFA induces tissue coagulative necrosis via delivery of electromagnetic energy to the patient. This is achieved by placing the patient within a closed-loop electrical circuit that incorporates an RF generator, an electrode applicator, and dispersive electrodes in the form of grounding pads that are placed on the patient. Within this closed-loop circuit, the RF generator creates a high-frequency alternating electrical field within the patient, and high electrical resistance within the tissues leads to ionic agitation as the ions within tissues attempt to align in the direction of the alternating electrical current. This ionic agitation results in friction, which in turn generates heat around the RF electrodes. In most instances, the heat that is generated exceeds 100 °C, which leads to coagulative necrosis (▶ Fig. 20.1).[10,11] RF electrode designs range from straight, nondeployable internally cooled electrodes to expandable electrodes. Similarly, treatment algorithms vary among manufacturers, but all have the common feature of achieving tissue necrosis through the application of electromagnetic energy.

20.2.2 Microwave Ablation

MWA (▶ Fig. 20.2; ▶ Fig. 20.3) also uses electromagnetic energy to achieve tissue destruction. With MWA, needles that are inserted into the patient act as antennas that receive electromagnetic energy in the range of 900 to 2,450 MHz.[12] In contrast to RF-induced agitation to induce heat, microwave energy in tissues results in rotation of water molecules within tissues. The rotational movement of water molecules generates frictional heat that then leads to coagulative necrosis.[13] Because an electrical circuit is not created within the patient as with RFA, MWA does not require the use of grounding pads. Currently available microwave devices do not employ internal cooling of antenna or perfusion options.

20.2.3 Cryoablation

Although not commonly used for liver tumor ablation, cryoablation is another thermal ablation option. In contrast to RFA and MWA, cryoablation achieves tissue necrosis by subjecting tissues to temperatures as low as −160 °C. This is accomplished by the circulation of high-pressure argon gas through the lumen of a cryoprobe. Through a thermodynamic process referred to as the Joule–Thomson effect, expansion of the argon gas within the cryoprobe results in tissue cooling.[14] When tissues are subjected to alternating freeze–thaw–freeze cycles, tissue destruction is achieved through different mechanisms. During freeze cycles, ice crystals form within the tissue; this increases osmotic pressure within tumor cells, which leads to cellular dehydration and disruption of cellular membranes, including those of intracellular organelles.[15,16] When tissue is subjected to the thaw cycle, the coalescence of ice crystals leads to cellular swelling and further disruption of cellular membranes. The ultimate result is tissue necrosis through cellular apoptosis. One of the limitations of cryoablation is a potentially devastating endotoxin-mediated post-treatment inflammatory response referred to as cryoshock, which is observed in approximately 1% of patients undergoing liver cryoablation and manifests as multi-organ failure and severe coagulopathy.[17,18] The cryoshock phenomenon may be associated with mortality rates as high as 18%.[18]

Table 20.1 Summary of ablation types

Ablation type	Pros	Cons
Radiofrequency ablation (RFA)	• Well studied • Highly effective for lesions ≤ 3 cm	• Limited efficacy as tumor size increases • Most tumors require multiple overlapping ablations
Microwave ablation	• Offers ability to generate large volumes of ablation in less time than RFA • Less influenced by adjacent blood vessels • Does not require grounding pads or antenna cooling	• Less studied than RFA • Limited clinical efficacy data
Cryoablation	• Offers ability to visualize iceball during treatment • Can be used to treat multiple lesions simultaneously	• Associated with risk of cryoshock • Limited ability to treat large lesions • Multiple probes required for larger lesions
Irreversible electroporation	• Nonthermal • May have a role for tumors near critical biliary or vascular structures	• Limited safety and clinical efficacy data • Requires general anesthesia

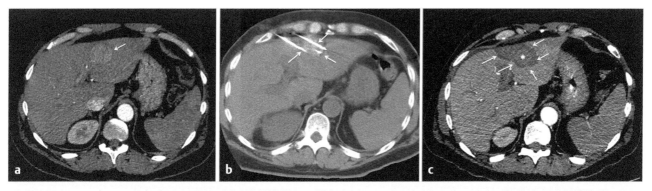

Fig. 20.1 Computed tomography (CT) imaging in patient with hepatocellular carcinoma (HCC). **(a)** Axial contrast-enhanced CT scan of the liver obtained during the arterial phase of imaging demonstrates an enhancing mass in the left hepatic lobe consistent with HCC (*white arrow*). **(b)** Axial unenhanced CT scan of the liver at the time of radiofrequency ablation (RFA). *White arrows* indicate RFA electrodes within tumor. **(c)** Axial contrast-enhanced CT scan of the liver obtained during the arterial phase of imaging 1 month after CT-guided RFA. *Asterisk* indicates treated tumor. *White arrows* indicate the ablative margin extending beyond the tumor margins.

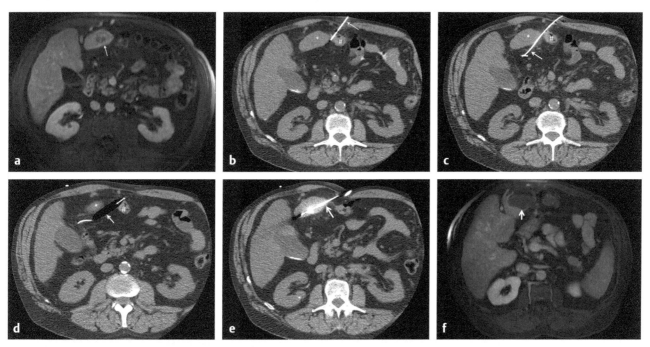

Fig. 20.2 Microwave ablation. **(a)** Coronal gadolinium-enhanced magnetic resonance imaging (MRI) of the liver demonstrating cholangiocarcinoma in segment III (*arrow*). **(b)** Axial unenhanced computed tomography (CT) scan at time of microwave ablation (MWA) that demonstrates a 19-gauge Ultrathin CHIBA needle (*white arrow*) placed between liver edge (*) and transverse colon (#) for attempted for balloon displacement. **(c)** Axial unenhanced CT scan at the time of MWA demonstrating a 0.035-inch guidewire (*white arrow*) advanced through the 19-gauge Ultrathin CHIBA needle placed between liver edge (asterisk) and transverse colon (asterisk). **(d)** Axial unenhanced CT at the time of MWA that demonstrates a 12-mm angiographic balloon (*white arrow*) that was advanced over the 0.035-inch guidewire, separating the liver edge (*) and transverse colon (#). **(e)** Axial unenhanced CT scan of the liver demonstrating microwave antenna in tumor (*arrow*). **(f)** Coronal contrast-enhanced MRI of the liver obtained 1 month after microwave ablation that demonstrates zone of ablation that encompasses tumor (*arrow*).

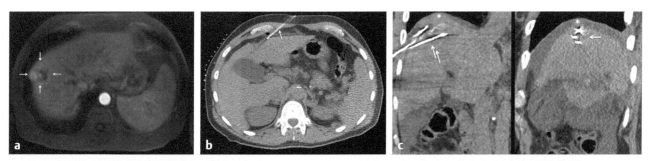

Fig. 20.3 Microwave ablation. **(a)** Axial gadolinium-enhanced magnetic resonance imaging (MRI) of the liver demonstrating hepatocellular carcinoma (HCC) in segment VIII (*white arrows*). **(b)** Axial computed tomography (CT) image of the liver at the time of microwave ablation. White arrow indicates 20-gauge needle used to instill 0.9% normal saline into the abdomen to displace the liver dome away from the diaphragm and lung. **(c)** Coronal and sagittal images of the liver at the time of microwave ablation demonstrating the microwave antennae in the lesion (*arrows*). Asterisk indicates fluid used to displace the liver away from the diaphragm and lung.

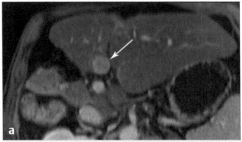
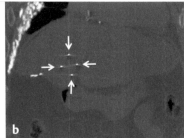
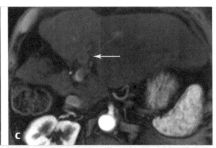

Fig. 20.4 Magnetic resonance imaging (MRI) in patient with hepatocellular carcinoma (HCC). **(a)** Axial gadolinium-enhanced MR image of the liver demonstrates a centrally located HCC (*white arrow*). **(b)** Axial unenhanced computed tomography (CT) scan of the liver demonstrating electrodes (*white arrows*) in tumor at time of electroporation. **(c)** Axial gadolinium-enhanced MRI scan of the liver demonstrating absence of enhancement of the centrally located tumor (*arrow*), indicating complete response.

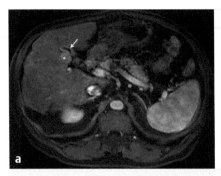
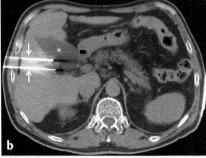
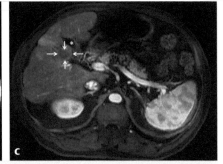

Fig. 20.5 Electroporation of hepatocellular carcinoma (HCC). **(a)** Axial gadolinium-enhanced magnetic resonance imaging (MRI) of the liver demonstrates HCC (*white arrow*) adjacent to the gallbladder (*asterisk*). **(b)** Axial unenhanced computed tomography (CT) scan of the liver at the time of electroporation demonstrating the electrodes (*white arrows*) in HCC adjacent to the gallbladder. **(c)** Axial gadolinium-enhanced MRI of the liver obtained 1 month after irreversible electroporation (IRE) demonstrating absence of enhancement of the HCC (*white arrows*) adjacent to the gallbladder (*asterisk*).

20.2.4 Irreversible Electroporation

IRE (▶ Fig. 20.4; ▶ Fig. 20.5), one of the newest ablation devices available for liver ablation, is generally considered to be a nonthermal form of ablation that achieves tissue necrosis through the repetitive delivery of short-duration, high-voltage electrical pulses to tissues.[19] The exposure of tissues to high electrical fields leads to irreversible disruption of cellular membranes, causing tissue necrosis through apoptosis. Because of the strong electrical pulses required, general anesthesia is necessary to achieve complete neuromuscular blockage. Additionally, synchronization between the delivery of electrical energy and the cardiac cycle is necessary to minimize the risk of cardiac dysrhythmias. A potential benefit of the nonthermal nature of IRE is that it is believed to preserve blood vessels and bile ducts, thus enabling treatment near vital structures.[19,20,21]

20.3 Preprocedural Evaluation

20.3.1 Patient Selection and Evaluation

Cases selected for ablation ideally should be reviewed in a multidisciplinary setting, as this allows experts in medical oncology, surgical oncology, radiation oncology, hepatology, and interventional radiology to contribute to clinical decision-making.[22,23] Once a case is selected for ablation, the interventional radiologist should conduct a thorough history and targeted physical examination. This helps identify patient factors that determine the appropriate type of sedation for the procedure (i.e., conscious sedation vs. general anesthesia), identifies any significant comorbidities and/or allergies, and allows the interventional radiologist to establish a relationship with the patient and discuss the goals of therapy.

20.3.2 Laboratory Assessment

As part of the patient workup, laboratory evaluations should be performed to assess for bleeding risks (complete blood count, prothrombin time, international normalized ratio [INR]) and underlying metabolic conditions that may affect the patient's ability to metabolize medications used during the procedure (blood urea nitrogen, creatinine). Elderly patients may require a recent electrocardiogram, especially those who will be treated with IRE.

For patients with hepatocellular carcinoma (HCC), assessment of underlying hepatic function with the Child–Turcotte–Pugh (CTP) score may help determine overall prognosis.[24] The CTP score is determined using a point system based on clinical factors (ascites, encephalopathy) and laboratory values (albumin, bilirubin, and INR) and classifies patients into one of three groups: group A (CTP score: 5 or 6), group B (CTP score: 7–9), or group C (CTP score: 10–15). Higher scores are associated with a lower life expectancy and an increase in procedure-related risks. Most patients treated with ablation fall into CTP groups A or B.

Several staging systems can be used to further stratify cases based on the underlying tumor type. Staging systems for HCC are numerous and include the Barcelona Clinic Liver Cancer Staging classification, the United Network for Organ Sharing, the Cancer of the Liver Italian Program classification, and the Hong Kong Liver Cancer staging system, among others.[25,26,27,28]

20.3.3 Imaging Review

An essential component of any ablation procedure is a thorough review of all relevant imaging of the patient. This typically includes ultrasound (US) examinations, computed tomography (CT) studies, magnetic resonance (MR) imaging studies, and/or positron emission tomography (PET) scans. Whenever possible, preablation CT or MR imaging should include contrast material for optimal identification of the tumor. Preprocedural imaging is necessary to assess tumor size and location and to determine the tumor's relationship to adjacent structures. Preprocedural imaging also provides a baseline against which postablation treatment response can be measured. Finally, physicians can use preprocedural images to make decisions about the ablation procedure, such as the need for particular patient positioning or the need for contrast on the day of the procedure to aid in tumor identification.

20.3.4 Selection of Imaging Guidance for Ablation

Any of the cross-sectioning imaging tools (US, CT, or MR imaging) available to interventional radiologists can be used to perform a liver ablation. US guidance offers the benefits of real-time imaging and lack of ionizing radiation but can be hampered by several factors, including liver heterogeneity and poor lesion detection, especially in the setting of cirrhosis. Also, ablated liver typically becomes echogenic during treatment, which renders electrode repositioning in or around the lesion difficult. Contrast-enhanced US may overcome some of these limitations, but this technique is not available in the United States.[29] CT allows better anatomic resolution than US with better identification of the probes and their relations to the tumor and adjacent structures. With CT fluoroscopy, probe placement times may be reduced while maintaining the overall high safety profile for liver RFA.[30] CT offers the additional benefit of gantry angulation, which can be especially useful for targeting lesions in the hepatic dome. With advances in computer software, navigational devices may also play an increased role in guiding liver ablations.[31,32,33]

20.4 Ablation Technique

All liver tumor ablations are performed with either intravenous procedural sedation or general anesthesia. The appropriate sedation technique is determined at the time of the initial consultation using the American Society of Anesthesiologists (ASA) physical status classification system as a guide.[34] Typically, intravenous procedural sedation is reserved for patients classified as ASA grade I or II; patients classified as grade III or higher require general anesthesia. All patients require continuous hemodynamic monitoring and oxygenation throughout the procedure.

Once the patient is properly sedated or anesthetized, preliminary images are obtained. For CT-guided procedures, it is often helpful to position the patient in the supine position with the arms extended above the head to eliminate streak artifact through the liver caused by the upper extremities. Baseline images depicting the tumor must be available in the procedure room for cross-reference at the time of the ablation. These images help localize the target, especially for lesions that are poorly detected without contrast, and are critical for CT-guided cases in which patients cannot receive contrast.

Once the tumor is localized, a suitable percutaneous trajectory to the lesion is identified and the overlying skin is prepared and draped using sterile techniques. The overlying skin and subcutaneous tissues are then anesthetized before the ablation probe is placed. With US, probe placement can be achieved in real time, whereas CT-guided procedures require probe placement, followed by confirmatory imaging with standard axial images or CT fluoroscopy. After the probe has been satisfactorily placed, ablation is carried out according to treatment algorithms determined by the device used and the size of the desired ablation. Overlapping ablations, if necessary, are determined by the tumor size and probe placements. With any of the ablation devices, a fundamental principle is to generate a volume of treated tissue that encompasses the tumor and extends beyond the tumor margins by at least 5 mm (▶ Fig. 20.1; ▶ Fig. 20.2; ▶ Fig. 20.3) to minimize the risk of incomplete treatment or tumor recurrence.[34]

After successful ablation of the tumor, the applicators are removed and immediate postprocedural scans are obtained to assess for procedure-related complications. Performing tract ablation while the probe is withdrawn may help minimize the risk of bleeding and/or tumor seeding.[35,36,37,38]

20.5 Clinical Outcomes

20.5.1 Hepatocellular Carcinoma

Local tumor ablation is considered first-line therapy for patients with early-stage HCC who are otherwise not surgical candidates.[39] HCC is probably the most frequently encountered liver tumor treated with ablation. RFA is highly effective for tumors smaller than 2 to 3 cm, with success rates approaching 90%.[40,41] Although most clinical studies have focused on the use of RFA for HCC,[42,43,44,45] emerging research suggests that MWA may offer clinical results comparable to those obtained with RFA. A recently published meta-analysis of the literature comparing RFA with MWA demonstrated similar efficacy for the two modalities with an apparent slight superiority of MWA for the treatment of tumors larger than 3 cm.[46] Another study that assessed RFA and MWA for the treatment of 109 tumors demonstrated a complete tumor ablation rate of 93%, a 3-year survival rate of 31%, and no difference in complications between the two modalities.[47] Other studies have demonstrated similar results, with complete ablation rates greater than 90% for tumors larger than 3 cm.[48,49] Overall, RFA and MWA appear to be equally effective for the treatment of HCC.

Emerging data suggest that IRE may also have a role in selected patients with HCC.[50,51,52] In a study of six patients, complete pathologic necrosis of HCC was observed in five of the patients treated with IRE, and this necrosis was confirmed in explanted livers after liver transplant.[52] Another study demonstrated that tumor proximity to the adjacent portal vein, hepatic veins, or hepatic arteries was not significantly associated with treatment response for HCC treated with IRE.[53] Because of its nonthermal mechanism of action, IRE may be well suited for the treatment of tumors near critical structures such as the gallbladder and central bile ducts (▶ Fig. 20.4; ▶ Fig. 20.5).[54]

20.5.2 Colorectal Metastases

Surgical resection is the primary treatment of choice for patients with metastatic liver disease from colorectal carcinoma. Unfortunately, only a minority of patients ever qualify for surgical resection; most patients are excluded because of the presence of extrahepatic disease, poor underlying liver function, or concurrent medical comorbidities.[55] Research assessing RFA for the treatment of colorectal liver metastases demonstrated median overall survival values ranging from 24 to 52 months.[56] As with HCC, RFA of colorectal metastases smaller than 3 cm is associated with favorable outcomes overall, but the risk of tumor recurrence increases as the tumor size increases. Ablation is thus currently favored to treat liver-dominant or liver-only disease for tumors limited in size and number.[57]

20.5.3 Complications

Complications associated with the ablation of liver tumors include hemoperitoneum, pneumothorax, and biliary injuries including stricture or biloma, as well as tumor seeding of the abdominal wall or peritoneum.[58] Patients with bilioenteric anastomoses are at increased risk of infectious complications.[59]

20.6 Conclusion

Several well-established and emerging ablation techniques are currently available to treat liver tumors. Current ablative techniques focus primarily on the management of HCC; the role of thermal ablation to treat metastatic disease continues to evolve and will likely define itself in the palliative setting. Newer, nonthermal techniques such as IRE may serve as additional treatment options for patients with tumors in otherwise challenging locations.

References

[1] Reynolds T. Researchers use radiofrequency ablation to "cook" and destroy human tumors. J Natl Cancer Inst. 1999; 91(11):909–910

[2] Wood TF, Rose DM, Chung M, Allegra DP, Foshag LJ, Bilchik AJ. Radiofrequency ablation of 231 unresectable hepatic tumors: indications, limitations, and complications. Ann Surg Oncol. 2000; 7(8):593–600

[3] Chong WK. Radiofrequency ablation of liver tumors. J Clin Gastroenterol. 2001; 32(5):372–374

[4] Gillams AR. Radiofrequency ablation in the management of liver tumours. Eur J Surg Oncol. 2003; 29(1):9–16

[5] Sutcliffe R, Maguire D, Ramage J, Rela M, Heaton N. Management of neuroendocrine liver metastases. Am J Surg. 2004; 187(1):39–46

[6] Schwartz M, Roayaie S, Konstadoulakis M. Strategies for the management of hepatocellular carcinoma. Nat Clin Pract Oncol. 2007; 4(7):424–432

[7] Zhang YJ, Liang HH, Chen MS, et al. Hepatocellular carcinoma treated with radiofrequency ablation with or without ethanol injection: a prospective randomized trial. Radiology. 2007; 244(2):599–607

[8] Siperstein AE, Berber E. Cryoablation, percutaneous alcohol injection, and radiofrequency ablation for treatment of neuroendocrine liver metastases. World J Surg. 2001; 25(6):693–696

[9] de Baere T, Deschamps F. New tumor ablation techniques for cancer treatment (microwave, electroporation). Diagn Interv Imaging. 2014; 95(7)(–)(8):677–682

[10] Goldberg SN, Gazelle GS, Dawson SL, Rittman WJ, Mueller PR, Rosenthal DI. Tissue ablation with radiofrequency: effect of probe size, gauge, duration, and temperature on lesion volume. Acad Radiol. 1995; 2(5):399–404

[11] Goldberg SN, Gazelle GS, Compton CC, Mueller PR, Tanabe KK. Treatment of intrahepatic malignancy with radiofrequency ablation: radiologic-pathologic correlation. Cancer. 2000; 88(11):2452–2463

[12] Brace CL, van der Weide DW, Lee FT, Laeseke PF, Sampson L. Analysis and experimental validation of a triaxial antenna for microwave tumor ablation. International Microwave Symposium Digest. Fort Worth, TX, 6–11 June, 2004;3:1437–1440

[13] Lubner MG, Brace CL, Hinshaw JL, Lee FT, Jr. Microwave tumor ablation: mechanism of action, clinical results, and devices. J Vasc Interv Radiol. 2010; 21(8) Suppl:S192–S203

[14] Niu LZ, Li JL, Xu KC. Percutaneous cryoablation for liver cancer. J Clin Transl Hepatol. 2014; 2(3):182–188

[15] Gage AA, Baust J. Mechanisms of tissue injury in cryosurgery. Cryobiology. 1998; 37(3):171–186

[16] Hanai A, Yang WL, Ravikumar TS. Induction of apoptosis in human colon carcinoma cells HT29 by sublethal cryo-injury: mediation by cytochrome c release. Int J Cancer. 2001; 93(4):526–533

[17] Seifert JK, Morris DL. World survey on the complications of hepatic and prostate cryotherapy. World J Surg. 1999; 23(2):109–113, discussion 113–114

[18] Joosten JJ, van Muijen GN, Wobbes T, Ruers TJ. Cryosurgery of tumor tissue causes endotoxin tolerance through an inflammatory response. Anticancer Res. 2003; 23 1A:427–432

[19] Scheffer HJ, Nielsen K, de Jong MC, et al. Irreversible electroporation for nonthermal tumor ablation in the clinical setting: a systematic review of safety and efficacy. J Vasc Interv Radiol. 2014; 25(7):997–1011, quiz 1011

[20] Cannon R, Ellis S, Hayes D, Narayanan G, Martin RC, II. Safety and early efficacy of irreversible electroporation for hepatic tumors in proximity to vital structures. J Surg Oncol. 2013; 107(5):544–549

[21] Silk MT, Wimmer T, Lee KS, et al. Percutaneous ablation of peribiliary tumors with irreversible electroporation. J Vasc Interv Radiol. 2014; 25(1):112–118

[22] Sørensen JB, Klee M, Palshof T, Hansen HH. Performance status assessment in cancer patients. An inter-observer variability study. Br J Cancer. 1993; 67(4):773–775

[23] Avadhani A, Tuite CM, Sun W. Evaluation of the cancer patient. In: Geschwind JH, Soulen MC, eds. Interventional Oncology Principles and Practice. Cambridge, UK: Cambridge University Press; 2008:23–27

[24] Child CG, Turcotte JG. Surgery and portal hypertension. In: Child CG, ed. The Liver and Portal Hypertension. Philadelphia, PA: Saunders; 1964:50–64

[25] Bruix J, Reig M, Sherman M. Evidence-based diagnosis, staging, and treatment of patients with hepatocellular carcinoma. Gastroenterology. 2016; 150(4):835–853

[26] Faria SC, Szklaruk J, Kaseb AO, Hassabo HM, Elsayes KM. TNM/Okuda/Barcelona/UNOS/CLIP International Multidisciplinary Classification of Hepatocellular Carcinoma: concepts, perspectives, and radiologic implications. Abdom Imaging. 2014; 39(5):1070–1087

[27] Kolly P, Reeves H, Sangro B, Knöpfli M, Candinas D, Dufour JF. Assessment of the Hong Kong Liver Cancer Staging System in Europe. Liver Int. 2016; 36(6):911–917

[28] Yau T, Tang VY, Yao TJ, Fan ST, Lo CM, Poon RT. Development of Hong Kong Liver Cancer staging system with treatment stratification for patients with hepatocellular carcinoma. Gastroenterology. 2014; 146(7):1691–700.e3

[29] Du J, Li HL, Zhai B, Chang S, Li FH. Radiofrequency ablation for hepatocellular carcinoma: utility of conventional ultrasound and contrast-enhanced ultrasound in guiding and assessing early therapeutic response and short-term follow-up results. Ultrasound Med Biol. 2015; 41(9):2400–2411

[30] Takaki H, Yamakado K, Nakatsuka A, et al. Frequency of and risk factors for complications after liver radiofrequency ablation under CT fluoroscopic guidance in 1500 sessions: single-center experience. AJR Am J Roentgenol. 2013; 200(3):658–664

[31] Spinczyk D. Towards the clinical integration of an image-guided navigation system for percutaneous liver tumor ablation using freehand 2D ultrasound images. Comput Aided Surg. 2015; 20(1):61–72

[32] Iwazawa J, Hashimoto N, Mitani T, Ohue S. Fusion of intravenous contrast-enhanced C-arm CT and pretreatment imaging for ablation margin assessment of liver tumors: A preliminary study. Indian J Radiol Imaging. 2012; 22(4):251–253

[33] Venkatesan AM, Kadoury S, Abi-Jaoudeh N, et al. Real-time FDG PET guidance during biopsies and radiofrequency ablation using multimodality fusion with electromagnetic navigation. Radiology. 2011; 260(3):848–856

[34] Keats AS. The ASA classification of physical status: a recapitulation. Anesthesiology. 1978; 49(4):233–236

[35] Shady W, Petre EN, Gonen M, et al. Percutaneous radiofrequency ablation of colorectal cancer liver metastases: factors affecting outcomes: a 10-year experience at a single center. Radiology. 2016; 278(2):601–611

[36] Kumar N, Gaba RC, Knuttinen MG, et al. Tract seeding following radiofrequency ablation for hepatocellular carcinoma: prevention, detection, and management. Semin Intervent Radiol. 2011; 28(2):187–192

[37] Conners D, Rilling W. Pleural tumor seeding following percutaneous cryoablation of hepatocellular carcinoma. Semin Intervent Radiol. 2011; 28(2):258–260

[38] Perkins JD. Seeding risk following percutaneous approach to hepatocellular carcinoma. Liver Transpl. 2007; 13(11):1603

[39] European Association For The Study Of The Liver, European Organisation For Research And Treatment Of Cancer. EASL-EORTC clinical practice guidelines: management of hepatocellular carcinoma [erratum in J Hepatol. 2012;56:1430]. J Hepatol. 2012; 56(4):908–943

[40] Livraghi T, Meloni F, Di Stasi M, et al. Sustained complete response and complications rates after radiofrequency ablation of very early hepatocellular carcinoma in cirrhosis: Is resection still the treatment of choice? Hepatology. 2008; 47(1):82–89

[41] Peng ZW, Zhang YJ, Chen MS, et al. Radiofrequency ablation with or without transcatheter arterial chemoembolization in the treatment of hepatocellular carcinoma: a prospective randomized trial. J Clin Oncol. 2013; 31(4):426–432

[42] Shi F, Tan Z, An H, Wang X, Xu Y, Wang S. Hepatocellular carcinoma ≤ 4 cm treated with radiofrequency ablation with or without percutaneous ethanol injection. Ann Hepatol. 2016; 15(1):61–70

[43] Kim GA, Shim JH, Kim MJ, et al. Radiofrequency ablation as an alternative to hepatic resection for single small hepatocellular carcinomas. Br J Surg. 2016; 103(1):126–135

[44] Poggi G, Tosoratti N, Montagna B, Picchi C. Microwave ablation of hepatocellular carcinoma. World J Hepatol. 2015; 7(25):2578–2589

[45] Hocquelet A, Balageas P, Laurent C, et al. Radiofrequency ablation versus surgical resection for hepatocellular carcinoma within the Milan criteria: a study of 281 Western patients. Int J Hyperthermia. 2015; 31(7):749–757

[46] Facciorusso A, Di Maso M, Muscatiello N. Microwave ablation versus radiofrequency ablation for the treatment of hepatocellular carcinoma: a systematic review and meta-analysis. Int J Hyperthermia. 2016; 32(3):339–344

[47] Yin XY, Xie XY, Lu MD, et al. Percutaneous thermal ablation of medium and large hepatocellular carcinoma: long-term outcome and prognostic factors. Cancer. 2009; 115(9):1914–1923

[48] Poggi G, Montagna B, DI Cesare P, et al. Microwave ablation of hepatocellular carcinoma using a new percutaneous device: preliminary results. Anticancer Res. 2013; 33(3):1221–1227

[49] Sun AX, Cheng ZL, Wu PP, et al. Clinical outcome of medium-sized hepatocellular carcinoma treated with microwave ablation. World J Gastroenterol. 2015; 21(10):2997–3004

[50] Cheng RG, Bhattacharya R, Yeh MM, Padia SA. Irreversible electroporation can effectively ablate hepatocellular carcinoma to complete pathologic necrosis. J Vasc Interv Radiol. 2015; 26(8):1184–1188

[51] Narayanan G, Froud T, Suthar R, Barbery K. Irreversible electroporation of hepatic malignancy. Semin Intervent Radiol. 2013; 30(1):67–73

[52] Cheung W, Kavnoudias H, Roberts S, Szkandera B, Kemp W, Thomson KR. Irreversible electroporation for unresectable hepatocellular carcinoma: initial experience and review of safety and outcomes. Technol Cancer Res Treat. 2013; 12(3):233–241

[53] Niessen C, Igl J, Pregler B, et al. Factors associated with short-term local recurrence of liver cancer after percutaneous ablation using irreversible electroporation: a prospective single-center study. J Vasc Interv Radiol. 2015; 26(5):694–702

[54] Dollinger M, Zeman F, Niessen C, et al. Bile duct injury after irreversible electroporation of hepatic malignancies: evaluation of MR imaging findings and laboratory values. J Vasc Interv Radiol. 2016; 27(1):96–103

[55] Adams RB, Aloia TA, Loyer E, Pawlik TM, Taouli B, Vauthey JN, Americas Hepato-Pancreato-Biliary Association, Society of Surgical Oncology, Society for Surgery of the Alimentary Tract. Selection for hepatic resection of colorectal liver metastases: expert consensus statement. HPB (Oxford). 2013; 15(2):91–103

[56] Mahnken AH, Pereira PL, de Baère T. Interventional oncologic approaches to liver metastases. Radiology. 2013; 266(2):407–430

[57] Lencioni R, de Baere T, Martin RC, Nutting CW, Narayanan G. Image-guided ablation of malignant liver tumors: recommendations for clinical validation of novel thermal and non-thermal technologies: a western perspective. Liver Cancer. 2015; 4(4):208–214

[58] Kang TW, Lim HK, Lee MW, et al. Long-term therapeutic outcomes of radiofrequency ablation for subcapsular versus nonsubcapsular hepatocellular carcinoma: a propensity score matched study. Radiology. 2016; 280(1):300–312

[59] Thomas KT, Bream PR, Jr, Berlin J, Meranze SG, Wright JK, Chari RS. Use of percutaneous drainage to treat hepatic abscess after radiofrequency ablation of metastatic pancreatic adenocarcinoma. Am Surg. 2004; 70(6):496–499

21 Pancreatic Cancer

Govindarajan Narayanan, Elizabeth Anne Hevert, and Shree Ramanan Venkat

21.1 Introduction

Pancreatic cancer is an uncommon condition, accounting for approximately 3% of all cancer cases in the United States; however, this disease is the third leading cause of cancer-related deaths.[1,2] Pancreatic cancer has a dismal prognosis with a median survival of approximately 4 to 6 months.[3] This prognosis is in part related to difficulties in diagnosis, with clinical symptoms that do not manifest until the later stages of the disease. Although mortality rates for the other major cancer types in the United States have decreased over the past decade, overall survival for patients with pancreatic cancer has not significantly improved despite technological improvements in diagnosis and surgical improvements in management.[1]

21.2 Types of Pancreatic Cancer

Pancreatic cancer can arise from the exocrine and endocrine portions of the pancreas. The majority of cases (96%) develop from the exocrine portion of the gland, which includes the ductal epithelium, the acinar cells, the connective tissue, and the lymphatics.[4] The remaining 4% arise from the endocrine portion of the pancreas or the islet cells; these cases are referred to as pancreatic neuroendocrine tumors.[5] Of the pancreatic exocrine neoplasms, approximately 90% are adenocarcinomas of the ductal epithelium.[6]

21.3 Epidemiology

It is estimated that more than 48,000 new cases of pancreatic cancer are diagnosed each year.[4] The incidence of pancreatic cancer is comparable between men and women but is remarkably higher in African Americans than in Caucasians.[4,7] An increased incidence of pancreatic cancer has also been observed in less developed countries, which is postulated to be related to the adoption of cancer-causing behaviors such as tobacco use (increases risk by 20%) and high-calorie diets.[4]

21.4 Risk Factors

Multiple modifiable and nonmodifiable risk factors have been implicated in the development of pancreatic cancer, and these factors may act in an additive or synergistic fashion. Research into these risk factors has provided insight into the disparities of cancer incidence among patients of different sexes and backgrounds.[8,9]

The modifiable risk factor most highly associated with pancreatic cancer is tobacco use, which has an attributable risk of approximately 20 to 25%.[7] Although smoking is often accompanied by excessive alcohol use, there is only a weak association between alcohol consumption and pancreatic cancer risk.[7] Type 2 diabetes is a moderate risk factor for pancreatic cancer; patients with long term (> 10 years) diabetes have a twofold increased risk of developing pancreatic cancer.[7,10] Obesity and dietary practices have also been suggested as modifiable risk factors but research into these factors has produced mixed results.[11] The risk of developing pancreatic cancer has also been related to chronic pancreatitis; patients with chronic pancreatitis have as high as a 14-fold increased risk of developing pancreatic cancer. The risk of cancer development among these patients increases linearly over time because of the accumulation of genetic mutations (e.g., mutations of the *KRAS* gene).[7,12,13]

21.5 Genetics

Investigations into the molecular genetics of pancreatic cancer have highlighted the highly complex and heterogeneous nature of this disease. Only 5 to 10% of pancreatic cancers are categorized as hereditary in nature, meaning that the vast majority of cases are sporadic.[7,12] The occurrence is believed to be due to an accumulation of germ line and somatic genetic mutations as dysplasia progresses to carcinoma.[12]

More than 90% of patients with pancreatic cancer have mutations in the *KRAS2* gene, which encodes a GTPase that mediates downstream signaling for growth factor receptors.[13] In addition to *KRAS* mutations, three-tumor suppressor genes are frequently mutated in the setting of pancreatic cancer. The tumor suppressor gene *CDKN2* encodes a cell cycle regulator and is inactivated in more than 90% of pancreatic cancer cases, leading to increased cell proliferation.[12] *P53* tumor suppressor gene mutations are encountered in approximately 75% of pancreatic cancer cases. In addition to this, somatic inactivation of SMAD4 occurs in approximately 55% of pancreatic cancer cases. The heterogeneity of this disease is further highlighted by the fact that although these four mutations are the most commonly encountered mutations in the setting of pancreatic adenocarcinoma, only 37% of patients have all the four mutations.[14] The activation of growth factors causes pancreatic stellate cells (myelofibroblasts) to produce the extensive desmoplastic reaction implicated in causing poor vascularization of the tumor.[12]

The genetic complexity of pancreatic cancer complicates the treatment of this disease and may partially explain the high incidence of chemotherapy and radiation resistance seen in this setting. However, this genetic complexity also offers possible future targets for molecular therapy.

21.6 Presentation

The signs and symptoms of pancreatic cancer are nonspecific and subtle in onset, frequently leading to a delay in diagnosis and more advanced stage at presentation. The median age of patients at diagnosis is 70 years.[1] One of the more commonly encountered clinical symptoms is abdominal pain; however, because of the vague nature of this complaint, it is commonly erroneously attributed to a different pathology. More than one-fourth of patients with pancreatic cancer will have no pain at diagnosis. Symptoms of pancreatic cancer, including significant weight loss, painless obstructive jaundice, ascites, and migratory thrombophlebitis, become more clinically apparent with more advanced disease.[4,12]

The laboratory findings in pancreatic cancer are also nonspecific; these findings may include normochromic anemia or thrombocytosis. As with the clinical presentation, laboratory findings are often not abnormal until the more advanced stages of the disease. Such abnormal findings may include elevations of bilirubin, alkaline phosphatase, and gamma-glutamyl transpeptidase levels in the setting of obstructive jaundice. Serum amylase and lipase levels are increased in less than half of patients with resectable pancreatic cancers and are increased in only one-fourth of patients with nonresectable tumors. The presence of liver metastasis may lead to mild elevations of aspartate aminotransferase and alanine aminotransferase levels.

Approximately 5% of patients with pancreatic cancer will initially present with acute pancreatitis; therefore, pancreatic cancer should be included in the differential diagnosis for an elderly patient with new-onset pancreatitis without other known precipitating factors. The sudden onset of type 2 diabetes mellitus in a patient aged more than 50 years may also suggest that pancreatic cancer is the underlying etiology for pancreatic dysfunction.[10]

Considerable research has been conducted to identify reliable biomarkers that will aid in early detection and provide information regarding prognosis and potential treatment response. At present, CA 19–9 is the only FDA-approved blood test for the assessment of pancreatic ductal adenocarcinoma. CA 19–9 is a sialylated oligosaccharide that is frequently found on circulating mucins in patients with cancer. Unfortunately, the antibody for CA 19–9 targets Lewis antigens with a specific fucosylation pattern; approximately 10% of patients have these antigens (Lewis a and b) and therefore cannot express CA 19–9 and will not test positive for CA 19–9 even in the setting of a high tumor burden.[12]

21.7 Imaging Diagnosis

The role of imaging in the setting of pancreatic cancer goes well beyond diagnosis and can include both disease staging and determination of resectability of local disease. Transabdominal ultrasonography (US) has limited utility in the diagnosis of pancreatic carcinoma because the pancreas can be obscured on these scans by overlying gas in the stomach or bowel. The overall sensitivity for the detection of pancreatic cancer with US is approximately 60 to 70%, and the sensitivity is considerably lower for smaller lesions.[15] Endoscopic US obviates the physical limitations of abdominal ultrasound through the use of a high-frequency transducer that is positioned within the stomach or duodenum in close proximity to the pancreas.[15] This technique has demonstrated superiority to computed tomography (CT) for the detection of pancreatic cancer, particularly for small tumors, and offers the diagnostic advantage of simultaneous US-guided biopsy and sampling of adjacent lymph nodes.[16]

The imaging mainstay for the assessment of suspected pancreatic cancer is CT. Advances in multidetector CT technology have dramatically improved the sensitivity of this modality for the detection of pancreatic cancer to approximately 97%.[15,17] One of the advantages of CT scanning is its accuracy in delineating the arterial and venous vascular involvement. This is important in the evaluation of locally advanced disease, as there is a distinct subset of tumor that blurs the distinction between resectable and locally advanced disease (deemed "tumors of borderline resectability" or borderline LAPC). Pancreatic adenocarcinomas on CT imaging are typically ill defined, hypovascular tumors that are poorly enhancing, appearing on arterial phase imaging as hypoattenuating lesions juxtaposed on the background of avidly enhancing normal pancreatic parenchyma. Approximately 5% of tumors are isodense to parenchyma on CT because of relatively lower tumor cellularity and a lesser degree of necrosis.[18]

Magnetic resonance imaging (MRI) offers soft tissue contrast superior to that of CT for pancreatic imaging. On MRI, the normal parenchyma demonstrates increased T1 signal intensity secondary to the high quantity of acinar proteins, and the pancreas demonstrates homogeneous avid arterial enhancement. The dense fibrous stroma of pancreatic adenocarcinoma results in hypointense T1 signal on T1 fat-saturation sequences; these hypovascular, poorly enhancing characteristics make the lesions more conspicuous on contrast-enhanced examinations.[15] Diffusion-weighted imaging is also helpful in identifying solid masses as compared with cystic masses. Due to the closely packed cellularity and dense fibrous stroma of pancreatic adenocarcinomas, these lesions will typically restrict diffusion and demonstrate low apparent diffusion coefficient (ADC) values.[19] MRI provides an advantage over CT in the setting of small tumors, particularly those smaller than 2 cm, and in the identification of the 5% of pancreatic cancers that are the same attenuation of background parenchyma on CT.[19]

Positron emission tomography (PET) using ^{18}F-FDG to serve as a marker for glucose metabolism can also be used to assess pancreatic cancer. The loss counts from attenuation as PET images are acquired results in increased noise and image distortion therefore integrated PET-CT scans are simultaneously acquired and co-registered, allowing for accurate localization of abnormal radiotracer uptake. PET-CT is useful in differentiating between benign and malignant pancreatic lesions, with a positive predictive value of 91%.[20] Unfortunately, PET-CT is associated with a high number of false negatives, and imaging resolution is poor for lesions sized smaller than 8 mm. However, PET-CT is effective in distinguishing between autoimmune pancreatitis, which demonstrates a diffuse radiotracer uptake pattern, and malignancies, which typically demonstrate a more focal area of radiotracer uptake.

21.8 Tumor Staging

Based on the TNM classification, tumors are categorized as locally resectable (stage I or II), locally advanced (stage III), or unresectable for metastatic disease (stage IV).[12] Approximately 20% of patients with pancreatic adenocarcinoma present with stage I or II disease.[4] T1 tumors are no more than 2 cm in size, whereas T2 tumors are larger than 2 cm in their greatest dimension. T3 disease describes tumor extension beyond the pancreas but not involving the celiac axis or superior mesenteric artery.[21]

Resectable tumors are traditionally those that do not involve the arterial or venous vasculature. Truly unresectable disease demonstrates greater than 180° involvement by the tumor of the superior mesenteric artery, greater than 180° involvement of the celiac or hepatic artery, and occlusion of the superior mesenteric vein/portal vein without surgical options for reconstruction.[15,21] Borderline resectable tumors include those tumors that involve less than 180° of the superior mesenteric artery circumference, short segment encasement or abutment of the hepatic artery, and short segment occlusion of the superior mesenteric vein /portal vein with technical options for surgical reconstruction.[17] Accurately distinguishing between these entities is of paramount importance to describe the tumor vessel interface, as the treatment strategies will differ accordingly. 3D reconstruction tools, including the generation of 3D maximum intensity projection (MIP) and 3D volume-rendered images, are being increasingly used for tumor staging with respect to vascular involvement. These tools also offer additional information that can be important for surgical planning.[22]

The presence of lymphadenopathy is becoming less important in the imaging evaluation of pancreatic adenocarcinoma, as peripancreatic lymph nodes are frequently resected with the specimen during surgery. Cases are rarely deemed unresectable at the time of surgery because of the presence of lymphadenopathy.

A significant factor contributing to the very poor prognosis in patients with pancreatic adenocarcinoma is the early extrapancreatic invasion of this disease and its tendency for metastatic spread. Pancreatic cancer first metastasizes to regional lymph nodes, with the liver serving as the most common primary site of metastatic disease. One of the characteristic modes of disease spread is perineural invasion resulting from malignant infiltration along the neural fascicles; neurotropic factors found within the pancreatic stroma appear to facilitate this process. Even small pancreatic cancers (< 2 cm) have demonstrated a high frequency of perineural invasion. The presence of extrapancreatic disease portends a worse prognosis, often resulting in positive surgical margins and increasing the likelihood of recurrence. Assessment for extrapancreatic disease should include evaluation for confluent soft tissue invasion along a known pathway of the peripancreatic neural plexus.[23]

A typical CT imaging finding in cases of liver metastasis from pancreatic adenocarcinoma is the presence of a hypovascular lesion that is usually best visualized during the portal venous phase.[15,22] MRI is substantially more sensitive for the detection of small liver metastases and can more readily differentiate between malignant and benign entities.[22] Metastatic lesions in the liver are typically hypointense on T1-weighted images and mildly hyperintense on T2-weighted images as opposed to cystic lesions, which demonstrate increased signal on fluid-sensitive sequences. Most metastatic lesions will demonstrate peripheral contrast enhancement on arterial phase imaging, which can help to delineate the pathology.[22] PET-CT has a sensitivity as high as 88% for the evaluation of metastatic disease.[20]

In the setting of metastatic disease, especially in the liver, US- or CT-guided biopsy may be performed. Endoscopic US is favored for biopsy of the primary lesion.[18] This technique used with fine needle aspiration has a negative predictive value of 100%.[15] Complications with this procedure are rarely reported (< 3%), with the greatest risks including bleeding and pancreatitis.[15]

21.9 Treatment

Consensus guidelines for pancreatic cancer suggest that the initial approach to disease evaluation should include diagnosis, staging, and evaluation of performance status followed by multidisciplinary treatment strategies including chemotherapy and/or radiotherapy combined with surgical resection or percutaneous ablative techniques.

21.9.1 Chemotherapy

As indicated above majority of patient present at advanced stages with approximately 35% of patients with pancreatic cancer present with locally advanced (stage III) disease more than 50% of patients present with metastatic disease. In these patients, chemotherapy-based regimens are the treatment of choice, with the patient's Eastern Cooperative Oncology Group (ECOG) performance status directing the choice of regimen. Despite the advances that have been made in chemotherapy, the average median survival for patients with metastatic disease is approximately 11.1 months with first-line FOLFIRINOX (leucovorin and fluorouracil plus irinotecan and oxaliplatin) therapy.[24] This is an improvement over the median survival in patients treated with gemcitabine, which is approximately 7 months.[24] In patients aged older than 75 years, the combination of gemcitabine and nab-paclitaxel has been shown to increase median survival to 8.5 months.[25] Current guidelines for patients with metastatic disease recommend the use of systemic chemotherapy. If FOLFIRINOX can be tolerated (common side effects include neutropenia, fatigue, diarrhea, neuropathy, and thrombocytopenia), this agent is favored over a regimen of gemcitabine plus nab-paclitaxel. Second-line therapy is not well defined in this patient population.

In patients with locally advanced disease, the goal of therapy is to downstage the disease to make the case eligible for resection. In a recent meta-analysis evaluating the use of FOLFIRINOX for locally advanced disease, the median overall survival was 24.2 months with FOLFIRINOX compared with 13 months with gemcitabine.[24] Rates of resection after treatment with FOLFIRINOX ranged from 0 to 43%.[24] Negative margins (R0) were achieved in 74% of the patients who underwent resection after receiving FOLFORINOX suggesting that there may be a role for neoadjuvant FOLFIRINOX even in resectable cases.[24,25] Multiple phase 2 trials exploring the role of FOLFIRINOX and nab-paclitaxel/gemcitabine in the neoadjuvant setting are currently under way for example the NEPAFOX and NEONAX studies.[26]

21.9.2 Surgery

When evaluating a patient with pancreatic cancer, the clinician must determine whether an adequate surgical resection with curative intent and allowing for negative surgical margins can be performed. Patient eligibility must be assessed, including the patient's performance status and the presence of any comorbidities.[27] Surgical margins are defined as R0 if there are no tumor cells within 1 mm of any surface, R1 if at least 1 tumor cell is visible within 1 mm of any surface, and R2 if the resection if incomplete macroscopically.[28] Margins are most commonly positive on the medial and posterior aspect.[28] The median survival in patients with R0 resections is as high as 25 months as opposed to 12 months in patients with R1 resections and 9.8 months in patients with R2 resections, with these lower survival times caused by high recurrence rates (mean, 66%).[29,30] The 5-year overall survival has been reported to be as high as 24% for curative surgery (R0) and as low as 4% for palliative resections (R1/R2).[30]

The most commonly performed operation is a pancreaticoduodenectomy, also known as the Kausch–Whipple procedure. This operation involves the removal of the pancreatic head, duodenum, gallbladder, and antrum of the stomach with surgical drainage of the distal pancreatic duct and biliary system accomplished through anastomosis to the jejunum. The overall mortality rate with a Whipple procedure is approximately 4 to 5%, with morbidity rates of 30 to 50%.[31,32,33] The most common postoperative complications include delayed gastric emptying (11–29%), postoperative pancreatic fistula (2–20%), postoperative abscess formation (9–13%), bile leak (2–8%), and postpancreatectomy hemorrhage (1–8%).[31,34,35]

Other variations of surgical management include the pylorus-sparing pancreaticoduodenectomy procedure, which is modified with the goal of improving nutritional deficiencies often encountered in patients after antrectomy.[30] A distal pancreatectomy is used in patients with tumors involving the body and the tail. A total pancreatectomy, which is a combination of these procedures, is reserved for large tumors and has the highest associated mortality rate.[30] The role of extended lymph node dissections in this patient population is debated.

Interventional radiology plays an integral role in the management of postoperative cases, particularly in managing the aforementioned post-procedural complications.[32] When postoperative fistulas and abscesses do not resolve with surgical drains, interventional radiologists may be consulted to place a percutaneous drainage catheter. Biliary leaks also often require percutaneous transhepatic cholangiogram and drainage and or stent placement, as altered anatomy renders access difficult for the endoscopist.[36] In the event of bleeding and visceral artery pseudoaneurysm formation angiography can resolve bleeding preventing need for reoperation. These interventions including drainage, biliary stenting and angiography help to prevent the need for surgical re-exploration in 85% of patients in one series of 129 patients with postoperative complications after pancreaticoduodenectomy.[32]

21.9.3 Adjuvant Therapy

Because of the high rates of positive margins and disease recurrence experienced by patients with pancreatic cancer treated with surgery alone, the disease management paradigm has shifted to embrace systemic treatment with the addition of adjuvant chemotherapy. Both gemcitabine and 5-FU-based regimens have been associated with improved disease-free survival and overall survival rates in patients with positive margins.[37] Gemcitabine is better tolerated and has a more favorable side effect profile then 5-FU-based regimens; however, no difference in efficacy has been demonstrated.[37]

The primary aim of adjuvant chemotherapy is systemic treatment, including treatment of hematogenous micrometastasis. However, the high rates of local recurrence seen with pancreatic cancer have led researchers to study whether there is a survival benefit with the addition of radiotherapy directed toward treating locoregional disease. As chemotherapy induces sensitization of tumor cells to radiotherapy, the combination of modalities could theoretically be more effective than either modality alone.[38] Several large trials have been conducted to compare the use of combined adjuvant chemotherapy and radiation versus adjuvant chemotherapy alone. Initial reports suggested that combination therapy was beneficial, with several later studies showing a nonsignificant trend toward improvement with combination therapy; the most recent trial found

that combination therapy was associated with a survival disadvantage.[37] These conflicting results have led to different treatment approaches in the United States and Europe; radiation therapy is added to adjuvant chemotherapy only in the United States.

21.9.4 Neoadjuvant Therapy

The use of neoadjuvant chemotherapy in the setting of potentially resectable tumors has been proposed to treat micrometastasis, increase the rate of negative margins (R0), and identify patients who would not benefit from surgical resection by either uncovering latent metastatic disease identified during the preoperative period or demonstrating progression of disease.[37,39] Although there is the possibility of a missed opportunity for surgical resection as a consequence of disease progression, there may be a paradoxical benefit for the patient who avoids a potentially morbid operation that may not correspond with a survival advantage. Studies have suggested that up to 25% of patients do not receive adjuvant chemotherapy after resection, most commonly because of postoperative complications or patient refusal.[40] In patients with locally advanced pancreatic cancer, the goal of neoadjuvant chemotherapy is to attempt to downstage the disease, as downstaging will offer an opportunity for resection. Combined chemoradiotherapy has been found to downstage disease in approximately 30% of patients with unresectable LAPC unable to be downstaged with FOLFIRINOX alone.[41] Possible regimens include gemcitabine, FOLFIRINOX, or 5-FU with the choice of treatment guided by the patient's performance status and ability to tolerate the side effects of treatment.[41] Full-dose FOLFIRINOX regimens have been associated with a median overall survival as high as 35 months in patients with unresectable/borderline resectable LAPC but included 11 patients who underwent resection.[42]

21.9.5 Palliative Care

The current standard of care for inoperable pancreatic cancer or metastatic pancreatic cancer includes interdisciplinary care that has been shown to improve quality of life, symptom intensity, mood, and resource consumption. Chemotherapy options are again guided by the patient's performance status.

In patients with a poor performance status, gemcitabine monotherapy is recommended, offering a median overall survival of 6.8 months.[43] In patients with a good performance status, FOLFIRINOX offers a median overall survival of 11.1 months.[41,43,44] Unfortunately, FOLFIRINOX therapy is often accompanied by side effects such as sensory neuropathy, diarrhea, thrombocytopenia, and neutropenia. For patients who cannot tolerate FOLFIRINOX, gemcitabine-based doublets with nab-paclitaxel or erlotinib can also provide an improvement in median overall survival over gemcitabine alone (up to 8.5 months).[43] In patients who cannot tolerate any chemotherapy, best supportive care includes a multidisciplinary approach (e.g., endoscopic or percutaneous stent placement to relieve symptoms such as obstructive jaundice, celiac plexus nerve blocks to alleviate pain, or gastrojejunostomy placement to allow for supplemental nutrition).

The use of stereotactic body radiation therapy in oligometastatic disease has expanded treatment to patients with limited disease resistant to or intolerant of chemotherapy.[45,46] For these patients, the interventional radiologist can be involved with either ablative or intra-arterial modalities.[47] For example, radio-embolization to control liver metastases has been reported in a limited series of patients with liver-dominant pancreatic cancer metastases with no response to chemotherapy.[48]

21.9.6 Image-Guided Treatments

Radiofrequency ablation (RFA) results in tissue destruction through the application of high-frequency alternating current that generates high local temperatures, leading to thermocoagulative necrosis. Early clinical applications of RFA from an open approach in the pancreas were associated with unacceptably high rates of morbidity (0–40%) and mortality (0–25%).[49] These complications were often the result of inadvertent damage to structures adjacent to the zone of ablation including the duodenum, normal pancreas, biliary tree, or peripancreatic vasculature. Active cooling of the major vessels and duodenum with saline during operative RFA reduces the incidence of these complications, but these techniques are not possible with the percutaneous approach.[50] Criticism regarding the use of RF systems has been focused on the potential for incomplete ablation, particularly near blood vessels because of the phenomenon of "heat sink effect" of local blood flow. RFA is also limited by increased impedance associated with tissue boiling and charring, as water vapor and charred tissue act as electrical insulators.[51] Despite these limitations, a phase 2 clinical trial assessing the safety of RFA in locally advanced pancreatic cancer has recently been completed, and results are forthcoming.[52]

Microwave ablation (MWA) is a form of dielectric heating based on an alternating electromagnetic field in which the tissue acts as the dielectric material. Water molecules in the tissue are forced to oscillate, with some bound molecules oscillating out of phase, causing energy to be converted to heat by molecular friction. Cellular death is achieved via coagulation necrosis. A pilot study in 10 patients with unresectable LAPC found that microwave ablation was feasible; however, therapy in this study was palliative, with success defined as a partial response.[53] Thermal injury is a concern with microwave ablation, with 1 patient in the pilot study demonstrating a delayed complication of pseudoaneurysm of the gastroduodenal artery.[53] This was treated by an endovascular approach.

Cryoablation is most commonly performed intraoperatively under US or CT guidance. Lesions smaller than 3 cm can be reliably frozen with a single, centrally placed probe, whereas larger tumors may require the placement of multiple probes or multiple treatment sessions. The most commonly utilized system uses argon gas and employs the double "freeze-thaw" cycle (5 minutes and 10 minutes, respectively). With this technique, it is recommended that clinicians maintain a 0.5-cm safety margin around adjacent vital structures.[49] Cryoablation has been found to induce antiangiogenesis and result in an immune response that likely has antitumor effects as well as providing pain control.[49,54] The surgical approach to cryoablation may be complicated by gastroparesis.[55] In a pilot study of 49 patients treated with cryoablation, pancreatitis occurred in six patients, hemorrhage occurred in three patients, and pancreatic leak and needle tract seeding occurred in one patient each.[56] The median overall survival in this study was 16.2 months.[56] In another study of 32 patients who were not surgical candidates because of the extent of disease or comorbidities, 27 patients reported greater than 50% reduction in pain, and 22 patients reported a 50% reduction in their consumption of pain medications.[57] Despite the presence of advanced disease in this group, the median overall survival was 12.6 months.[54,57] Current investigations of cryoablation are focusing on combining cryotherapy with brachytherapy and immunotherapy.[54]

High-intensity focused US (HIFU) is a noninvasive method of ablation that uses US energy focused on the tumor to induce thermal denaturation of tissue without affecting surrounding organs. In one series, HIFU was performed in 13 patients with the goal of relieving pain; 10 of the 13 patients reported at least partial pain relief, but follow-up was limited to just 6 months.[58] In another series, MR-guided HIFU performed in seven patients found that the treatment was feasible and effective for pain management, but again, there was no long-term follow up.[59] In a larger series, 43 patients treated with HIFU demonstrated a median overall survival of 13 months, with major complications including severe pancreatitis causing gastrointestinal bleeding and two grade III skin burns requiring plastic surgery.[60] Although complications such as pancreatitis and hemorrhage have been reported with other modalities, skin burns are unique to this procedure.

Irreversible electroporation (IRE) differs from the aforementioned ablative techniques, as this procedure triggers cell death while preserving the extracellular matrix.[61] IRE is a predominantly nonthermal ablative technique in which the delivery of targeted millisecond, high-voltage electrical pulses induces cell membrane permeability through the generation of defects on a nanoscale in the lipid bilayer.[62] This technique, long used for improving intracellular drug delivery, can result in irreversible permeabilization of the cell membrane when sufficient energy pulses are used, thus resulting in apoptosis.[63] Previous studies have demonstrated the safety and efficacy of this treatment modality in proximity to vessels, and IRE has been shown to be effective in the ablation of tumor tissue up to the margin of blood vessels without vessel damage.[63] The safety of IRE treatment of tumors adjacent to the bile ducts has also been demonstrated.[64] IRE can be used in patients with pancreatic cancer who have been treated with multiple lines of chemotherapy with the goal of disease control or in patients with locally advanced pancreatic cancer that has been stable over time. In such patients, intraoperative or percutaneous IRE in combination with standard chemotherapy and/or chemoradiation therapy has been found to lead to improved progression-free survival and overall survival rates versus chemotherapy or chemoradiation alone.[45,65,66]

The surgical approach to IRE can include IRE alone or resection with margin accentuation with IRE.[66] In a series of 200 patients with locally advanced pancreatic cancer who were treated with 4 to 6 weeks of chemotherapy or chemoradiation before the intervention, the median overall survival in patients undergoing IRE alone was 23.2 months, and the median overall survival in those undergoing IRE and resection was 24.9 months.[67] Complications were reported in 37% of patients, with three deaths reported in the IRE-alone group; one death was related to a duodenal ulcer and upper gastrointestinal bleed, one was caused by liver failure, and one was caused by a pulmonary embolus.[67]

Percutaneous Irreversible Electroporation

More than 5 years of experience at the University of Miami has led to the development of a unique approach to the treatment of pancreatic cancer: using IRE in a percutaneous approach. Indications for percutaneous IRE include treating disease localized to the pancreas with a palliative intent when the patient cannot tolerate chemotherapy, downstaging locally advanced disease to allow for curative surgery, and treating recurrence after surgery. Anatomic contraindications to this treatment include overlying colon or obscuring varices. Additionally, patients with a poor performance status (ECOG > 2) cannot tolerate this intervention.

Evaluation in these patients begins with a multidisciplinary approach. A biopsy is required to confirm active disease, and imaging should up obtained within a month of evaluation, including triple-phase contrast-enhanced CT or MRI of the abdomen to evaluate the extent of local disease, involvement of adjacent vessels, and presence of liver metastases (▶ Fig. 21.1). PET-CT can be used to help stage the disease; however, not all cases are FDG avid (▶ Fig. 21.2).

Important laboratory screening includes a coagulation profile, complete blood count, and a comprehensive metabolic panel focusing on renal and liver function. The patient also requires anesthesia clearance, as the procedure is performed under general anesthesia. CA 19–9 levels should be obtained to monitor response after the procedure.

Before the procedure, the patient is asked to undergo bowel preparation to decrease the chance of the colon obscuring the approach to the pancreas. If varices obscure the approach, then proximal splenic artery embolization can be used to decrease supply. Although IRE can be performed safely close to peribiliary tumors, in patients with incompetent ampulla due to prior surgery, extended antibiotic coverage should be offered to decrease the risk of infection. Chemotherapy must be timed to allow adequate bone marrow recovery before intervention.

On the day of the procedure, a preintubation CT scan is performed to ensure a safe window to the tumor. If the window is clear, general anesthesia is induced. A Foley catheter and a nasogastric tube are placed. The latter allows opacification of the bowel with contrast, as well as insufflation of the stomach to push the colon caudally. Preprocedural antibiotics are administered, and defibrillator pads are placed. A triple-phase CT scan of the abdomen is performed with approximately 65 mL of contrast followed by a 65-mL saline bolus. This allows for delineation of critical structures and assessment of tumor extent. Breath holds are synchronized with the anesthesia team to ensure that alignment is maintained.

Before the probes are inserted, the tips of the probes are exposed to 1.0 or 1.5 cm, depending on the required ablation zone. Under CT fluoroscopic guidance, the 19-gauge probes (which are available in two lengths, 15 and 25 cm) are placed in a parallel orientation no more than 2.2 cm apart and no closer than 1.0 cm (▶ Fig. 21.3). Up to six probes may be used at a given time.

An AccuSync (Accusync Medical Research Corporation, Milford, CT) device is used to gate the patient's electrocardiogram and to detect the R wave and send a signal, allowing the Nanoknife (Angiodynamics, Queensbury, NY) to fire the electrical pulses after a 0.05-s delay. The device is set to deliver 70-microsecond high-voltage (1500–3000 V) direct-current (25–45 A) electrical pulses. After a round of 10 test pulses are sent between the paired unipolar electrodes, another 60 pulses are performed to complete the ablation. The voltage settings can be adjusted in the setting of high current as needed.

After ablation is complete, a contrast-enhanced scan is performed, using the remaining 65 mL of contrast followed by a saline bolus. This allows immediate assessment of the ablation zone and the integrity of the surrounding vessels. Small gas bubbles are commonly seen in the treatment zone secondary to hydrolysis (▶ Fig. 21.3). Immediate postprocedural follow-up also includes setting the nasogastric tube to low intermittent

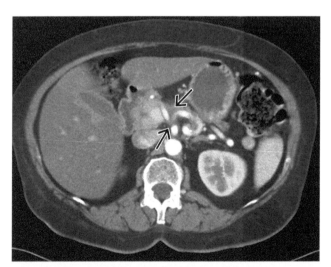

Fig. 21.1 Contrast enhanced axial CT images revealing hypoattenuating mass encasing the celiac axis and superior mesenteric vein (SMV) (*black arrows*) in a 62-year-old woman with biopsy proven locally advanced pancreatic cancer treated with chemotherapy and radiation. (Reproduced with permission from Narayanan et al.[65])

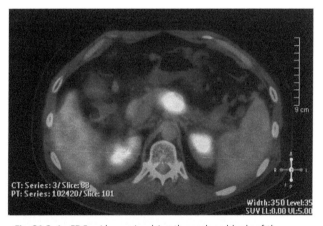

Fig. 21.2 An FDG avid mass involving the neck and body of the pancreas in a 41-year-old male with biopsy proven locally advanced disease is shown on this axial fused PET-CT image. In the two years prior to his referral to IR, his therapy included FOLFIRINOX complicated by thrombocytopenia and radiation.

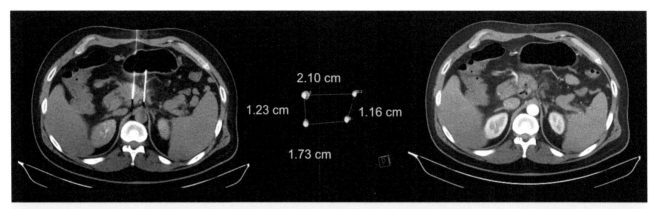

Fig. 21.3 Parallel CT guided probe placement is shown in axial CT image, which is accompanied by 3D reconstruction confirms satisfactory treatment configuration to cover desired lesion. Gas in the in the tumor bed located in the pancreatic body from hydrolysis is demonstrated on this contrast enhanced axial CT image obtained immediately after ablation of the case of the 41-year-old male whose PET-CT images are seen in ▶ Fig. 21.2.

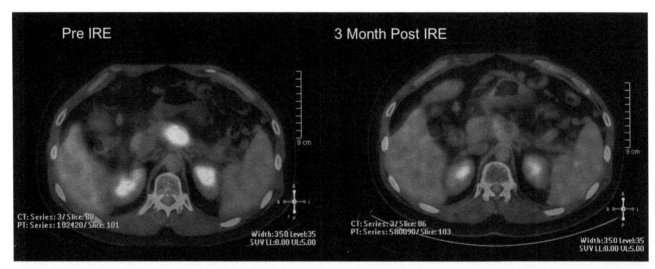

Fig. 21.4 A PET-CT obtained 3 months after IRE demonstrates dramatic response in comparison with prior images in the case of the 41-year-old male shown in ▶ Fig. 21.2 and ▶ Fig. 21.3. His CA 19–9 was never elevated.

suction. The patient's diet is not advanced until amylase and lipase levels are found to be normal or to normalize. Pain is managed with a patient-controlled analgesia pump until oral medications can be tolerated. Oral antibiotic prophylaxis is continued.

After 4 weeks, a triple-phase CT scan should be obtained to assess for complications. Chemotherapy should be resumed in the interval. After 3 months, a follow-up PET-CT scan should be obtained to assess response; CA 19–9 levels should also be monitored (▶ Fig. 21.4). Ablation can be repeated if necessary.

Currently, there are no high-level guidelines from any expert body regarding surveillance practices after potentially curative surgical resection. The National Comprehensive Cancer Network provides the most direction, suggesting that physicians should perform a physical examination and obtain a history, draw blood to assess CA 19–9, and perform CT imaging every 3 to 6 months for up to 2 years after surgery.[67] Early detection of recurrence may improve survival outcomes, allowing implementation of therapeutic advances. CA 19–9 levels have profound prognostic significance; a review of the National Cancer Database demonstrated that elevated CA 19–9 levels (above 37 U/mL) were associated with decreased survival at all stages of disease.[68] This finding not only highlights the importance of following CA 19–9 levels but also suggests the potential use of this factor to risk stratify patients.[38] The normalization of CA 19–9 levels within 6 months of surgery has also been found to be an independent predictor of improved survival.[69]

The first human data on the use of percutaneous IRE in pancreatic cancer was obtained from 14 patients who received a total of 15 treatments.[65] This was followed by a retrospective review of 43 patients who underwent 50 percutaneous IRE procedures, including 30 patients with local advanced pancreatic cancer and 13 patients with metastatic pancreatic cancer.[44] The median overall survival was 16.2 months in patients with locally advanced pancreatic cancer and 8.6 months in patients with metastatic pancreatic cancer. Two patients were downstaged to surgery, and both underwent R0 resections (▶ Fig. 21.5).[67] No deaths were directly related to the procedure.[44]

A recent retrospective evaluation of percutaneous IRE in the management of unresectable LAPC included 50 patients

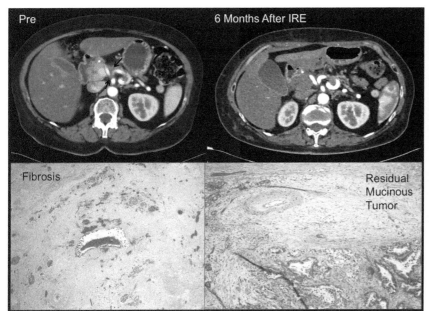

Fig. 21.5 The 62-year-old female with locally advanced disease shown in ▶ Fig. 21.1 was downstaged with IRE as demonstrated by decreased encasement of celiac axis on 6-month follow-up contrast enhanced axial CT image. Due to response to treatment, the patient was able to undergo distal pancreatectomy and splenectomy. Evaluation of the specimen revealed negative margins, extensive fibrosis, and minimal residual intraductal mucinous cancer. (Reproduced with permission from Narayanan et al.[65])

demonstrated an improved median overall survival of 27 months.[70] In patients with tumors less than 3 cm median, overall survival increased to 33.8 months from time of diagnosis and 16.2 months from time of IRE.[70] These studies demonstrate the prolonged survival with percutaneous IRE in selected patients with localized pancreatic cancer. Further studies are needed to identify ideal candidates and the best time course in which to intervene; some studies are already recruiting patients.[71]

21.10 Conclusion

Pancreatic cancer is a complex disease with a poor prognosis despite advances in therapy. The radiologist plays an integral role in the diagnosis, staging, and determination of resectability of this disease. The interventional radiologist's role in managing pancreatic cancer has expanded beyond the treatment of complications from resection to the treatment of locally advanced and metastatic disease, and this role continues to evolve.

References

[1] Howlader NNA, Krapcho M, Miller D, et al. Cronin KA (ed). SEER Cancer Statistics Review, 1975–2013. Bethesda, MD: National Cancer Institute.; 2016 [cited 2016 05/24/16]; based on November 2015 SEER data submission, posted to the SEER web site, April 6.]. Available at: http://seer.cancer.gov/csr/1975_2013/

[2] Sarfati D, Koczwara B, Jackson C. The impact of comorbidity on cancer and its treatment. CA Cancer J Clin. 2016; 66(4):337–350

[3] Yeo TP, Lowenfels AB. Demographics and epidemiology of pancreatic cancer. Cancer J. 2012; 18(6):477–484

[4] American Cancer Society. Cancer Facts & Figures 2015. Atlanta, GA: American Cancer Society; 2015

[5] Grozinsky-Glasberg S, Mazeh H, Gross DJ. Clinical features of pancreatic neuroendocrine tumors. J Hepatobiliary Pancreat Sci. 2015; 22(8):578–585

[6] Makarova-Rusher OV, Ulahannan S, Greten TF, Duffy A. Pancreatic Squamous Cell Carcinoma: A Population-Based Study of Epidemiology, Clinicopathologic Characteristics and Outcomes. Pancreas. 2016; 45(10):1432–1437

[7] Raimondi S, Maisonneuve P, Lowenfels AB. Epidemiology of pancreatic cancer: an overview. Nat Rev Gastroenterol Hepatol. 2009; 6(12):699–708

[8] Bao Y, Michaud DS, Spiegelman D, et al. Folate intake and risk of pancreatic cancer: pooled analysis of prospective cohort studies. J Natl Cancer Inst. 2011; 103(24):1840–1850

[9] Seo JY, Masamune A, Shimosegawa T, Kim H. Protective effect of lycopene on oxidative stress-induced cell death of pancreatic acinar cells. Ann N Y Acad Sci. 2009; 1171:570–575

[10] Huxley R, Ansary-Moghaddam A, Berrington de González A, Barzi F, Woodward M. Type-II diabetes and pancreatic cancer: a meta-analysis of 36 studies. Br J Cancer. 2005; 92(11):2076–2083

[11] Batty GD, Kivimaki M, Morrison D, et al. Risk factors for pancreatic cancer mortality: extended follow-up of the original Whitehall Study. Cancer Epidemiol Biomarkers Prev. 2009; 18(2):673–675

[12] Hidalgo M. Pancreatic cancer. N Engl J Med. 2010; 362(17):1605–1617

[13] Löhr M, Klöppel G, Maisonneuve P, Lowenfels AB, Lüttges J. Frequency of K-ras mutations in pancreatic intraductal neoplasias associated with pancreatic ductal adenocarcinoma and chronic pancreatitis: a meta-analysis. Neoplasia. 2005; 7(1):17–23

[14] Wood LD, Hruban RH. Genomic landscapes of pancreatic neoplasia. J Pathol Transl Med. 2015; 49(1):13–22

[15] Pietryga JA, Morgan DE. Imaging preoperatively for pancreatic adenocarcinoma. J Gastrointest Oncol. 2015; 6(4):343–357

[16] Vitali F, Pfeifer L, Janson C, et al. Quantitative perfusion analysis in pancreatic contrast enhanced ultrasound (DCE-US): a promising tool for the differentiation between autoimmune pancreatitis and pancreatic cancer. Z Gastroenterol. 2015; 53(10):1175–1181

[17] Lopez NE, Prendergast C, Lowy AM. Borderline resectable pancreatic cancer: definitions and management. World J Gastroenterol. 2014; 20(31):10740–10751

[18] Balachandran A, Bhosale PR, Charnsangavej C, Tamm EP. Imaging of pancreatic neoplasms. Surg Oncol Clin N Am. 2014; 23(4):751–788

[19] Wang Y, Miller FH, Chen ZE, et al. Diffusion-weighted MR imaging of solid and cystic lesions of the pancreas. Radiographics. 2011; 31(3):E47–E64

[20] Kauhanen SP, Komar G, Seppänen MP, et al. A prospective diagnostic accuracy study of 18F-fluorodeoxyglucose positron emission tomography/computed tomography, multidetector row computed tomography, and magnetic resonance imaging in primary diagnosis and staging of pancreatic cancer. Ann Surg. 2009; 250(6):957–963

[21] Morana G, Cancian L, Pozzi Mucelli R, Cugini C. Staging cancer of the pancreas. Cancer Imaging. 2010; 10 Spec no A:S137–S141

[22] Raman SP, Horton KM, Fishman EK. Multimodality imaging of pancreatic cancer-computed tomography, magnetic resonance imaging, and positron emission tomography. Cancer J. 2012; 18(6):511–522

[23] Deshmukh SD, Willmann JK, Jeffrey RB. Pathways of extrapancreatic perineural invasion by pancreatic adenocarcinoma: evaluation with 3D volume-rendered MDCT imaging. AJR Am J Roentgenol. 2010; 194(3):668–674

[24] Suker M, Beumer BR, Sadot E, et al. FOLFIRINOX for locally advanced pancreatic cancer: a systematic review and patient-level meta-analysis. Lancet Oncol. 2016; 17(6):801–810

[25] Kamisawa T, Wood LD, Itoi T, Takaori K. Pancreatic cancer. Lancet. 2016; 388 (10039):73–85

[26] Wong J, Solomon NL, Hsueh CT. Neoadjuvant treatment for resectable pancreatic adenocarcinoma. World J Clin Oncol. 2016; 7(1):1–8

[27] Callery MP, Chang KJ, Fishman EK, Talamonti MS, William Traverso L, Linehan DC. Pretreatment assessment of resectable and borderline resectable pancreatic cancer: expert consensus statement. Ann Surg Oncol. 2009; 16(7):1727–1733

[28] Esposito I, Kleeff J, Bergmann F, et al. Most pancreatic cancer resections are R1 resections. Ann Surg Oncol. 2008; 15(6):1651–1660

[29] Schlitter AM, Esposito I. Definition of microscopic tumor clearance (r0) in pancreatic cancer resections. Cancers (Basel). 2010; 2(4):2001–2010

[30] Bachmann J, Michalski CW, Martignoni ME, Büchler MW, Friess H. Pancreatic resection for pancreatic cancer. HPB (Oxford). 2006; 8(5):346–351

[31] Gervais DA, Fernandez-del Castillo C, O'Neill MJ, Hahn PF, Mueller PR. Complications after pancreatoduodenectomy: imaging and imaging-guided interventional procedures. Radiographics. 2001; 21(3):673–690

[32] Sohn TA, Yeo CJ, Cameron JL, et al. Pancreaticoduodenectomy: role of interventional radiologists in managing patients and complications. J Gastrointest Surg. 2003; 7(2):209–219

[33] Malgras B, Duron S, Gaujoux S, et al. Early biliary complications following pancreaticoduodenectomy: prevalence and risk factors. HPB (Oxford). 2016; 18(4):367–374

[34] Bassi C, Dervenis C, Butturini G, et al. International Study Group on Pancreatic Fistula Definition. Postoperative pancreatic fistula: an international study group (ISGPF) definition. Surgery. 2005; 138(1):8–13

[35] Wente MN, Veit JA, Bassi C, et al. Postpancreatectomy hemorrhage (PPH): an International Study Group of Pancreatic Surgery (ISGPS) definition. Surgery. 2007; 142(1):20–25

[36] Brown DB, Narayanan G. Interventional radiology and the pancreatic cancer patient. Cancer J. 2012; 18(6):591–601

[37] Smaglo BG, Pishvaian MJ. Postresection chemotherapy for pancreatic cancer. Cancer J. 2012; 18(6):614–623

[38] Abrams RA. Evolving concepts regarding the use of radiotherapy in the adjuvant management of periampullary pancreatic adenocarcinoma. Cancer J. 2012; 18(6):624–632

[39] Lee JC, Ahn S, Paik KH, et al. Clinical impact of neoadjuvant treatment in resectable pancreatic cancer: a systematic review and meta-analysis protocol. BMJ Open. 2016; 6(3):e010491

[40] Evans DB, Byrd DR, Mansfield PF. Preoperative chemoradiotherapy for adenocarcinoma of the pancreas. Rationale and technique. Am J Clin Oncol. 1991; 14(4):359–364

[41] Hosein PJ, Macintyre J, Kawamura C, et al. A retrospective study of neoadjuvant FOLFIRINOX in unresectable or borderline-resectable locally advanced pancreatic adenocarcinoma. BMC Cancer. 2012; 12:199

[42] Khushman M, Dempsey N, Maldonado JC, et al. Full dose neoadjuvant FOLFIRINOX is associated with prolonged survival in patients with locally advanced pancreatic adenocarcinoma. Pancreatology. 2015; 15(6):667–673

[43] Ghosn M, Kourie HR, El Karak F, Hanna C, Antoun J, Nasr D. Optimum chemotherapy in the management of metastatic pancreatic cancer. World J Gastroenterol. 2014; 20(9):2352–2357

[44] Venkat S, Hosein PJ, Narayanan G. Percutaneous approach to irreversible electroporation of the pancreas: miami protocol. Tech Vasc Interv Radiol. 2015; 18(3):153–158

[45] Gurka MK, Kim C, He AR, et al. Stereotactic body radiation therapy (SBRT) combined with chemotherapy for unresected pancreatic adenocarcinoma. Am J Clin Oncol. 2017; 40(2):152–157

[46] Tree AC, Khoo VS, Eeles RA, et al. Stereotactic body radiotherapy for oligometastases. Lancet Oncol. 2013; 14(1):e28–e37

[47] Bhatia SS, Arya R, Narayanan G. Niche applications of irreversible electroporation. Tech Vasc Interv Radiol. 2015; 18(3):170–175

[48] Cianni R, Urigo C, Notarianni E, et al. Radioembolisation using yttrium 90 (Y-90) in patients affected by unresectable hepatic metastases. Radiol Med (Torino). 2010; 115(4):619–633

[49] Keane MG, Bramis K, Pereira SP, Fusai GK. Systematic review of novel ablative methods in locally advanced pancreatic cancer. World J Gastroenterol. 2014; 20(9):2267–2278

[50] Pezzilli R, Serra C, Ricci C, et al. Radiofrequency ablation for advanced ductal pancreatic carcinoma: is this approach beneficial for our patients? A systematic review. Pancreas. 2011; 40(1):163–165

[51] Wright AS, Lee FT, Jr, Mahvi DM. Hepatic microwave ablation with multiple antennae results in synergistically larger zones of coagulation necrosis. Ann Surg Oncol. 2003; 10(3):275–283

[52] van Hillegersberg R. Safety Study of Radiofrequency Ablation of Locally Advanced Pancreatic Cancer (RFA of LAPC) [cited 2016 July 28, 2016.]; Available from: https://clinicaltrials.gov/ct2/show/NCT01628458

[53] Carrafiello G, Ierardi AM, Fontana F, et al. Microwave ablation of pancreatic head cancer: safety and efficacy. J Vasc Interv Radiol. 2013; 24(10):1513–1520

[54] Luo XM, Niu LZ, Chen JB, Xu KC. Advances in cryoablation for pancreatic cancer. World J Gastroenterol. 2016; 22(2):790–800

[55] Dong K, Li B, Guan QL, Huang T. Analysis of multiple factors of postsurgical gastroparesis syndrome after pancreaticoduodenectomy and cryotherapy for pancreatic cancer. World J Gastroenterol. 2004; 10(16):2434–2438

[56] Xu KC, Niu LZ, Hu YZ, et al. A pilot study on combination of cryosurgery and (125)iodine seed implantation for treatment of locally advanced pancreatic cancer. World J Gastroenterol. 2008; 14(10):1603–1611

[57] Niu L, He L, Zhou L, et al. Percutaneous ultrasonography and computed tomography guided pancreatic cryoablation: feasibility and safety assessment. Cryobiology. 2012; 65(3):301–307

[58] Marinova M, Rauch M, Mücke M, et al. High-intensity focused ultrasound (HIFU) for pancreatic carcinoma: evaluation of feasibility, reduction of tumour volume and pain intensity. Eur Radiol. 2016; 26(11):4047–4056

[59] Anzidei M, Marincola BC, Bezzi M, et al. Magnetic resonance-guided high-intensity focused ultrasound treatment of locally advanced pancreatic adenocarcinoma: preliminary experience for pain palliation and local tumor control. Invest Radiol. 2014; 49(12):759–765

[60] Vidal-Jove J, Perich E, del Castillo MA. Ultrasound guided high intensity focused ultrasound for malignant tumors: The Spanish experience of survival advantage in stage III and IV pancreatic cancer. Ultrason Sonochem. 2015; 27:703–706

[61] Davalos RV, Mir IL, Rubinsky B. Tissue ablation with irreversible electroporation. Ann Biomed Eng. 2005; 33(2):223–231

[62] Narayanan G, Froud T, Suthar R, Barbery K. Irreversible electroporation of hepatic malignancy. Semin Intervent Radiol. 2013; 30(1):67–73

[63] Narayanan G, Bhatia S, Echenique A, Suthar R, Barbery K, Yrizarry J. Vessel patency post irreversible electroporation. Cardiovasc Intervent Radiol. 2014; 37(6):1523–1529

[64] Silk MT, Wimmer T, Lee KS, et al. Percutaneous ablation of peribiliary tumors with irreversible electroporation. J Vasc Interv Radiol. 2014; 25(1):112–118

[65] Narayanan G, Hosein PJ, Arora G, et al. Percutaneous irreversible electroporation for downstaging and control of unresectable pancreatic adenocarcinoma. J Vasc Interv Radiol. 2012; 23(12):1613–1621

[66] Gonzalez-Beicos A, Venkat S, Songrug T, et al. Irreversible electroporation of hepatic and pancreatic malignancies: radiologic-pathologic correlation. Tech Vasc Interv Radiol. 2015; 18(3):176–182

[67] Castellanos JA, Merchant NB. Intensity of follow-up after pancreatic cancer resection. Ann Surg Oncol. 2014; 21(3):747–751

[68] Bergquist JR, Puig CA, Shubert CR, et al. Carbohydrate antigen 19-9 elevation in anatomically resectable, early stage pancreatic cancer is independently associated with decreased overall survival and an indication for neoadjuvant therapy: A National Cancer Database Study. J Am Coll Surg. 2016; 223(1):52–65

[69] Williams JL, Kadera BE, Nguyen AH, et al. CA 19-9 normalization during pre-operative treatment predicts longer survival for patients with locally progressed pancreatic cancer. J Gastrointest Surg. 2016; 20(7):1331–1342

[70] Narayanan G, Hosein PJ, Beulaygue IC, et al. Percutaneous image-guided irreversible electroporation for the treatment of unresectable, locally advanced pancreatic adenocarcinoma. J Vasc Interv Radiol. 2017; 28(3):342–348

[71] Meijerink M. PANFIRE Study: irreversible electroporation (IRE) to treat locally advanced pancreatic carcinoma (PANFIRE). ClinicalTrials.gov. [cited 2016 July 28, 2016]; Available from: https://clinicaltrials.gov/ct2/show/NCT01939665?term=pancreatic+ire&rank=2

22 Embolization of Liver Tumors: Technical Challenges and Anatomic Considerations

David S. Shin and Siddharth A. Padia

22.1 Introduction

At the time of presentation, many patients with primary and metastatic liver malignancy are outside the transplant criteria (e.g., Milan criteria) or have portal hypertension that renders surgery high risk. Therefore, minimally invasive, catheter-based techniques serve an important treatment role in selected patients with liver malignancy. In current practice, the predominantly used endovascular therapeutic options are transarterial chemoembolization and yttrium-90 (^{90}Y) radioembolization. The fundamental goal in catheter-based techniques is the targeted delivery of therapeutic agents in locally high concentration within the tumor bed via embolic vectors, such as ethiodized oil, particles, and microspheres. The key to success in liver tumor embolization is familiarity with the hepatic arterial anatomy to enable accurate identification and selection of the arteries feeding the tumor and to avoid nontarget embolization.

When surgically placed intra-arterial chemotherapy infusion catheters were used in the early days of liver-directed therapy, a higher rate of complications was noted in the presence of variant arterial anatomy.[1,2] Gastroduodenal erosions and ulcerations have been reported after transarterial embolization of hepatocellular carcinoma; these effects are postulated to be due to reflux of embolic agents into the right gastric artery and/or gastroduodenal artery (GDA).[3,4,5] The risk of hollow viscus injury is potentially much higher with ^{90}Y radioembolization. Inadvertent extrahepatic infusion of even a very small number of ^{90}Y microspheres can potentially cause erosion, ulceration, and even perforation of the stomach and duodenum.[6,7,8,9] Furthermore, because ^{90}Y-induced gastrointestinal injury is centered at the serosal surface, it may not respond to medical therapy, can be difficult to assess by endoscopy, and may require surgical intervention.[8,10]

These reports of complications highlight the importance of mastering the standard and variant arterial anatomy, primarily to prevent nontarget embolization. The following discussion reviews the basic angiographic techniques of endovascular liver tumor embolization with special attention to the relevant hepatic and extrahepatic arterial anatomy.

22.2 Basic Angiographic Techniques

All liver tumor embolization procedures begin with diligent angiographic evaluation to detect the visceral arterial anatomy, confirm portal vein patency, identify variant anatomy, find relevant extrahepatic vessels, and assess tumor vascularity. For ^{90}Y radioembolization, this "mapping" angiogram occurs as a separate session 1 to 2 weeks before the infusion procedure and may involve prophylactic embolization of native vessels (e.g., the GDA and right gastric artery) to avoid nontarget delivery of ^{90}Y.

In a typical angiographic evaluation for liver tumor embolization, extensive review of preprocedural cross-sectional imaging, especially the arterial phase, is performed to familiarize the interventional radiologist with the proximal hepatic arterial vasculature. For cases in which high-quality arterial phase computed tomography (CT) or magnetic resonance (MR) imaging is not available for review, an initial aortogram can be performed with a multisidehole catheter to delineate the proximal mesenteric branch vessels. Otherwise, after common femoral arterial access is obtained, initial selection of the superior mesenteric artery (SMA) is performed with a 4- or 5-French diagnostic catheter (▶ Fig. 22.1). Typical injection is at a rate of 3 mL/s for a total of 24 to 30 mL of contrast agent. The presence of replaced hepatic artery from the SMA is assessed (i.e., replaced/accessory right hepatic artery [RHA], replaced proper hepatic artery, or replaced common hepatic artery). Imaging is carried out to the venous phase to evaluate the patency of the central portal veins. Next, the celiac trunk is selected and injected at a rate of 4 mL/s for a total of 15 mL of contrast agent. The hepatic arterial anatomy is interrogated with attention to the presence of replaced/accessory left hepatic artery (LHA), middle hepatic artery, and inferior phrenic arteries. A microcatheter is then coaxially advanced to the common or proper hepatic artery and injected at 4 mL/s for a total of 12 mL. At this point, the GDA, right gastric artery, and any supraduodenal branches should be localized. Subsequently, the LHA and RHA are selected and interrogated with power injection to assess for tumor vascularity and

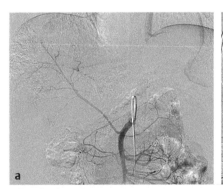
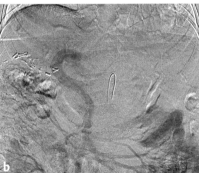
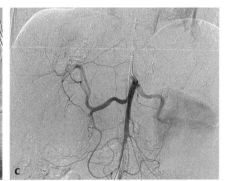

Fig. 22.1 Superior mesenteric artery. (**a**) Angiogram of the SMA shows a replaced RHA originating from the SMA. (**b**) Delayed SMA imaging opacifies the portal vein with right portal vein thrombosis. (**c**) SMA angiogram shows a replaced common hepatic artery to the SMA.

extrahepatic vessels. C-arm cone-beam CT—a technique of reconstructing cross-sectional images from a single rotational fluoroscopic acquisition—is often used in conjunction with planar angiography to increase diagnostic sensitivity and assess tortuous vessel anatomy.

22.3 Anatomy

22.3.1 Conventional Hepatic Arterial Anatomy

In a patient with conventional hepatic arterial anatomy (▶ Fig. 22.2), the celiac artery arises from the ventral surface of the abdominal aorta near the level of the T12 vertebral body. The celiac trunk shortly gives rise to the left gastric artery, which courses superiorly; the splenic artery, which courses to the left; and the common hepatic artery, which courses to the right. This "conventional" celiac trunk anatomy is observed in only approximately 60% of cases.[11] Numerous variations of celiac branching exist, including the presence of separate origins of the main branch vessels directly from the aorta. The common hepatic artery becomes the proper hepatic artery after it gives off the GDA. At the porta hepatis, the proper hepatic artery divides into the LHA and RHA, which supply the respective lobes.

Hepatic parenchymal anatomy is surgically defined by eight Couinaud segments, each with its own portal pedicle that consists of a segmental hepatic artery, portal vein, and bile duct.[12] In conventional arterial anatomy, the RHA feeds hepatic segments V to VIII, and the LHA feeds segments II to IV. Arterial supply to segment IV is variable and may arise as a distinct branch from the proximal RHA or from the RHA/LHA bifurcation (i.e., trifurcation). By convention, this artery is then termed the middle hepatic artery. The caudate lobe (i.e., segment I) is distinct anatomically from the right and left lobes. In a large series of chemoembolization of caudate hepatocellular carcinomas, Miyayama et al[13] found that the segment I artery most commonly arises from the RHA, followed by the LHA, the anterior division of the RHA, and the posterior division of the RHA

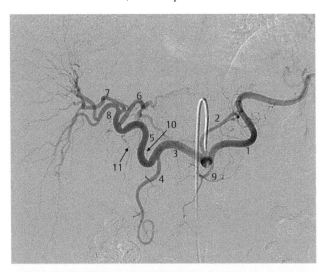

Fig. 22.2 Conventional celiac artery anatomy. 1, splenic artery; 2, left gastric artery; 3, common hepatic artery; 4, GDA; 5, proper hepatic artery; 6, LHA; 7, posterior RHA; 8, anterior RHA; 9, dorsal pancreatic artery; 10, right gastric artery; 11, cystic artery.

in almost equal frequency. The variable origin and tiny vessel caliber make it quite challenging to identify and select the caudate artery during tumor embolization.

22.3.2 Common Hepatic Artery Variants

Replaced/Accessory Right Hepatic Artery

A replaced hepatic artery occurs when an entire lobe is supplied by an aberrantly originating artery, whereas an accessory hepatic artery occurs when a portion of the involved lobe is supplied by an aberrant vessel. An accessory hepatic artery is generally considered to supply a unique portion of the liver, rather than being a redundant vessel.[14] The replaced or accessory RHA, which occurs in 10 to 30% of the population, arises from the SMA in almost all cases, usually as the first major branch (▶ Fig. 22.1a).[7] When accessory, an aberrant RHA usually supplies the posterior half of the right lobe (i.e., segments VI and VII). On cross-sectional imaging, the aberrant artery can be seen coursing between the main portal vein and the inferior vena cava.

Replaced/Accessory Left Hepatic Artery

In 12 to 21% of the population, an artery feeding the left hepatic lobe arises from the left gastric artery.[7] The common trunk of the aberrant LHA and the left gastric artery is conventionally termed the gastrohepatic trunk (▶ Fig. 22.3a). The presence of this anatomic variant poses a challenge for embolization of left lobar tumors. Not infrequently, multiple extrahepatic branches, including the inferior phrenic, inferior esophageal, and accessory left gastric arteries, can originate from the gastrohepatic trunk.[8,10] Therefore, embolization via the replaced/accessory LHA poses a risk of iatrogenic gastric ulcers. On cross-sectional imaging, the fissure for the ligamentum venosum is an important anatomic landmark; a vascular structure coursing through it may represent the replaced/accessory left hepatic artery, accessory left gastric artery, or inferior esophageal artery (▶ Fig. 22.3b).[10] When treating via the gastrohepatic trunk, the horizontal segment coursing to the right side of the abdomen may have several perforating branches (▶ Fig. 22.3c–f). Branches arising from this horizontal portion should be assumed to perfuse extrahepatic structures. Therefore, embolization should be performed from a location that is distal to the horizontal portion, and reflux must be avoided.

Double Hepatic Artery

The double hepatic artery is seen in approximately 1% of the population. This represents a variant in which there are two separate origins of the hepatic artery from the aorta. This variant can alternatively be thought of as an accessory RHA arising directly from the aorta. An aberrant artery, such as the replaced/accessory RHA or double hepatic artery, should be suspected whenever the celiac arteriography does not opacify the entire liver. Because of rich intrahepatic collateralization, a tumor can be supplied by branches from both hepatic arteries.

Celiac Stenosis

Although not an embryogenic anatomic variant, celiac stenosis represents an important anatomic abnormality with significant

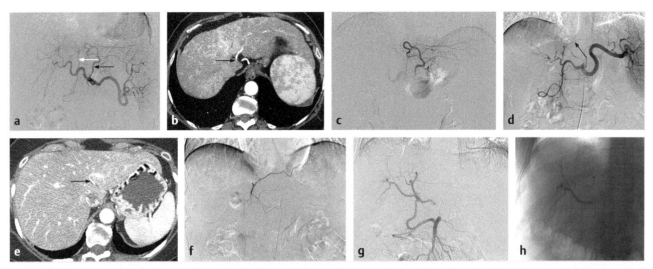

Fig. 22.3 Celiac artery variants. **(a)** Gastrohepatic trunk (*black arrow*) with an accessory LHA originating from the left gastric artery. A separate middle hepatic artery (*white arrow*) supplies segment IV. **(b)** Contrast-enhanced CT demonstrates a vessel in the fissure for ligamentum venosum (*black arrow*). When present, this represents a replaced/accessory LHA, accessory left gastric artery, or inferior esophageal artery. **(c)** Angiogram of the gastrohepatic trunk shows several proximal branches perfusing the stomach with distal branches perfusing segments II and III of the left hepatic lobe. **(d)** Celiac angiogram shows a vessel coursing to the left side of the abdomen (*arrow*), initially thought to be the LHA. **(e)** Contrast-enhanced CT demonstrates a vessel in the fissure for ligamentum venosum (*black arrow*). **(f)** Selective angiogram of the vessel in question shows perfusion of the gastric fundus, compatible with an accessory left gastric artery. **(g)** SMA angiogram shows retrograde flow through the GDA, consistent with celiac stenosis. **(h)** In this case, catheterization of the RHA was performed via the SMA and GDA.

implications for liver tumor embolization. Celiac stenosis is most commonly caused by atherosclerosis and median arcuate ligament compression. The two entities can often be distinguished by evaluating patient demographics and cross-sectional imaging appearance. On angiography, hemodynamically significant stenosis is suspected when selective SMA injection demonstrates a robust pancreaticoduodenal arcade with retrograde flow into the GDA and filling of the hepatic arteries (▶ Fig. 22.3g). To pursue hepatic tumor embolization, it is possible to navigate a flexible microcatheter through the pancreaticoduodenal arcade and retrogradely catheterize the GDA to gain access to the liver from the SMA (▶ Fig. 22.3h).[10] In cases of symptomatic atherosclerotic celiac stenosis, one could also consider treating the stenosis with a stent before proceeding with embolization via celiac access.

22.3.3 Important Extrahepatic Arteries

Right Gastric Artery

The right gastric artery is one of the most important vessels to identify, especially for ^{90}Y radioembolization (▶ Fig. 22.4a). Its origin is variable but typically occurs along the proper hepatic artery (in approximately 50% of the population) or the LHA (in approximately 20% of the population).[15,16] It anastomoses to the left gastric artery via an arterial arcade along the lesser curvature of the stomach (▶ Fig. 22.4b). The collateralization between the two gastric arteries is robust and is often evident during hepatic angiogram as the characteristic intermixing of opacified and unopacified blood along the lesser curvature. Embolization of the right gastric artery can sometimes be quite challenging because of its small caliber relative to the proper or common hepatic artery and its typical acute angulation of origin. We have found that smaller-caliber curved-tip microcatheters (i.e.,

45-degree angle, 2.3-French distal outer diameter) can facilitate successful catheterization. When the direct catheterization of the right gastric artery is difficult, retrograde selection and embolization via the left gastric artery can be performed (▶ Fig. 22.4c–e).[17]

Gastroduodenal Artery

The largest extrahepatic vessel in the celiac artery territory is the GDA (▶ Fig. 22.5a). It supplies the stomach, duodenum, and pancreas via multiple branches (▶ Fig. 22.5b). Routine prophylactic embolization of the GDA before radioembolization has been advocated to minimize the possibility of gastrointestinal delivery of [90]Y. This is especially recommended when the planned infusion position is fairly proximal (e.g., lobar infusion). When the GDA is embolized, it is important to embolize up to the origin of the vessel because miniscule early branches can hypertrophy in the setting of incomplete embolization, leading to nontarget embolization (▶ Fig. 22.5c,d).[8] Retrograde flow of the GDA, as seen in cases of celiac stenosis (see above), obviates the need for prophylactic embolization because embolic agents will not enter the GDA and its branches from the hepatic artery side.

Pancreaticoduodenal Arcade

The pancreaticoduodenal arcade is a complex network of arterial anastomoses between the celiac axis and the SMA that supply the head and uncinate process of the pancreas and the proximal duodenum. Within this anastomotic network, there are a few named vessels that require attention during angiography, including retroduodenal and supraduodenal arteries (▶ Fig. 22.6), to prevent iatrogenic pancreatitis and duodenal ulceration.[7,18,19] The posterior superior pancreaticoduodenal

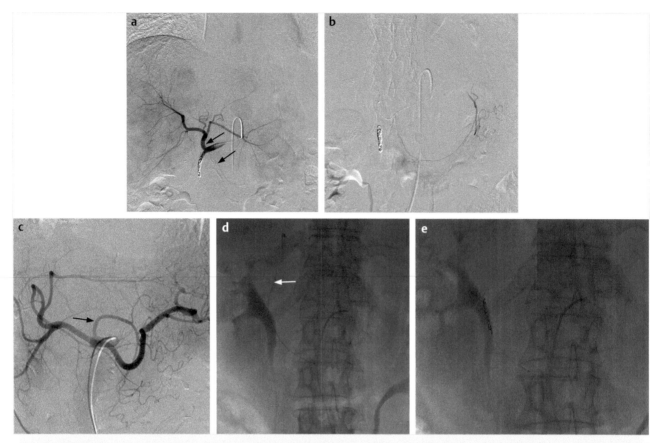

Fig. 22.4 Right gastric artery. **(a)** Angiogram of the common hepatic artery shows a faint vessel (*black arrows*) arising from the proper hepatic artery, consistent with the right gastric artery. The GDA has been coiled. **(b)** Selective angiography of the right gastric artery shows its course along the lesser curvature of the stomach with communication to the left gastric artery. **(c)** Celiac angiogram fails to demonstrate the origin of the right gastric artery. However, the left gastric artery (*black arrow*) is prominent. **(d)** Catheterization of the left gastric artery facilitates selection of the right gastric artery via the lesser curvature, with identification of the right gastric artery origin (*arrow*). **(e)** Coil embolization of the right gastric artery was performed.

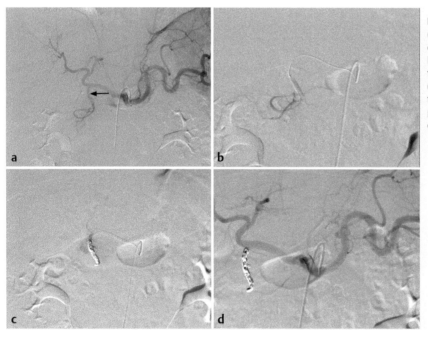

Fig. 22.5 Gastroduodenal artery. **(a)** The GDA (*arrow*) is usually the first major branch from the common hepatic artery. **(b)** The GDA typically bifurcates into the right gastroepiploic artery and the superior pancreaticoduodenal arcade. **(c)** After coil embolization, one must ensure that there is complete occlusion, including all small perforators. **(d)** This often necessitates embolizing to the origin of the vessel.

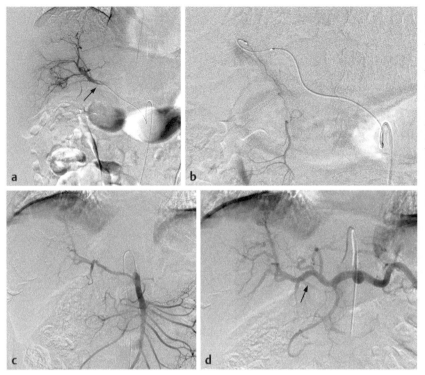

Fig. 22.6 Supraduodenal and retroduodenal arteries. **(a)** Angiogram of the RHA shows a small vessel (*arrow*) coursing in an inferior-medial direction. **(b)** Selective catheterization of this vessel confirms it as a supraduodenal artery, with eventual communication to the gastroduodenal arcade. **(c)** SMA angiogram shows the first branch perfusing the liver via communication to the RHA distribution, initially suggestive of a replaced or accessory RHA. **(d)** However, celiac angiogram in the same patient shows perfusion of the same RHA distribution. The communicating vessel between the celiac artery and SMA is shown (*arrow*). These findings are consistent with a retroduodenal artery.

artery is typically the first major branch of the GDA; however, it may arise from various branches of the hepatic artery (in 15% of the population).[20] This vessel is also referred to as the retroduodenal artery[21] and may form a prominent direct collateral pathway between a hepatic artery and the SMA. The anterior superior pancreaticoduodenal artery is one of the terminal branches of the GDA.[14] The inferior pancreaticoduodenal artery is usually the first branch of the SMA, and its branches anastomose with those of the superior pancreaticoduodenal arteries. The supraduodenal artery is highly variable in its origin and may arise from the GDA (in 27% of the population), common hepatic artery (in 20% of the population), LHA (in 20% of the population), or RHA (in 13% of the population).[7,22] In addition, several supraduodenal vessels may be present. These often hypertrophy if prophylactic embolization of the GDA is performed.

Cystic Artery

In the vast majority of cases (up to 95%), the cystic artery originates from the RHA (▶ Fig. 22.2).[23] Much less common origins include the LHA, common hepatic artery, and GDA.[24] In cases of the replaced RHA (see below), the main or accessory cystic artery almost always originates from this aberrant artery.[7] Inadvertent infusion of therapeutic agents into the cystic artery may result in chemical/radiation acute cholecystitis, and in rare cases may require operative management.[7] Furthermore, delivery of chemoembolic agents to the gallbladder may increase the risk of postembolization syndrome and lengthen hospitalization after hepatic chemoembolization.[25] Despite these risks, prophylactic coil embolization before chemoembolization or radioembolization is rarely warranted, as the toxicity from radiation- or chemotherapy-induced cholecystitis is usually transient. In many cases, infusion can be performed from a position in the RHA distal to the origin of the cystic artery takeoff.

Occasionally, the RHA may have a relatively early bifurcation into anterior and posterior divisions, with the cystic artery origin in close proximity to the bifurcation. In this situation, multivessel selective infusion of therapeutic agents can be performed (i.e., single infusion to the anterior RHA and single infusion to the posterior RHA) to avoid the cystic artery while appropriately covering the entire right hepatic lobe.

Falciform Artery

The falciform artery runs within the falciform ligament, which represents a double fold of peritoneum anterior to the left hepatic lobe, dividing it into the medial and lateral segments (▶ Fig. 22.7).[7] Its branches anastomose with the terminal branches of the internal mammary and inferior epigastric arteries to supply the anterior abdominal wall.[10] It arises from the LHA or middle hepatic artery, and may be single or double.[26] Although rare, inadvertent infusion of ^{90}Y microspheres to this artery may result in abdominal pain, skin necrosis, and rash.[24] Although not always seen angiographically, the classic appearance of the falciform artery is an L-shaped vessel that arises from the LHA, courses inferiorly and to the right initially, then curves toward the umbilicus.

Inferior Phrenic Artery

The right inferior phrenic artery is a common source of extrahepatic parasitization of blood flow, particularly for large tumors in the hepatic dome (▶ Fig. 22.8).[10] When a hepatic dome tumor is incompletely stained on a selective RHA injection or inadequately treated by a prior embolization, parasitization by this vessel should be suspected. Identification and selection of the right inferior phrenic artery is required for proper endovascular treatment planning. In appropriately selected patients,

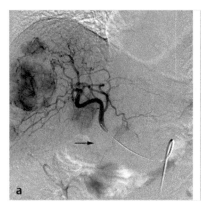
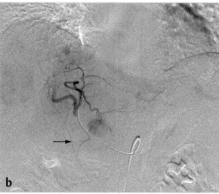

Fig. 22.7 Falciform artery. **(a)** Angiogram of the proper hepatic artery shows an extrahepatic vessel coursing in an inferior-medial direction (*arrow*). **(b)** Selective LHA angiogram confirms that this is the falciform artery (*arrow*).

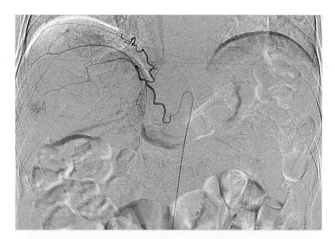

Fig. 22.8 Right inferior phrenic artery. Angiogram of the right inferior phrenic artery demonstrates perfusion to tumors in the posterior right hepatic lobe.

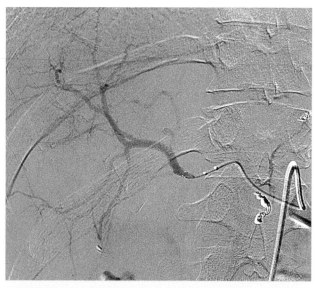

Fig. 22.9 Antireflux catheter. In this patient who had been recently treated with biologic agents for colorectal cancer, RHA flow was diminished, with risk of reflux into extrahepatic branches. A Surefire antireflux catheter was used to promote antegrade flow.

chemoembolization can be considered via the parasitized right inferior phrenic artery.[27]

22.4 Techniques to Avoid Nontarget Embolization

The main goal of prophylactic embolization before radioembolization is to prevent nontarget ^{90}Y delivery to the hollow viscus. Hepaticoenteric anastomoses are identified and embolized with coils to prune any gastrointestinal inflows.[28] The most commonly embolized arteries during the mapping angiogram are the GDA and right gastric artery, especially in the setting of lobar radioembolization. For a more selective embolization at a segmental or subsegmental level, we have found that routine prophylactic embolization of these vessels is not required. If a microcatheter can be placed at a sufficiently distal location remote from any gastrointestinal circulation and adequate forward flow is confirmed on contrast injection, then it is safe to proceed with the ^{90}Y delivery without prior embolization of the extrahepatic arteries.

In certain situations, it may be advantageous to use a special catheter that is designed to promote directional flow during infusion of embolic agents. The Surefire Infusion System (Surefire Medical, Inc., Westminster, CO) is one such device. This system features an expandable tip at the distal end of the microcatheter that collapses in forward flow and expands in reverse flow to reduce reflux (▶ Fig. 22.9). Another device is the IsoFlow infusion catheter (Vascular Designs, Inc., San Jose, CA), which employs 2 occlusion balloons along the microcatheter to isolate and target a particular arterial branch for embolization.

22.5 Challenging Scenario: Tumors with Multiple Supplies

Sometimes a tumor is supplied by multiple segmental arteries (▶ Fig. 22.10). A classic example is a tumor that is in the arterial watershed zone of the liver near the Cantlie line (i.e., the anatomic plane that separates the left and right lobes). Such a tumor can be supplied by the middle hepatic artery or the segment IV artery from the LHA, as well as from the segment VIII artery from the RHA. One study found that tumors located across the Cantlie line showed a significantly higher viability rate after unilateral chemoembolization than after bilateral chemoembolization.[29] In other words, when a watershed tumor is

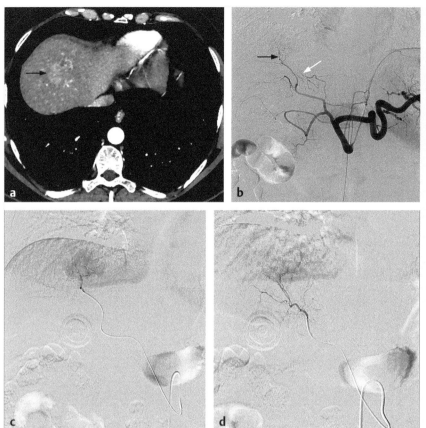

Fig. 22.10 Multiple feeding arteries. **(a)** Contrast-enhanced CT shows a tumor (*arrow*) at the junction of the right and left hepatic lobes. **(b)** Celiac angiogram shows possible perfusion of the tumor from both the segment VIII RHA (*black arrow*) and the segment IV artery (*white arrow*). **(c)** Selective angiography of the segment VIII RHA shows tumor hypervascularity. **(d)** Selective angiography of the segment IV artery also shows tumor hypervascularity. In this case, both vessels were treated.

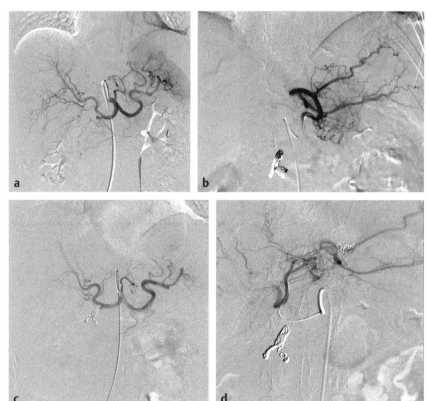

Fig. 22.11 Flow redistribution. **(a)** In a patient with bilobar hypovascular colon cancer metastases to the liver, celiac angiogram shows a gastrohepatic trunk with the replaced LHA originating from the left gastric artery. **(b)** Angiogram of the gastrohepatic trunk shows multiple small perforating gastric vessels with two larger horizontal branches perfusing segments II and III of the liver. **(c)** Coil embolization of the left gastric trunk was performed to induce redistribution of arterial flow from the RHA to the LHA. The GDA was also embolized. **(d)** Selective catheterization of the middle hepatic artery now shows communication to the segment II and III branches of the replaced LHA.

treated only from one side, the efficacy of embolization is decreased. Therefore, it is important to interrogate potential dual arterial supplies for tumors in the watershed zones and to deliver embolic agents via both feeders.

A hepatic tumor may also parasitize arterial supply from extrahepatic arteries. For example, a tumor located subjacent to the right hemidiaphragm in the hepatic dome may have inflows from the right inferior phrenic artery in addition to the segment VII or VIII supply. In such cases, the extrahepatic vessel can be embolized to restore exclusively intrahepatic arterial supply to the tumor.[30] This preparatory process before embolization is referred to as consolidation or flow redistribution (▶ Fig. 22.11). The goal is to simplify the tumor supply to only intrahepatic arteries that can later be easily embolized using standard techniques.

22.6 Summary and Pearls

- Catheter-based embolization techniques have an important role in the treatment of primary and metastatic liver tumors in selected patients.
- Nontarget delivery of embolic agents can result in serious gastrointestinal complications, including erosion, ulceration, and perforation.
- Meticulous catheter techniques and in-depth knowledge of vascular anatomy are required for safe and effective endovascular procedures.
- Common hepatic arterial variants include the replaced/accessory RHA from the SMA, the replaced/accessory LHA from the left gastric artery, and the double hepatic artery from the aorta.
- Important extrahepatic vessels arising from the hepatic arteries include the right gastric artery, pancreaticoduodenal arteries, cystic artery, falciform artery, and inferior phrenic artery.
- Prophylactic extrahepatic embolization, selective catheter position, antireflux infusion system, and flow redistribution are some of the strategies used to reduce nontarget radioembolization.

References

[1] Allen PJ, Stojadinovic A, Ben-Porat L, et al. The management of variant arterial anatomy during hepatic arterial infusion pump placement. Ann Surg Oncol. 2002; 9(9):875–880

[2] Campbell KA, Burns RC, Sitzmann JV, Lipsett PA, Grochow LB, Niederhuber JE. Regional chemotherapy devices: effect of experience and anatomy on complications. J Clin Oncol. 1993; 11(5):822–826

[3] Ishigaki H, Suto T, Sasaki D, et al. [Factors of gastric lesions following after transcatheter arterial embolization for primary hepatoma]. Nippon Shokakibyo Gakkai Zasshi. 1990; 87(1):57–61

[4] Leung TK, Lee CM, Chen HC. Anatomic and technical skill factor of gastroduodenal complication in post-transarterial embolization for hepatocellular carcinoma: a retrospective study of 280 cases. World J Gastroenterol. 2005; 11(10):1554–1557

[5] Tsuchigame T, Takahashi M, Watanabe O, et al. [Pathogenesis and prevention of gastrointestinal complications following transcatheter arterial embolization]. Nippon Igaku Hoshasen Gakkai Zasshi. 1990; 50(7):798–803

[6] Lau WY, Ho S, Leung TW, et al. Selective internal radiation therapy for nonresectable hepatocellular carcinoma with intra-arterial infusion of 90yttrium microspheres. Int J Radiat Oncol Biol Phys. 1998; 40(3):583–592

[7] Liu DM, Salem R, Bui JT, et al. Angiographic considerations in patients undergoing liver-directed therapy. J Vasc Interv Radiol. 2005; 16(7):911–935

[8] Paprottka PM, Jakobs TF, Reiser MF, Hoffmann RT. Practical vascular anatomy in the preparation of radioembolization. Cardiovasc Intervent Radiol. 2012; 35(3):454–462

[9] Yip D, Allen R, Ashton C, Jain S. Radiation-induced ulceration of the stomach secondary to hepatic embolization with radioactive yttrium microspheres in the treatment of metastatic colon cancer. J Gastroenterol Hepatol. 2004; 19 (3):347–349

[10] Lewandowski RJ, Sato KT, Atassi B, et al. Radioembolization with 90Y microspheres: angiographic and technical considerations. Cardiovasc Intervent Radiol. 2007; 30(4):571–592

[11] Uflacker R. Atlas of Vascular Anatomy: An Angiographic Approach. Baltimore, MD: Williams and Wilkins; 1997

[12] Fong Y, Blumgart LH. Hepatic resection. In: Souba WW, Fink MP, Jurkovich GJ, et al, eds. ACS Surgery: Principles and Practice. 6th ed. Hamilton, Ontario: WebMD, Inc; 2007:766–784

[13] Miyayama S, Yamashiro M, Hattori Y, et al. Angiographic evaluation of feeding arteries of hepatocellular carcinoma in the caudate lobe of the liver. Cardiovasc Intervent Radiol. 2011; 34(6):1244–1253

[14] Valji K. The Practice of Interventional Radiology. Philadelphia, PA: Elsevier Saunders; 2012

[15] VanDamme JP, Bonte J. Vascular Anatomy in Abdominal Surgery. New York, NY: Thieme; 1990

[16] Yamagami T, Nakamura T, Iida S, Kato T, Nishimura T. Embolization of the right gastric artery before hepatic arterial infusion chemotherapy to prevent gastric mucosal lesions: approach through the hepatic artery versus the left gastric artery. AJR Am J Roentgenol. 2002; 179(6):1605–1610

[17] Hashimoto M, Heianna J, Tate E, Kurosawa R, Nishii T, Mayama I. The feasibility of retrograde catheterization of the right gastric artery via the left gastric artery. J Vasc Interv Radiol. 2001; 12(9):1103–1106

[18] Carr BI, Zajko A, Bron K, Orons P, Sammon J, Baron R. Phase II study of Spherex (degradable starch microspheres) injected into the hepatic artery in conjunction with doxorubicin and cisplatin in the treatment of advanced-stage hepatocellular carcinoma: interim analysis. Semin Oncol. 1997; 24(2) Suppl 6:S6–S97, S6–S99

[19] Choplin RH, Gelfand DW, Hunt TH. Gastric perforation from hepatic artery infusion chemotherapy. Gastrointest Radiol. 1983; 8(2):133–134

[20] Van Damme JP, Van der Schueren G, Bonte J. Vascularisation du pancreas: proposition de nomenclature PNA et angioarchitecture des ilots. C R Assoc Anat. 1968; 139:1184–1192

[21] Song SY, Chung JW, Kwon JW, et al. Collateral pathways in patients with celiac axis stenosis: angiographic-spiral CT correlation. Radiographics. 2002; 22(4):881–893

[22] Bianchi HF, Albanèse EF. The supraduodenal artery. Surg Radiol Anat. 1989; 11(1):37–40

[23] Ottery FD, Scupham RK, Weese JL. Chemical cholecystitis after intrahepatic chemotherapy. The case for prophylactic cholecystectomy during pump placement. Dis Colon Rectum. 1986; 29(3):187–190

[24] Arora R, Soulen MC, Haskal ZJ. Cutaneous complications of hepatic chemoembolization via extrahepatic collaterals. J Vasc Interv Radiol. 1999; 10 (10):1351–1356

[25] Leung DA, Goin JE, Sickles C, Raskay BJ, Soulen MC. Determinants of postembolization syndrome after hepatic chemoembolization. J Vasc Interv Radiol. 2001; 12(3):321–326

[26] Baba Y, Miyazono N, Ueno K, et al. Hepatic falciform artery. Angiographic findings in 25 patients. Acta Radiol. 2000; 41(4):329–333

[27] Xu HB, Yan XQ. Diagnosis and therapy for primary hepatic carcinoma: transcatheter inferior phrenic arteriography and chemoembolization. J Tongji Med Univ. 1993; 13(3):186–189

[28] Wang DS, Louie JD, Sze DY. Intra-arterial therapies for metastatic colorectal cancer. Semin Intervent Radiol. 2013; 30(1):12–20

[29] Chou CT, Huang YC, Lee CW, Lee KW, Chen YL, Chen RC. Efficacy of transarterial chemoembolization for hepatocellular carcinoma in interlobar watershed zone of liver: comparison of unilateral and bilateral chemoembolization. J Vasc Interv Radiol. 2012; 23(8):1036–1042

[30] Abdelmaksoud MH, Louie JD, Kothary N, et al. Embolization of parasitized extrahepatic arteries to reestablish intrahepatic arterial supply to tumors before yttrium-90 radioembolization. J Vasc Interv Radiol. 2011; 22(10): 1355–1362

23 Yttrium-90 Radioembolization of Malignant Liver Tumors

Christopher A. Molvar and Robert J. Lewandowski

23.1 Introduction

The liver is a frequent site of metastatic disease, often of colorectal origin (metastatic colorectal cancer [mCRC]), and is also a site of lethal primary malignancy. Hepatocellular carcinoma (HCC) is the most common primary hepatic tumor and the third most common cause of cancer mortality. Surgery offers a cure for primary and secondary hepatic tumors; however, many patients are not candidates for surgical resection, and so palliative treatments dominate. Hepatic yttrium-90 (^{90}Y) radioembolization is an evolving palliative treatment option offering new promise to patients with often limited treatment choices. As with other transarterial therapies, radioembolization relies on the dual blood supply of the liver. More specifically, malignant tumors are primarily supplied by the hepatic artery, whereas the background nontumorous liver is primarily supplied by the portal vein. Therefore, radioembolization delivers high-dose internal radiation to the tumor while sparing much of the nontumorous liver. This chapter will review patient selection, technique, and outcomes of hepatic radioembolization for primary and select secondary tumor types.

23.2 Patient Selection and Indications

^{90}Y radioembolization is a potent treatment option for patients with unresectable liver-dominant disease who have preserved liver function and performance status. Treatment goals are varied but may include improved survival and improved quality of life, including symptomatic relief. This technique may also be used for neoadjuvant applications.

Radioembolization is currently performed with small microspheres that deliver yttrium-90, a beta-emitting isotope. These microspheres emit high-energy, low-penetration radiation (approximately 2.5 mm) to the tumor while sparing the surrounding liver parenchyma. Pathologic studies after radioembolization have demonstrated a relative 50- to 70-fold greater microsphere density at the tumor periphery compared to the density in the background liver parenchyma.[1]

Two radioactive microspheres are commercially available; these microspheres differ in the type of ^{90}Y carrier used. TheraSphere (BTG International, London, UK) is a glass microsphere that is 20 to 30 microns in size and has a high specific activity (2500 Bq per sphere) at calibration. SIR-Spheres (Sirtex Medical, Sydney, Australia) are resin microspheres similar in size to TheraSphere microspheres but with a lower specific activity (50 Bq per sphere). Despite these technical differences, response rates for hepatic tumors treated with these two types of microspheres appear to be equivalent. TheraSphere was approved in 1999 by the Food and Drug Administration (FDA) under a Humanitarian Device Exemption for the treatment of unresectable HCC,[2] and the SIR-Spheres microsphere was granted approval in 2002 for the treatment of mCRC.[3]

For HCC, patient eligibility parallels eligibility for chemoembolization, including unresectable liver-dominant disease with preserved liver function (Child–Pugh class A or B) and performance status (Eastern Cooperative Oncology Group [ECOG] score, 0–2). The microembolic nature of radioembolization also allows for its use in patients with portal vein thrombosis (PVT), thus limiting the risk of ischemic hepatitis.[4]

The fundamental patient selection criteria for radioembolization in secondary liver tumors match those described for HCC. Eligible patients typically have unresectable liver-dominant tumor after standard-of-care chemotherapy. Some patients require palliative therapy for painful bulky tumors. Many modern chemotherapeutic regimens are associated with liver toxicity, including chemotherapy-associated steatohepatitis (seen with irinotecan) and veno-occlusive disease (seen with oxaliplatin). As such, preservation of hepatic function is critical to patient selection. Biologic anticancer agents such as bevacizumab make the vasculature more prone to injury. Recent use of these agents increases the risk of vascular dissection and rupture, which can prevent the use of transarterial treatment. Careful microcatheter and microwire manipulation are required for patients exposed to systemic anticancer therapies.[5]

Special considerations are made for patients lacking a competent sphincter of Oddi, often because of the presence of bilioenteric anastomosis or a biliary stent. Hepatic artery embolization in this setting is known to markedly increase the risk of hepatic abscess.[6] Recent evidence suggests that a prolonged course of antibiotics and the use of radioembolization rather than chemoembolization may lower the risk of hepatic abscess in these patients.[7,8]

23.3 Contraindications

Appropriate patient selection is paramount to limiting adverse radioembolization outcomes. Regardless of tumor type, maintenance of performance status is critical. An ECOG score greater than 2 predicts poor treatment outcomes and represents a relative contraindication to therapy. Similarly, patients with extensive and progressive extrahepatic tumor should not undergo treatment. Cases in which more than 75% of the liver parenchyma has been replaced by tumor are at significant risk of hepatic decompensation. If treatment of these patients is undertaken, it should be carefully staged with sublobar administrations. Moreover, cases of advanced cirrhosis and liver dysfunction, as seen with Child–Pugh class C patients, are typically not eligible for embolization because of competing risk of death from liver failure. Liver function tests should be within normal limits for patients with hepatic metastasis, unless the majority of the liver is replaced by tumor.[5] Prior exposure of the liver to external beam radiation may lead to increased toxicity with radioembolization.[9]

Patients clinically eligible for radioembolization undergo planning angiography and ^{99m}Tc-macroaggregated albumin

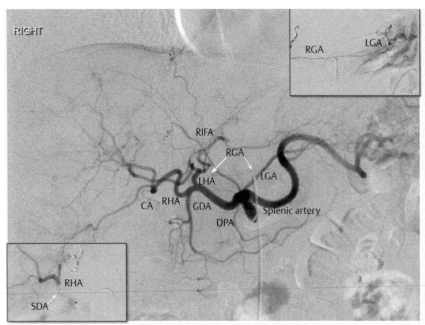

Fig. 23.1 Celiac trunk DSA. Contrast visualization of the splenic artery, left gastric artery (LGA), dorsal pancreatic artery (DPA), gastroduodenal artery (GDA), right gastric artery (RGA), left hepatic artery (LHA), right hepatic artery (RHA), cystic artery (CA), and right inferior phrenic artery (RIFA). Note the variant origin of the GDA, distal to the LHA. Inset views show the RGA (retrograde opacification via the LGA) and supraduodenal artery (SDA) with bowel enhancement (*). Coil embolization of a small terminal left hepatic artery branch was performed for therapeutic flow consolidation.

(MAA) administration. This may reveal absolute contraindications to radioembolization such as uncorrectable hepatoenteric arterial communications and significant hepatopulmonary shunting. Nontarget radiation can lead to gut ulceration (sometimes necessitating surgery), pancreatitis, and radiation pneumonitis. The lungs can tolerate 30 Gray (Gy) per treatment and 50 Gy cumulatively.[10] Additional caution should therefore be exercised when treating patients with underlying pulmonary disease.

23.4 Technique

Before a patient is treated with radioembolization therapy, planning angiography with MAA administration is performed to delineate tumor perfusion and quantify arterial-venous shunting. Meticulous power-injected digital subtraction angiography (DSA) of the visceral and hepatic vasculature is essential. An abdominal aortogram should also be considered if recent cross-sectional imaging did not include an arterial phase; this will aid in visceral catheter selection and identification of extrahepatic tumor supply. The superior mesenteric artery should be assessed for evidence of possible hepatic perfusion, such as a replaced or accessory right hepatic artery or retrograde flow in the gastroduodenal artery (GDA) as is seen with hemodynamically significant celiac stenosis and tumor sump. Delayed images can be used to identify portal vein patency and flow dynamics (hepatopetal). The celiac artery should be catheterized to assess hepatic and intestinal arterial flow, and the common and proper hepatic arteries should be evaluated, along with branch supply to the left and right lobes of the liver. The use of microcatheters and high contrast injection rates (2–3 mL/s for 8–12 mL) is compulsory. It is critical to identify the position of the gastroduodenal and right gastric arteries, the latter of which often arises from the proximal left hepatic artery. Depending on flow dynamics and the intended site of ^{90}Y microsphere infusion, embolization of branch vessels

supplying the intestine should also be considered to prevent nontarget microsphere deposition. Early in an operator's experience, aggressive prophylactic embolization of such branch vessels is commonly employed. Embolization should include the vessel origin to minimize the risk of collateral formation and recanalization, especially if staged therapy is planned. The incidence of gastroduodenal ulceration after radioembolization ranges from 0.7 to 28.6%, with a weighted mean incidence of 4.8%.[11] With experience, routine prophylactic coil embolization of the GDA and right gastric artery can be reconsidered, especially when glass microspheres are used.[12] The cystic, supraduodenal, falciform, accessory left gastric, and right/left inferior phrenic arteries should also be identified (▶ Fig. 23.1). These vessels can be embolized to prevent nontarget embolization or to redistribute therapeutic flow.[13]

The planning angiogram concludes with the administration of MAA. Typically, a microcatheter is placed at the site(s) of intended treatment and a dose of 4 to 5 mCi is infused intraarterially. MAA closely mimics the size, and hence, distribution of ^{90}Y microspheres. This distribution is assessed with planar or single-photon emission computed tomography (SPECT) gamma cameras. A lung shunt fraction (LSF) is calculated (total lung counts/[total lung counts + total liver counts]) given inherent arterial venous connections in liver tumors, which shunt blood to the lungs. Determination of this shunt fraction allows estimation of the lung dose before radioembolization. In addition, scintigraphy, especially SPECT-computed tomography (CT), can detect other instances of nontarget deposition, including gut deposition. When nontarget deposition is identified, angiographic images should be carefully reviewed, with possible repeat angiography and MAA administration after correction of hepatoenteric communications.

Cone-beam CT (CBCT) produces CT-like images in an angiography suite and thus provides information about tissue perfusion in 3 dimensions. In a recent radioembolization study, CBCT was able to identify potentially hazardous instances of nontarget embolization and/or incomplete tumor perfusion that were

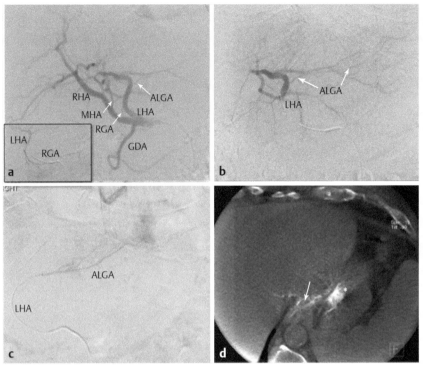

Fig. 23.2 Variant anatomy. **(a)** Common hepatic DSA. Note the variant middle hepatic artery (MHA) with origin off the proper hepatic artery and accessory left gastric artery (ALGA) with origin off the LHA. Inset view shows the RGA with origin off the proximal LHA. **(b)** Microcatheter cannulation in the LHA with contrast opacification of the ALGA. **(c)** Microcatheter placement in the ALGA with DSA demonstrating gastric enhancement and **(d)** CBCT with visualization of gastric (*) and inferior esophageal (*arrow*) perfusion.

not detected on DSA.[14] Delivery of ^{90}Y microspheres without recognition of these vascular patterns can lead to ulcers or incomplete tumor coverage (▶ Fig. 23.2). Instead, CBCT in this study resulted in additional embolization or altered microcatheter treatment positions in one-third of patients, allowing for safe and complete tumor therapy.

Patients who meet the criteria for radioembolization typically return on a separate day for treatment. Single-session radioembolization, in which MAA administration and ^{90}Y microsphere infusion occur on the same day, is a novel concept that has demonstrated feasibility and safety in a pilot study.[15] Radioembolization is considered an outpatient procedure given the lack of macroscopic vessel occlusion and hence the occurrence of only mild postembolization syndrome.

In the radioembolization procedure, a microcatheter is placed into a treatment vessel and a prescribed dose of ^{90}Y microspheres is infused per the manufacturer's guideline. The recommended activity for TheraSphere radioembolization ranges from 80 to 150 Gy, with 120 Gy representing a dose target that balances safety and efficacy. Assuming a uniform distribution of ^{90}Y microspheres, together with a known LSF and liver mass, a TheraSphere dose is calculated. There are several methods for calculating SIR-Spheres dosing, including the body surface area (BSA) and partition models.[3] Both methods assume a uniform distribution of ^{90}Y microspheres and require a known LSF and liver mass and estimation of tumor burden. Activity calculators are available from both manufacturers.

23.5 Outcomes

23.5.1 Hepatocellular Carcinoma

HCC claims more than half a million lives annually.[16] Surveillance programs can lead to early diagnosis of HCC; however, only approximately half of the population at risk receives appropriate screening, resulting in frequent presentation of disease without curative options.[17] More specifically, only approximately 10% of patients with HCC receive therapy with curative intent[18]; thus, most patients are treated with palliative intent. This treatment is often catheter based, namely transarterial chemoembolization (TACE) and ^{90}Y radioembolization.[19] TACE has demonstrated improved survival among patients with HCC in randomized controlled trials and is considered the standard of care for appropriately selected patients with unresectable HCC according to the Barcelona Clinic Liver Cancer (BCLC) staging system, which is endorsed by the American Association for the Study of Liver Diseases.[20,21,22,23] Radioembolization is not recognized by the BCLC staging system; nevertheless, this therapy has received regulatory approval and acknowledgment by NCCN Clinical Practice Guidelines in Oncology (NCCN Guidelines®) for the treatment of HCC (Category 2A; ▶ Table 23.1).[24,25]

Table 23.1 The NCCN categories of evidence

Category 1	Based on high level of evidence, there is uniform NCCN consensus that the intervention is appropriate
Category 2A	Based on lower-level evidence, there is uniform NCCN consensus that the intervention is appropriate
Category 2B	Based on lower-level evidence, there is NCCN consensus that the intervention is appropriate
Category 3	Based on any level of evidence, there is major NCCN disagreement that the intervention is appropriate

Source: Adapted with permission from the NCCN Clinical Practice Guidelines in Oncology (NCCN Guidelines) © 2017 National Comprehensive Cancer Network, Inc. All rights reserved. The NCCN Guidelines and illustrations herein may not be reproduced in any form for any purpose without the express written permission of NCCN. To view the most recent and complete version of the NCCN Guidelines, go online to NCCN.org. The NCCN Guidelines are a work in progress that may be refined as often as new significant data becomes available.

Over the past decade, significant advancement in the science of radioembolization has occurred, along with technical standardization. Radioembolization is now a routine procedure yielding predictable results.[18] Numerous well-controlled studies have documented the safety and tumoricidal effect of ^{90}Y microspheres. In a single-center prospective 5-year cohort study of 291 patients treated with glass radioembolization in 2010, the intricate interaction between tumor characteristics and the degree of hepatic dysfunction was highlighted.[26] As expected, survival was negatively affected by liver dysfunction (survival in patients with Child–Pugh class A, 17.2 months; Child–Pugh class B, 7.7 months). Moreover, time to progression (TTP) was also affected by Child–Pugh class and the presence of PVT (TTP in patients with Child–Pugh class A or B without PVT, 15.5 and 13 months, respectively; Child–Pugh class A or B with PVT, 5.6 and 5.9 months, respectively). These data compare favorably with the results of the Sorafenib Hepatocellular Carcinoma Assessment Randomized Protocol (SHARP), in which sorafenib therapy yielded a TTP of 5.5 months with an overall survival of 10.7 months in a principally Child–Pugh class A population.[27]

Survival and prognostic factors were recently assessed in a retrospective multicenter European registry of 325 patients with unresectable HCC treated with resin radioembolization.[28] The median overall survival was 12.8 months, and survival was significantly influenced by BCLC stage (survival in patients with BCLC stage A, 24.4 months; BCLC stage B, 16.9 months; BCLC stage C, 10 months). The reproducible data achieved among the eight participating centers highlight the technical feasibility of the procedure.[18]

A phase 2 study by Mazzaferro et al[29] assessed the efficacy and safety of radioembolization in patients with intermediate (BCLC-B) and advanced stage HCC (BCLC-C). The median TTP was 11 months, with a median overall survival of 15 months. The authors concluded that radioembolization is a competitive treatment option with a manageable toxicity profile. This study also further validates the reproducible outcomes of radioembolization in select patients, including those with vascular invasion.

No randomized trial has compared radioembolization with TACE for the treatment of HCC; more than 1,000 patients would need to enroll in such a trial to identify significant differences between the two treatments.[30] To date, several comparative effectiveness trials have evaluated radioembolization and TACE with regard to efficacy and their effects on downstaging and quality of life. A large comparative effectiveness study published in 2011 matched 122 patients treated with TACE with 123 patients treated with ^{90}Y radioembolization.[30] Radioembolization resulted in a significantly longer TTP (13.3 months) versus TACE (8.4 months; $p = 0.046$). However, overall survival with the two techniques was not statistically different (TACE, 17.4 months; radioembolization, 20.5 months; $p = 0.232$), likely because of competing risks of death from HCC and cirrhosis.

TACE is a recognized method for downstaging from United Network for Organ Sharing (UNOS) T3 disease to T2 disease.[31] When this downstaging is successful, patients are considered for transplant and granted a Model for End-Stage Liver Disease (MELD) upgrade for HCC. In one study, the downstaging efficacy of TACE and radioembolization was evaluated in 86 patients with T3 disease.[32] Downstaging to UNOS T2 was achieved in 31% of TACE-treated patients and 58% of radioembolization-treated patients ($p = 0.023$). The median TTP was 12.8 months for TACE

and 33.3 months for radioembolization ($p = 0.005$). These results demonstrate that radioembolization outperforms TACE for downstaging UNOS T3 disease to T2 disease, thus expanding the pool of patients considered for curative transplant.

Primary liver tumors are associated with a diminished quality of life. Disease presentation at an advanced stage means that most patients are treated with palliative intent. Because affected patients have a reduced life expectancy, quality of life becomes equally as important as overall survival.[33] In a prospective study, health-related quality of life was compared in patients treated with TACE or ^{90}Y radioembolization. Despite the more advanced disease in patients treated with radioembolization, several quality of life metrics were significantly better, and overall quality of life reached near-significant improvement in patients treated with radioembolization versus those treated with TACE ($p = 0.055$).

As shown in these comparative effectiveness trials, radioembolization outperforms TACE in select patients with regard to TTP, downstaging to transplant, and maintenance of quality of life. Additionally, many investigators now consider ^{90}Y radioembolization a preferred therapy for patients with advanced BCLC B and early BCLC C disease.[18]

23.5.2 Metastatic Colorectal Cancer

Colorectal cancer is the second most commonly diagnosed cancer and the liver is the most common site of metastatic disease in patients with this cancer type, occurring in 20 to 30% of patients at presentation and in up to 60% of patients over the course of their disease.[34,35,36] The majority of patients with mCRC will die because of this disease burden.[37] Complete surgical resection offers the best chance of long-term survival, with 5-year survival rates of approximately 50%.[38] However, only approximately 25% of patients with liver mCRC are candidates for resection at presentation.[39] Moreover, for patients who have undergone resection, tumor recurrence rates approach 50%.[40] For unresectable mCRC, systemic chemotherapy is the standard first-line treatment. Despite significant advances in systemic chemotherapy and biologic agents, most patients with mCRC eventually develop progressive disease.[35] [90]Y radioembolization offers a powerful local treatment for patients with advanced liver mCRC.

Several nonrandomized cohort studies have assessed the benefits of radioembolization in advanced mCRC. Lewandowski et al[41] reported prospective data from 214 patients treated with glass radioembolization for unresectable liver mCRC refractory to standard-of-care therapy. The median overall survival after radioembolization was 10.6 months. On univariate/multivariate analysis, independent predictors of survival included prior exposure to two or fewer cytotoxic agents, which supports the use of radioembolization treatment earlier in the course of disease. Most toxicities with radioembolization were transient and controlled with symptom relief. A recent large retrospective study assessed the use of resin radioembolization in 302 patients with unresectable, chemorefractory mCRC, including patients with extrahepatic disease.[42] The median survival was 10.5 months in this heavily pretreated cohort with an advanced burden of disease. Consistent with previous reports, most complications were minor and resolved without intervention. Overall, these results compare favorably with systemic salvage

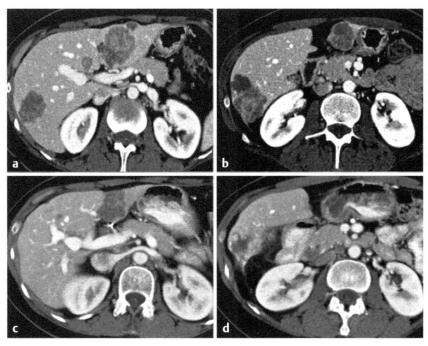

Fig. 23.3 A 42-year-old woman with liver mCRC treated with resection of the primary tumor and multiple lines of chemotherapy, including bevacizumab, with progression of liver disease and rising carcinoembryonic antigen (CEA). **(a,b)** Contrast-enhanced CT of bilobar mCRC. Patient was treated with sequential bilobar glass radioembolization. **(c,d)** Six months after radioembolization, contrast-enhanced CT demonstrates partial response with decreased size of bilobar lesions, along with decreased CEA.

studies, in which median survival has ranged from 3 to 7 months.[43,44]

National Comprehensive Cancer Network (NCCN®) considers radioembolization for mCRC a category 2A recommendation in select patients with chemotherapy-refractory, liver-dominant disease (▶ Table 23.1). According to the European Society for Medical Oncology (ESMO) practice guidelines, resin radioembolization is generally recommended for liver-limited mCRC failing chemotherapy based on retrospective and case-control studies (▶ Fig. 23.3).

Randomized controlled trials are needed to better define the role of radioembolization in the treatment of mCRC. The results of one such study, SIRFLOX, were recently reported. This study was designed to assess the efficacy and safety of combining folinic acid, fluorouracil, and oxaliplatin (FOLFOX) ±bevacizumab with or without resin radioembolization as first-line treatment for patients with unresectable liver-only or liver-dominant tumor burden. The primary end point was progression-free survival (PFS) based on Response Evaluation Criteria in Solid Tumors (RECIST). A total of 530 patients were randomized; 40% had extrahepatic disease. The addition of resin radioembolization to standard chemotherapy failed to improve overall PFS, although the median liver PFS was significantly extended (chemotherapy plus radioembolization, 20.5 months; chemotherapy alone, 12.6 months, *p* = 0.002). The addition of radioembolization was associated with acceptable toxicity. An overall survival analysis combining data from sister trials is awaited.[45] These investigations seek to determine the appropriate integration of radioembolization, as a proven safe and efficacious treatment, into treatment regimens for one of the most common causes of cancer death.[46]

23.5.3 Neuroendocrine Tumors

Neuroendocrine tumors (NETs) arise from neural and endocrine organs throughout the body, most commonly the gastrointestinal

system and pancreas. The World Health Organization (WHO) classifies well-differentiated gastroenteropancreatic NETs into low-grade and intermediate-grade tumors; most poorly differentiated tumors are considered high-grade tumors based on mitotic count/Ki-67 proliferative index.[47] Well-differentiated tumors of the digestive system are traditionally called carcinoid and pancreatic neuroendocrine (islet cell) tumors. These tumors are often indolent, even in the setting of metastatic disease, and thus are labeled "cancers in slow motion."[48]

The clinical presentation of NETs often occurs in the setting of metastatic disease, resulting from tumor biochemical activity or bulk symptoms. Symptoms of hormonal excess from islet cell and carcinoid tumors are often well controlled with somatostatin analogs (specifically, octreotide and lanreotide).[49]

Radioembolization is a potent local therapeutic option for liver metastatic NET (mNET), especially for low-grade tumors with hormonal symptoms or tumors that progress on long-acting somatostatin analogues. Treatment with ^{90}Y microspheres is effective for both tumor control and symptom relief.[50] As with other arterial therapies, ^{90}Y device selection for the treatment of liver mNET is institution-specific, level 1 evidence guiding patient selection and timing of treatment has not been established. However, radioembolization is an NCCN category 2B option for those considering a hepatic-directed therapy for hepatic-predominant metastatic gastrointestinal NET, if disease progression after treatment (▶ Table 23.1).[25]

A recent meta-analysis of resin radioembolization for liver mNET demonstrated a pooled response rate of 50%, a disease control rate of 86%, and improved overall survival for patients responding to therapy versus nonresponders. These rates compare favorably with the rates observed for somatostatin analogs, cytotoxic chemotherapy, and newer biologic therapies.[51] Yang et al[52] performed a comparative review of radioembolization, bland embolization, and chemoembolization for the treatment of unresectable liver mNET. The three transarterial therapies demonstrated comparable efficacy in terms of tumor response, symptom palliation, and patient survival. Side effect profiles vary among the techniques; however, there were no significant differences in the rate of major complications.

23.6 Complications

Radioembolization has a favorable toxicity profile but knowledge of potential complications is still essential. Appropriate patient selection through the use of a multidisciplinary approach can improve outcomes and decrease the risk of complications. Moreover, meticulous pretreatment angiography is critical to minimizing adverse advents. The most common side effect of radioembolization is transient fatigue, occurring in approximately 80% of patients, likely due to low-dose radiation effects on the liver parenchyma.[53] This effect is self-limited and abated by a tapering course of oral steroids. Other potential complications are discussed in the following sections.

23.6.1 Postembolization Syndrome

Postembolization syndrome, which has been reported after chemoembolization, is rare after radioembolization. Patients with this condition may experience mild right upper quadrant or generalized abdominal discomfort that is typically responsive to nonprescription analgesics.[5]

23.6.2 Gastroenteritis/Gastrointestinal Ulcer

Gastrointestinal complications occur because of hepatoenteric arterial communications with resultant extrahepatic microsphere deposition. It is essential that these vascular connections are identified and possibly embolized before microsphere infusion. Review of the left hepatic arteriogram should allow for identification of the accessory left gastric and inferior esophageal arteries.[5] The falciform artery is also commonly seen arising from the left hepatic artery; if technically feasible, this artery should be embolized with coils. Alternatively, ice can be applied to the anterior abdomen before microsphere infusion to cause thermal vasoconstriction, thus preventing periumbilical skin injury.[54]

Prophylactic use of gastric acid suppression is recommended after ^{90}Y microsphere infusion. If gut ulceration is suspected, endoscopy with biopsy should be performed to confirm the diagnosis. Overall, treatment with surgical resection is required in 0.4% of cases.[55]

23.6.3 Biliary Injury

Given the small size of ^{90}Y microspheres, they can enter the peribiliary plexus and cause injury due to ischemia or radiation.[56] Possible injuries include bile duct stricture, cholangitis, biliary necrosis, and biloma. As mentioned, violation of the sphincter of Oddi markedly increases the risk of intrahepatic abscess formation.[6] Radioembolization in the setting of biliary obstruction caused by a tumor is safe assuming a lack of acute cholangitis and near-normal serum bilirubin.[57] In general, cirrhosis is protective against biliary complications because of a robust peribiliary vascular plexus.[58]

Radiation cholecystitis requiring cholecystectomy is rare (< 2%). However, imaging findings of gallbladder inflammation are common and may be accompanied by right upper quadrant pain.[59] Identifying the cystic artery and infusing microspheres distal to its origin will prevent injury.

23.6.4 Radioembolization-Induced Liver Disease

Radioembolization-induced liver disease (REILD) is a potentially life-threatening complication of radioembolization that occurs in approximately 4% of cases, usually 4 to 8 weeks after therapy.[5] REILD is characterized by ascites, elevated alkaline phosphatase level, thrombocytopenia, and veno-occlusive-type disease on biopsy.[60] REILD is caused by overexposure of the hepatic parenchyma to radiation; based on studies of external beam radiation, the normal liver tolerance for radiation is approximately 30 Gy.[61] Previous exposure to external beam radiation may lead to increased liver toxicity with radioembolization.[9] Moreover, repeat whole-liver radioembolization is a significant risk factor for the development of REILD.[62]

Routine assessment of liver function is recommended after radioembolization to screen for manifestations of REILD and hepatic dysfunction. In a single-center evaluation of resin radioembolization, liver function toxicity (grades 1–4) was seen in 58% of infusions. Grade 3 or higher toxicities occurred in 9% of infusions, which is similar to the 9.8% incidence of grade 3 toxicities reported with glass microspheres.[59,63] Grade 3 or higher biliary toxicities are more common in patients with metastatic disease than with HCC because of the previously mentioned protective effect of cirrhosis and the frequent use of hepatotoxic chemotherapy in patients with metastatic disease.[59]

23.6.5 Hepatic Fibrosis/Portal Hypertension

Hepatic fibrosis and/or portal hypertension may occur after radioembolization. In a study of patients with secondary hepatic malignancy treated with bilobar radioembolization, a mean decrease in liver volume of 11.8% and mean increase in splenic volume of 27.9% were identified.[64] Radioembolization may yield imaging changes of portal hypertension; however, clinical sequelae, namely thrombocytopenia and variceal bleeding, are rare.[5]

23.6.6 Radiation Pneumonitis

Radiation pneumonitis occurs rarely when standard dosimetry models are used, as these techniques limit the delivery of radiation to the lung to 30 Gy per treatment and 50 Gy cumulatively.[10] When radiation pneumonitis does occur, it can manifest as a bat-wing-type consolidation on imaging.[65]

23.6.7 Lymphopenia

Lymphopenia is a possible sequela of radioembolization, given the sensitivity of lymphocytes to radiation. A decrease in lymphocyte count of more than 25% can occur with glass radioembolization; however, no opportunistic infection has been described.[66,67]

23.7 Advances and New Concepts

With increasing clinical experience, the potential uses for radioembolization are expanding, including into new areas such as radiation segmentectomy and radiation lobectomy. Although these concepts have not been tested in a diverse multicenter setting, they represent a technological evolution that lays the foundation for future rigorous testing.

23.7.1 Radiation Segmentectomy

According to the BCLC staging system, resection and ablation are curative treatment options for HCC tumors 3 cm or smaller.[21] Ablation is considered high risk when the lesion is located in close proximity to critical structures.[68] Combining microcatheter technology and the localized radiation emission properties of ^{90}Y microspheres, highly selective radioembolization, or radiation segmentectomy, is a novel treatment alternative to ablation for high-risk tumor locations (▶ Fig. 23.4).

A recent study assessed the efficacy of radiation segmentectomy in solitary HCC tumors that were not amenable to ablation or resection.[69] Patients in this study were treatment naïve and had solitary HCC tumors that were 5 cm or smaller. Radiation segmentectomy was defined as ^{90}Y microsphere infusion limited to 2 or fewer Couinaud segments. Dosing was achieved by infusing a calculated lobar dose (120–150 Gy) into a segmental tumor-feeding vessel. With this technique, segmental doses are higher than lobar doses by the ratio of lobar to segmental liver volumes. This methodology minimizes radiation to the nontumorous liver parenchyma while delivering ablation-type tumor doses. Among the 99 patients with imaging follow-up, complete response was achieved in 47%, partial response in 39%, and stable disease in 12% according to modified RECIST (mRECIST) criteria. The median TTP was 33.1 months. Approximately one-third of the study patients underwent transplant after radiation segmentectomy, allowing for radiology-pathology correlation. Pathology revealed 90 to 100% tumor necrosis in all patients. More complete tumor necrosis was observed when the radiation dose to the segment exceeded 190 Gy ($p = 0.03$), suggesting that this level could be used as a threshold dose for radiation segmentectomy.

Achieving complete pathologic necrosis with radiofrequency ablation is dependent on the lesion size and location. In one study, complete pathologic necrosis was achieved in 65.7% of lesions treated with radiofrequency ablation, with a mean lesion size of 2.5 cm.[70] These data provide a framework for evaluating the 52% complete pathologic necrosis rate for radiation segmentectomy in lesions up to 5 cm in size.[69] Notably, radiation segmentectomy also avoids transhepatic tumor puncture and eliminates the potential risk of tumor tract seeding inherent to radiofrequency ablation.

23.7.2 Radiation Lobectomy

In contrast to radiation segmentectomy in which lobar radiation doses are delivered sublobar, radiation lobectomy describes changes after the lobar delivery of therapy. The ipsilateral atrophy and contralateral hypertrophy seen with lobar radioembolization comprise the atrophy-hypertrophy complex.[71] Radiation lobectomy is described in patients with right lobe disease that is potentially amenable to curative resection but has been excluded because of a small future liver remnant (FLR), often expressed as a percent ratio of the whole liver volume. Traditionally, these patients are treated with portal vein embolization (PVE), resulting in redirection of portal flow, with subsequent FLR hypertrophy and surgical resection. The required FLR varies based on underlying liver pathology, from approximately 20% (normal) to 40% (cirrhosis).[72,73] Because many intrahepatic tumors are primarily supplied by the hepatic artery, PVE does not provide local tumor control. Instead, proangiogenic factors after PVE may lead to tumor progression, including an increased chance of contralateral hepatic metastasis.[74,75,76,77,78] Radiation lobectomy is a single procedure that provides local tumor control with initiation of the atrophy-hypertrophy complex and can be used as a bridge to resection. Studies have demonstrated a slower rate of portal flow diversion with radiation lobectomy than with PVE, which may limit proangiogenic tumor progression.[71] A biologic test of time inherent to this slow portal flow diversion can identify patients best suited for resection.[18,71]

Vouche et al[79] performed a comprehensive time-dependent analysis of liver volumes after lobar radioembolization. In this study, 83 patients met the inclusion criteria, including isolated

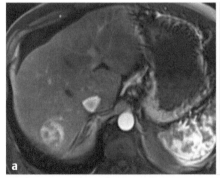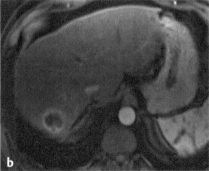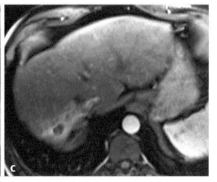

Fig. 23.4 A 54-year-old man with hepatitis C cirrhosis complicated by HCC. (a) Arterial phase MR imaging demonstrates 4-cm hypervascular lesion in segment 7 with washout on delayed images, consistent with HCC. Given the subdiaphragmatic tumor location, the decision was made to preform radiation segmentectomy. A ^{90}Y microsphere dose of > 200 Gy was infused into segment 7. (b) Arterial phase MR image obtained 1 month after radioembolization demonstrates lack of central enhancement with thin residual rim enhancement and decreased lesion size, compatible with a complete response by mRECIST. (c) Arterial phase MR image obtained 4 months after treatment shows further decreased size of HCC with lack of enhancement and atrophy of segment 7 with reactive enhancement.

right lobe tumor not amenable to immediate resection. Patients were treated with radiation lobectomy using glass ^{90}Y microspheres for right lobe HCC, colorectal cancer, and cholangiocarcinoma. A significant decrease in right lobe volume, together with hypertrophy of the left lobe, was seen 1 month after treatment, resulting in a 7% increase in the FLR ($p < 0.001$). After more than 9 months, the median percent FLR hypertrophy had reached 45% ($p < 0.001$). Similarly, Theyson et al[80] reported time-dependent changes of cirrhotic liver volumes after lobar radioembolization for HCC. At 6 months after right lobe treatment, the left lobe volume had increased by 30.8% ($p < 0.01$), confirming compensatory hypertrophy even with background cirrhosis. Future studies comparing long-term outcomes with PVE versus radiation lobectomy are warranted.

23.8 Posttreatment

Radioembolization is performed as an outpatient procedure because of its favorable toxicity profile. After four half-lives, or approximately 2 weeks, the majority of yttrium-90 has decayed. Physicians at the interventional oncology clinic see patients at this time to assess for adverse events and to plan for additional treatment, as most whole-liver therapies are carried out as sequential lobar therapies. Changes in biochemical parameters and performance status are recorded to ensure that there are no contraindications to continued therapy. Cross-sectional imaging is performed at approximately 1 month to assess response in the treated lobe, to identify possible complications, and to establish a new baseline for the untreated lobe. Once treatment of the liver is complete, serial imaging should occur at 3-month intervals, often together with assessment of relevant tumor markers and liver function.

23.9 Conclusion

Radioembolization offers a minimally invasive, safe, and efficacious treatment option for primary and secondary liver tumors. Treatment is palliative; however, technical advances such as radiation segmentectomy and neoadjuvant applications such as radiation lobectomy and downstaging have expanded the population of patients who can be treated with curative intent. Supportive data are improving, and radioembolization is now recognized by NCCN as a treatment option for a variety of tumor types. Future studies should continue to refine patient selection and timing of therapy.

References

[1] Campbell AM, Bailey IH, Burton MA. Analysis of the distribution of intra-arterial microspheres in human liver following hepatic yttrium-90 microsphere therapy. Phys Med Biol. 2000; 45(4):1023–1033

[2] TheraSphere Yttrium-90 Microspheres Package Insert, MDS Nordion. Kanata. 2004

[3] SIR-Spheres Yttrium-90 Microsphere Package Insert, SIRTeX Medical. Lane Cove. 2004

[4] Kulik LM, Carr BI, Mulcahy MF, et al. Safety and efficacy of 90Y radiotherapy for hepatocellular carcinoma with and without portal vein thrombosis. Hepatology. 2008; 47(1):71–81

[5] Riaz A, Awais R, Salem R. Side effects of yttrium-90 radioembolization. Front Oncol. 2014; 4:198

[6] Kim W, Clark TW, Baum RA, Soulen MC. Risk factors for liver abscess formation after hepatic chemoembolization. J Vasc Interv Radiol. 2001; 12(8): 965–968

[7] Cholapranee A, van Houten D, Deitrick G, et al. Risk of liver abscess formation in patients with prior biliary intervention following yttrium-90 radioembolization. Cardiovasc Intervent Radiol. 2015; 38(2):397–400

[8] Khan W, Sullivan KL, McCann JW, et al. Moxifloxacin prophylaxis for chemoembolization or embolization in patients with previous biliary interventions: a pilot study. AJR Am J Roentgenol. 2011; 197(2):W343–5

[9] Lam MG, Abdelmaksoud MH, Chang DT, et al. Safety of 90Y radioembolization in patients who have undergone previous external beam radiation therapy. Int J Radiat Oncol Biol Phys. 2013; 87(2):323–329

[10] Ho S, Lau WY, Leung TW, Chan M, Johnson PJ, Li AK. Clinical evaluation of the partition model for estimating radiation doses from yttrium-90 microspheres in the treatment of hepatic cancer. Eur J Nucl Med. 1997; 24(3):293–298

[11] Naymagon S, Warner RR, Patel K, et al. Gastroduodenal ulceration associated with radioembolization for the treatment of hepatic tumors: an institutional experience and review of the literature. Dig Dis Sci. 2010; 55(9):2450–2458

[12] Hamoui N, Minocha J, Memon K, et al. Prophylactic embolization of the gastroduodenal and right gastric arteries is not routinely necessary before radioembolization with glass microspheres. J Vasc Interv Radiol. 2013; 24 (11):1743–1745

[13] Abdelmaksoud MH, Louie JD, Kothary N, et al. Consolidation of hepatic arterial inflow by embolization of variant hepatic arteries in preparation for yttrium-90 radioembolization. J Vasc Interv Radiol. 2011; 22(10):1364–1371. e1

[14] Louie JD, Kothary N, Kuo WT, et al. Incorporating cone-beam CT into the treatment planning for yttrium-90 radioembolization. J Vasc Interv Radiol. 2009; 20(5):606–613

[15] Gates VL, Marshall KG, Salzig K, Williams M, Lewandowski RJ, Salem R. Outpatient single-session yttrium-90 glass microsphere radioembolization. J Vasc Interv Radiol. 2014; 25(2):266–270

[16] El-Serag HB. Hepatocellular carcinoma and hepatitis C in the United States. Hepatology. 2002; 36(5) Suppl 1:S74–S83

[17] Kim WR, Gores GJ, Benson JT, Therneau TM, Melton LJ, III. Mortality and hospital utilization for hepatocellular carcinoma in the United States. Gastroenterology. 2005; 129(2):486–493

[18] Salem R, Mazzaferro V, Sangro B. Yttrium 90 radioembolization for the treatment of hepatocellular carcinoma: biological lessons, current challenges, and clinical perspectives. Hepatology. 2013; 58(6):2188–2197

[19] Molvar C, Lewandowski R. Yttrium-90 Radioembolization of Hepatocellular Carcinoma-Performance, Technical Advances, and Future Concepts. Semin Intervent Radiol. 2015; 32(4):388–397

[20] Llovet JM, Brú C, Bruix J. Prognosis of hepatocellular carcinoma: the BCLC staging classification. Semin Liver Dis. 1999; 19(3):329–338

[21] Llovet JM, Burroughs A, Bruix J. Hepatocellular carcinoma. Lancet. 2003; 362 (9399):1907–1917

[22] Llovet JM, Real MI, Montaña X, et al. Barcelona Liver Cancer Group. Arterial embolisation or chemoembolisation versus symptomatic treatment in patients with unresectable hepatocellular carcinoma: a randomised controlled trial. Lancet. 2002; 359(9319):1734–1739

[23] Lo CM, Ngan H, Tso WK, et al. Randomized controlled trial of transarterial lipiodol chemoembolization for unresectable hepatocellular carcinoma. Hepatology. 2002; 35(5):1164–1171

[24] Thomas MB, Jaffe D, Choti MM, et al. Hepatocellular carcinoma: consensus recommendations of the National Cancer Institute Clinical Trials Planning Meeting. J Clin Oncol. 2010; 28(25):3994–4005

[25] NCCN Clinical Practice Guidelines in Oncology. (NCCN Guidelines Version 2.2016) for hepatobiliary cancers. © 2016 National Comprehensive Cancer Network, Inc. Available at: www.NCCN.org. Accessed January 5, 2017

[26] Salem R, Lewandowski RJ, Mulcahy MF, et al. Radioembolization for hepatocellular carcinoma using Yttrium-90 microspheres: a comprehensive report of long-term outcomes. Gastroenterology. 2010; 138(1):52–64

[27] Llovet JM, Ricci S, Mazzaferro V, et al. SHARP Investigators Study Group. Sorafenib in advanced hepatocellular carcinoma. N Engl J Med. 2008; 359(4): 378–390

[28] Sangro B, Carpanese L, Cianni R, et al. European Network on Radioembolization with Yttrium-90 Resin Microspheres (ENRY). Survival after yttrium-90 resin microsphere radioembolization of hepatocellular carcinoma across Barcelona clinic liver cancer stages: a European evaluation. Hepatology. 2011; 54(3):868–878

[29] Mazzaferro V, Sposito C, Bhoori S, et al. Yttrium-90 radioembolization for intermediate-advanced hepatocellular carcinoma: a phase 2 study. Hepatology. 2013; 57(5):1826–1837

[30] Salem R, Lewandowski RJ, Kulik L, et al. Radioembolization results in longer time-to-progression and reduced toxicity compared with chemoembolization in patients with hepatocellular carcinoma. Gastroenterology. 2011; 140(2):497–507.e2

[31] Hanje AJ, Yao FY. Current approach to down-staging of hepatocellular carcinoma prior to liver transplantation. Curr Opin Organ Transplant. 2008; 13(3):234–240

[32] Lewandowski RJ, Kulik LM, Riaz A, et al. A comparative analysis of transarterial downstaging for hepatocellular carcinoma: chemoembolization versus radioembolization. Am J Transplant. 2009; 9(8):1920–1928

[33] Salem R, Gilbertsen M, Butt Z, et al. Increased quality of life among hepatocellular carcinoma patients treated with radioembolization, compared with chemoembolization. Clin Gastroenterol Hepatol. 2013; 11(10):1358–1365.e1

[34] Mahnken AH, Pereira PL, de Baère T. Interventional oncologic approaches to liver metastases. Radiology. 2013; 266(2):407–430

[35] Wang DS, Louie JD, Sze DY. Intra-arterial therapies for metastatic colorectal cancer. Semin Intervent Radiol. 2013; 30(1):12–20

[36] Weiss L, Grundmann E, Torhorst J, et al. Haematogenous metastatic patterns in colonic carcinoma: an analysis of 1541 necropsies. J Pathol. 1986; 150(3):195–203

[37] Geoghegan JG, Scheele J. Treatment of colorectal liver metastases. Br J Surg. 1999; 86(2):158–169

[38] Wei AC, Greig PD, Grant D, Taylor B, Langer B, Gallinger S. Survival after hepatic resection for colorectal metastases: a 10-year experience. Ann Surg Oncol. 2006; 13(5):668–676

[39] Khatri VP, Chee KG, Petrelli NJ. Modern multimodality approach to hepatic colorectal metastases: solutions and controversies. Surg Oncol. 2007; 16(1):71–83

[40] Bhattacharjya S, Aggarwal R, Davidson BR. Intensive follow-up after liver resection for colorectal liver metastases: results of combined serial tumour marker estimations and computed tomography of the chest and abdomen - a prospective study. Br J Cancer. 2006; 95(1):21–26

[41] Lewandowski RJ, Memon K, Mulcahy MF, et al. Twelve-year experience of radioembolization for colorectal hepatic metastases in 214 patients: survival by era and chemotherapy. Eur J Nucl Med Mol Imaging. 2014; 41(10):1861–1869

[42] Saxena A, Meteling B, Kapoor J, Golani S, Morris DL, Bester L. Is Yttrium-90 Radioembolization a Viable Treatment Option for Unresectable, Chemorefractory Colorectal Cancer Liver Metastases? A Large Single-Center Experience of 302 Patients. Ann Surg Oncol. 2015; 22(3):794–802

[43] Wasan H, Kennedy A, Coldwell D, Sangro B, Salem R. Integrating radioembolization with chemotherapy in the treatment paradigm for unresectable colorectal liver metastases. Am J Clin Oncol. 2012; 35(3):293–301

[44] Seidensticker R, Denecke T, Kraus P, et al. Matched-pair comparison of radioembolization plus best supportive care versus best supportive care alone for chemotherapy refractory liver-dominant colorectal metastases. Cardiovasc Intervent Radiol. 2012; 35(5):1066–1073

[45] van Hazel GA, Heinemann V, Sharma NK, et al. SIRFLOX: Randomized phase III trial comparing first-line mFOLFOX6 (plus or minus bevacizumab) versus mFOLFOX6 (plus or minus bevacizumab) plus selective internal radiation therapy in patients with metastatic colorectal cancer. J Clin Oncol. 2016; 34(15):1723–1731

[46] Molvar C, Lewandowski RJ. Intra-Arterial Therapies for Liver Masses: Data Distilled. Radiol Clin North Am. 2015; 53(5):973–984

[47] Bosman FT, Carneiro F, Hruban RH, Theise ND. WHO Classification of Tumours of the Digestive System. IARC Press. 2010;

[48] Moertel CG. Karnofsky memorial lecture. An odyssey in the land of small tumors. J Clin Oncol. 1987; 5(10):1502–1522

[49] Rindi G, Wiedenmann B. Neuroendocrine neoplasms of the gut and pancreas: new insights. Nat Rev Endocrinol. 2011; 8(1):54–64

[50] Memon K, Lewandowski RJ, Mulcahy MF, et al. Radioembolization for neuroendocrine liver metastases: safety, imaging, and long-term outcomes. Int J Radiat Oncol Biol Phys. 2012; 83(3):887–894

[51] Devcic Z, Rosenberg J, Braat AJ, et al. The efficacy of hepatic 90Y resin radioembolization for metastatic neuroendocrine tumors: a meta-analysis. J Nucl Med. 2014; 55(9):1404–1410

[52] Yang TX, Chua TC, Morris DL. Radioembolization and chemoembolization for unresectable neuroendocrine liver metastases - a systematic review. Surg Oncol. 2012; 21(4):299–308

[53] Lewandowski RJ, Thurston KG, Goin JE, et al. 90Y microsphere (TheraSphere) treatment for unresectable colorectal cancer metastases of the liver: response to treatment at targeted doses of 135–150 Gy as measured by [18F] fluorodeoxyglucose positron emission tomography and computed tomographic imaging. J Vasc Interv Radiol. 2005; 16(12):1641–1651

[54] Wang DS, Louie JD, Kothary N, Shah RP, Sze DY. Prophylactic topically applied ice to prevent cutaneous complications of nontarget chemoembolization and radioembolization. J Vasc Interv Radiol. 2013; 24(4):596–600

[55] Murthy R, Brown DB, Salem R, et al. Gastrointestinal complications associated with hepatic arterial Yttrium-90 microsphere therapy. J Vasc Interv Radiol. 2007; 18(4):5:53–561, quiz 562

[56] Liu DM, Salem R, Bui JT, et al. Angiographic considerations in patients undergoing liver-directed therapy. J Vasc Interv Radiol. 2005; 16(7):911–935

[57] Gaba RC, Riaz A, Lewandowski RJ, et al. Safety of yttrium-90 microsphere radioembolization in patients with biliary obstruction. J Vasc Interv Radiol. 2010; 21(8):1213–1218

[58] Demachi H, Matsui O, Kawamori Y, Ueda K, Takashima T. The protective effect of portoarterial shunts after experimental hepatic artery embolization in rats with liver cirrhosis. Cardiovasc Intervent Radiol. 1995; 18(2):97–101

[59] Atassi B, Bangash AK, Lewandowski RJ, et al. Biliary sequelae following radioembolization with Yttrium-90 microspheres. J Vasc Interv Radiol. 2008; 19(5):691–697

[60] Riaz A, Lewandowski RJ, Kulik LM, et al. Complications following radioembolization with yttrium-90 microspheres: a comprehensive literature review. J Vasc Interv Radiol. 2009; 20(9):1121–1130–, quiz 1131

[61] Russell AH, Clyde C, Wasserman TH, Turner SS, Rotman M. Accelerated hyperfractionated hepatic irradiation in the management of patients with liver metastases: results of the RTOG dose escalating protocol. Int J Radiat Oncol Biol Phys. 1993; 27(1):117–123

[62] Lam MG, Louie JD, Iagaru AH, Goris ML, Sze DY. Safety of repeated yttrium-90 radioembolization. Cardiovasc Intervent Radiol. 2013; 36(5):1320–1328

[63] Piana PM, Gonsalves CF, Sato T, et al. Toxicities after radioembolization with yttrium-90 SIR-spheres: incidence and contributing risk factors at a single center. J Vasc Interv Radiol. 2011; 22(10):1373–1379

[64] Jakobs TF, Saleem S, Atassi B, et al. Fibrosis, portal hypertension, and hepatic volume changes induced by intra-arterial radiotherapy with 90yttrium microspheres. Dig Dis Sci. 2008; 53(9):2556–2563

[65] Leung TW, Lau WY, Ho SK, et al. Radiation pneumonitis after selective internal radiation treatment with intraarterial 90yttrium-microspheres for inoperable hepatic tumors. Int J Radiat Oncol Biol Phys. 1995; 33(4):919–924

[66] Salem R, Lewandowski RJ, Atassi B, et al. Treatment of unresectable hepatocellular carcinoma with use of 90Y microspheres (TheraSphere): safety, tumor response, and survival. J Vasc Interv Radiol. 2005; 16(12):1627–1639

[67] Carr BI. Hepatic arterial 90Yttrium glass microspheres (Therasphere) for unresectable hepatocellular carcinoma: interim safety and survival data on 65 patients. Liver Transpl. 2004; 10(2) Suppl 1:S107–S110

[68] Crocetti L, de Baere T, Lencioni R. Quality improvement guidelines for radiofrequency ablation of liver tumours. Cardiovasc Intervent Radiol. 2010; 33(1):11–17

[69] Vouche M, Habib A, Ward TJ, et al. Unresectable solitary hepatocellular carcinoma not amenable to radiofrequency ablation: multicenter radiology-pathology correlation and survival of radiation segmentectomy. Hepatology. 2014; 60(1):192–201

[70] Lu DS, Yu NC, Raman SS, et al. Percutaneous radiofrequency ablation of hepatocellular carcinoma as a bridge to liver transplantation. Hepatology. 2005; 41(5):1130–1137

[71] Gaba RC, Lewandowski RJ, Kulik LM, et al. Radiation lobectomy: preliminary findings of hepatic volumetric response to lobar yttrium-90 radioembolization. Ann Surg Oncol. 2009; 16(6):1587–1596

[72] Kubota K, Makuuchi M, Kusaka K, et al. Measurement of liver volume and hepatic functional reserve as a guide to decision-making in resectional surgery for hepatic tumors. Hepatology. 1997; 26(5):1176–1181

[73] Zorzi D, Laurent A, Pawlik TM, Lauwers GY, Vauthey JN, Abdalla EK. Chemotherapy-associated hepatotoxicity and surgery for colorectal liver metastases. Br J Surg. 2007; 94(3):274–286

[74] Belghiti J, Benhaïm L. Portal vein occlusion prior to extensive resection in colorectal liver metastasis: a necessity rather than an option! Ann Surg Oncol. 2009; 16(5):1098–1099

[75] Pamecha V, Glantzounis G, Davies N, Fusai G, Sharma D, Davidson B. Long-term survival and disease recurrence following portal vein embolisation prior to major hepatectomy for colorectal metastases. Ann Surg Oncol. 2009; 16(5):1202–1207

[76] Pamecha V, Levene A, Grillo F, Woodward N, Dhillon A, Davidson BR. Effect of portal vein embolisation on the growth rate of colorectal liver metastases. Br J Cancer. 2009; 100(4):617–622

[77] Azoulay D, Castaing D, Smail A, et al. Resection of nonresectable liver metastases from colorectal cancer after percutaneous portal vein embolization. Ann Surg. 2000; 231(4):480–486

[78] Hoekstra LT, van Lienden KP, Verheij J, van der Loos CM, Heger M, van Gulik TM. Enhanced tumor growth after portal vein embolization in a rabbit tumor model. J Surg Res. 2013; 180(1):89–96

[79] Vouche M, Lewandowski RJ, Atassi R, et al. Radiation lobectomy: time-dependent analysis of future liver remnant volume in unresectable liver cancer as a bridge to resection. J Hepatol. 2013; 59(5):1029–1036

[80] Theysohn JM, Ertle J, Müller S, et al. Hepatic volume changes after lobar selective internal radiation therapy (SIRT) of hepatocellular carcinoma. Clin Radiol. 2014; 69(2):172–178

24 Liver Transplant Complications: Diagnosis and Management

Mikin V. Patel and Brian Funaki

24.1 Introduction

Orthotopic liver transplantation (LT) is the treatment of choice for end-stage hepatic disease. Over the years, improvements in surgical techniques, organ preservation therapies, and detection of postoperative complications have improved post-LT care such that 1-, 5-, and 10-year patient survival rates have increased to 88, 80, and 74%, respectively.[1,2] However, vascular and biliary complications continue to persist at an estimated rate of 25 to 27%.[3] Interventional radiology is an essential component of a successful LT program because it provides minimally invasive solutions to potentially lethal complications, typically precluding the need for major surgery or retransplantation.[3,4,5,6,7]

24.2 Vascular Complications

In LT patients with hepatic failure, bile leak, gastrointestinal bleeding, or sepsis, vascular complications are a primary diagnostic consideration, and prompt treatment is needed to salvage the graft in such cases.[8,9,10] Vascular complications occur in approximately 8 to 15% of LT patients; the incidence of arterial complications is approximately 5 to 10%; portal venous complications occur in 3 to 5% and outflow venous complications in < 2%.[11] Clinical and biochemical markers are generally nonspecific, so diagnosis requires imaging, usually with Doppler ultrasound (US), contrast-enhanced computed tomography (CT), or magnetic resonance (MR) imaging.[3,8]

24.2.1 Arterial Complications

Arterial complications include hepatic artery thrombosis (HAT), hepatic artery stenosis (HAS), and hepatic artery pseudoaneurysm (HAP), with incidences of 0.8 to 9.3%, 1.9 to 16.6%, and 0 to 3%, respectively.[11,12]

Hepatic Artery Thrombosis

Despite the use of modern surgical techniques for LT, patients undergoing this procedure are at risk of developing thrombosis at the arterial anastomosis. Multiple etiologies have been proposed for HAT, including differences in size of donor and recipient vessels, prolonged cold ischemia time, previous transcatheter arterial chemoembolization, variant arterial anatomy, and positive donor cytomegalovirus serology.[13,14] HAT can readily be diagnosed with Doppler US; on US, HAT will present as absent flow in the proper hepatic and intrahepatic arteries. CT and MR can also be used to perform contrast angiography, which will demonstrate abrupt cutoff of the hepatic artery, usually at the site of anastomosis.

Clinically, HAT is generally divided into early (< 30 days after LT) and late (> 30 days after LT) thrombosis, although this definition may vary. Early HAT invariably leads to devastating complications such as liver parenchymal necrosis, biliary necrosis, and sepsis if not treated. These patients face a mortality rate of 33.3% and are usually urgently listed for retransplantation.[14,15] Given the limited donor pool, however, revascularization is frequently attempted, with endovascular techniques emerging as the less invasive treatments of choice.[12,16,17,18,19] Prompt revascularization within 7 or 14 days of HAT yields graft survival rates of 81 and 62%, respectively, but graft survival drops to 0% if revascularization is delayed beyond 14 days.[18]

Late HAT can remain clinically silent for months or years with an insidious course characterized by cholangitis, relapsing fevers, and bacteremia with nonspecific symptoms.[20,21] Arterial collaterals develop from the diaphragm, retroperitoneum, and the omentum as early as 2 weeks after LT, which explains why late HAT does not present with the devastating symptoms seen with early HAT.[12,22,23] As with early HAT, however, endovascular revascularization is a viable treatment option, yielding graft survival rates of 50%.[18]

The first successful attempts at endovascular treatment of HAT began in 1989 with intra-arterial thrombolytic (IAT) infusion of urokinase (UK).[24] Since then, the use of IAT for HAT has been further studied and refined, yielding promising outcomes (▶ Table 24.1).[16,19,25,26,27,28,29,30,31,32,33,34,35,36] Larger reviews have found that IAT was successful in 47 of 69 (68%) patients, with complications occurring in 18 (26%) patients, 3 of which were fatal.[12] The risks of IAT include bleeding and rethrombosis of the hepatic artery; however, IAT has been used safely and effectively as early as 4 hours after transplant.[33] Nevertheless, before beginning IAT, the treatment team must be prepared to address hemorrhagic complications with termination of IAT, supportive blood products, and endovascular or surgical hemostasis as needed. Of note, recent research has raised concerns about the safety and efficacy of IAT, with a recanalization rate of 46% and a major complication rate of 42%.[36]

IAT for HAT (▶ Fig. 24.1) entails selective catheterization of the hepatic artery stump using a microcatheter, so knowledge of the patient's anatomy and vascular anastomosis is critical. Infusion of thrombolytic drugs is initiated once the hepatic artery is selectively catheterized and the catheter is advanced to or within the thrombus. Although there is no consensus on dose and duration for IAT, alteplase (t-PA) infusion at 0.25 mg/h can be used for 12 to 14 hours with bolus infusions as deemed necessary. Use of the pulse-spray technique is encouraged because it may be able to reestablish flow in a single treatment and can prevent the need for overnight thrombolytic infusion. To limit bleeding risk, thrombolytic dosing should be monitored regularly through evaluation of fibrinogen levels. Adjunctive heparin is frequently used, with a target partial thromboplastin time of 1.25 to 1.5 times control. IAT success is determined by periodic evaluation with hepatic arteriography until the terminal branches of the hepatic artery are visualized. IAT is usually terminated if thrombus persists after 36 to 48 hours of therapy. Often, underlying stenosis is also present and must be corrected to avoid rethrombosis. For cases in which percutaneous

Table 24.1 Hepatic artery thrombosis treatment by endovascular interventions

Study	N	Time from transplant	Intervention	Technical success, n/N	Complication/hemorrhage, n/N
Cotroneo et al (2002)[25]	2	120 d	UK	2/2	Not reported
Zhou et al (2005)[19]	8	2 to 19 d	UK	8/8	5/8
Wang et al (2005)[26]	9	16 h to 10 d	UK	7/9	1/9
Kim et al (2006)[27]	2	4 to 6 h	UK	2/2	1/2
Li et al (2007)[28]	9		UK	6/9	2/9
Saad et al (2007)[29]	5	7 to 71 d	UK/t-PA	1/5	1/5
Boyvat et al (2008)[30]	9	6 h to 10 d	UK/t-PA	9/9	Not reported
Yang et al (2008)[31]	3		UK	1/3	1/3
López-Benítez et al (2008)[32]	1	3 d	UK	1/1	Not reported
Jeon et al (2008)[33]	4	1 to 13 d	UK	2/4	2/4
Singhal et al (2010)[34]	1		t-PA	1/1	Not reported
Wu et al (2011)[35]	2	2 to 3 d	UK	1/2	Not reported
Abdelaziz et al (2012)[16]	11	1 to 11 d	SK/t-PA	9/11	2/11
Kogut et al (2015)[36]	26		UK/t-PA	12/26	11/26

Abbreviations: SK, streptokinase; t-PA, alteplase; UK, urokinase.

techniques fail, surgical thrombectomy or retransplantation is the next step.

Hepatic Artery Stenosis

Post-LT HAS is insidious in onset; a high level of clinical suspicion and expert imaging are necessary for diagnosis. Early recognition and intervention can be important in HAS, as this condition often progresses to HAT and ischemic organ damage.[22,37] HAS typically occurs at or near the surgical anastomosis and is thought to be secondary to technical factors such as clamp injury, kinked vessels, faulty anastomotic suture placement, and differences in vessel caliber.[5,15,38] In the setting of graft rejection, however, HAS may be the result of severe hepatic dysfunction rather than its underlying cause.[39] Furthermore, the body may compensate for a slowly developing stenosis with collateral formation.[38] Ultimately, in patients with severe or late minimal hepatic dysfunction, intervention for isolated HAS may not affect graft survival and may not be warranted.

Doppler US is the method of choice for the diagnosis of HAS. Findings on US include focal increase in peak systolic velocity at the site of stenosis in the hepatic artery of two to three times the prestenosis velocity. Additional findings include poststenosis turbulent flow and the tardus-parvus intrahepatic waveform, with acceleration time greater than 8 ms and resistive index less than 0.5. When clinical suspicion for HAS is high, CT or MR angiography should be performed, as these modalities are more accurate in demonstrating narrowing of the hepatic artery.[2]

The mainstay of endovascular treatment for HAS is percutaneous transluminal angioplasty (PTA) with or without stent placement (▶ Table 24.2).[37,40,41,42,43,44,45,46,47,48,49,50,51,52,53,54,55] Technical success rates of endovascular treatment for HAS (81–100%) are comparable to those of surgical revision (78–100%).[3,15,56] Overall, case series have demonstrated technical success rates of 90 and 98% and complication incidences of 16 and 19% with PTA and PTA plus stent placement, respectively.[57] Recurrent stenosis after PTA can be addressed by repeat PTA with or without stent placement, yielding 95 to 100% hepatic artery patency with 82 and 88% 5-year graft and patient survival rates, respectively.[41,58] Short focal lesions respond better to endovascular treatment than long segment or multifocal stenoses.[37,39] The major complications of endovascular HAS treatment include rupture, dissection, and

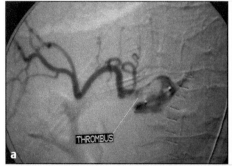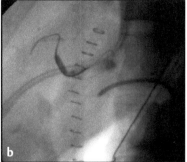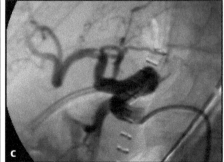

Fig. 24.1 Endovascular treatment of hepatic artery thrombosis. **(a)** Hepatic arteriography in a 38-year-old man 10 days after LT shows an occluded segment with thrombus. IAT was performed with a microcatheter using an initial pulse of t-PA followed by overnight infusion. **(b)** This patient was also found to have underlying stenosis, which was treated with balloon angioplasty. **(c)** Completion angiography demonstrates technical success with patent hepatic artery. Two months after thrombolysis, the patient developed recurrent HAT and underwent revision LT.

Table 24.2 Hepatic artery stenosis treatment by endovascular interventions

Study	N	Intervention	Technical success, n/N	Complications, n/N	Reintervention/ retransplant, n/N
Saad et al (2005)[37]	41	PTA	33/41	5/41	5/41
Huang et al (2006)[40]	14	Stent	12/14	Not reported	1/14
Kodama et al (2006)[41]	14	PTA	13/14	2/14	4/13
Ueno et al (2006)[42]	26	Stent	26/26	6/26	8/26
Huang et al (2007)[43]	11	Stent	11/11	0/11	1/11
Shaikh et al (2007)[44]	1	Stent	1/1	0/1	0/1
Zhao et al (2007)[45]	4	PTA, 1	1/1	0/1	0/1
		Stent, 3	3/3	0/3	0/3
da Silva et al (2008)[46]	8	PTA, 2	2/2	0/2	0/2
		Stent, 6	6/6	0/6	4/6
Jiang et al (2008)[47]	1	Stent	1/1	0/1	0/1
Chen et al (2009)[48]	20	PTA, 4	4/4	0/4	1/3
		Stent, 16	16/16	0/16	8/13
Maruzzelli et al (2010)[49]	15	PTA, 6	6/6	1/6	2/6
		Stent, 9	9/9	1/9	0/9
Kim et al (2011)[50]	3	PTA	3/3	0/3	0/3
Laštovičková and Peregrin (2011)[51]	18	PTA, 4	4/4	1/4	0/3
		Stent, 14	14/14	0/14	2/13
Sabri et al (2011)[52]	25	PTA, 21	20/21	3/21	9/25
		Stent, 4	4/4	0/4	
Steinbrück et al (2011)[53]	1	PTA	1/1	0/1	0/1
Frongillo et al (2013)[54]	10	PTA + stent	10/10	Not reported	Not reported
Hamby et al (2013)[55]	23	PTA, 10	22/23	Not reported	10/23
		Stent, 13			

Abbreviation: PTA, percutaneous transluminal angioplasty.

technical failure. Although there is often concern about anastomotic rupture, PTA has been performed as soon as 10 or even 3 days after LT.[5,40]

Endovascular treatment for HAS (▶ Fig. 24.2) begins by accessing and crossing the area of stenosis. The transstenotic pressure gradient can be measured to document a significant (> 10 mm Hg) gradient. A low-profile PTA balloon, usually 3 to 6 mm in diameter, is used to treat the stenosis. Heparin administration is standard before PTA, and a small amount of nitroglycerine can also be infused to prevent spasm. Patients should be observed and treated with anticoagulation overnight after PTA.

Metallic stents can be placed if patency is not adequately restored after PTA. Research has demonstrated generally comparable results for PTA with and without stent placement in HAS after LT.[57] In patients treated with stent placement, antiplatelet therapy should be considered, with recommendations varying from 30 days to > 1 year after the procedure.[52,55,57] Restenosis of previously treated HAS can be treated with repeat PTA or stent placement. Ultimately, in cases of HAS that cannot be treated with endovascular approaches, surgical therapies are indicated.

Hepatic Artery Pseudoaneurysm

HAP occurs less frequently than HAT or HAS and its etiology varies by location; intrahepatic HAP is often a result of

iatrogenic injury, whereas extrahepatic HAP at the anastomosis is commonly mycotic.[4,5] Patients with HAP typically present with hemobilia, hepatic artery occlusion, or unexplained graft dysfunction. Prompt treatment is warranted because HAP can lead to hemoperitoneum, massive gastrointestinal bleeding, or hemobilia, especially in the post-LT setting, in which the risk of rupture is much higher.[59]

HAP can be identified on Doppler US as a cystic structure near the hepatic artery with turbulent internal flow. The pseudoaneurysm can also be readily demonstrated on contrast-enhanced CT or MR angiography.

Multiple percutaneous strategies have been employed in treating HAP, including endovascular coil embolization and stent graft placement (▶ Table 24.3).[60,61,62,63,64,65] Technical success rates for endovascular treatment of HAP are very good (89%), with adequate preservation of underlying hepatic arterial flow.[15] For cases in which endovascular treatment is not feasible, direct percutaneous puncture of the pseudoaneurysm with thrombin injection has been successfully performed.[66] The major complication of endovascular HAP treatment is hepatic artery occlusion with subsequent graft ischemia.

The choice of endovascular treatment of HAP depends on the angiographic appearance of the pseudoaneurysm. Most cases of HAP can be selected with a microcatheter and selectively embolized using detachable coils. If the neck of the pseudoaneurysm cannot be accessed, placement of covered stent grafts or flow-diverting stents can be attempted; however, this

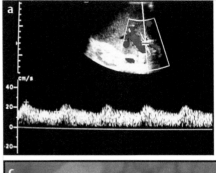
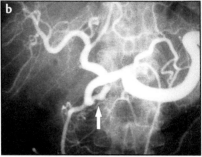
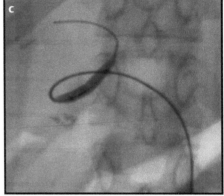
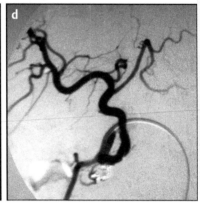

Fig. 24.2 Endovascular treatment of hepatic artery stenosis. **(a)** Doppler US in a 42-year-old man with elevated liver enzymes after LT shows tardus-parvus waveform suggestive of HAS. **(b)** Angiogram shows a focal stenosis of the hepatic artery (*arrow*). **(c)** An intra-arterial dose of heparin was given, and the stenotic lesion was crossed and treated with PTA. The decision was made to treat with PTA only and not with primary stent placement. **(d)** Angiography 5 years after PTA demonstrates patent hepatic artery without recurrent stenosis.

procedure is often difficult. Stent grafts should be reserved as a temporizing measure, as they may serve as infectious niduses in the setting of a mycotic aneurysm.[65] In cases of severe acute HAP hemorrhage, endovascular embolization can be used to sacrifice the hepatic artery, stabilize the patient, and facilitate subsequent surgical retransplantation.[59,67]

24.2.2 Portal Venous Complications

Portal Vein Stenosis

Although portal vein stenosis (PVS) is a relatively uncommon complication of LT, it occurs more frequently in the setting of pediatric LT, with an incidence ranging from 7 to 27%.[68,69,70] In cases of living-related LT, the donor portal venous segment is often relatively short and larger than the recipient portal vein. The consequent need for surgical plication of the donor portal vein and the use of interposition grafts to reduce tension on the anastomosis are risk factors for the development of PVS.[69,71] PVS occurring within 6 months of LT is relatively rare and is thought to be the result of technical factors; most PVS cases occur more than 6 months after LT and are due to scarring and fibrosis with neointimal hyperplasia.[68,72] PVS can manifest with symptoms of portal hypertension including ascites, gastrointestinal hemorrhage, and splenomegaly; however, most cases of PVS are detected on routine screening imaging.[73] Therefore, the decision to treat PVS must be made after carefully evaluating all available clinical information and should be weighed against the option of active surveillance.

On Doppler US, PVS appears as a more than three- to fourfold increase in flow velocity relative to the prestenotic segment at the site of stenosis. Additional findings on US include poststenosis dilation or increased number and size of collateral vessels in the hepatic hilum. CT or MR angiography can depict narrowing of the portal vein, as well.

The earliest attempts at endovascular treatment of PVS began around 1990 with PTA and stent placement[74]; multiple reports and small case series since have described successful endovascular treatment of PVS (▶ Table 24.4).[71,75,76,77,78,79] Overall, primary patency rates approach 36 to 71% at 2 to 3 years after PTA and up to 100% at 3 to 5 years after stent placement for PVS.[69,70,71] Complications of endovascular PVS treatment are relatively rare and include portal thrombosis and bleeding, either into the peritoneum or at the access site.

Endovascular treatment for PVS (▶ Fig. 24.3) generally begins with a transhepatic puncture into a secondary or tertiary branch of the portal vein via the right subcostal or left

Table 24.3 Hepatic artery pseudoaneurysm treatment by endovascular interventions

Study	N	Intervention	Technical success, n/N	Normal flow on follow-up, n/N
Banga et al (2005)[60]	2	Stent	2/2	1/1
Ginat et al (2009)[61]	1	Stent	1/1	1/1
Ou et al (2011)[62]	1	Embolization	1/1	1/1
Chen and Frenette (2012)[63]	1	Embolization	1/1	Not reported
Lu et al (2012)[64]	1	Stent	1/1	1/1
Saad et al (2013)[65]	12	Embolization, 4	3/4	8/12
		Stent, 8	7/8	

Table 24.4 Portal vein stenosis treatment by endovascular interventions

Study	N	Intervention	Technical success, n/N	Complications, n/N	Long-term patency, n/N
Funaki et al (2000)[71]	25	PTA, 7 Stent, 12 Failure, 6	19/25	2/25 (thrombosis)	19/19
Park et al (2005)[75]	6	PTA	6/6	1/6 (access bleed)	5/6
Shibata et al (2005)[76]	45	PTA	35/45	Not reported	34/35
Ko et al (2007)[77]	9	Stent	7/9	2/9 (hemoperitoneum) 1/9 (hepatic artery pseudoaneurysm)	6/6
Wei et al (2009)[78]	16	Stent	16/16	Not reported	16/16
Schneider et al (2011)[79]	2	PTA, 1 Stent, 1	2/2	0/2	2/2

Abbreviation: PTA, percutaneous transluminal angioplasty.

subxiphoid approach depending on graft orientation. Once the PVS is crossed, pressure is measured, with a gradient higher than 5 mm Hg considered significant. Before PTA is performed, an intravenous heparin bolus is administered to reduce the risk of thrombosis. Balloon dilation is then performed using a balloon matching the size of the allograft portal vein. If post-PTA venogram demonstrates a residual stenosis, a self-expanding metallic stent is recommended. Although only one-third of patients with PVS may require stent placement at the time of primary intervention, another third will require repeat angioplasty with subsequent stent placement within 31 months of the primary intervention.[71] There is theoretical concern about the use of stents in pediatric patients, as the stents do not grow with the patient and may complicate future surgery. However,

case reports have described stent patency of more than 20 years in pediatric patients with stents placed for PVS.[39] Some researchers have suggested the use of balloon-expandable stents in this patient population, as these stents can be postdilated to larger diameters as needed in the future.[3] In all patients, surgical treatment for refractory cases of PVS involves resection of the stenotic segment with reanastomosis.

Portal Vein Thrombosis

Portal vein thrombosis (PVT) after LT is rare, occurring in less than 4% of patients. This complication is believed to result from hypercoagulable states, stasis of portal venous flow, high intrasinusoidal pressure in graft rejection, or underlying PVS.[69] PVT

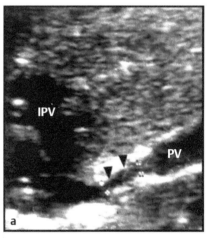
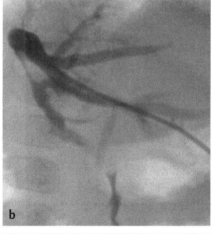
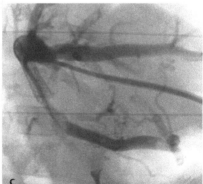
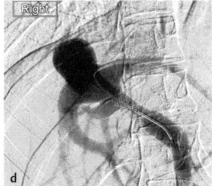

Fig. 24.3 Endovascular treatment of portal vein stenosis. **(a)** US image in a 2-year-old boy who presented 4 months after LT with elevated liver enzymes and ascites. There is focal stenosis of the portal vein (PV) just proximal to its bifurcation (*arrowheads*). Note the poststenotic dilation of the left portal vein (LPV). **(b)** Portal venography confirms US findings and demonstrates PVS. After PTA and stent placement **(c)**, portal venography shows a patent portal vein. **(d)** Twenty years later, the portal vein remains patent. Stent placement in pediatric patients with PVS can be safe and effective over the long term.

within 30 days of LT comprises more than 80% of cases and is more likely to cause graft loss than PVT occurring more than 30 days after LT, which may be asymptomatic.[80] Thrombus extending into the mesenteric veins can be devastating especially in the acute setting, leading to bowel necrosis and peritonitis in up to two-thirds of cases.[81] Therefore, treatment of PVT must be tailored to each individual clinical scenario. Potential treatments range from conservative anticoagulation to more aggressive endovascular and surgical procedures.

Imaging is critical to confirm, evaluate the extent of, and identify secondary complications of PVT. US may show an echogenic filling defect in the portal vein or lack of flow with Doppler imaging. Enhanced CT or MR can show intraluminal filling defects and may help to identify the extent of thrombus.

Endovascular treatment of PVT involves accessing the thrombus and then performing mechanical or pharmacologic thrombolysis. There are only scattered case reports of percutaneous PVT treatment, and techniques vary widely among institutions; therefore, conclusions regarding technical success rates, complications, and longevity of successful procedures cannot be drawn. Best estimates based on the limited available data suggest technical success rates of 55 to 70%, with mid- to long-term patency rates of 50 to 60%.[70,82]

Various approaches have been described for the endovascular treatment of PVT, including transhepatic or transjugular access with a range of pharmacologic agents and mechanical thrombectomy devices (► Fig. 24.4). Percutaneous transhepatic access of the portal vein can be obtained quickly using US guidance and has been used for successful pharmacologic thrombolysis.[82] The transjugular approach is generally more involved and takes more time, possibly requiring anesthesia for the patient, but offers a number of potential benefits.[72] Transjugular access is larger in caliber, allowing the use of larger platforms for thrombectomy devices such as the Trellis (ev3; Plymouth, MN), Trerotola (Arrow; Reading, PA), or suction thrombectomy catheters.[83,84,85] Transjugular access also has the benefit of a lower bleeding risk, and this technique establishes a route for transjugular intrahepatic portosystemic shunt (TIPS) creation if needed to treat portal hypertension.[86] Ultimately, many patients with PVT require PTA and stent placement, as well.[73] Nevertheless, percutaneous treatment of PVT has shown promise as an effective alternative to surgery.

24.2.3 Outflow Venous Complications

Venous outflow obstruction after LT is rare but can occur at the level of the hepatic vein or inferior vena cava (IVC). Early outflow obstruction is generally due to tight anastomosis, donor–recipient size mismatch, abnormal twisting of the veins, or the presence of an intimal flap; late outflow obstruction develops as a result of fibrosis or intimal hyperplasia.[3,87] On Doppler US, a triphasic waveform is normally seen in the hepatic vein. A persistent monophasic waveform is a sensitive but nonspecific finding of outflow stenosis.[8] Direct signs of outflow stenosis include focal stricture on US, CT, or MR imaging. Secondary findings include prestenotic dilation of the hepatic veins or mosaic perfusion of the liver parenchyma. Ultimately, identification of stenosis on venography and a pressure gradient greater than 5 mm Hg generally warrant treatment.[88,89]

Hepatic Vein Stenosis

Hepatic venous stenosis (HVS) occurs after LT with an incidence of less than 1%. Patients with this complication typically present late, on average 37 months after LT.[68] HVS generally manifests clinically as ascites, splenomegaly, abdominal fullness, or variceal bleeding with biochemical abnormalities indicating hepatic dysfunction.

Good results have been reported for endovascular treatment of HVS with PTA and stent placement, including technical success rates of 94 to 100% and long-term patency rates of 80, 65, and 60% at 3, 6, and 12 months, respectively.[90] Complications of the procedure are usually minor and include hypotension or arrhythmia.[90] The most significant complication is stent migration, which can lead to devastating consequences if untreated.[91,92]

Treatment of HVS can begin from internal jugular, femoral, or transhepatic approaches (► Fig. 24.5). Jugular and femoral approaches are preferred, as placement of a transhepatic sheath followed by anticoagulation may carry a higher risk of complications.[93] In the setting of hepatic vein occlusion, however, US-guided transhepatic access is preferred. Once the stenosis is crossed, PTA is performed with a slightly oversized balloon. The target posttreatment pressure gradient is less than 3 mm Hg. Case reports have also described the successful use of cutting balloons to treat HVS, although this technique has not been well studied.[94] A subset of patients respond to venoplasty alone; however, repeat PTA is often required to achieve long-term patency.[95]

In adult patients, stent placement can be considered after initial PTA. Many clinicians prefer balloon-expanded stents in HVS, as these stents allow precise placement and offer greater radial strength.[87] In pediatric patients, however, stent placement is reserved for cases of numerous recurrences of HVS after PTA. When stents are placed in pediatric patients, the largest possible stent diameter and shortest stent length should be used to accommodate future growth and to allow for potential repeat transplantation.

IVC Stenosis

IVC stenosis occurs in less than 3% of transplant recipients. These patients typically present with lower extremity edema in addition to findings of HVS.[68] Of note, these patients can present in a fulminant state as the stenosis both triggers and is worsened by ascites.

Endovascular treatment of IVC stenosis is associated with very favorable technical success and long-term patency rates.[91,93,96] Unlike HVS, however, IVC stenosis generally does not respond to angioplasty alone. Most stenoses require stent placement, particularly those that occur early after LT. IVC stenosis in these patients is largely due to surgical technique, graft migration, or graft torsion, etiologies that require stent placement.[96]

IVC stenoses are usually accessed from a jugular or femoral approach (► Fig. 24.6). If the patient is within 1 month of LT, a conservative choice of balloon diameter (maximum, 16 mm) is recommended for PTA to avoid anastomotic rupture. Also, the time during which the balloon is inflated should be limited as the reduced blood flow to the heart can lead to hypotension.

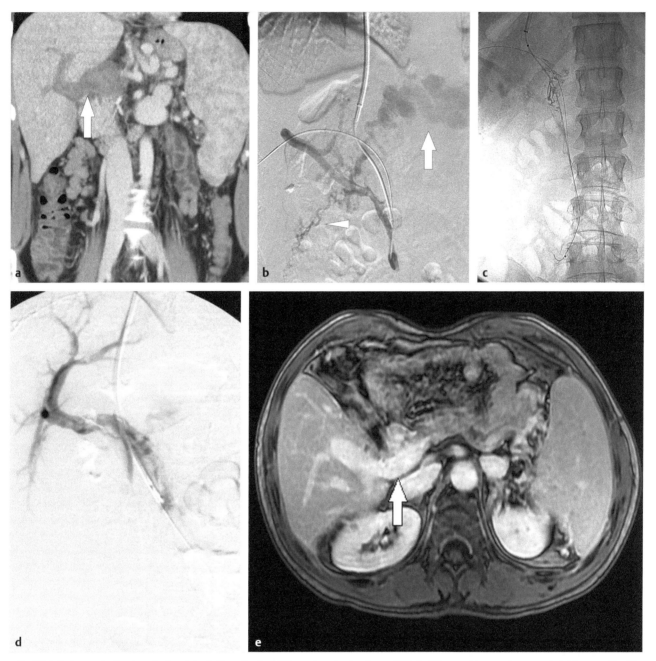

Fig. 24.4 Endovascular treatment of portal vein thrombosis. **(a)** Coronal contrast-enhanced CT of a 26-year-old man who presented 4.8 years after LT with elevated liver enzymes and intermittent gastrointestinal hemorrhage. Nonopacified and enlarged portal vein (*arrow*) indicates PVT. **(b)** Transjugular transhepatic injection of the superior mesenteric vein shows portomesenteric thrombosis with opacification of mesenteric collaterals (*arrowhead*) and large gastric varices (*arrow*). A microwire was initially introduced percutaneously into the thrombosed portomesenteric system to serve as a target for transjugular transhepatic access. **(c)** A Trellis device was advanced through the area of thrombosis. **(d)** Remaining intrahepatic thrombus was cleared by pulling the clot into the right portal vein with a balloon catheter and aspirating through the sheath. This resulted in markedly improved intrahepatic portal patency. **(e)** Contrast-enhanced MR imaging 34 months after the procedure demonstrates widely patent portal system (*arrow*).

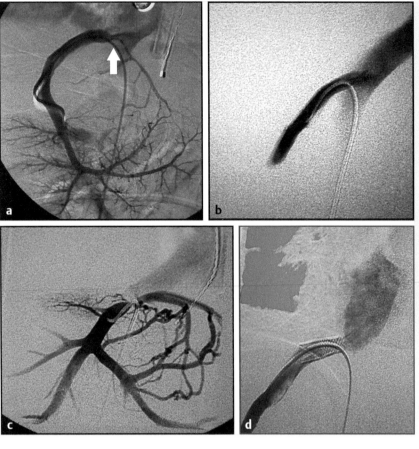

Fig. 24.5 Endovascular treatment of hepatic vein stenosis. **(a)** A 4-year-old girl presented with elevated liver enzymes and ascites 4 months after LT. Femoral approach venography demonstrates a focal HVS (*arrow*). **(b)** Lesion was initially treated with PTA with technical success and resolution of stenosis on post-PTA venogram. **(c)** The patient returned with recurrent HVS 6 months later. **(d)** After repeat PTA, a stent was placed with good technical result. The 3-year follow-up identified no clinical recurrence.

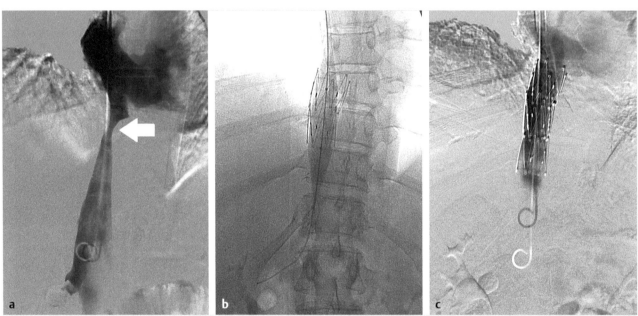

Fig. 24.6 Endovascular treatment of inferior vena cava stenosis. **(a)** A 52-year-old man presented with elevated liver enzymes and ascites 15 days after LT. Initial venogram demonstrates IVC stenosis (*arrow*) with pressure gradient of 10 mm Hg. **(b)** Gianturco stents were placed via the transjugular approach and expanded with a balloon to treat the stenosis. **(c)** Completion venography demonstrates improvement in the IVC stenosis and a pressure gradient that had decreased to < 2 mm Hg.

Stents with open interstices such as the Gianturco stent (Cook; Bloomington, IN) are less likely to obstruct hepatic venous outflow and are recommended for primary stent placement to reduce the risk of "jailing" hepatic veins. Placement from a jugular approach is preferred so that if the stent unexpectedly moves forward during deployment, it is still deployed safely within the IVC.

24.3 Biliary Complications

Biliary tract complications have decreased in frequency as transplant techniques have improved but are still among the most common complications after LT, occurring at an incidence of 15 to 25%.[3,4,5] Bile leaks are the most common biliary complication in living-donor LT with an incidence of 17.1%, whereas strictures are the most common complication in deceased-donor LT with an incidence of 7.5%.[97]

Biliary complications can be either vascular or nonvascular in etiology. The donor biliary system relies heavily on hepatic arterial supply after LT because collateral circulation is compromised during transplantation. Therefore, complications such as HAT or HAS can cause ischemic complications of the biliary tract including strictures, occlusions, leaks, and abscesses.[98] Nonvascular biliary tract complications are usually due to surgical technique but also manifest as strictures, obstructions, and leaks. Rarely, biliary complications are due to medical conditions such as graft-versus-host disease, recurrent primary sclerosing cholangitis, infections, and drug toxicity; these underlying conditions must be addressed.

The most common biliary anastomoses in LT are choledocho-choledochostomy with a T-tube and Roux-en-Y choledochojejunostomy. Early post-LT biliary complications can be effectively evaluated with T-tube cholangiography. However, once this access is removed, noninvasive imaging is generally the first step for evaluation of a patient who presents with clinical and biochemical findings of biliary complication. US and CT are frequently used, but MR cholangiography is the most sensitive imaging modality for outlining the post-LT biliary anatomy and identifying complications.[8] Endoscopic retrograde cholangiopancreatography is often performed for diagnostic purposes and is also often used to treat complications. In LT patients with Roux-en-Y choledochojejunostomy, the anatomy may be too difficult to traverse endoscopically; in such cases, percutaneous techniques are the next line of treatment.

24.3.1 Biliary Stricture

Anastomotic biliary strictures are the most common complication of LT. Surgical revision of biliary strictures is successful in two-thirds of cases but exposes patients to high morbidity, with a recent series reporting a morbidity rate of 58%.[99] Percutaneous or endoscopic treatments are less likely to cause complications and are very effective, with 65 to 71% of patients responding.[100,101] Minimally invasive options do generally commit the patient to long-term external drainage or repeat procedures, so management must be carefully coordinated with the transplant team to optimize long-term results.

Treatment of biliary stricture begins with percutaneously accessing the biliary system and navigating the stricture (▶ Fig. 24.7). The stricture is then dilated with balloon cholangioplasty, and an internal–external biliary drainage (IEBD) catheter is placed. Placement of dual IEBD catheters from both the left and right hepatic lobes or even two smaller catheters through the same tract may provide better long-term results.[102] Percutaneous placement of covered stents to maintain patency has been studied with modest results; a study comparing stent placement to biliary catheter placement found 70% clinical success in the stent group versus 95% in the catheter group.[103]

24.3.2 Biliary Leak

Biliary leaks usually occur at the biliary anastomosis and result in perihepatic or peritoneal collections. If leaks occur early after LT, surgical repair or reconstruction should be the primary therapeutic consideration. For cases of complete anastomotic breakdown or small leaks occurring from an otherwise intact extrahepatic biliary system, endovascular or percutaneous treatments can successfully divert drainage to allow healing or temporize the patient's symptoms.

Treatment of biliary leaks primarily involves diversion of biliary drainage via endoscopic placement of a stent or percutaneous placement of an IEBD catheter. For smaller leaks, this can be the definitive treatment that allows the biliary tract to heal, although this may take several months. Even in cases that ultimately require surgical reconstruction, an IEBD catheter can stabilize and alleviate the patient's symptoms while facilitating future creation of a Roux-en-Y hepaticojejunostomy (▶ Fig. 24.8).[98]

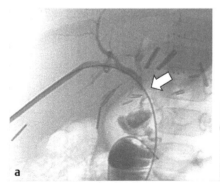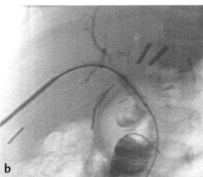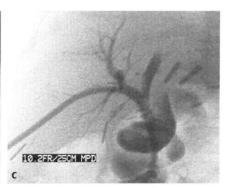

Fig. 24.7 Percutaneous treatment of biliary stricture. **(a)** A 4-year-old boy with a biliary-enteric stricture (*arrow*) 2 months after LT. **(b)** Balloon dilatation was performed to a diameter of 6 mm. **(c)** Follow-up cholangiogram shows immediate resolution of the stricture; an IEBD was placed. This catheter was removed at 1 month after cholangiographic demonstration of persistent patency.

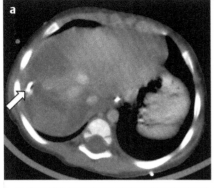
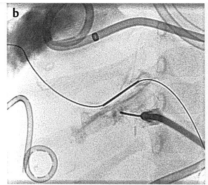
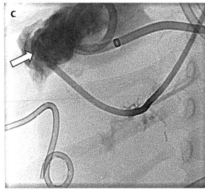
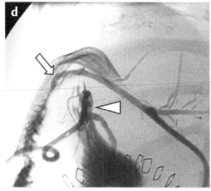

Fig. 24.8 Management of bile leak. **(a)** Ductal leak in a 24-year-old man 3 days after LT. Axial CT images show a percutaneous drainage catheter (*arrow*) within a large fluid collection adjacent to graft. **(b)** Injection of the pigtail catheter demonstrated reflux from a biloma into a bile duct. US and fluoroscopic guidance was used to access this bile duct, and a wire was passed across the cut edge of the liver into the biloma. **(c)** An IEBD catheter was placed extending from the duct into the biloma (*arrow*). **(d)** Surgical reconstruction was then performed by cutting the newly placed pigtail from the abdominal side and performing a new anastomosis to the Roux-en-Y using the protruding straight portion (*arrow*) as a guide. A separate IEBD (*arrowhead*) is shown.

24.4 Conclusion

Interventional radiology offers various treatment options for both vascular and nonvascular complications after LT. In many situations, nonsurgical interventions have become the first line of treatment. Therefore, interventional radiology is an essential component of any successful LT program.

References

[1] Organ Procurement and Transplantation Network. Available at: https://optn.transplant.hrsa.gov/data/view-data-reports/national-data/. December 25, 2015. Accessed January 2, 2016

[2] García-Criado A, Gilabert R, Bargalló X, Brú C. Radiology in liver transplantation. Semin Ultrasound CT MR. 2002; 23(1):114–129

[3] Ng S, Tan KA, Anil G. The role of interventional radiology in complications associated with liver transplantation. Clin Radiol. 2015; 70(12):1323–1335

[4] Karani JB, Yu DF, Kane PA. Interventional radiology in liver transplantation. Cardiovasc Intervent Radiol. 2005; 28(3):271–283

[5] Amesur NB, Zajko AB. Interventional radiology in liver transplantation. Liver Transpl. 2006; 12(3):330–351

[6] Miraglia R, Maruzzelli L, Caruso S, et al. Interventional radiology procedures in adult patients who underwent liver transplantation. World J Gastroenterol. 2009; 15(6):684–693

[7] Miraglia R, Maruzzelli L, Caruso S, et al. Interventional radiology procedures in pediatric patients with complications after liver transplantation. Radiographics. 2009; 29(2):567–584

[8] Caiado AH, Blasbalg R, Marcelino AS, et al. Complications of liver transplantation: multimodality imaging approach. Radiographics. 2007; 27(5):1401–1417

[9] Quiroga S, Sebastià MC, Margarit C, Castells L, Boyé R, Alvarez-Castells A. Complications of orthotopic liver transplantation: spectrum of findings with helical CT. Radiographics. 2001; 21(5):1085–1102

[10] Nghiem HV. Imaging of hepatic transplantation. Radiol Clin North Am. 1998; 36(2):429–443

[11] Pérez-Saborido B, Pacheco-Sánchez D, Barrera-Rebollo A, et al. Incidence, management, and results of vascular complications after liver transplantation. Transplant Proc. 2011; 43(3):749–750

[12] Singhal A, Stokes K, Sebastian A, Wright HI, Kohli V. Endovascular treatment of hepatic artery thrombosis following liver transplantation. Transpl Int. 2010; 23(3):245–256

[13] Silva MA, Jambulingam PS, Gunson BK, et al. Hepatic artery thrombosis following orthotopic liver transplantation: a 10-year experience from a single centre in the United Kingdom. Liver Transpl. 2006; 12(1):146–151

[14] Bekker J, Ploem S, de Jong KP. Early hepatic artery thrombosis after liver transplantation: a systematic review of the incidence, outcome and risk factors. Am J Transplant. 2009; 9(4):746–757

[15] Chen J, Weinstein J, Black S, Spain J, Brady PS, Dowell JD. Surgical and endovascular treatment of hepatic arterial complications following liver transplant. Clin Transplant. 2014; 28(12):1305–1312

[16] Abdelaziz O, Hosny K, Amin A, Emadeldin S, Uemoto S, Mostafa M. Endovascular management of early hepatic artery thrombosis after living donor liver transplantation. Transpl Int. 2012; 25(8):847–856

[17] Nikeghbalian S, Kazemi K, Davari HR, et al. Early hepatic artery thrombosis after liver transplantation: diagnosis and treatment. Transplant Proc. 2007; 39(4):1195–1196

[18] Scarinci A, Sainz-Barriga M, Berrevoet F, et al. Early arterial revascularization after hepatic artery thrombosis may avoid graft loss and improve outcomes in adult liver transplantation. Transplant Proc. 2010; 42(10):4403–4408

[19] Zhou J, Fan J, Wang JH, et al. Continuous transcatheter arterial thrombolysis for early hepatic artery thrombosis after liver transplantation. Transplant Proc. 2005; 37(10):4426–4429

[20] Gunsar F, Rolando N, Pastacaldi S, et al. Late hepatic artery thrombosis after orthotopic liver transplantation. Liver Transpl. 2003; 9(6):605–611

[21] Leonardi MI, Boin I, Leonardi LS. Late hepatic artery thrombosis after liver transplantation: clinical setting and risk factors. Transplant Proc. 2004; 36(4):967–969

[22] Wozney P, Zajko AB, Bron KM, Point S, Starzl TE. Vascular complications after liver transplantation: a 5-year experience. AJR Am J Roentgenol. 1986; 147(4):657–663

[23] Oh CK, Pelletier SJ, Sawyer RG, et al. Uni- and multi-variate analysis of risk factors for early and late hepatic artery thrombosis after liver transplantation. Transplantation. 2001; 71(6):767–772

[24] Hidalgo EG, Abad J, Cantarero JM, et al. High-dose intra-arterial urokinase for the treatment of hepatic artery thrombosis in liver transplantation. Hepatogastroenterology. 1989; 36(6):529–532

[25] Cotroneo AR, Di Stasi C, Cina A, et al. Stent placement in four patients with hepatic artery stenosis or thrombosis after liver transplantation. J Vasc Interv Radiol. 2002; 13(6):619–623

[26] Wang XH, Yan LN, Zhang F, et al. Early experiences on living donor liver transplantation in China: multicenter report. Chin Med J (Engl). 2006; 119 (12):1003–1009

[27] Kim BW, Won JH, Lee BM, Ko BH, Wang HJ, Kim MW. Intraarterial thrombolytic treatment for hepatic artery thrombosis immediately after living donor liver transplantation. Transplant Proc. 2006; 38(9):3128–3131

[28] Li ZW, Wang MQ, Zhou NX, Liu Z, Huang ZQ. Interventional treatment of acute hepatic artery occlusion after liver transplantation. Hepatobiliary Pancreat Dis Int. 2007; 6(5):474–478

[29] Saad WE, Davies MG, Saad NE, et al. Catheter thrombolysis of thrombosed hepatic arteries in liver transplant recipients: predictors of success and role of thrombolysis. Vasc Endovascular Surg. 2007; 41(1):19–26

[30] Boyvat F, Aytekin C, Harman A, Sevmiş S, Karakayali H, Haberal M. Endovascular stent placement in patients with hepatic artery stenoses or thromboses after liver transplant. Transplant Proc. 2008; 40(1):22–26

[31] Yang Y, Li H, Fu BS, et al. Hepatic artery complications after orthotopic liver transplantation: interventional treatment or retransplantation? Chin Med J (Engl). 2008; 121(20):1997–2000

[32] López-Benítez R, Schlieter M, Hallscheidt PJ, et al. Successful arterial thrombolysis and percutaneous transluminal angioplasty for early hepatic artery thrombosis after split liver transplantation in a four-month-old baby. Pediatr Transplant. 2008; 12(5):606–610

[33] Jeon GS, Won JH, Wang HJ, Kim BW, Lee BM. Endovascular treatment of acute arterial complications after living-donor liver transplantation. Clin Radiol. 2008; 63(10):1099–1105

[34] Singhal A, Mukherjee I, Stokes K, Wright HI, Sebastian A, Kohli V. Continuous intraarterial thrombolysis for early hepatic artery thrombosis following liver transplantation: case report. Vasc Endovascular Surg. 2010; 44(2):134–138

[35] Wu L, Zhang J, Guo Z, et al. Hepatic artery thrombosis after orthotopic liver transplant: a review of the same institute 5 years later. Exp Clin Transplant. 2011; 9(3):191–196

[36] Kogut MJ, Shin DS, Padia SA, Johnson GE, Hippe DS, Valji K. Intra-arterial thrombolysis for hepatic artery thrombosis following liver transplantation. J Vasc Interv Radiol. 2015; 26(9):1317–1322

[37] Saad WE, Davies MG, Sahler L, et al. Hepatic artery stenosis in liver transplant recipients: primary treatment with percutaneous transluminal angioplasty. J Vasc Interv Radiol. 2005; 16(6):795–805

[38] Rinaldi P, Inchingolo R, Giuliani M, et al. Hepatic artery stenosis in liver transplantation: imaging and interventional treatment. Eur J Radiol. 2012; 81(6):1110–1115

[39] Lorenz J, Funaki B. Endovascular management of vascular complications of liver transplantation. Paper presented at: Digestive Disease Interventions; October 2015; Boston, MA

[40] Huang M, Shan H, Jiang Z, et al. The use of coronary stent in hepatic artery stenosis after orthotopic liver transplantation. Eur J Radiol. 2006; 60(3): 425–430

[41] Kodama Y, Sakuhara Y, Abo D, et al. Percutaneous transluminal angioplasty for hepatic artery stenosis after living donor liver transplantation. Liver Transpl. 2006; 12(3):465–469

[42] Ueno T, Jones G, Martin A, et al. Clinical outcomes from hepatic artery stenting in liver transplantation. Liver Transpl. 2006; 12(3):422–427

[43] Huang Q, Zhai RY, Dai DK. Interventional treatment of hepatic artery stenosis after orthotopic liver transplantation with balloon-expandable coronary stent. Transplant Proc. 2007; 39(10):3245–3250

[44] Shaikh F, Solis J, Bajwa T. Hepatic artery stenosis after liver transplant, managed with percutaneous angioplasty and stent placement. Catheter Cardiovasc Interv. 2007; 69(3):369–371

[45] Zhao DB, Shan H, Jiang ZB, et al. Role of interventional therapy in hepatic artery stenosis and non-anastomosis bile duct stricture after orthotopic liver transplantation. World J Gastroenterol. 2007; 13(22):3128–3132

[46] da Silva RF, Raphe R, Felício HC, et al. Prevalence, treatment, and outcomes of the hepatic artery stenosis after liver transplant. Transplant Proc. 2008; 40(3):805–807

[47] Jiang XZ, Yan LN, Li B, et al. Arterial complications after living-related liver transplantation: single-center experience from West China. Transplant Proc. 2008; 40(5):1525–1528

[48] Chen GH, Wang GY, Yang Y, et al. Single-center experience of therapeutic management of hepatic artery stenosis after orthotopic liver transplantation. Report of 20 cases. Eur Surg Res. 2009; 42(1):21–27

[49] Maruzzelli L, Miraglia R, Caruso S, et al. Percutaneous endovascular treatment of hepatic artery stenosis in adult and pediatric patients after liver transplantation. Cardiovasc Intervent Radiol. 2010; 33(6):1111–1119

[50] Kim SJ, Yoon YC, Park JH, Oh DY, Yoo YK, Kim DG. Hepatic artery reconstruction and successful management of its complications in living donor liver transplantation using a right lobe. Clin Transplant. 2011; 25(6): 929–938

[51] Laštovičková J, Peregrin J. Percutaneous transluminal angioplasty of hepatic artery stenosis in patients after orthotopic liver transplantation: mid-term results. Cardiovasc Intervent Radiol. 2011; 34(6):1165–1171

[52] Sabri SS, Saad WE, Schmitt TM, et al. Endovascular therapy for hepatic artery stenosis and thrombosis following liver transplantation. Vasc Endovascular Surg. 2011; 45(5):447–452

[53] Steinbrück K, Enne M, Fernandes R, et al. Vascular complications after living donor liver transplantation: a Brazilian, single-center experience. Transplant Proc. 2011; 43(1):196–198

[54] Frongillo F, Grossi U, Lirosi MC, et al. Incidence, management, and results of hepatic artery stenosis after liver transplantation in the era of donor to recipient match. Transplant Proc. 2013; 45(7):2722–2725

[55] Hamby BA, Ramirez DE, Loss GE, et al. Endovascular treatment of hepatic artery stenosis after liver transplantation. J Vasc Surg. 2013; 57(4):1067–1072

[56] Orons PD, Zajko AB, Bron KM, Trecha GT, Selby RR, Fung JJ. Hepatic artery angioplasty after liver transplantation: experience in 21 allografts. J Vasc Interv Radiol. 1995; 6(4):523–529

[57] Rostambeigi N, Hunter D, Duval S, Chinnakotla S, Golzarian J. Stent placement versus angioplasty for hepatic artery stenosis after liver transplant: a meta-analysis of case series. Eur Radiol. 2013; 23(5):1323–1334

[58] Sommacale D, Aoyagi T, Dondero F, et al. Repeat endovascular treatment of recurring hepatic artery stenoses in orthotopic liver transplantation. Transpl Int. 2013; 26(6):608–615

[59] Fistouris J, Herlenius G, Bäckman L, et al. Pseudoaneurysm of the hepatic artery following liver transplantation. Transplant Proc. 2006; 38(8):2679–2682

[60] Banga NR, Kessel DO, Patel JV, et al. Endovascular management of arterial conduit pseudoaneurysm after liver transplantation: a report of two cases. Transplantation. 2005; 79(12):1763–1765

[61] Ginat DT, Saad WE, Waldman DL, Davies MG. Stent-graft placement for management of iatrogenic hepatic artery branch pseudoaneurysm after liver transplantation. Vasc Endovascular Surg. 2009; 43(5):513–517

[62] Ou HY, Concejero AM, Yu CY, et al. Hepatic arterial embolization for massive bleeding from an intrahepatic artery pseudoaneurysm using N-butyl-2-cyanoacrylate after living donor liver transplantation. Transpl Int. 2011; 24 (3):e19–e22

[63] Chen WC, Frenette C. Hepatic artery pseudoaneurysm: a rare cause of gastrointestinal bleeding in a post liver transplant patient. J Gastrointestin Liver Dis. 2012; 21(2):125

[64] Lu NN, Huang Q, Wang JF, Wei BJ, Gao K, Zhai RY. Treatment of post-liver transplant hepatic artery pseudoaneurysm with balloon angioplasty after failed stent graft placement. Clin Res Hepatol Gastroenterol. 2012; 36(6): e109–e113

[65] Saad WE, Dasgupta N, Lippert AJ, et al. Extrahepatic pseudoaneurysms and ruptures of the hepatic artery in liver transplant recipients: endovascular management and a new iatrogenic etiology. Cardiovasc Intervent Radiol. 2013; 36(1):118–127

[66] Patel JV, Weston MJ, Kessel DO, Prasad R, Toogood GJ, Robertson I. Hepatic artery pseudoaneurysm after liver transplantation: treatment with percutaneous thrombin injection. Transplantation. 2003; 75(10):1755–1757

[67] Marshall MM, Muiesan P, Srinivasan P, et al. Hepatic artery pseudoaneurysms following liver transplantation: incidence, presenting features and management. Clin Radiol. 2001; 56(7):579–587

[68] Buell JF, Funaki B, Cronin DC, et al. Long-term venous complications after full-size and segmental pediatric liver transplantation. Ann Surg. 2002; 236 (5):658–666

[69] Saad WE. Portal interventions in liver transplant recipients. Semin Intervent Radiol. 2012; 29(2):99–104

[70] Ueda M, Egawa H, Ogawa K, et al. Portal vein complications in the long-term course after pediatric living donor liver transplantation. Transplant Proc. 2005; 37(2):1138–1140

[71] Funaki B, Rosenblum JD, Leef JA, et al. Percutaneous treatment of portal venous stenosis in children and adolescents with segmental hepatic transplants: long-term results. Radiology. 2000; 215(1):147–151

[72] Saad WE. Liver transplant-related vascular disease. In: Geshwind J-F, Dake MD, eds. Abrams' Angiography: Interventional Radiology. 3rd ed. Philadelphia, PA: Lippincott Williams & Wilkins; 2012:924–951

[73] Woo DH, Laberge JM, Gordon RL, Wilson MW, Kerlan RK, Jr. Management of portal venous complications after liver transplantation. Tech Vasc Interv Radiol. 2007; 10(3):233–239

[74] Olcott EW, Ring EJ, Roberts JP, Ascher NL, Lake JR, Gordon RL. Percutaneous transhepatic portal vein angioplasty and stent placement after liver transplantation: early experience. J Vasc Interv Radiol. 1990; 1(1):17–22

[75] Park KB, Choo SW, Do YS, Shin SW, Cho SG, Choo IW. Percutaneous angioplasty of portal vein stenosis that complicates liver transplantation: the mid-term therapeutic results. Korean J Radiol. 2005; 6(3):161–166

[76] Shibata T, Itoh K, Kubo T, et al. Percutaneous transhepatic balloon dilation of portal vein stenosis in patients with living donor liver transplantation. Radiology. 2005; 235(3):1078–1083

[77] Ko GY, Sung KB, Yoon HK, Lee S. Early posttransplantation portal vein stenosis following living donor liver transplantation: percutaneous transhepatic primary stent placement. Liver Transpl. 2007; 13(4):530–536

[78] Wei BJ, Zhai RY, Wang JF, Dai DK, Yu P. Percutaneous portal venoplasty and stenting for anastomotic stenosis after liver transplantation. World J Gastroenterol. 2009; 15(15):1880–1885

[79] Schneider N, Scanga A, Stokes L, Perri R. Portal vein stenosis: a rare yet clinically important cause of delayed-onset ascites after adult deceased donor liver transplantation: two case reports. Transplant Proc. 2011; 43 (10):3829–3834

[80] Khalaf H. Vascular complications after deceased and living donor liver transplantation: a single-center experience. Transplant Proc. 2010; 42(3): 865–870

[81] Kumar S, Sarr MG, Kamath PS. Mesenteric venous thrombosis. N Engl J Med. 2001; 345(23):1683–1688

[82] Durham JD, LaBerge JM, Altman S, et al. Portal vein thrombolysis and closure of competitive shunts following liver transplantation. J Vasc Interv Radiol. 1994; 5(4):611–615, discussion 616–618

[83] Lorenz JM, Bennett S, Patel J, Van Ha TG, Funaki B. Combined pharmacomechanical thrombolysis of complete portomesenteric thrombosis in a liver transplant recipient. Cardiovasc Intervent Radiol. 2014; 37(1):262–266

[84] Baccarani U, Gasparini D, Risaliti A, et al. Percutaneous mechanical fragmentation and stent placement for the treatment of early posttransplantation portal vein thrombosis. Transplantation. 2001; 72(9): 1572–1582

[85] Carnevale FC, Borges MV, Moreira AM, Cerri GG, Maksoud JG. Endovascular treatment of acute portal vein thrombosis after liver transplantation in a child. Cardiovasc Intervent Radiol. 2006; 29(3):457–461

[86] Cherukuri R, Haskal ZJ, Naji A, Shaked A. Percutaneous thrombolysis and stent placement for the treatment of portal vein thrombosis after liver transplantation: long-term follow-up. Transplantation. 1998; 65(8):1124–1126

[87] Darcy MD. Management of venous outflow complications after liver transplantation. Tech Vasc Interv Radiol. 2007; 10(3):240–245

[88] Raby N, Karani J, Thomas S, O'Grady J, Williams R. Stenoses of vascular anastomoses after hepatic transplantation: treatment with balloon angioplasty. AJR Am J Roentgenol. 1991; 157(1):167–171

[89] Borsa JJ, Daly CP, Fontaine AB, et al. Treatment of inferior vena cava anastomotic stenoses with the Wallstent endoprosthesis after orthotopic liver transplantation. J Vasc Interv Radiol. 1999; 10(1):17–22

[90] Kubo T, Shibata T, Itoh K, et al. Outcome of percutaneous transhepatic venoplasty for hepatic venous outflow obstruction after living donor liver transplantation. Radiology. 2006; 239(1):285–290

[91] Weeks SM, Gerber DA, Jaques PF, et al. Primary Gianturco stent placement for inferior vena cava abnormalities following liver transplantation. J Vasc Interv Radiol. 2000; 11(2, Pt 1):177–187

[92] Guimarães M, Uflacker R, Schönholz C, Hannegan C, Selby JB. Stent migration complicating treatment of inferior vena cava stenosis after orthotopic liver transplantation. J Vasc Interv Radiol. 2005; 16(9):1247–1252

[93] Lorenz JM, Van Ha T, Funaki B, et al. Percutaneous treatment of venous outflow obstruction in pediatric liver transplants. J Vasc Interv Radiol. 2006; 17(11, Pt 1):1753–1761

[94] Narumi S, Hakamada K, Totsuka E, et al. Efficacy of cutting balloon for anastomotic stricture of the hepatic vein. Transplant Proc. 2004; 36(10): 3093–3095

[95] Totsuka E, Hakamada K, Narumi S, et al. Hepatic vein anastomotic stricture after living donor liver transplantation. Transplant Proc. 2004; 36(8):2252–2254

[96] Lorenz JM, van Beek D, Funaki B, et al. Long-term outcomes of percutaneous venoplasty and Gianturco stent placement to treat obstruction of the inferior vena cava complicating liver transplantation. Cardiovasc Intervent Radiol. 2014; 37(1):114–124

[97] Duailibi DF, Ribeiro MA, Jr. Biliary complications following deceased and living donor liver transplantation: a review. Transplant Proc. 2010; 42(2): 517–520

[98] Lorenz JM. The role of interventional radiology in the multidisciplinary management of biliary complications after liver transplantation. Tech Vasc Interv Radiol. 2015; 18(4):266–275

[99] Reichman TW, Sandroussi C, Grant DR, et al. Surgical revision of biliary strictures following adult live donor liver transplantation: patient selection, morbidity, and outcomes. Transpl Int. 2012; 25(1):69–77

[100] Anderson CD, Turmelle YP, Darcy M, et al. Biliary strictures in pediatric liver transplant recipients - early diagnosis and treatment results in excellent graft outcomes. Pediatr Transplant. 2010; 14(3):358–363

[101] Lee SH, Ryu JK, Woo SM, et al. Optimal interventional treatment and long-term outcomes for biliary stricture after liver transplantation. Clin Transplant. 2008; 22(4):484–493

[102] Gwon DI, Sung KB, Ko GY, Yoon HK, Lee SG. Dual catheter placement technique for treatment of biliary anastomotic strictures after liver transplantation. Liver Transpl. 2011; 17(2):159–166

[103] Kim J, Ko GY, Sung KB, et al. Percutaneously placed covered retrievable stents for the treatment of biliary anastomotic strictures following living donor liver transplantation. Liver Transpl. 2010; 16(12):1410–1420

25 Islet Cell Transplantation

Ashley Altman and Jonathan M. Lorenz

25.1 Introduction

Islet cell transplantation (ICT) continues to evolve as a minimally invasive alternative to whole pancreas transplantation for the treatment of select patients with type 1 diabetes mellitus. Earlier success in preventing adverse hypoglycemic events has led to continued research and improvement in the rate of sustained insulin independence, the holy grail of diabetes research. The clinical success of ICT now approaches that of gold-standard whole pancreas transplantation without the serious complications associated with major surgery. The need for immunosuppressive medication after ICT currently limits its application to a subset of diabetic patients with severe, end-stage, type 1 diabetes. However, ongoing research to optimize organ selection, organ procurement, islet cell isolation, and immunosuppressive therapy may lead to further improvements in clinical success and the broadening of the application of ICT.

25.2 Evolution of ICT and Current Practice

Approximately 11 to 22 million people worldwide are affected by type 1 diabetes mellitus. Patients with type 1 diabetes suffer from an inability to produce sufficient quantities of insulin because of a deficiency in pancreatic β-cells from either an autoimmune or idiopathic cause, resulting in chronic hyperglycemia. Hyperglycemia results in a multitude of long-term adverse consequences including microvascular and macrovascular injury, ultimately causing nephropathy, neuropathy, retinopathy, and atherosclerotic/cardiovascular disease. Hyperglycemia has traditionally been controlled by a combination of oral medications and insulin injections, both of which are accompanied by the life-threatening risk of hypoglycemic episodes. ICT is the process of allotransplantation of cadaveric donor islet cells to a recipient for the purposes of ameliorating or curing the symptoms and complications associated with diabetes and achieving long-term insulin independence. By providing a physiologic hormonal response via the body's natural feedback mechanism, ICT and pancreatic transplantation have provided a means to control hyperglycemia while reducing the risk of hypoglycemia.

In the United States, ICT is currently offered as part of research protocols, but in many countries, ICT is offered as a standard therapeutic option. The procedure, which is described in detail later in this chapter, is an intensive, multistep process involving organ procurement by an on-call transplant surgery team, enzymatic and mechanical islet cell isolation from the donor graft, quality assurance testing for contamination and cell count adequacy, simultaneous induction of immune suppression of the recipient candidate, and, ultimately, transhepatic infusion into the recipient portal vein by interventional radiologists.

The first steps toward insulin independence were made in 1966 when the first whole pancreas transplant was performed.[1] ICT became a possibility in the late 1960s when a collagenase-based isolation protocol was developed. The development of the islet cell transfer protocol has undergone continued evolution since the first animal studies were performed in 1972,[2] but advancements beginning in 1989 led to significant milestones in ICT research such as marked reductions in hypoglycemic episodes, consequential improvements in quality of life, and increasingly sustained periods of reduced or no insulin requirements.[3,4] However, the studies performed during the 1980s and 1990s showed only a transient reduction of insulin requirement, with most patients returning to complete insulin dependence within 3 to 5 years, requiring additional ICTs to overcome this obstacle.[5,6,7] In 2000, Shapiro et al showed greater than 1-year, complete insulin independence in seven patients after ICT using a glucocorticoid-free immunosuppression regimen.[8] Since 2000, the protocol for ICT has been modified numerous times, with improved results largely owing to optimized steroid-free immunosuppression regimens and patient/donor selection.

Currently, widespread adoption of ICT and whole pancreas transplant is limited by the availability of donor organs. Ongoing research continues to explore the possibility of harvesting β-cell transplants from human pluripotent stem cells, which would largely circumvent this obstacle.[9] Progress continues to be made in the realm of immunosuppressant regimens and the use of new transplant sites other than portal access.

25.3 Indications

25.3.1 Medical Therapy

ICT is most appropriate for patients in whom insulin therapy has failed to adequately control blood glucose. These patients have a high risk of clinical complications and poor quality of life. Despite its limitations in this delicate population, insulin therapy is still a standard treatment approach. Typical therapy involves subcutaneous insulin injections administered at least three times daily or the use of a continuous infusion pump. Despite optimization of the insulin regimen using standard protocols, patients still face a high risk of nephropathy, neuropathy, retinopathy, peripheral vascular disease, and cardiovascular disease. Regimens of intensive insulin therapy decrease the risk of these complications but increase the risk of hypoglycemic events, as exogenous administration cannot approximate physiologic feedback mechanisms. Moreover, intensive insulin therapy is only appropriate for highly motivated patients who are compliant with frequent blood glucose monitoring and nutritional counseling. Because ICT candidates suffer from the principal complaint of hypoglycemic unawareness, intensive insulin therapy is quite limited as an alternative treatment approach.

25.3.2 Whole Pancreas Transplantation versus ICT

Pancreas transplantation is the main surgical alternative to ICT and is the gold standard for appropriate candidates. Whole pancreas transplants may be performed in isolation or concomitantly with renal transplant for patients in renal failure; uremic patients are currently treated with whole pancreas or combined pancreas and kidney transplants. The goals of these transplants are to normalize blood glucose levels while minimizing adverse events related to hypoglycemic episodes and to eventually eliminate exogenous insulin dependence.

ICT offers a number of distinct advantages over whole pancreas transplant. The main advantage of ICT is the ability to intervene earlier in the course of the disease by using a minimally invasive technique with a substantially reduced risk of morbidity; in contrast, the reported complication rate for whole pancreas transplant is as high as 36%.[10] A larger percentage of the donor population qualifies for ICT, resulting in shorter wait times. Additionally, because ICT is a minimally invasive procedure, patients have shorter hospital stays, typically ranging from 24 to 48 hours for observation and reoptimization of management of blood glucose levels. Pain is minimal and easily controlled, and recovery typically occurs within a few days. Poor surgical candidates such as those with peripheral vascular disease may undergo ICT in most cases.

Whole pancreas transplantation requires cadaveric harvest followed by open creation of vascular and bowel anastomoses typically to the iliac vessels and jejunum; permanent immunosuppression is then required. As a result, the surgery is associated with significant morbidity. The most common complication leading almost invariably to early postoperative graft loss is vascular thrombosis, which occurs in 3 to 10% of patients.[11] Other common complications include duodenal leak, peripancreatic fluid collections, graft pancreatitis, graft site and wound infections, hemorrhage, and sepsis. Reoperations to resect, reanastomose, or retransplant are not uncommon, occurring in 24 to 36% of patients because of technical failures.[10] Mortality rates are 3% at 1 year and 8% at 3 years after simultaneous pancreas and kidney transplants, and these rates are similar for patients undergoing pancreas transplant alone or pancreas-after-kidney transplant.[12] One- and three-year graft failure rates range from 11 to 20% and 20 to 40%, respectively.[13]

In contrast, major complications with ICT are relatively uncommon. The most common complication after ICT is intraperitoneal and subcapsular hemorrhage, with an incidence rate reaching up to 13%.[14] The risk of bleeding is associated with the total number of ICTs performed and with the dose of heparin used.[14] Another main complication is nonocclusive portal vein thrombosis, which occurs in less than 5% of patients.[15] Other complications include transient liver enzyme elevation, abdominal pain, severe hypoglycemia, and graft loss. Bleeding after ICT is almost always minor and can be managed conservatively. However, bleeding complications in the early postoperative period after ICT threaten graft viability, as the postprocedural anticoagulation necessary for graft survival is usually terminated.

25.4 Procedure

25.4.1 Donor Selection and Tissue Isolation

As with pancreas transplantation, ICT begins with the best attempt at optimal harvesting of the donor organ by minimizing cold ischemic time, maximizing donor matching, and optimizing both donor and recipient characteristics. The criteria for ideal donor selection are currently up for debate; however, donor age and body mass index have been previously reported to be critical factors.[16] The donor pancreas is harvested in such a way as to preserve the organ capsule and the connection to the duodenum. Cold ischemia time is limited to 12 hours. After arriving at the transplant center, the donor organ is treated with proteolytic collagenase through the main pancreatic duct. The next step is tissue digestion in the Ricordi chamber, in which the tissue is dissolved and dissected using multiple metallic beads that help to break down the fibrous septal tissue. Finally, the β-cells are isolated using density centrifugation. The cells are washed and maintained in temperature-controlled culture media for 12 to 72 hours until the time of transplant.

25.4.2 Patient Selection

Candidates for ICT include patients with longstanding type 1 diabetes mellitus (> 5 years), absence of endogenous C-peptide secretion, intermittent severe undetected hypoglycemic episodes, or worsening diabetes-related complications despite intensive insulin therapy. Most patients have normal renal function or have already undergone a renal transplant.

Contraindications to ICT typically include age less than 18 years, untreated diabetic retinopathy, portal hypertension, active infection, substance abuse, pregnancy, severe uncontrolled hypertension, severe cardiac disease, macroalbuminurea, renal insufficiency, and noncompliance with immunosuppression. Relative contraindications include obesity and relative insulin resistance.[17] Patients are typically treated with antibiotics and antivirals as well as a lymphocyte-depleting agent such as antithymocyte globulin or alemtuzumab before ICT.

25.4.3 Transplant

The isolated donor acinar cells are infused percutaneously via the portal vein in the interventional angiography suite under moderate conscious sedation and real-time cardiopulmonary monitoring (▶ Fig. 25.1). Under ultrasound guidance, percutaneous access into a third-order branch of the right portal vein is achieved using a small 21-gauge needle. A microwire is placed through the needle, over which a 4- to 6-French catheter or vascular sheath is placed transhepatically and into the main portal vein. Systemic heparin is then infused (typically 5,000 U). The portal venous pressure is measured; an elevated pressure (> 20 mm Hg) is a contraindication to proceeding. The islet cells are maintained in a preparation solution that is heparinized (70 U/kg) and infused via gravity over the span of a few hours. The portal pressure is intermittently measured; if at any time the pressure becomes greater than 22 mm Hg for longer than 10 minutes, the infusion should be ceased. After infusion, the tract is embolized with coils and/or Gelfoam or microfibrillary collagen paste under fluoroscopic guidance to minimize bleeding. The catheter is subsequently withdrawn.

25.4.4 Posttransplant

Directly after ICT, patients are admitted for 24 to 48 hours and maintained on a constant heparin infusion to prevent portal vein thrombosis. At discharge, the heparin is changed to subcutaneous

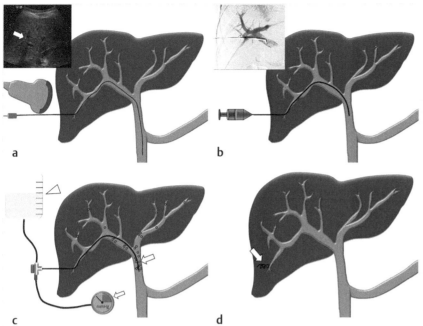

Fig. 25.1 ICT procedure in interventional radiology. **(a)** Under direct ultrasound guidance, a 21-gauge needle is advanced into a peripheral portal vein branch, and a microwire is advanced to the main portal vein. The inset ultrasound image shows the needle tip (*arrow*) nearing the portal branch without traversing other large vessels. **(b)** A small (typically 4 French) catheter is advanced over the wire to the main portal vein. The inset image shows minimal contrast injection to demonstrate adequate catheter placement. **(c)** Islet cells (*large arrow*) are infused into the main portal vein from a gravity bag (*arrowhead*). A closed system with a stopcock can allow intermittent monitoring of portal pressure (*small arrow*) during infusion. **(d)** Tract embolization using coils (*arrow*) follows completion of infusion. Other embolization agents have also been described for this purpose.

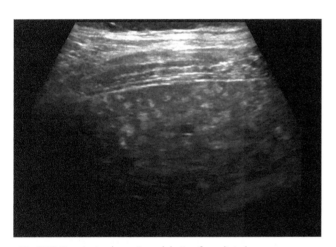

Fig. 25.2 Transient echogenic nodularity of no clinical consequence may be observed on ultrasound examinations after ICT in a minority of cases.

enoxaparin and aspirin for at least 1 week. Strict glucose control is crucial in the recovery period, as apoptotic cells release insulin into the bloodstream. Patients continue to self-administer insulin to maintain fasting blood glucose levels under 140 mg/dL and postprandial blood glucose levels under 180 mg/dL. Insulin therapy is continued for at least 1 month to aid graft uptake and reduce cellular stress, with gradual tapering and eventual cessation of exogenous insulin shortly thereafter. Doppler ultrasound of the liver is obtained at 1 day and 1 week after the procedure to assess portal vein patency. Transient echogenic nodules may be seen in a minority of cases, but this finding has no clinical consequence (▶ Fig. 25.2). After ICT, patients must continue a life-long immunosuppression regimen to prevent graft rejection. Maintenance therapy consists of calcineurin inhibitors and mycophenolate mofetil.[18] Finally, many patients require multiple rounds of ICT (up to three) to achieve therapeutic results.

25.5 Outcomes

25.5.1 Clinical Success

Clinical data continue to support whole pancreas transplants as the gold-standard treatment for patients with β-cell deficiency. The 5-year patient survival rate after combined kidney and pancreas transplants is above 80%, with a 5-year graft survival rate above 70% and an average addition of 4.6 life years per transplant recipient.[19,20] Patients with a solitary pancreas transplant or a pancreas-after-kidney transplant have similar 5-year survival rates but lower 5-year graft survival rates (62–65% and 50–58%, respectively).[21] The reasons for this discrepancy are unclear but may be related to an increased rate of early graft thrombosis or variations in immunosuppression regimens. Limited long-term follow-up after ICT is available, but 5-year patient survival of 94.6% was reported in a single-center observational study of 112 patients.[22]

While whole pancreas transplants suffer from a high complication and graft loss rate due to technical factors, patients who undergo ICT may fail to achieve long-term insulin independence because of a gradual "burnout" effect with progressive decrease in function over time. Encouragingly, the Collaborative Islet Transplant Registry has reported an increase in 3-year insulin independence from 2002 to 2010 (from 27 to 44%, respectively).[23] Other centers have reported 5-year insulin independence rates of greater than 50%, with a rate of 40% after a single infusion.[24] This may be in part related to improved isolation and purification techniques.

The primary determinant of ICT success on a case-by-case basis is the total number of transplanted β-cells, or the islet equivalent. Multiple donor organs or multiple rounds of infusion may be needed to achieve a high islet equivalent. However, several recent studies have shown the ability to attain insulin independence after a single infusion.[24,25]

Complications related to chronic immunosuppression are common to both ICT and pancreas transplants, but patients with type 1 diabetes at any level of glycemic control who already take immunosuppressive medication are potential candidates for ICT. Currently, ICT research protocols in the United States include a study arm of renal transplant patients. Such patients have no increased risk involving immunosuppressive medication and are poor candidates for whole pancreas transplant.

25.6 Conclusion

Pancreatic ICT is a minimally invasive, safe therapy for patients with severe longstanding type 1 diabetes mellitus, with an increasing amount of data supporting the long-term efficacy of this treatment. ICT restores normal β-cell function, resulting in a physiologic response to hyperglycemia, long-term insulin independence, and a reduction in hypoglycemic episodes. ICT is currently limited in scope to large centers with established research protocols; the use of this treatment is also limited by the scarcity of available donor organs. Furthermore, lifelong immunosuppression is currently required after ICT is performed. More work is needed to reduce graft loss and host rejection over time. Continued research in the areas of pancreatic stem cell harvest and autotransplant will also remain of high interest in the future as possible cures for type 1 diabetes.

References

[1] Kelly WD, Lillehei RC, Merkel FK, Idezuki Y, Goetz FC. Allotransplantation of the pancreas and duodenum along with the kidney in diabetic nephropathy. Surgery. 1967; 61(6):827–837

[2] Ballinger WF, Lacy PE. Transplantation of intact pancreatic islets in rats. Surgery. 1972; 72(2):175–186

[3] Lake SP, Bassett PD, Larkins A, et al. Large-scale purification of human islets utilizing discontinuous albumin gradient on IBM 2991 cell separator. Diabetes. 1989; 38 Suppl 1:143–145

[4] Scharp DW, Lacy PE, Santiago JV, et al. Insulin independence after islet transplantation into type I diabetic patient. Diabetes. 1990; 39(4):515–518

[5] Warnock GL, Kneteman NM, Ryan EA, et al. Continued function of pancreatic islets after transplantation in type I diabetes. Lancet. 1989; 2(8662):570–572

[6] Socci C, Falqui L, Davalli AM, et al. Fresh human islet transplantation to replace pancreatic endocrine function in type 1 diabetic patients. Report of six cases. Acta Diabetol. 1991; 28(2):151–157

[7] Ricordi C, Tzakis AG, Carroll PB, et al. Human islet isolation and allotransplantation in 22 consecutive cases. Transplantation. 1992; 53(2): 407–414

[8] Shapiro AM, Lakey JR, Ryan EA, et al. Islet transplantation in seven patients with type 1 diabetes mellitus using a glucocorticoid-free immunosuppressive regimen. N Engl J Med. 2000; 343(4):230–238

[9] Piran M, Enderami SE, Piran M, Sedeh HS, Seyedjafari E, Ardeshirylajimi A. Insulin producing cells generation by overexpression of miR-375 in adipose-derived mesenchymal stem cells from diabetic patients. Biologicals. 2017; 46: 23–28

[10] Reddy KS, Stratta RJ, Shokouh-Amiri MH, Alloway R, Egidi MF, Gaber AO. Surgical complications after pancreas transplantation with portal-enteric drainage. J Am Coll Surg. 1999; 189(3):305–313

[11] Gruessner AC, Sutherland DE. Pancreas transplant outcomes for United States (US) cases as reported to the United Network for Organ Sharing (UNOS) and the International Pancreas Transplant Registry (IPTR). Clin Transpl. 2008:45–56

[12] Redfield RR, Rickels MR, Naji A, Odorico JS. Pancreas transplantation in the modern era. Gastroenterol Clin North Am. 2016; 45(1):145–166

[13] Gruessner RW, Sutherland DE, Gruessner AC. Mortality assessment for pancreas transplants. Am J Transplant. 2004; 4(12):2018–2026

[14] Villiger P, Ryan EA, Owen R, et al. Prevention of bleeding after islet transplantation: lessons learned from a multivariate analysis of 132 cases at a single institution. Am J Transplant. 2005; 5(12):2992–2998

[15] Ryan EA, Paty BW, Senior PA, et al. Five-year follow-up after clinical islet transplantation. Diabetes. 2005; 54(7):2060–2069

[16] Takita M, Naziruddin B, Matsumoto S, et al. Body mass index reflects islet isolation outcome in islet autotransplantation for patients with chronic pancreatitis. Cell Transplant. 2011; 20(2):313–322

[17] Ludwig B, Ludwig S, Steffen A, Saeger HD, Bornstein SR. Islet versus pancreas transplantation in type 1 diabetes: competitive or complementary? Curr Diab Rep. 2010; 10(6):506–511

[18] Wisel SA, Braun HJ, Stock PG. Current outcomes in islet versus solid organ pancreas transplant for β-cell replacement in type 1 diabetes. Curr Opin Organ Transplant. 2016; 21(4):399–404

[19] Gruessner RW, Gruessner AC. The current state of pancreas transplantation. Nat Rev Endocrinol. 2013; 9(9):555–562

[20] Rana A, Gruessner A, Agopian VG, et al. Survival benefit of solid-organ transplant in the United States. JAMA Surg. 2015; 150(3):252–259

[21] Kandaswamy R, Skeans MA, Gustafson SK, et al. OPTN/SRTR 2013 Annual Data Report: pancreas. Am J Transplant. 2015; 15 Suppl 2:1–20

[22] Wilson GC, Sutton JM, Abbott DE, et al. Long-term outcomes after total pancreatectomy and islet cell autotransplantation: is it a durable operation? Ann Surg. 2014; 260(4):659–665, discussion 665–667

[23] Squifflet JP, Gruessner RW, Sutherland DE. The history of pancreas transplantation: past, present and future. Acta Chir Belg. 2008; 108(3):367–378

[24] Al-Adra DP, Gill RS, Imes S, et al. Single-donor islet transplantation and long-term insulin independence in select patients with type 1 diabetes mellitus. Transplantation. 2014; 98(9):1007–1012

[25] Hering BJ, Kandaswamy R, Ansite JD, et al. Single-donor, marginal-dose islet transplantation in patients with type 1 diabetes. [erratum in JAMA. 2005;293:1594]. JAMA. 2005; 293(7):830–835

26 Percutaneous Enteral Access

Jonathan M. Lorenz

26.1 Introduction

Percutaneous enteral access (PEA) devices are key components in the management of a wide variety of conditions requiring long-term enteral nutrition, gastroenteric decompression, and gastroenteric diversion. PEA devices, which are placed routinely by radiologists, gastroenterologists, and surgeons, include percutaneous gastrostomy tubes (pGTs), gastrojejunostomy tubes (pGJTs), and jejunostomy tubes (pJTs). Given the ease of placement of PEA devices using minimally invasive options, it is not surprising that their use has steadily increased.[1] This chapter reviews the indications for PEA device placement, the devices that are available, placement techniques, aftercare, and the management of complications related to these devices.

Enteric access options include temporary access through bloodless anatomic pathways if the device is required for less than 4 to 6 weeks and permanent access through a percutaneous pathway if the device is required for a longer interval.[2] Temporary options include nasally or orally placed tubes terminating in the stomach, duodenum, or jejunum. Minimally invasive permanent options are the focus of this chapter and include pGTs, pGJTs, and pJTs placed endoscopically, usually by a gastroenterologist, or with imaging guidance, usually by a radiologist. In terms of nomenclature, recommendations from the Society of Interventional Radiology (SIR) Standards of Practice guidelines will be followed in this chapter.[3] The terms "transoral" (also called "pull-type") placement and "transabdominal" (also called "push-type") placement will be used to describe the route of tube advancement through the abdominal wall. As a given provider may be skilled in a variety of placement techniques, specific medical disciplines will be replaced by the general terms "imaging-guided" and "endoscopic" when describing techniques of placement.

26.2 Indications

In general, indications for PEA include long-term enteral nutrition, gastroenteric decompression, and gastroenteric diversion. The latter two indications are widely accepted, but controversy exists regarding the possible overuse of percutaneous enteral nutrition.[4] For some conditions, published results show that the benefits clearly outweigh the risks, but for others, PEA is commonly used despite no clear benefit.

For the decompression of malignant and nonmalignant gastrointestinal (GI) obstruction, PEA is an accepted, standard option with measurable benefits.[5,6,7] Depending on the clinical presentation and indication for device placement, this application can improve quality of life (QoL), improve survival, prevent immediate morbidity and mortality, and obviate the need for surgical intervention.[8] Examples include definitive treatment of postoperative abdominal adhesions and palliative decompression of cancers such as gynecological malignancies.[5,6,7,9] Another well-established application is the diversion of GI contents and formula from a benign or malignant esophageal, gastric, or intestinal fistula to promote healing and to facilitate enteral feeding.

For functional impairment or mechanical obstruction of the upper GI tract that prevents swallowing, PEA for enteral nutrition improves QoL and survival for select indications.[10] Benign examples include esophageal strictures and neurological conditions such as stroke, traumatic brain injury, amyotrophic lateral sclerosis, and neuromuscular disorders in children. Malignant examples include head and neck and esophageal cancer, although the use of PEA devices in patients with these conditions has been associated with a higher procedural risk.[11] In some cases, impairment in swallowing results in aspiration pneumonia; published studies have reported mixed results with PEA devices used to prevent this condition in high-risk patients.[12,13] Some research found that PEA devices offer no clinical benefit in preventing aspiration pneumonia, and PEA itself can be complicated by aspiration both during placement and during feeding.[14] For patients with other indications for PEA and documented aspiration pneumonia, conversion from a pGT to a pGJT or pJT may mitigate or prevent this complication.[15]

For select chronic conditions that cause failure to thrive, PEA can improve QoL and reduce morbidity. Examples include Crohn's disease in children, metabolic disorders, and benign anatomic causes for food intolerance such as superior mesenteric artery syndrome (▶ Fig. 26.1).[16] On the other hand, when failure to thrive results from anorexia, published results argue in favor of prioritizing medical and psychiatric therapies with an occasional application of PEA.[17] Furthermore, little clinical benefit has been demonstrated with PEA for impaired feeding or failure to thrive associated with cachexia caused by terminal cancer with a poor prognosis for long-term survival, dementia-related loss of cognitive function, or permanent vegetative states.[18,19] Patients with poor or absent cognitive function may lack the ability for self-determination, and the decision by caregivers to place PEA devices in such cases is controversial as this procedure may actually prolong suffering rather than improve QoL. In many of these cases, nonmedical influences such as medicolegal pressure, input from family members and caregivers, and instructions left by patients in living wills win out over published evidence, leading to the placement of a PEA device.

For most indications, pGT is the most commonly used PEA device as this type is easy to place and replace, comes in a variety of models to fit most access needs, and has a decades-long track record of technical and clinical success. However, clinical and anatomic considerations may indicate the need for additional or separate small bowel access via a pGJT or pJT. Small bowel access may be indicated to prevent vomiting and aspiration pneumonia in patients with other indications for PEA. Examples include high-risk patients with a history of gastroesophageal reflux and patients on ventilators requiring enteral nutrition. Published meta-analyses support this indication.[15,20,21] Other indications for small bowel access include extension of PEA beyond a GI fistula or obstruction for enteral nutrition, decompression, or diversion. Small bowel PEA facilitates delivery of medications and formula distal to the fistula. In such cases, a dual-lumen pGJT is helpful to allow gastric suction concurrently with small bowel feeding.

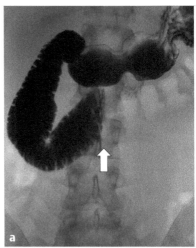
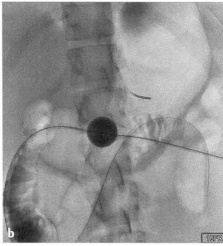

Fig. 26.1 A 22-year-old woman with a history of marked weight loss presented with pain, bilious vomiting, and difficulty gaining weight. **(a)** Upper GI barium study showed craniocaudal, midline compression of the third duodenal segment (*arrow*). Further imaging supported the diagnosis of superior mesenteric artery syndrome. **(b)** A pGJT was placed for gastric decompression through the gastric port and enteral feeding through the jejunal port. Subsequent weight gain resulted in an increase in the aortomesenteric arterial angle and resolution of the compression. The tube was removed after 8 months.

26.3 Placement Options

Imaging-guided PEA device placement requires no endoscope and instead makes use of fluoroscopy and occasionally ultrasound (US) and computed tomography (CT). Standard imaging-guided PEA requires initial advancement of a small nasogastric catheter to facilitate gastric insufflation for percutaneous puncture, but initial gastric puncture using a skinny needle for insufflation can bypass this requirement.[22] Endoscopic PEA requires the patient to be a candidate for endoscopy and to be thin enough to allow successful transillumination of the abdominal wall to guide gastric puncture. Most published reports show no difference in success and complication rates for endoscopic and imaging-guided PEA.[9,23,24] In addition, minimally invasive options are associated with comparable success rates and lower complication rates compared to surgical options[25,26,27] and can be performed under conscious sedation rather than general anesthesia in most cases. Therefore, depending on local expertise, surgical PEA device placement is usually reserved as a secondary option when other options fail or are infeasible. A major advantage of imaging-guided PEA is the ability to place tubes when endoscopic PEA fails or is infeasible, as in patients with severe facial and neck fractures, esophageal strictures, severe mucositis, head and neck tumors, or morbid obesity that prevents endoscopic transillumination (see "Techniques of Placement"). In addition, imaging-guided PEA avoids the complications of endoscopy itself such as esophageal perforation. On the other hand, advantages of endoscopic over imaging-guided PEA include bedside placement in immobile patients, the absence of exposure to ionizing radiation, and the ability to directly visualize GI pathology that may alter or contraindicate the procedure such as peptic ulcer disease and varices. Ultimately, both of these placement options are viable in most cases; in select cases, clinical and anatomic considerations may determine the appropriateness of imaging-guided, endoscopic, or surgical PEA.

In terms of the route of advancement through the skin, two basic options exist: transoral PEA, which involves pulling the tube from the mouth through the abdominal wall, and transabdominal PEA, which involves pushing the tube directly through the abdominal wall (see "Techniques of Placement"). The main advantage of transabdominal over transoral PEA is the option for PEA even when conditions prevent the advancement of large-bore, bumper-retained tubes through the upper GI tract. Examples include patients with esophageal strictures or bulky head and neck tumors. Head and neck cancer is a relative contraindication to transoral PEA because of published reports of metastatic seeding of the stomal site resulting from cancer cells that adhere to the tube as it traverses the region of the primary tumor (▶ Fig. 26.2).[28] The only obstacle to transabdominal PEA is the lack of a safe window for gastric puncture. The main advantage of transoral over transabdominal PEA is the routine placement of tubes that are large bore and bumper retained, leading to fewer long-term complications such as clogging and dislodgment.[29,30] For the two advancement routes, procedure-related complication rates are similar.[9,23,24,29]

In some cases, surgical PEA may be preferable to minimally invasive alternatives. Recurrent large-volume ascites impedes stomal tract formation and is associated with peristomal leakage of ascites when minimally invasive methods are attempted; surgical gastropexy may be preferable in such cases. Interposed colon or liver during attempts at imaging-guided or endoscopic PEA may necessitate surgical PEA. In some cases, congenital or acquired conditions profoundly affect the position of the stomach and adjacent structures and may necessitate surgical PEA. Examples include extensive gastric pathology, partial gastrectomy, and gastric bypass.

26.4 Device Options

26.4.1 Small-Bore versus Large-Bore Devices

PEA devices are distinguished by two key factors: diameter and type of internal retainer. Regarding diameter, tubes less than or equal to 14 French are considered small bore. Debate exists among authors regarding placement of small-bore versus large-bore devices. For most enteral feeding indications, large-bore tubes are just as easy to place, have similar rates of procedure-related complications, and are tolerated just as well as small-bore tubes, but with fewer long-term complications such as clogging or dislodgment. A retrospective series comparing 88 small-bore pGTs to 72 large-bore pGTs found that small-bore pGTs had more complications (17 vs. 5.6%) and were less likely

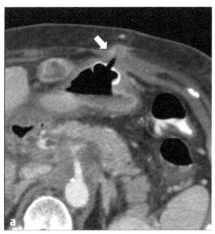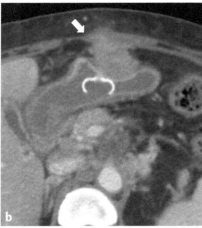

Fig. 26.2 A 66-year-old man with a history of head and neck cancer needed long-term enteric nutrition. **(a)** CT with contrast obtained 2 months after transoral pGT placement showed soft tissue (*arrow*) surrounding the bumper-retained pGT. **(b)** Five months after placement, a soft-tissue mass (*arrow*) displaced the stomach, consistent with metastatic seeding of the pGT tract. Transabdominal pGT placement is preferred in patients with head and neck cancer to avoid this uncommon complication.

to meet their feeding goal.[30] Additionally, small-bore pGTs were more prone to long-term dysfunction. Despite such results, published procedural and long-term complication rates for both small- and large-bore tubes are within acceptable limits.[3] In addition, small-bore tubes have their advantages. Small, pigtail-retained pGTs can be placed quickly with minimal or no serial dilatation, making them especially suitable for gastric decompression or for difficult cases such as pJT placement or CT-guided pGT placement.

26.4.2 Internal Retainers

Internal retainers include balloon-, locking-loop-, and Malecot-retained tubes that are placed transabdominally and bumper-retained tubes that are placed transorally. The transorally placed bumper-retained pGT, the mainstay of percutaneous endoscopic gastrostomy, has been tested for decades and has proven itself to be highly durable.[5,7,9,27] Unlike pigtail and balloon retainers, the bumper cannot be inadvertently "unlocked" by patients or caregivers and requires strong traction force for removal in most cases. As expected, published rates of dislodgment are low. Funaki et al[29] retrospectively reviewed long-term complication rates for bumper-retained and balloon-retained pGTs and found a significantly lower rate of dislodgment for the former. In addition, procedure-related complications such as peristomal leakage, peritoneal leakage, and pneumoperitoneum are uncommon with bumper-retained tubes as the use of over sized peel-away sheaths and serial dilatation is unnecessary for placement. This feature makes bumper-retained pGTs suitable for feeding within 4 hours of placement in most cases as opposed to 12- to 24-hour delays for other devices. Unlike bumper-retained tubes, balloon-, locking-loop-, and Malecot-retained tubes are advanced transabdominally under fluoroscopic guidance. Their main advantage over bumper-retained tubes is their suitability for patients with contraindications to endoscopy or transoral advancement of large-bore tubes.

26.4.3 Low-Profile Tubes

Another variation in PEA is the low-profile tube, also called a "button" tube. Its primary benefit is to reduce tampering and dislodgment in children and high-risk adults, but patients often favor this option for its cosmetic benefit. Low-profile tubes have

a small external flange that doubles as an access port, eliminating the long external tube associated with other options. Low-profile tubes are manufactured with balloon-, bumper-, and locking-loop-retainers, as well as single- or double-lumen options for gastric and jejunal access.

26.5 Screening and Preparation

26.5.1 General Considerations

A patient referred for PEA device placement should undergo initial screening for the appropriateness of the clinical indication, the optimal PEA option for the indication, and considerations that may dictate a specific technique and provider. Attention is then turned to eligibility for device placement. Contraindications vary from relative to absolute depending on the type and severity, and include uncorrectable coagulopathy, hemodynamic instability, peritonitis, bowel ischemia, marked ascites, ileus or mechanical obstruction (if for enteral nutrition), the absence of an option for long-term tube management (either by the patient or by a caregiver), and the absence of a safe window for stomal creation. Patients should be screened for the need for general anesthesia versus conscious sedation and the presence of an adequate oral airway the day before the procedure. Cessation of intake by mouth after midnight should be ordered to minimize the risk of aspiration and infection.[14]

26.5.2 Infection

Infection is a relative contraindication to device placement unless the patient has the absolute contraindication of peritonitis. Fever and local infections remote from the stomal site do not preclude pGT placement; if possible, bacteremia should be treated to resolution before device placement. Ventriculoperitoneal shunt is a relative contraindication, as placement of a pGT increases the risk of shunt infection and ascending meningitis.[31] Prophylactic periprocedural antibiotics have been shown to decrease postprocedural infection rates[32,33] and should be chosen to cover cutaneous pathogens, although patients covered with antibiotics for other conditions usually do not require additional coverage. A meta-analysis of 11 prospective randomized trials demonstrated that prophylactic antibiotics significantly reduce peristomal infections after primary PEA placement.[32]

26.5.3 Safe Needle Pathway

A history of GI infection, inflammation, or obstruction and a history of surgical procedures such as gastric resection or bypass may alter the position and relationships of abdominal structures and affect the feasibility and method of PEA device placement. In addition, a variety of congenital or acquired conditions may affect the risk and feasibility of the procedure. The main concern is gastric displacement from an acceptable puncture site or interposition of structures or pathology between the puncture site and the gastric lumen. Gastric displacement occurs with large GI hernias, intrathoracic stomachs, previous GI surgery, previous abdominal surgery with resultant disruption of the gastric ligaments, and GI malrotation. Potentially interposed normal structures include the colon, small bowel, liver, or vasculature such as gastric or mesenteric arteries and varices; pathologic structures include tumors of the abdominal wall, peritoneum, or stomach; hernias; local infections; burns; and surgical wounds. To minimize the risk of nontarget puncture, all relevant past radiologic and endoscopic studies should be reviewed, although new imaging is usually not indicated. Some providers routinely administer 100 to 200 mL oral barium contrast the night before the procedure to distinguish the colon during fluoroscopically guided gastric puncture, but this practice is optional as low complication rates have been described when this step is omitted.[29] Careful evaluation of frontal fluoroscopy at the time of gastric puncture is almost always sufficient to avoid colon puncture. Additional measures include obtaining a lateral fluoroscopic view or injecting contrast through a skinny needle along the expected stomal tract under fluoroscopic guidance to expose interposed bowel or liver. Interposed vasculature and solid structures may necessitate direct US guidance of gastric puncture.

26.5.4 Ascites

Published reports have described success with PEA in the presence of ascites, but the degree of ascites and the timing of reaccumulation likely influence the outcome.[34] Ascites causes poor tract maturation and separation of the stomach wall from the anterior abdominal wall after primary pGT placement. This places the patient at risk for leakage of ascites along the tract and leakage of stomach contents into the peritoneum with resultant peritonitis. For ascites that surrounds the expected stomal site, a trial of paracentesis and repeat US after 1 week is warranted to rule out rapid reaccumulation. Consult for surgical PEA is indicated for cases with rapid reaccumulation of large volume ascites.

26.5.5 Bleeding Risk

In terms of screening for bleeding risk, the Clinical Practice Guidelines of the SIR and American Gastroenterological Association Institute rate PEA as moderate risk.[35] SIR recommends correction of the international normalized ratio (INR) if this value is greater than 1.5, transfusion of platelets if the platelet count is less than 50,000/μL, withholding of clopidogrel for 5 days before the procedure, and withholding of one therapeutic dose of low-molecular-weight heparin before the procedure. Aspirin need not be held. The American Society for Gastrointestinal Endoscopy rates PEA as high risk and recommends cessation of warfarin for 5 days with conversion to intravenous (IV) low-molecular-weight heparin, which is then stopped the morning of the procedure.[36] Clopidogrel can be stopped 7 days before the procedure and substituted with aspirin. Warfarin and clopidogrel can be restarted the evening of and the morning after the procedure, respectively. Although it is not necessary to obtain other laboratory values other than INR and platelet level, it is prudent to assess all existing coagulation and hematology values to establish the risk level for informed consent.

26.6 Techniques of Placement

The two basic methods for minimally invasive PEA device placement are defined by the route of tube advancement: transoral and transabdominal. Each of these methods can be performed using endoscopic or imaging guidance. Multiple variations of these methods have been described, but two commonly used techniques are described below. Gastropexy sutures are used variably among practitioners, more commonly for transabdominal placement, but associated complications make their use controversial.

26.6.1 Transoral Gastrostomy

The transoral technique (▶ Fig. 26.3) can be performed using either imaging or endoscopic guidance. For imaging-guided transoral placement, 1-mg IV glucagon is administered to tighten the pyloric sphincter and stall peristalsis.[29] The stomach is insufflated with air through a preexisting nasogastric tube or through a small, 5-French multipurpose angiographic catheter placed immediately before the procedure. The movement and position of the stomach and colon are monitored fluoroscopically during insufflation. The abdomen and peritoneum are anesthetized with a local injection of lidocaine, and a small incision is made. Under fluoroscopy, the midbody of the stomach is punctured with an 18-G needle angled toward the antrum to allow for conversion to a pGJT if indicated. Deviation from this tract orientation can cause delayed retraction of the jejunal component into the gastric lumen. Access to the esophagus is achieved using a standard guidewire; a 10-French sheath is then advanced over this wire into the esophagus, and the wire is advanced out the mouth. The loop snare provided in bumper-retained pGT kits is attached to the abdominal end of the wire and pushed through the sheath as the wire is pulled out of the mouth. The snare exits the mouth and is attached to a loop on the pGT. The snare is pulled from the abdominal end, which pulls the pGT through the esophagus and out the stomal tract until its bumper is against the inner gastric wall. The external flange is advanced until it is slightly loose (2–5 mm over the skin surface) to decrease the risk of pressure-related complications of the skin and tract.[25] The position of the flange should allow for in-and-out excursion of the tube by 1 cm. The external tube length at the skin surface should be documented if marked on the pGT. Feeding can typically be initiated after 4 hours.

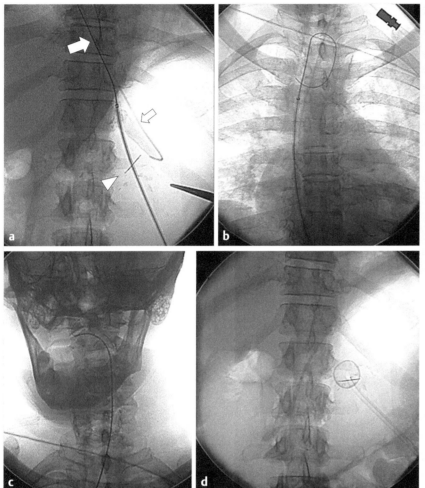

Fig. 26.3 Imaging-guided transoral pGT placement. **(a)** Under fluoroscopic monitoring and guidance, the stomach is insufflated with air through a nasogastric tube (*small arrow*), the midbody is punctured, an optional gastropexy suture is placed (*arrowhead*), a separate puncture is made with an 18-G needle, a wire is advanced into the esophagus (*large arrow*), and a long 10-French sheath is placed. **(b)** Wire and sheath are advanced to the upper esophagus. **(c)** Wire is advanced out of the mouth for guidance of snare advancement entering the abdomen and exiting the mouth. **(d)** Snare is attached to a loop on the pGT dilator and the pGT is pulled down the esophagus until the bumper is against the anterior gastric wall.

For endoscopic transoral placement, after endoscopic access to the stomach is achieved, the stomach is insufflated with air and the puncture site is chosen by a combination of transillumination from the gastric lumen and endoscopic observation of a finger indenting the abdominal wall at the point of transillumination. The abdomen and peritoneum are anesthetized with a local injection of lidocaine, and a small incision is made. The lidocaine needle is often advanced into the gastric lumen to verify the absence of bowel transgression by a combination of air aspiration and endoscopic visualization of the needle. The stomach is punctured with a small trocar, and a wire is passed into the lumen, grasped endoscopically, and pulled out of the mouth. This wire is used to advance a snare from the abdominal wall out of the mouth. This snare is attached to a pGT, and the snare and pGT are pulled out of the abdominal wall until the bumper is juxtaposed to the inner gastric wall. The tube is then prepared and used as described for imaging-guided transoral placement.

26.6.2 Transabdominal Gastrostomy

The transabdominal technique (▶ Fig. 26.4) is most commonly performed using fluoroscopic guidance, but in some cases, CT guidance is required. As in imaging-guided transoral placement, 1-mg IV glucagon is administered, and the stomach is insufflated. The abdomen and peritoneum are anesthetized with a local injection of lidocaine, and a small incision is made. The midbody of the stomach is optionally tacked against the abdominal wall with three to four gastropexy sutures based on operator preference, a separate puncture is made using an 18-G needle angled toward the antrum, and a standard guidewire is advanced into the stomach. For small-bore, locking-loop catheters, the pGT is advanced over the wire into the stomach. Serial dilatation may be required to facilitate pGT advancement, but this is often avoided to prevent leakage when the pGT is placed for decompression. For balloon-retained catheters, serial dilatation is performed over a wire, a peel-away sheath is advanced over the wire into the gastric lumen, and the pGT is advanced over the wire and through the peel-away sheath. The balloon is inflated, the sheath is removed, and the external flange is advanced over the skin surface as described for transoral placement. The required peel-away sheath is typically four French sizes larger than the pGT, which creates a theoretical increased risk of leakage. This overdilation prompts most providers to leave gastropexy sutures in place for 10 to 14 days and delay feeding for 12 to 24 hours. A one-step method has been described to speed up the placement of balloon-retained pGTs and obviate the need for serial dilators and peel-away sheaths. After the placement of gastropexy sutures and achievement of wire access into the gastric lumen, a 16-French balloon-retained pGT mounted on a 9-mm angioplasty balloon is

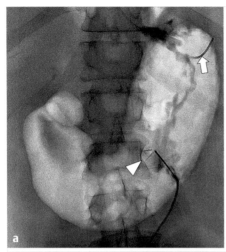
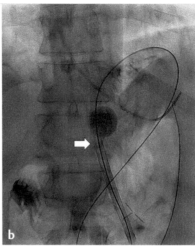

Fig. 26.4 Imaging-guided transabdominal pGT placement. **(a)** Under fluoroscopic monitoring and guidance, the stomach is insufflated with air through a nasogastric tube (*arrow*), three to four gastropexy sutures are placed (*arrowhead*), and the midbody of the stomach is punctured with an 18-G needle. **(b)** A stiff guidewire is advanced into the stomach, a tract is dilated, a peel-away sheath is placed, and a balloon-retained pGT is advanced into the stomach over the wire and through the sheath. The balloon is inflated just beyond the tip of the peel-away sheath (*arrow*), and the sheath is removed. **(c)** The balloon is retracted against the anterior gastric wall and secured.

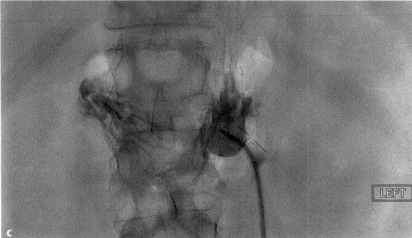

advanced over the wire. The angioplasty balloon is advanced across the stomal tract first and inflated. The pGT is then advanced across the stomal tract behind the deflating angioplasty balloon.

CT guidance of PEA can be used for cases that fail or are infeasible using standard fluoroscopic imaging guidance. This option is a primary choice for patients who have undergone operations that prevent insufflation or alter gastric size, including distal antrectomy, Billroth II, and gastric bypass.

26.6.3 Gastrojejunostomy

Small bowel PEA can be achieved by primary or secondary placement of a pGJT using either the transoral or the transabdominal method. For transoral placement, a bumper-retained pGT is converted to a pGJT without the discomfort of removal of the original pGT. This is accomplished by advancement of a jejunal extension tube through the pGT. The final result is a dual lumen tube with ports for both gastric and jejunal access. For transabdominal placement, a pGJT can be placed primarily using the technique for transabdominal pGT described above, or an existing pGT can be exchanged over a wire under fluoroscopic guidance for a pGJT. Transabdominal pGJT placement results in either a single larger lumen terminating in the jejunum or two smaller lumens for both gastric and jejunal access. Low-profile tubes are typically placed by exchanging a standard tube over a

wire after a 4- to 6-week period of tract maturation. Before this exchange, careful measurement of stomal length is required to select and order the correct device.

26.6.4 Direct Percutaneous Jejunostomy

Direct pJT placement can be performed using either endoscopic or imaging guidance. The endoscopic technique involves the performance of jejunoscopy followed by the application of the endoscopic techniques described above for transoral pGT placement: transillumination, finger indentation, and testing of the expected stomal tract using a skinny needle. The skinny needle is grasped with a snare to stabilize the jejunum for trocar puncture, a wire is advanced into the jejunum, and a pJT is placed using either the transabdominal or transoral technique. For imaging-guided pJT placement, an angiographic catheter from the nasal or oral approach is used to catheterize the proximal jejunum. A jejunal target is then punctured under fluoroscopic guidance by targeting rapidly insufflated intraluminal air or a large balloon. US-guided puncture is possible if the jejunal loop is rapidly filled with saline. Gastropexy anchors are commonly used for pJTs because leakage is common. Placement pJTs is usually performed using the transabdominal technique described for pGTs. Small-bore pigtail tubes are popular for pJT options as they require minimal serial dilatation.

26.7 Postprocedural Management and Aftercare

26.7.1 Feeding

Daily follow-up immediately after PEA and long-term aftercare are critical. Delayed complications far outnumber procedure-related complications. The first considerations are often the timing and rate of feeding initiation and the formula used. Post-procedure orders should be written for a nutrition consultation to customize the feeding regimen and assess tolerance levels. In adults, feeding 2 to 4 hours after bumper-retained pGT placement has been described without increased complication rates.[37,38,39,40,41,42] For locking-loop- and balloon-retained pGTs, it is common to wait 12 to 24 hours after placement before feeding initiation, as published support for earlier feeding regimens is lacking. Patients should be fed upright (30–45 degrees) to avoid reflux and aspiration,[43,44] and feeding should be terminated during procedures that require the patient to lie flat. Commercially prepared formula should be used at the rates designated by the manufacturer to avoid infection, clogging, or compromise of appropriate nutritional and electrolyte support.[45]

26.7.2 Daily Evaluation and Care

Formal education of patients, family members, and all other potential caregivers should be performed before patient discharge. Discussion should include the importance of regular dressing changes for the first month, after which dressing is not required for uncomplicated tubes. Washing of hands with soap and water should precede daily assessment; this daily assessment should include stomal site examination, stomal site cleaning with soap and water (after the first month), tube position examination, tube rotation, tube movement in and out, and tube flushes. The tube length marked at the skin should be compared to the documented length at the time of placement. External flange rotation prevents skin complications, and movement in and out can be used to evaluate for buried bumper syndrome (described below) or inadvertent tube dislodgment. The tube should be freely injectable with 50 mL without inducing pain. Tap water is sufficient for most patients, whereas sterile water is occasionally used for immunocompromised patients. When obstruction of the tube is encountered, injection of water is recommended over alternative options.[46] The smaller the diameter and the longer the tube (e.g., pGJTs), the more prone to obstruction, particularly by ground medications and protein-based formulas.[47,48]

26.7.3 Imaging Evaluation

Imaging after PEA device placement is not routinely necessary but should be considered to evaluate signs and symptoms of infection or in cases of pain on movement and flushing. Injection of water-soluble contrast under fluoroscopy can exclude leakage and verify correct positioning of the retainer within the gastric lumen, but increasing abdominal distention, signs of infection, and an immobile PEA device on physical examination may necessitate evaluation with CT. Radiographic free air is seen in more than one-third of patients after PEA device

placement, but this occurrence rarely needs follow-up in the absence of other signs of complications.[2]

26.7.4 Exchange

Routine exchange of most PEA devices is not necessary, although practices vary based on provider opinion and a case-by-case assessment of the risk of complications. When left in place for extended periods, most tubes will eventually degrade from overuse and yeast infection. Bumper-retained pGTs will typically last for years, so exchange is reserved for cases of complications such as corrosion, deformity, or leakage of the tube. These devices can be exchanged over a wire under fluoroscopy with transabdominal advancement of either a balloon-retained or bumper-retained replacement tube. Balloon-retained tubes require more frequent replacement and exchange because of an increased incidence of dislodgment from accidental balloon deflation or rupture. Many practitioners exchange locking-loop tubes every 3 months, a downside of these devices. Balloon-retained and locking-loop pGTs can be replaced "blind" at bedside by trained personnel, whereas exchange of pGJTs is best performed under fluoroscopic guidance. Finally, removal of PEA devices should be performed only after tract maturation, which occurs in 14 days in most immunocompetent patients but may take more than 30 days in immunocompromised patients.

26.8 Management of Complications

Major procedure-related complications occur in less than 5% of patients undergoing PEA device placement, but delayed complication rates exceed 30% in some studies.[3] The earliest complications are typically related to vascular injury, bowel perforation, conscious sedation, or general anesthesia. Patients with poor renal function, poor airway protection, chronic malnutrition, and cardiopulmonary disease may be at risk for oversedation and aspiration during tube placement; in such cases, general anesthesia may be warranted.

26.8.1 Bleeding

Bleeding complications are often detected during serial dilation or after tube placement and generally manifest as hematoma formation, abdominal distention, altered hemodynamic status, or blood aspirated from the newly placed tube. Bleeding occurs in less than 0.5% of cases and may result from preexisting peptic ulcer disease, gastritis, arterial injury, or transgression of varices.[49] Arterial injury most commonly involves the gastroepiploic artery, but branches of the left gastric, splenic, gastroduodenal, and superior epigastric arteries (▶ Fig. 26.5) can also be affected. Persistent bleeding should prompt arterial embolization. Adequate gastric insufflation during tube placement minimizes the risk of this complication by displacing the gastroepiploic artery caudal to the puncture site. Other arterial injuries often result from puncture locations that vary from the standard midbody location, either inadvertently or because of limited options. The left gastric artery and its branches can be injured by a high puncture near the lesser curvature or cardia, and the gastroduodenal artery and its branches can be injured

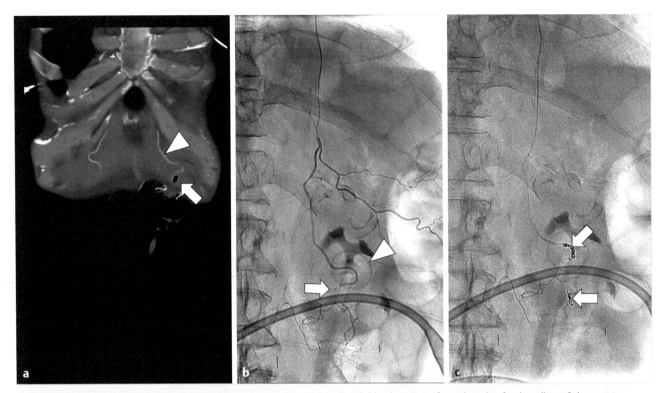

Fig. 26.5 A 72-year-old man presented 1 day after transoral pGT placement with bloody aspirate from the tube, focal swelling of the anterior abdominal wall, and bleeding at the stomal site. **(a)** Coronal-reformatted CT with contrast showed the superior epigastric artery (*arrowhead*) immediately juxtaposed to the pGT (*arrow*). **(b)** Selective superior epigastric arteriography showed arterial vasospasm (*arrow*) adjacent to the pGT (*arrowhead*). **(c)** Successful embolization of the superior epigastric artery cranial and caudal to the abnormal segment was performed using coils (*arrows*).

by antral puncture (▶ Fig. 26.6). Transgression of known varices can be avoided by using techniques that provide visualization of varices during puncture, typically either endoscopic or CT-guided tube placement.

26.8.2 Abdominal Distention

Abdominal distention in the first few days after tube placement should progressively diminish but may indicate either ileus or peritoneal leakage. Ileus should be suspected when feeds are not tolerated and when patients experience persistent generalized abdominal discomfort and distention. In such cases, the stomach should be decompressed through the pGT either by placement of the tube to gravity drainage or to low intermittent suction, and serial abdominal examinations should be performed. Peritoneal leakage results from a perforated viscus or an incompetent tract caused by factors such as overdilation, ineffective gastropexy, or the presence of ascites at the stomal site. If serial abdominal examinations reveal increasing distention or significant pain, feeding should be terminated and the pGT should be used for gastric decompression; radiography or CT evaluation may be indicated. Pneumoperitoneum is not uncommon after pGT placement and typically resolves spontaneously, but severe cases may be managed with a temporary abdominal drain in conjunction with low intermittent gastric suction through the pGT. In more minor cases, imaging options include water-soluble contrast injection of the pGT under

fluoroscopy or CT to assess tube location, peristomal leakage, and infection. More serious findings include peritoneal signs, frank sepsis that may indicate colonic perforation, and the development of peritoneal air–fluid levels.[50] Such signs should prompt surgical consultation.

26.8.3 Misplacement or Early Dislodgment

Misplacement or dislodgment within the first few weeks of tube placement can be inconsequential or can result in severe pain, peritonitis, and infection of the anterior abdominal wall. Misplacement can range from inadvertent peritoneal placement to transgression of organs such as the colon (▶ Fig. 26.7). In the case of peritoneal placement, the pGT can be removed in most cases, but if feeding has been initiated, the pGT can be maintained and placed to suction. In the case of colonic placement or transgression, removal should be postponed for at least 2 weeks to allow the tract to mature. The occurrence of sepsis or peritoneal signs should prompt surgical consultation. If dislodgment is suspected, feeding should be stopped and the abdomen should be assessed immediately. Imaging may be indicated; options include CT, endoscopy, and water-soluble contrast injection under fluoroscopy. Replacement of the tube is often possible during fluoroscopic and endoscopic evaluation, even within the first week after placement.

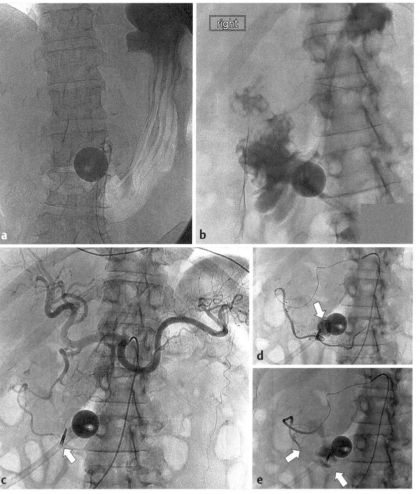

Fig. 26.6 A 47-year-old woman presented with intermittent midepigastric pain, nonbilious vomiting, and stomal bleeding 3 days after balloon-retained pGT placement. **(a)** Abdominal radiograph showed that the stomal site was unusually distal, and the pGT entered the antrum rather than the midbody. This location predisposed the patient to intermittent gastric outlet obstruction and bleeding from the gastroduodenal artery. **(b)** Under fluoroscopy, the pGT was retracted and injected with water-soluble contrast material. The distal antrum and duodenum immediately opacified, indicating that intermittent balloon-related gastric outlet obstruction was causing the patient's symptoms. **(c)** After bleeding increased, the patient underwent endoscopy that failed to control the source; she was referred for angiography. Selective celiac arteriography showed an endoscopic clip (*arrow*) placed at the gastroduodenal artery adjacent to the pGT tract. **(d)** Superselective gastroduodenal arteriogram showed extravasation at that location (*arrow*). **(e)** The extravasation was terminated after placement of proximal and distal vascular plugs (*arrows*).

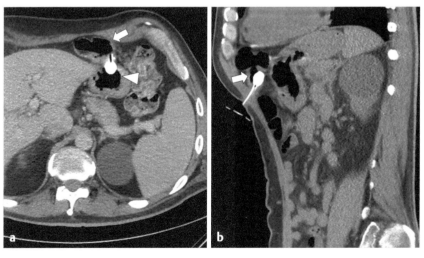

Fig. 26.7 Fecal aspirate was noted from a balloon-retained pGT 2 days after placement; the patient was otherwise asymptomatic. **(a)** The pGT transgressed the colon (*arrow*) and terminated in the stomach (*arrowhead*). **(b)** The complication was managed by retracting the pGT into the colon (*arrow*). The tube was left in place for 4 weeks to allow tract formation and then removed without sequelae.

26.8.4 Peristomal Complications

Peristomal complications may occur in the immediate postprocedural period or as a delayed complication. Severe peristomal pain soon after PEA placement can be caused by ischemia or perforation of the adjacent stomach resulting from an overly tight external flange or a complication of gastropexy sutures.

The result can be gastric necrosis, gastric perforation, peristomal abscess formation, and peritoneal leakage with peritonitis. Tight gastropexy sutures cause intractable pain and may erode through the gastric lumen into the adjacent abdominal wall. When pain related to gastropexy sutures is encountered, early release of the sutures may prevent these sequelae. Delayed peristomal complications are often related to the external

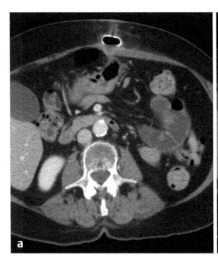
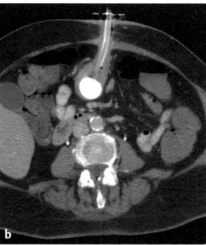

Fig. 26.8 Delayed abdominal pain occurred after transoral pGT placement. **(a)** CT showed inadvertent retraction of a bumper-retained pGT into the anterior abdominal wall 2 months after placement. Pain was noted during attempts to flush the tube with water. **(b)** The tube was exchanged over a wire for a balloon-retained pGT.

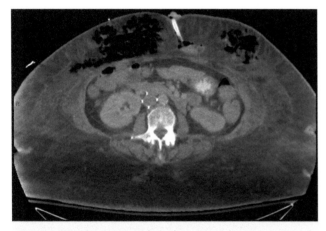

Fig. 26.9 CT without contrast showed extensive subcutaneous gas and irregularity of the anterior abdominal musculature caused by late pGT displacement and subsequent attempts at enteral feeding. Surgical debridement was required.

flange or bolster.[51] Complications include peristomal excoriation, ulceration, leakage, and stomal enlargement. The risk is increased for diabetic patients, patients on high-dose corticosteroids, and patients with poor nutritional status. When stomal enlargement occurs, treatment options include slowing the rate of feeding, using gastric decompression through the pGT between feedings, and, in some cases, converting from pGT to pGJT to facilitate decompression of the stomach concurrently with feeding into the jejunal port. A common peristomal issue is exuberant granulation tissue formation, which is usually inconsequential but can be reduced by simple debridement, application of topical steroids, or treatment with silver nitrate sticks.[52,53]

26.8.5 Delayed Dislodgment and Clogging

The most common delayed complications of PEA are dislodgment and clogging. Balloon-retained tubes dislodge earlier than bumper-retained tubes because of degradation and rupture of

the balloon or inadvertent balloon deflation by caregivers. Complete removal should prompt replacement as soon as possible, typically within a few days. When a tract has matured for more than 30 days, bedside replacement can be performed by trained personnel, although fluoroscopic replacement is preferred. A Foley catheter is occasionally used by clinic or emergency room staff to preserve a tract before definitive tube replacement, but a Foley balloon lacks an external flange, and migration with gastric outlet obstruction may occur if the Foley is left in place for more than a few days. A painful, uninjectable tube may indicate either a dislodged tube (▶ Fig. 26.8) or the related condition of buried bumper or buried balloon syndrome, which results from progressive impaction of the internal retention device within hypertrophied gastric mucosa.[54] This uncommon condition was originally described for transorally placed bumper retainers, but it can occur with both balloon- and bumper-retained tubes. Continued use of a buried or dislodged tube for enteral feeding can result in complications ranging from minor local infections to severe necrotizing fasciitis (▶ Fig. 26.9). Clogging is more commonly seen with small-bore and longer tubes such as pGJTs.[30] If water injection will not clear the tube, other options include biopsy brushes, balloons, wires, or tube exchange.

26.8.6 Bowel Obstruction

Bowel obstruction can result from transgression of an intervening bowel loop during placement or misplacement/migration of the internal retainer resulting in gastric outlet obstruction (▶ Fig. 26.6) or small bowel obstruction. The retainer can serve as a lead point for intussusception or volvulus in rare cases (▶ Fig. 26.10).

26.9 Conclusion

PEA devices are standard tools for the management of a wide range of conditions, and a broad variety of device and placement options are available and can be tailored on a case-by-case basis. When patients are carefully selected and screened, minimally invasive PEA is safe and effective for reducing morbidity and improving survival and QoL, depending on the

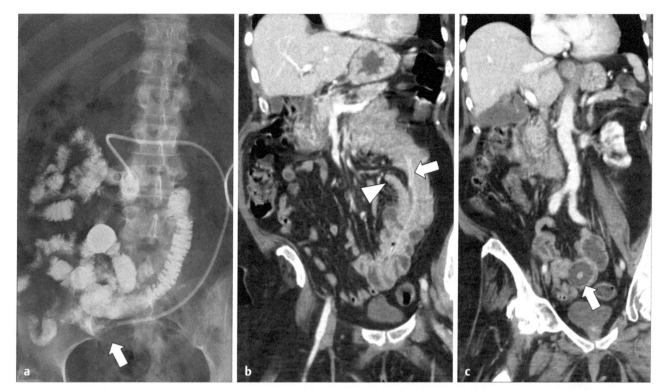

Fig. 26.10 A 78-year-old man presented with crampy abdominal pain after replacement of an inadvertently displaced pGT in the emergency department. A Foley catheter lacking an external retention flange was used as a temporary pGT. **(a)** Abdominal radiography showed migration of the inflated Foley balloon (*arrow*) into the caudal abdomen. **(b)** Coronal-reformatted CT with contrast showed a small bowel to small bowel intussusception (*arrowhead*) of the segment containing the Foley catheter (*arrow*). Mesenteric fat was displaced into a small bowel segment. **(c)** The balloon (*arrow*) was in the distal jejunum. Subsequently, under fluoroscopic guidance, the Foley catheter was deflated and removed over a wire, the intussusception spontaneously resolved within a few minutes, and a standard, balloon-retained pGT was placed over the wire.

indication. Careful education of caregivers regarding daily evaluation and maintenance of PEA devices is paramount to minimize and manage complications.

References

[1] Mendiratta P, Tilford JM, Prodhan P, Curseen K, Azhar G, Wei JY. Trends in percutaneous endoscopic gastrostomy placement in the elderly from 1993 to 2003. Am J Alzheimers Dis Other Demen. 2012; 27(8):609–613

[2] Stroud M, Duncan H, Nightingale J, British Society of Gastroenterology. Guidelines for enteral feeding in adult hospital patients. Gut. 2003; 52 Suppl 7:vii1–vii12

[3] Itkin M, DeLegge MH, Fang JC, et al. Interventional Radiology and American Gastroenterological Association, American Gastroenterological Association Institute, Canadian Interventional Radiological Association, Cardiovascular and Interventional Radiological Society of Europe. Multidisciplinary practical guidelines for gastrointestinal access for enteral nutrition and decompression from the Society of Interventional Radiology and American Gastroenterological Association (AGA) Institute, with endorsement by Canadian Interventional Radiological Association (CIRA) and Cardiovascular and Interventional Radiological Society of Europe (CIRSE). J Vasc Interv Radiol. 2011; 22(8):1089–1106

[4] Niv Y, Abuksis G. Indications for percutaneous endoscopic gastrostomy insertion: ethical aspects. Dig Dis. 2002; 20(3–4):253–256

[5] Marks WH, Perkal MF, Schwartz PE. Percutaneous endoscopic gastrostomy for gastric decompression in metastatic gynecologic malignancies. Surg Gynecol Obstet. 1993; 177(6):573–576

[6] Gowen GF. Long tube decompression is successful in 90% of patients with adhesive small bowel obstruction. Am J Surg. 2003; 185(6):512–515

[7] Felsher J, Chand B, Ponsky J. Decompressive percutaneous endoscopic gastrostomy in nonmalignant disease. Am J Surg. 2004; 187(2):254–256

[8] Sartori S, Trevisani L, Tassinari D, et al. Cost analysis of long-term feeding by percutaneous endoscopic gastrostomy in cancer patients in an Italian health district. Support Care Cancer. 1996; 4(1):21–26

[9] Silas AM, Pearce LF, Lestina LS, et al. Percutaneous radiologic gastrostomy versus percutaneous endoscopic gastrostomy: a comparison of indications, complications and outcomes in 370 patients. Eur J Radiol. 2005; 56(1):84–90

[10] Skelly RH. Are we using percutaneous endoscopic gastrostomy appropriately in the elderly? Curr Opin Clin Nutr Metab Care. 2002; 5(1):35–42

[11] Grant DG, Bradley PT, Pothier DD, et al. Complications following gastrostomy tube insertion in patients with head and neck cancer: a prospective multi-institution study, systematic review and meta-analysis. Clin Otolaryngol. 2009; 34(2):103–112

[12] Light VL, Slezak FA, Porter JA, Gerson LW, McCord G. Predictive factors for early mortality after percutaneous endoscopic gastrostomy. Gastrointest Endosc. 1995; 42(4):330–335

[13] Finucane TE, Bynum JP. Use of tube feeding to prevent aspiration pneumonia. Lancet. 1996; 348(9039):1421–1424

[14] Larson DE, Burton DD, Schroeder KW, DiMagno EP. Percutaneous endoscopic gastrostomy. Indications, success, complications, and mortality in 314 consecutive patients. Gastroenterology. 1987; 93(1):48–52

[15] Heyland DK, Drover JW, MacDonald S, Novak F, Lam M. Effect of postpyloric feeding on gastroesophageal regurgitation and pulmonary microaspiration: results of a randomized controlled trial. Crit Care Med. 2001; 29(8):1495–1501

[16] Israel DM, Hassall E. Prolonged use of gastrostomy for enteral hyperalimentation in children with Crohn's disease. Am J Gastroenterol. 1995; 90(7):1084–1088

[17] Malfi G, Agnello E, Da Pont MC, et al. Chronic anorexia nervosa: enteral nutrition via percutaneous endoscopic gastrostomy and liaison psychiatry. Minerva Gastroenterol Dietol. 2006; 52(4):431–435

[18] Schurink CA, Tuynman H, Scholten P, et al. Percutaneous endoscopic gastrostomy: complications and suggestions to avoid them. Eur J Gastroenterol Hepatol. 2001; 13(7):819–823

[19] Amann W, Mischinger HJ, Berger A, et al. Percutaneous endoscopic gastrostomy (PEG). 8 years of clinical experience in 232 patients. Surg Endosc. 1997; 11(7):741–744

[20] Heyland DK, Montalvo M, MacDonald S, Keefe L, Su XY, Drover JW. Total parenteral nutrition in the surgical patient: a meta-analysis. Can J Surg. 2001; 44(2):102–111

[21] Marik PE, Zaloga GP. Gastric versus post-pyloric feeding: a systematic review. Crit Care. 2003; 7(3):R46–R51

[22] de Baere T, Chapot R, Kuoch V, et al. Percutaneous gastrostomy with fluoroscopic guidance: single-center experience in 500 consecutive cancer patients. Radiology. 1999; 210(3):651–654

[23] Rustom IK, Jebreel A, Tayyab M, England RJ, Stafford ND. Percutaneous endoscopic, radiological and surgical gastrostomy tubes: a comparison study in head and neck cancer patients. J Laryngol Otol. 2006; 120(6):463–466

[24] Bankhead RR, Fisher CA, Rolandelli RH. Gastrostomy tube placement outcomes: comparison of surgical, endoscopic, and laparoscopic methods. Nutr Clin Pract. 2005; 20(6):607–612

[25] Chung RS, Schertzer M. Pathogenesis of complications of percutaneous endoscopic gastrostomy. A lesson in surgical principles. Am Surg. 1990; 56 (3):134–137

[26] Ho CS, Yee AC, McPherson R. Complications of surgical and percutaneous nonendoscopic gastrostomy: review of 233 patients. Gastroenterology. 1988; 95(5):1206–1210

[27] Nicholson FB, Korman MG, Richardson MA. Percutaneous endoscopic gastrostomy: a review of indications, complications and outcome. J Gastroenterol Hepatol. 2000; 15(1):21–25

[28] Lee DS, Mohit-Tabatabai MA, Rush BF, Jr, Levine C. Stomal seeding of head and neck cancer by percutaneous endoscopic gastrostomy tube placement. Ann Surg Oncol. 1995; 2(2):170–173

[29] Funaki B, Peirce R, Lorenz J, et al. Comparison of balloon- and mushroom-retained large-bore gastrostomy catheters. AJR Am J Roentgenol. 2001; 177 (2):359–362

[30] Kuo YC, Shlansky-Goldberg RD, Mondschein JI, et al. Large or small bore, push or pull: a comparison of three classes of percutaneous fluoroscopic gastrostomy catheters. J Vasc Interv Radiol. 2008; 19(4):557–563, quiz 564

[31] Sane SS, Towbin A, Bergey EA, et al. Percutaneous gastrostomy tube placement in patients with ventriculoperitoneal shunts. Pediatr Radiol. 1998; 28(7):521–523

[32] Lipp A, Lusardi G. A systematic review of prophylactic antimicrobials in PEG placement. J Clin Nurs. 2009; 18(7):938–948

[33] Cosmulescu MP, Russell JN. Antibiotic prophylaxis considering patient outcome from percutaneous endoscopic gastrostomy. Rev Med Chir Soc Med Nat Iasi. 2011; 115(3):686–691

[34] Ryan JM, Hahn PF, Mueller PR. Performing radiologic gastrostomy or gastrojejunostomy in patients with malignant ascites. AJR Am J Roentgenol. 1998; 171(4):1003–1006

[35] Malloy PC, Grassi CJ, Kundu S, et al. Standards of Practice Committee with Cardiovascular and Interventional Radiological Society of Europe (CIRSE) Endorsement. Consensus guidelines for periprocedural management of coagulation status and hemostasis risk in percutaneous image-guided interventions. J Vasc Interv Radiol. 2009; 20(7) Suppl:S240–S249

[36] Eisen GM, Baron TH, Dominitz JA, et al. American Society for Gastrointestinal Endoscopy. Guideline on the management of anticoagulation and antiplatelet therapy for endoscopic procedures. Gastrointest Endosc. 2002; 55(7):775–779

[37] Stein J, Schulte-Bockholt A, Sabin M, Keymling M. A randomized prospective trial of immediate vs. next-day feeding after percutaneous endoscopic gastrostomy in intensive care patients. Intensive Care Med. 2002; 28(11):1656–1660

[38] Bechtold ML, Matteson ML, Choudhary A, Puli SR, Jiang PP, Roy PK. Early versus delayed feeding after placement of a percutaneous endoscopic gastrostomy: a meta-analysis. Am J Gastroenterol. 2008; 103(11):2919–2924

[39] Brown DN, Miedema BW, King PD, Marshall JB. Safety of early feeding after percutaneous endoscopic gastrostomy. J Clin Gastroenterol. 1995; 21(4):330–331

[40] Choudhry U, Barde CJ, Markert R, Gopalswamy N. Percutaneous endoscopic gastrostomy: a randomized prospective comparison of early and delayed feeding. Gastrointest Endosc. 1996; 44(2):164–167

[41] McCarter TL, Condon SC, Aguilar RC, Gibson DJ, Chen YK. Randomized prospective trial of early versus delayed feeding after percutaneous endoscopic gastrostomy placement. Am J Gastroenterol. 1998; 93(3):419–421

[42] Szary NM, Arif M, Matteson ML, Choudhary A, Puli SR, Bechtold ML. Enteral feeding within three hours after percutaneous endoscopic gastrostomy placement: a meta-analysis. J Clin Gastroenterol. 2011; 45(4):e34–e38

[43] Bankhead R, Boullata J, Brantley S, et al. A.S.P.E.N. Board of Directors. Enteral nutrition practice recommendations. JPEN J Parenter Enteral Nutr. 2009; 33 (2):122–167

[44] Metheny N. Turning tube feeding off while repositioning patients in bed. Crit Care Nurse. 2011; 31(2):96–97

[45] Klek S, Szybinski P, Sierzega M, et al. Commercial enteral formulas and nutrition support teams improve the outcome of home enteral tube feeding. JPEN J Parenter Enteral Nutr. 2011; 35(3):380–385

[46] Wilson MF, Haynes-Johnson V. Cranberry juice or water? A comparison of feeding-tube irrigants. Nutr Support Serv. 1987; 7:23–24

[47] Fortunato JE, Darbari A, Mitchell SE, Thompson RE, Cuffari C. The limitations of gastro-jejunal (G-J) feeding tubes in children: a 9-year pediatric hospital database analysis. Am J Gastroenterol. 2005; 100(1):186–189

[48] Marcuard SP, Perkins AM. Clogging of feeding tubes. JPEN J Parenter Enteral Nutr. 1988; 12(4):403–405

[49] Mamel JJ. Percutaneous endoscopic gastrostomy. Am J Gastroenterol. 1989; 84(7):703–710

[50] Taheri MR, Singh H, Duerksen DR. Peritonitis after gastrostomy tube replacement: a case series and review of literature. JPEN J Parenter Enteral Nutr. 2011; 35(1):56–60

[51] McClave SA, Jafri NS. Spectrum of morbidity related to bolster placement at time of percutaneous endoscopic gastrostomy: buried bumper syndrome to leakage and peritonitis. Gastrointest Endosc Clin N Am. 2007; 17(4):731–746

[52] Warriner L, Spruce P. Managing overgranulation tissue around gastrostomy sites. Br J Nurs. 2012; 21(5):S14–S16, S18, S20 passim

[53] Lynch CR, Fang J. Prevention and management of complications of percutaneous endoscopic gastrostomy (PEG) tubes. Pract Gastroenterol. 2004; 28:66–77

[54] El AZ, Arvanitakis M, Ballarin A, Devière J, Le Moine O, Van Gossum A. Buried bumper syndrome: low incidence and safe endoscopic management. Acta Gastroenterol Belg. 2011; 74(2):312–316

27 Image-Guided Colorectal Obstruction Management

Horacio R. V. D'Agostino, David H. Ballard, Paul A. Jordan, Kenneth Manas, Antonio Mainar, and Miguel A. De Gregorio

27.1 Introduction

Benign or malignant acute colorectal obstruction is typically managed with emergency surgery. For patients who can tolerate the procedure, right colonic obstruction is managed with a right conventional or extended colectomy. Surgery for acute left colonic obstruction usually consists of an operation that may include resection and creation of an ostomy. Despite advances in ostomy care, avoidance of the colostomy is still desirable, as the presence of an ostomy affects patient well-being. A colostomy is also associated with increased morbidity at the time of the procedure and when the colostomy is reversed. The additional surgery required for colostomy closure leads to a prolonged hospital stay and an increase in the overall costs for colonic obstruction management.

Currently, transanal stent placement is a mainstream procedure used to manage colonic obstruction. The complexity of deploying a colonic stent is influenced by the location of the obstructive lesion, the length of intestine involved, and the presence of complications such as associated fistula or small bowel obstruction. Lesions located in the left colon from the rectosigmoid junction up to the splenic flexure are the most amenable for transanal stent placement. In cases of colonic obstruction that are not amenable for surgery and cannot be managed by retrograde placement of a stent, a decompressive percutaneous cecostomy is indicated (▶ Fig. 27.1, ▶ Fig. 27.2).

In this chapter, we focus on percutaneous cecostomy and transanal stent placement for image-guided management of colonic obstruction. Percutaneous cecostomy is generally performed by interventional radiologists. However, as with many other procedures initiated by interventional radiologists, colonic stent placement is currently performed by gastroenterologists and surgeons, as well. In an ideal situation, interventional radiologists, gastroenterologists, and surgeons can work together to manage cases of colonic obstruction, combining their expertise to provide optimal patient care.

27.2 Percutaneous Cecostomy

27.2.1 Background

Percutaneous cecostomy consists of percutaneous insertion of a catheter through the anterior abdominal wall within the lumen of the cecum to decompress distal colonic obstruction. This procedure is often used in cases that are not amenable for surgery or in which transanal stent placement has failed. Occasionally, another limb of the colon (e.g., right or transverse colon) will be more accessible, and these sites can be accessed in a manner similar to that used in percutaneous cecostomy; in such cases, the procedure is termed percutaneous colostomy.[1]

Percutaneous cecostomy was first described in 1986 by Casola et al[2] in a case of massive cecal dilatation secondary to obstruction; in this case, lower endoscopy could not traverse the obstruction. A subsequent report in 1987 by Haaga et al[3] described the use of percutaneous cecostomy for decompression of Ogilvie's syndrome (▶ Fig. 27.3). The indications and uses for this procedure subsequently expanded, and this technique is now considered an effective treatment for neurogenic motility disorders causing chronic constipation with overflow fecal incontinence, chronic nonobstructive colonic dilatation (e.g., Ogilvie's syndrome), and refractory cases of large bowel obstruction.[1,4,5] When percutaneous cecostomy is used for chronic constipation with overflow fecal incontinence (typically in patients with a central neurologic disease such as spina bifida), the catheter is used for elective anterograde enema flushes. In this chapter, we focus on the use of percutaneous cecostomy for the treatment of colonic obstruction; other uses are described in detail elsewhere.[4,6]

Cecal perforation is an absolute contraindication for percutaneous cecostomy. Relative contraindications are similar to those for percutaneous catheter insertion, including coagulopathy and prolonged dilatation of the cecum that may cause ischemia of the cecal wall. In such cases, careful evaluation of the acute

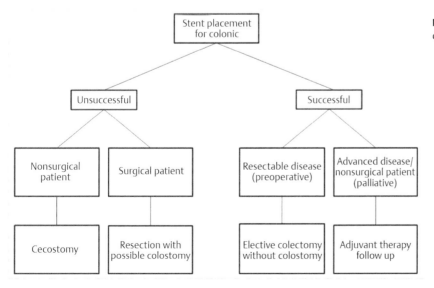

Fig. 27.1 Basic algorithm for cecostomy and colonic stent placement.

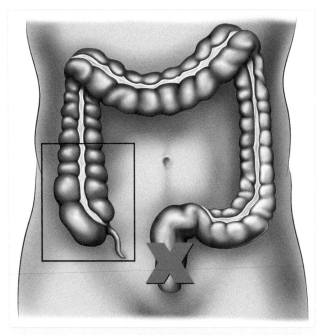

Fig. 27.2 Lesion location and transanal stent placement. No stents are to be placed distal to the rectosigmoid angle (*crossed*). The colors indicate the progressive complexity from less complex distally (*green*) to more complex proximally (*yellow*, *orange*, and *red* [no stents]) for transanal colonic stent placement. The square on the cecum and ascending colon indicates the location for cecostomy.

abdomen is necessary, as emergent surgical exploration may be required.

27.2.2 Procedure

Patient Evaluation and Preparation

Patient evaluation includes an assessment of the patient's general condition and comorbidities. Routine hematologic, metabolic, and coagulation panels should be obtained. Additional cardiovascular or respiratory evaluation may be necessary for frail patients with a history of acute or chronic cardiorespiratory insufficiency. Usually, these patients have undergone plain radiography or computed tomography (CT) of the abdomen for imaging evaluation of their disease and for treatment planning.

Patient preparation for percutaneous cecostomy is usually minimal. Patients with colonic obstruction should be fasting and should have a nasogastric tube in place. Oral or rectal bowel preparations are not necessary; however, when percutaneous cecostomy is used for chronic constipation or fecal incontinence, various bowel regimens are advocated.

Procedural sedation or monitored anesthesia care is sufficient for patients undergoing percutaneous cecostomy. Intravenous conscious sedation (midazolam and fentanyl) and local anesthesia (lidocaine 1%) are the authors' preferences.

Image Guidance

C-arm fluoroscopy can clearly identify the location of the cecum and is reliably accurate for percutaneous cecostomy performance. Some colleagues have used CT for percutaneous cecostomy guidance. Ultrasound can be useful in preventing injury to the epigastric vessels and may be needed to identify a fluid-filled cecum and to guide bowel puncture.

Materials Needed

- General tray.
- Percutaneous sutures (Saf-T-Pexy T-fasteners [Kimberly-Clark] or Brown-Mueller T-fasteners).
- Access needle: Seldinger thin-wall 19 gauge.
- Guidewires: Amplatz 0.038-inch, 4- to 7-cm floppy tip.
- Dilators: 7 to 14 French (Fr) or coaxial dilator (Kimberly-Clark).
- Catheters: Multipurpose locking pigtail catheter 10.2- to 14-Fr suffices for gas and liquid stools decompression. Catheters with larger diameters may be needed for cecostomy colonic decompression if catheters with smaller diameters are unable to decompress the dilated cecum (▶ Fig. 27.4)
- Drainage bag connected to the catheter for evacuation of gas and liquid stools. An ostomy bag leaving the catheter inside may be necessary for evacuation of enteric content with particles or liquid stools

Technique

- Identification of the cecum: The previous imaging studies are reviewed to confirm that the dilated cecum is against the abdominal wall with the bowel not intervening. An

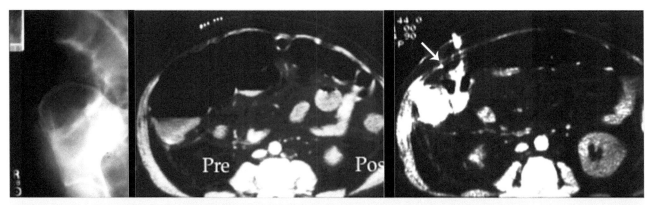

Fig. 27.3 Percutaneous cecostomy for decompression in a 68-year-old man with Ogilvie's syndrome. In this patient, CT guidance and percutaneous sutures to the anterior abdominal wall were used (*arrow*).

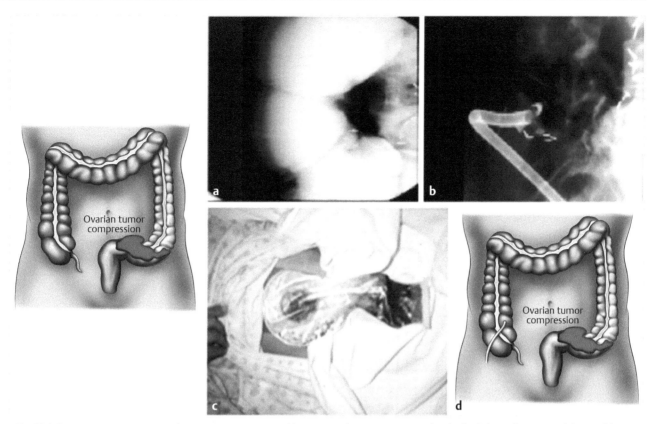

Fig. 27.4 Percutaneous cecostomy with cecopexy in a 46-year-old woman with ovarian cancer and multiple abdominal surgeries. **(a)** A small bowel follow-through caused acute obstruction from external tumor involvement of the sigmoid colon. Transanal endoscopy failed to decompress the colon, and the patient had excruciating pain. **(b)** Cecostomy decompressed the colon with insertion of a 24-Fr Malecot catheter. **(c,d)** The catheter was exchanged for a balloon catheter. The patient lived for 6 months after the cecostomy.

abdominal fluoroscopic survey is used to identify the cecum and its most accessible portion for cecopexy and percutaneous cecostomy catheter insertion. Supplemental ultrasound is used to identify the location of the epigastric vessels and to guide puncture of a fluid-filled cecum. CT guidance may be necessary if the cecum's position does not seem consistent with its position on the preprocedural CT scan.

- Cecopexy and percutaneous cecostomy access: Under image guidance, the anterior wall of the cecum is fixed to the anterior abdominal wall with three percutaneous sutures. Once the cecum is anchored to the abdominal wall, the lumen of the cecum is accessed in the center of the cecopexy using the Seldinger needle. The guidewire is then inserted and directed distally in the ascending colon. The enterocutaneous tract is dilated by serial dilatation or by the use of a coaxial dilator to the diameter of the catheter to be inserted. The cecostomy catheter is placed approximately 10 to 15 cm into the cecum and ascending colon over the guidewire. Aspiration through the catheter is performed to determine whether evacuation of the cecum is effective. If evaluation is not effective, a larger diameter catheter may need to be inserted. Once evacuation is achieved, the catheter is secured in place to the skin with two sutures. Some authors advocate placing the catheter tip within the luminal gas rather than within fecal material. An ostomy appliance is placed over the catheter or a drainage bag is connected to the proximal catheter.

27.2.3 Postprocedural Care

After percutaneous cecostomy, the patient should be followed up to assess for effective decompression, catheter status, and the presence of complications. As soon as the patient is eliminating gas and liquid stools through the cecostomy, the nasogastric tube should be removed and oral intake of fluids should be resumed. Nutrition by mouth should be advanced to tolerance and according to the ultimate management of the colonic obstruction. Patients who are able to have their obstruction corrected with surgery will be prepared for the procedure. Those patients who cannot have their obstruction resolved may have the cecostomy for life.

On a long-term basis, fecal material may clog the catheter, requiring flushing with normal saline. Exchanges are needed when the catheter has hardened because of stool residue, dislodgement, migration, dysfunction, or occlusion.

27.2.4 Complications

Major complications of percutaneous cecostomy include peritonitis and abdominal wall infection. The latter occurred in 1 patient of 27 (3.7%) in one series[1]; a pericecal abscess occurred in 1 patient of 23 (5%) in another series.[7] Minor complications include leakage around the tube, transient pain, and catheter dislodgement.[1,7]

27.2.5 Comments about Percutaneous Cecostomy

Percutaneous cecostomy is usually performed by interventional radiologists. This technique is a safe palliative procedure for colonic obstruction in appropriately selected patients. Such patients include those with lesions on the right or transverse colon that are not amenable for surgery and cases in which colonic stenting failed (i.e., failure to deploy, obstruction, or migration).

Whereas colonic stents have been studied in multiple randomized trials, including a Cochrane review pooled analysis,[8,9,10,11,12,13,14,15,16,17] the data for percutaneous cecostomy are relatively rare and have all come from small retrospective series,[1,4,5] including only one dedicated series in patients with colonic obstruction.[1] Although more studies are needed to support the use of this technique, percutaneous cecostomy currently plays an important role in the management of colonic obstruction in appropriately selected patients.

27.3 Transanal Stent Placement

27.3.1 Background

Transanal stent placement is an image-guided minimally invasive intervention that relieves colonic obstruction by transorificial placement of a stent through the obstructed colonic segment.

After the idea of placing a transanal nasogastric tube for left colonic decompression was introduced in 1986, several techniques were suggested for the nonoperative management of colonic obstruction, including the first report of a transanal stent insertion in 1990.[18,19] Two years later, Keen and Orsay[20] placed a 24-Fr thoracostomy tube in a patient to relieve a malignant rectosigmoid obstruction; they proposed preoperative insertion of such a functional stent for malignant colonic obstruction with the objective of managing comorbidities and preparing the colon for elective surgery in an attempt to avoid colostomy. Additional reports of cases of transanal stent placement followed. In 1994, Tejero et al[21] reported using transanal stent placement for malignant colonic obstruction in two patients. The authors later reported on the results of a large series designed to substantiate this technique and described outcomes when colonic stents were used as a bridge to surgical resection or as palliative relief for colonic obstruction.[22,23]

Indications for transanal colonic stents now include the preoperative or palliative management of benign and malignant colonic obstruction and the treatment of selected patients who have fistulas between the colon and the small bowel, urinary tract, or skin. Transanal stenting can therefore serve as either a bridge to surgery or a palliative measure for patients who are not surgical candidates.[24] Preoperative colonic stent placement resolves colonic obstruction temporarily while the patient is assessed and prepared for surgery. The patient's general condition and comorbidities are improved with stenting, and imaging provides information on the nature and extent of the disease. If surgery is the best treatment option, the colon is prepared for resection and primary anastomoses is carried out without leaving a colostomy (▶ Fig. 27.5, ▶ Fig. 27.6). Palliative transanal stent placement, on the other hand, maintains colonic patency in patients who are not surgical candidates. In a randomized controlled trial comparing stenting with surgical management as palliative measures for patients with colonic obstruction, patients who underwent transanal colonic stenting demonstrated a faster return to their diet, had a shorter hospital stay, and were less likely to need an ostomy (▶ Fig. 27.7).

Absolute contraindications to transanal stent placement include colonic perforation, multifocal colonic obstruction, and tumors involving the distal rectum. Placement of a stent in patients with this latter condition may cause tenesmus; anal incontinence; or stent migration, dislodgement, and expulsion.

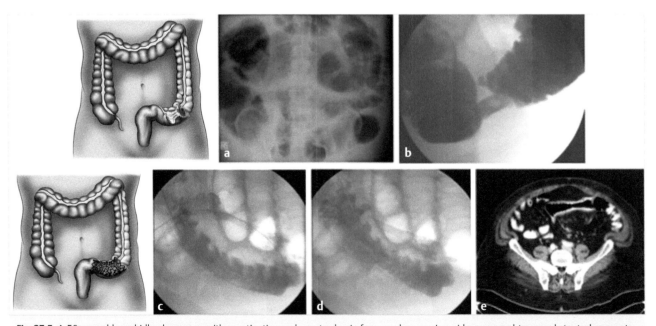

Fig. 27.5 A 56-year-old morbidly obese man with constipation and proctorrhagia from apple-core sigmoid cancer and transanal stent placement. **(a)** Plain film of the abdomen showing intestinal obstruction. **(b)** Diagnostic enema revealing the obstructive apple-core lesion location. **(c,d)** Stent placement. **(e)** Staging CT scan showing the stent fully deployed and resolution of the intestinal obstruction.

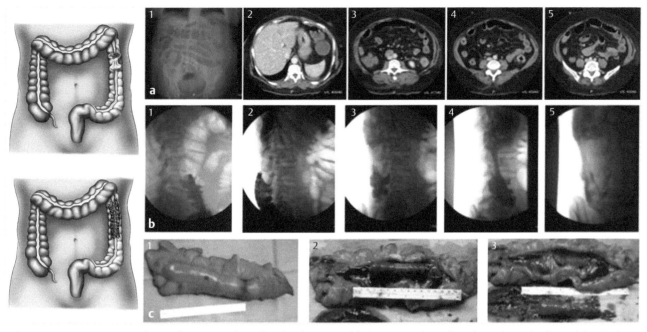

Fig. 27.6 Preoperative transanal stent placement with combined endoscopy and fluoroscopy guidance for a descending colon lesion. **(a)** 1–5, plain scanogram of the abdomen revealing large bowel obstruction and sequential images showing proximal dilated colon, the tumor with ulceration, and postobstructive empty descending colon. **(b)** 1–5, stent placement (see text). **(c)** 1–3, operative specimen.

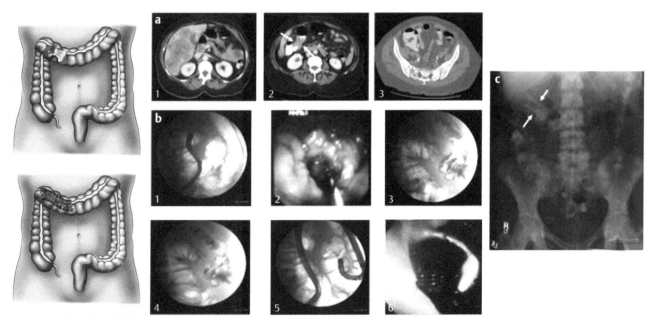

Fig. 27.7 Palliative transanal stent placement with combined endoscopy and fluoroscopy guidance for a hepatic flexure colon lesion. **(a)** CT scan of the abdomen showing liver metastases (1), apple core lesion in the hepatic flexure (2, *arrows*), and diffuse bony metastases in the sacrum and pelvis (3). **(b)** (1,2) Endoscope in the transverse colon with jagwire through the tumor. (3,4) Stent placement. (5) Endoscopic evaluation of resolution of the obstruction. (6) Liquid stools flowing through the stent. **(c)** Delayed postoperative film showing the stent fully expanded (*arrows*).

Relative contraindications include long-segment tumors and tumors proximal to the splenic flexure; retrograde transanal stent placement is more technically demanding in patients with these conditions.[25,26]

27.3.2 Procedure

Patient Evaluation and Preparation

Patients evaluated for colonic stent placement undergo routine preprocedural laboratory assessments (American College of Radiology/Society of Interventional Radiology laboratory guidelines and plain and CT abdominal imaging). CT imaging is essential, as a scan of the abdomen and pelvis will depict the obstructive lesion location and whether there are single or multiple lesions. CT can also help to determine whether the lesion is benign or malignant and can provide information about the regional and distant extension of the disease (adenopathy and metastases, respectively) and about the presence of complications (perforation or fistulas). Patients may also undergo a water-soluble contrast enema so that the distal obstruction site can be identified; this procedure can also demonstrate whether the obstruction is partial or complete and whether the lesion is benign or malignant.

Patients undergoing transanal stent placement are usually fasting and have a nasogastric tube in place for intestinal decompression. Patient preparation for the procedure may therefore involve stabilizing any comorbidities and improving the general condition of the patient with hydration, electrolyte replacement, and blood transfusion as needed. Oral contrast is contraindicated. If a barium enema has been performed, cleansing enemas are indicated to remove the barium from the colonic lumen, as the barium would interfere with transanal stent placement.

Transanal stent placement is a transorificial intervention and does not involve major trauma. This procedure can be carried out with continuous vital sign monitoring and intravenous conscious sedation (midazolam and fentanyl). However, patients who are older or in poor health may benefit from controlled deep sedation for this emergency intervention; the use of deep sedation by anesthesiologists is becoming more popular and commonplace for colonic stent placement.

Image Guidance

Transanal stent placement can be accomplished by fluoroscopic guidance alone or through a combination of fluoroscopy and colonoscopy. Although some interventionists prefer the systematic use of fluoroscopy guidance, a combination of endoscopy and C-arm fluoroscopy guidance is most effective for colonic stent deployment. The addition of colonoscopy reduces procedural time and radiation exposure to the patient and the interventional radiology team. Fluoroscopy guidance alone is mostly used in cases of distal left colon lesions down to the rectosigmoid angle.

Materials

Glide and stiff guidewires and seeking catheters are used to navigate the colon and negotiate the stricture/obstruction. Lesions in the distal transverse colon, splenic flexure, and proximal left colon require longer guidewires, guiding catheters, and sheaths. These lesion locations also benefit most from endoscopic guidance for navigating to the stricture/obstruction. Except for longer sheaths, guidewires, and colonic stents, most of the materials needed to place colorectal stents are already available in a well-equipped interventional radiology laboratory. Adjunct endoscopy guidance streamlines the use of this equipment, as the scope rapidly reaches the obstructing lesion in a retrograde fashion. Fluoroscopy-guided transanal stent placement also requires the availability of sheaths of various lengths to correct the flexible curvature of the colon navigated until reaching the obstructing lesion.

A variety of bare and covered stents can be used for transanal stent placement. We prefer uncovered metallic stents that are flared at one or both ends to minimize the chance of migration. Most colonic stents are nitinol self-expandable wire lattice tubular structures with various diameters and lengths. We prefer a stent diameter of approximately 22 to 25 mm or larger. As an example, Wallstents and Wallflex (Boston Scientific, Natick, MA) have diameters ranging from 22 to 30 mm with an expanded length of 60 to 120 mm. Wallstents have sharp wires at both ends that may cause injury or perforation, whereas Wallflex have smooth ends. Wallflex are loaded on a 10-Fr delivery system that is 175 to 220 cm long. These delivery systems require the use of long 0.035-inch, 500-cm stiff guidewires (i.e., Super Stiff Guidewire H965180011, Boston Scientific), stiff jagwires, or similar. The stent length should be equal to the length of the obstruction plus 1 to 2 cm proximally and distally as measured by contrast injection and fluoroscopic imaging. According to package labeling, nitinol stents can be used in a magnetic resonance environment.

Technique

The patient should be placed in the left lateral decubitus position to ensure patient comfort and to facilitate endoscope introduction and fluoroscopy-guided maneuvers. Alternatively, the patient can be positioned supine with the legs open for fluoroscopy-guided stent placement, but this positioning is more uncomfortable for both patient and operator.

- Access to the distal end of the obstruction: The rectosigmoid junction is straightforward to reach by fluoroscopy or endoscopy alone. Further retrograde navigation through the colonic lumen up to the distal end of the stricture/obstruction is more efficient with the endoscope than with interventional radiology materials.
- Distal end of the colonic stricture/obstruction imaging: Once the catheter or the scope has reached the stricture/obstruction, water-soluble contrast is injected to provide a landmark where the distal end of the lesion is located. This will enable the operator to determine whether there is partial or complete obstruction and whether a fistula is present (Fig. 27.6b [1]).
- Stricture/obstruction negotiation: A glidewire is usually used to negotiate the stricture/obstruction under fluoroscopy or endoscopy guidance alone or with both modalities.
- Proximal end of the colonic stricture/obstruction imaging: Contrast is injected through a catheter or the endoscope to image the proximal end of the stricture/obstructive lesion (▶ Fig. 27.6b [2,3]).

- Measurement of the extent of the lesion and stent length selection: The distal and proximal ends of the lesion are identified by the contrast previously injected. The lesion extent is measured between the two reference points where normal colonic mucosal pattern is identified proximally and distally from the lesion. The stent length is based on this measurement plus at least 1 to 2 cm on each end.
- Stent deployment over a guidewire and immediate evaluation of results: An appropriate-length stiff guidewire suitable for the stent delivery system is inserted through a catheter placed across the lesion into the dilated colon proximal to the negotiated stricture/obstruction. The stent delivery system may slide over the guidewire, achieving the desired deployment location without obstacles. However, when stenting proximal lesions, it may be beneficial to insert a dilator sheath system to keep the colon straight and facilitate the stent reaching position and deployment. Once the stent has been placed satisfactorily across the lesion, it is carefully deployed under direct image monitoring. If the stent length selection and deployment are assertive, the deployed stent will progressively expand, showing a narrowed central waist or hourglass appearance at the level of the stricture/obstruction (▶ Fig. 27.6b [4,5]). The stent position must be evaluated at this time in case additional stents are needed to cover beyond both ends of the strictured length to accomplish the desired colonic decompression. A successful transanal stent placement results in retained enteric fluid filling of the stent and is usually followed by a spontaneous intestinal evacuation on the procedure table (▶ Fig. 27.7b [6]).

Note that dilatation of the deployed colonic stent is contraindicated. This maneuver is associated with a high risk of uncontrolled bowel perforation.

27.3.3 Postprocedural Care

A multidisciplinary approach involving the patient's surgeon, gastroenterologist, and interventionist is needed for optimal management of colorectal stent cases. Surgical candidates are evaluated for surgery during their admission for stent placement or are discharged, with surgery performed at a later time. If the procedure was considered palliative and no surgery will be performed, short- and long-term follow-up directions should be given to the patient.

Patients with cancer who have colonic stents placed may have routine follow-up with the oncologist, whereas those rare patients with benign colonic strictures should have follow-up with the gastroenterologist or surgeon. Serial imaging may be conducted when a recurrence or worsening of baseline obstructive symptoms occurs. In such cases, a CT scan of the abdomen and colonoscopy are warranted for evaluation and further stent revision.

27.3.4 Dietary Recommendations

Once the colonic obstruction is alleviated by the stent, the patient is started on clear liquids and progressively advanced to a bland low-residue diet. The dietary goal is for the patient to have soft stools that will not block the stent. Plenty of fluids, mild laxatives, and small enemas may be used to prevent enteral content stent impaction. Abundant information regarding dietary and general recommendations for patients with colonic stents is provided on several websites specifically designed for patients with enteral stents placed. These instructions are essential for patients who have undergone palliative colonic stenting.

27.3.5 Complications

Major complications of colonic stenting include stent obstruction (2.1–9.9%), stent migration (2.1–9.8%), perforation (3.6–5.9%), bleeding (4.5%), and death (1%). Overall, the 30-day mortality is approximately 2.3% in patients undergoing transanal stent placement. Minor complications include self-limited bleeding, transient pain, temporary incontinence, and fecal impaction.[16,25,26]

27.3.6 Transanal Stent Placement

Optimally, transanal stent placement is performed using endoscopy and fluoroscopy guidance combined, as advancing wires and catheters in the lumen of the colon is technically challenging when fluoroscopy alone is used. Guidewires, catheters, and sheaths that coil against the colonic wall may take a long time to reach the stricture/obstructive lesion, which increases radiation exposure. The use of endoscopy allows the obstructive lesion to be reached much more quickly. At this time, an injection of contrast through the scope channel and fluoroscopy can image the distal end of the obstruction. The use of endoscopy/fluoroscopy alone or combined is usually able to negotiate the colonic stricture/obstruction. Lesions in the transverse colon proximal to the splenic flexure are difficult to reach and will definitively benefit from endoscopic assistance to reach the obstructive lesion and straighten the colon, thus facilitating stent deployment.

To proceed with a combined fluoroscopy–endoscopic approach for colonic stents, we suggest two practical options. The first is to work with gastroenterologists or surgeons and perform a combined transanal stent placement. This is a practical approach that fosters a positive interaction among the disciplines. This approach, while less demanding logistically, may be challenging depending on local culture. The other alternative is for interventionists to train on colonoscopy and perform the stent placement procedure without the assistance of other specialists. However, this option may not be logistically feasible for most interventionists.

27.4 Acknowledgments

The authors would like to express our appreciation to the residents, technologists, and nurses that participated in our procedures. Additional appreciation to Ms. Lory Tubbs for the professional diagrams used in the chapter.

References

[1] Tewari SO, Getrajdman GI, Petre EN, et al. Safety and efficacy of percutaneous cecostomy/colostomy for treatment of large bowel obstruction in adults with cancer. J Vasc Interv Radiol. 2015; 26(2):182–188

[2] Casola G, Withers C, vanSonnenberg E, Herba MJ, Saba RM, Brown RA. Percutaneous cecostomy for decompression of the massively distended cecum. Radiology. 1986; 158(3):793–794

[3] Haaga JR, Bick RJ, Zollinger RM, Jr. CT-guided percutaneous catheter cecostomy. Gastrointest Radiol. 1987; 12(2):166–168

[4] Chait PG, Shlomovitz E, Connolly BL, et al. Percutaneous cecostomy: updates in technique and patient care. Radiology. 2003; 227(1):246–250

[5] vanSonnenberg E, Varney RR, Casola G, et al. Percutaneous cecostomy for Ogilvie syndrome: laboratory observations and clinical experience. Radiology. 1990; 175(3):679–682

[6] Marker DR, Perosi N, Ul Haq F, Morefield W, Mitchell S. Percutaneous cecostomy in adult patients: safety and quality-of-life results. J Vasc Interv Radiol. 2015; 26(10):1526–1532.e1

[7] Maginot TJ, Cascade PN. Abdominal wall cellulitis and sepsis secondary to percutaneous cecostomy. Cardiovasc Intervent Radiol. 1993; 16(5):328–331

[8] Cheung HY, Chung CC, Tsang WW, Wong JC, Yau KK, Li MK. Endolaparoscopic approach vs conventional open surgery in the treatment of obstructing left-sided colon cancer: a randomized controlled trial. Arch Surg. 2009; 144(12):1127–1132

[9] Park S, Cheon JH, Park JJ, et al. Comparison of efficacies between stents for malignant colorectal obstruction: a randomized, prospective study. Gastrointest Endosc. 2010; 72(2):304–310

[10] Pirlet IA, Slim K, Kwiatkowski F, Michot F, Millat BL. Emergency preoperative stenting versus surgery for acute left-sided malignant colonic obstruction: a multicenter randomized controlled trial. Surg Endosc. 2011; 25(6):1814–1821

[11] van Hooft JE, Bemelman WA, Oldenburg B, et al. collaborative Dutch Stent-In study group. Colonic stenting versus emergency surgery for acute left-sided malignant colonic obstruction: a multicentre randomised trial. Lancet Oncol. 2011; 12(4):344–352

[12] Ho KS, Quah HM, Lim JF, Tang CL, Eu KW. Endoscopic stenting and elective surgery versus emergency surgery for left-sided malignant colonic obstruction: a prospective randomized trial. Int J Colorectal Dis. 2012; 27(3):355–362

[13] Ahlström H, Feltelius N, Nyman R, Hällgren R. Magnetic resonance imaging of sacroiliac joint inflammation. Arthritis Rheum. 1990; 33(12):1763–1769

[14] Young CJ, De-Loyde KJ, Young JM, et al. Improving quality of life for people with incurable large-bowel obstruction: randomized control trial of colonic stent insertion. Dis Colon Rectum. 2015; 58(9):838–849

[15] Sloothaak DA, van den Berg MW, Dijkgraaf MG, et al. collaborative Dutch Stent-In study group. Oncological outcome of malignant colonic obstruction in the Dutch Stent-In 2 trial. Br J Surg. 2014; 101(13):1751–1757

[16] Sagar J. Colorectal stents for the management of malignant colonic obstructions. Cochrane Database Syst Rev. 2011(11):CD007378

[17] Fiori E, Lamazza A, De Cesare A, et al. Palliative management of malignant rectosigmoidal obstruction. Colostomy vs. endoscopic stenting. A randomized prospective trial. Anticancer Res. 2004; 24(1):265–268

[18] Lelcuk S, Ratan J, Klausner JM, Skornick Y, Merhav A, Rozin RR. Endoscopic decompression of acute colonic obstruction. Avoiding staged surgery. Ann Surg. 1986; 203(3):292–294

[19] Dohmoto M, Rupp KD, Hohlbach G. [Endoscopically-implanted prosthesis in rectal carcinoma]. Dtsch Med Wochenschr. 1990; 115(23):915

[20] Keen RR, Orsay CP. Rectosigmoid stent for obstructing colonic neoplasms. Dis Colon Rectum. 1992; 35(9):912–913

[21] Tejero E, Mainar A, Fernández L, Tobío R, De Gregorio MA. New procedure for the treatment of colorectal neoplastic obstructions. Dis Colon Rectum. 1994; 37(11):1158–1159

[22] Mainar A, De Gregorio Ariza MA, Tejero E, et al. Acute colorectal obstruction: treatment with self-expandable metallic stents before scheduled surgery-results of a multicenter study. Radiology. 1999; 210(1):65–69

[23] de Gregorio MA, Mainar A, Tejero E, et al. Acute colorectal obstruction: stent placement for palliative treatment–results of a multicenter study. Radiology. 1998; 209(1):117–120

[24] Baron TH. Expandable metal stents for the treatment of cancerous obstruction of the gastrointestinal tract. N Engl J Med. 2001; 344(22):1681–1687

[25] Katsanos K, Sabharwal T, Adam A. Stenting of the lower gastrointestinal tract: current status. Cardiovasc Intervent Radiol. 2011; 34(3):462–473

[26] de Gregorio MA, Mainar A, Rodriguez J, et al. Colon stenting: a review. Semin Intervent Radiol. 2004; 21(3):205–216

28 Obesity and Bariatric Embolization

Charles Y. Kim

28.1 Introduction

Recently, the interventional radiology literature has included reports about treating obesity with an endovascular method that involves the disruption of ghrelin secretion.[1] This procedure entails percutaneous transarterial embolization of the gastric fundus, which is the site of the highest concentration of ghrelin-secreting cells in the body. Because the left gastric artery serves as the predominant supply to the gastric fundus, this artery has been targeted in a number of studies, and as such this procedure has been referred to as "left gastric artery embolization." However, because other arteries to the gastric fundus may also be embolized and because the left gastric artery is often embolized for the treatment of acute gastric bleeding, the term "bariatric embolization" has been introduced to more accurately describe this procedure when performed specifically for the treatment of obesity. Embolization of the gastric fundus has been shown to decrease serum ghrelin levels in animals and induce relative weight loss.[1] Because ghrelin is the only hormone known to cause hunger, it is hypothesized that decreasing serum ghrelin levels may decrease hunger and food intake, thereby inducing weight loss. This chapter will review the clinical significance of obesity, the pathophysiology of hunger, and the existing preclinical and clinical data on bariatric embolization for the treatment of obesity.

28.2 Obesity

Obesity has become one of the most concerning and growing health problems in the world. In 2008, more than 1.4 billion adults were overweight, with a body mass index (BMI) of 25 or greater. A total of 500 million were obese, with a BMI of 30 or higher.[2] Thus, 11% of the world's population met the criteria for obesity. The rate of obesity is growing, with an incidence that has nearly doubled since 1980. In 1997, the World Health Organization (WHO) designated obesity as a global epidemic.[3] This marked the first time in history that a noninfectious entity was labeled as an epidemic, which emphasizes the increasing prevalence of obesity and its critical effect on global health.[3]

The health implications of obesity are vast. Obesity is ranked as the fifth leading risk for mortality globally and has been strongly linked to numerous comorbidities, including type 2 diabetes, hyperlipidemia, hypertension, obstructive sleep apnea, heart disease, stroke, asthma, cancer, and depression.[2,4] The risk that obesity imparts on these comorbidities is substantial, including an 18-fold higher prevalence of diabetes and a 72% higher relative risk of coronary artery disease. In aggregate, these obesity-related comorbidities have been reported to be responsible for more than 2.5 million deaths per year worldwide.[4] Life expectancy is profoundly decreased by obesity; a 25-year-old morbidly obese man can expect a 22% reduction in lifespan.[5] In fact, an expert panel convened by the National Institutes of Health (NIH) stated that for the first time in history, the steadily improving worldwide life expectancy could level off or even decline within the first half of this century, specifically as the result of the increasing prevalence of obesity.[6]

The fundamental cause of obesity is an energy imbalance, with more calories being consumed than expended. The global rise in obesity can be attributed at least in part to the increased intake of high-calorie and high-fat foods and a decrease in physical activity related to increasingly sedentary lifestyles resulting from modernization and automation. However, numerous additional etiologies and pathologies are also known to be responsible for obesity.

28.3 Regulation of Hunger

The hormonal regulation of hunger is complex and is primarily governed by hunger-inhibiting hormones.[7] Mechanical and chemical factors associated with meals stimulate enteroendocrine cells, resulting in signals transmitted neurally through vagal nerves and/or circulating hormones. The end result is modulation of hunger in the central nervous system. Short-term hunger modulation in response to meals is largely due to cholecystokinin. Longer-term regulation of energy balance and weight is controlled largely by the effects of insulin and leptin. Interestingly, although more than 40 hormones have been shown to inhibit appetite, only one hormone, ghrelin, has been shown to stimulate appetite.[7]

28.3.1 Ghrelin

Ghrelin was first identified and reported in the literature in 1999 as an endogenous ligand for the growth hormone secretagogue receptor.[8] Since then, ghrelin has been the focus of a multitude of investigations. Ghrelin has been shown to be a peptide hormone that is secreted primarily from the mucosa of the gastrointestinal tract from a distinct endocrine cell type. The concentration of ghrelin-secreting cells is highest in the gastric fundus, with progressively decreasing concentrations in the small and large intestine.[9] Ghrelin is also expressed in the pancreatic islets, hypothalamus, and pituitary gland. Ghrelin receptors are predominantly expressed in the arcuate and ventromedial nuclei and in the hippocampus, with much lesser quantities in many peripheral organs.[8]

While the functionality of ghrelin is multifactorial and complex, one of its primary functions is stimulation of appetite. Ghrelin directly stimulates appetite and induces positive energy balance, resulting in body weight gain. In addition to stimulating appetite, ghrelin has also been shown to increase levels of circulating growth hormone, adrenocorticotropic hormone, cortisol, prolactin, and glucose.[9] Because of the unique nature of this hormone and its effect on appetite, multiple approaches to modulate ghrelin production and binding have been attempted; however, none to date have been shown to be clinically practical or effective, including a ghrelin vaccine and intraventricular and large intraperitoneal delivery of ghrelin antagonists in rats.[10,11,12,13]

28.3.2 Gastric Distribution of Ghrelin

The distribution of ghrelin-expressing cells has been reported in two separate studies.[14,15] Whereas Kim et al[14] analyzed gastric specimens from patients with gastric cancer undergoing total gastrectomy, Goitein et al[15] analyzed resected gastric specimens from patients undergoing sleeve gastrectomy, which entails a vertical resection of most of the stomach volume, including the entire fundus, most of the gastric body, and part of the antrum. In both studies, polymerase chain reaction analysis of ghrelin mRNA and immunostaining for ghrelin-expressing cells were performed throughout the resected specimen. In both studies, ghrelin mRNA and ghrelin-expressing cells were identified throughout the entire stomach; however, the concentration of ghrelin mRNA and ghrelin-expressing cells was statistically highest in the gastric fundus and lowest in the gastric antrum. Kim et al[14] reported a ghrelin-to-actin mRNA ratio of 0.78 in the fundus, 0.20 in the body, and 0.07 in the antrum, reflecting a ghrelin concentration level that was 10 times higher in the fundus than in the antrum. Goitein et al[15] similarly reported a ghrelin-to-ribosomal mRNA ratio in the fundus, body, and antrum of 0.043, 0.026, and 0.015, respectively, reflecting a ghrelin concentration level that was approximately three times higher in the fundus than in the antrum.

28.4 Treatment Options for Obesity

The mainstay of conservative therapy for obesity includes both diet and exercise regimens. Although these regimens have proven effective in the short term, both have been shown to be difficult to maintain in the long term.[16] Plasma ghrelin levels have been shown to increase sharply shortly before meals, correlating with hunger that occurs just before meal consumption.[17] Conversely, ghrelin levels decrease shortly after each meal, correlating with the satiation of hunger after food consumption. Diet regimens to induce weight loss have been shown to be difficult to sustain because of an increase in hunger.[16] Thus, it may not be surprising that dieting induces a 24% increase in the 24-hour ghrelin profile ($p = 0.006$).[17] This elevated ghrelin secretion may be a reason why dieting can be highly challenging to maintain over the long term.

Pharmacologic modulation of hunger would be perhaps the ultimate means of controlling appetite and weight. However, despite tremendous efforts in this arena, current pharmacotherapeutics can achieve only modest levels of weight loss (range of 2.0–6.5 kg of sustained weight loss).[17]

Although bariatric surgery has been shown to result in substantial degrees of sustained weight loss, the surgical risk in this patient population is significant. Alterations in ghrelin levels also occur with bariatric surgery. Research has demonstrated a 27% increase in serum ghrelin levels after gastric banding, which may be undesirable if it results in increased hunger.[18] The effect of roux-en-Y gastric bypass on serum ghrelin is somewhat controversial. Although some studies have demonstrated a decrease in serum ghrelin, other studies have shown ghrelin levels to be unchanged.[19,20,21] However, with sleeve gastrectomy, the levels of serum ghrelin have been shown in multiple studies to be markedly decreased (by approximately 60%).[20,21]

In fact, ghrelin levels have been shown to be significantly decreased as long as 5 years after surgery.[22] Because the majority of the gastric fundus is removed during sleeve gastrectomy, a large proportion of ghrelin-secreting cells are also removed. This may be one of the primary reasons why sleeve gastrectomy is the most effective of the bariatric surgeries and, conversely, may explain why surgeries that have no gastric tissue resection, such as gastric banding, have relatively poorer efficacy.

28.5 Gastric Artery Chemical Embolization

Arepally et al[23] introduced the concept of endovascular destruction of ghrelin-producing cells by minimally invasive catheter-directed techniques in 2007. In their pilot study, the authors demonstrated that infusion of sodium morrhuate into the left gastric artery of swine resulted in elevated serum ghrelin levels at low doses but decreased serum ghrelin levels at moderate doses. At high doses, death resulted secondary to gastric necrosis and perforation. The researchers went on to perform gastric artery chemical embolization with moderate doses in a larger number of swine and compared these subjects with a control arm, analyzing differences in serum ghrelin levels and weights over a 4-week period.[24] Again, the serum ghrelin levels in treated animals were shown to be significantly decreased compared to the levels in controls. In these growing swine, the mean weight was statistically lower at 3 and 4 weeks compared to the weight of untreated controls. However, the mean serum ghrelin levels among treated swine had increased by 51% at 4 weeks, suggesting that the treatment effect may be transient.

28.6 Preclinical Bariatric Embolization

Although sodium morrhuate demonstrated promise in studies of swine, using this agent in humans would be difficult. This sclerotherapy agent was typically used to injure the endothelium of varicose veins. The distribution of flow and extent of treatment with this liquid agent can be difficult to control. The appropriate amount to administer would also be difficult to ascertain given variability in stomach size and vascularity. In the treatment of veins, a well-described complication of sodium morrhuate is pulmonary arterial injury and respiratory failure resulting from excessive passage into the systemic venous circulation.[25] Given that the gastric venous return is to the liver, hepatic injury with acute hepatic failure and eventual cirrhosis is a major theoretical concern if this agent is used in humans. However, transmural necrosis and perforation are the most worrisome complications with infusion into the gastric arteries.[23]

To impair ghrelin-secreting cells in the gastric fundus in a manner that is more benign, controllable, and potentially easily translatable to human trials, Paxton et al[1] investigated the use of particle embolization to induce gastric fundal ischemia, referring to the procedure as "bariatric embolization." Because the initial results by Arepally et al[23] were achieved using a highly toxic substance, the smallest commercially available particles (40-μm diameter calibrated microspheres) were chosen to induce maximal ischemia in these studies. Using a swine model, the authors performed particle embolization of all four arteries supplying the gastric fundus to stasis. Subsequently, groups in Italy[26] and China[27] published similar preclinical investigations on bariatric embolization and obtained similar results but with additional important information, which is discussed below. In aggregate, a wealth of information was learned about the efficacy, mechanism, and complications of this procedure over the course of several years, which formed the basis of eventual bariatric embolization in humans.

28.6.1 Effect of Bariatric Embolization on Ghrelin Levels and Weight

The ability of particle embolization to impart significant decreases in serum ghrelin levels and weight has been demonstrated in three separate preclinical studies. In the study by Paxton et al,[1] particle embolization of all four arteries to the gastric fundus led to significantly lower ghrelin levels over an 8-week period in the treated swine than in animals that underwent a sham procedure ($p = 0.004$). Weights at the end of the study were also significantly lower in treated animals ($p = 0.025$). Diana et al[26] performed embolization of the left and right gastroepiploic arteries in swine using 100- to 300-μm particles with coils and observed a significant decrease in serum ghrelin levels ($p = 0.036$); weight changes were not assessed. Bawudun et al[27] conducted a similarly designed study in a canine model, in which the left gastric artery was embolized with 500- to 700-μm polyvinyl alcohol (PVA) particles. Over an 8-week period, plasma ghrelin levels and body weight were significantly decreased in treated subjects versus controls ($p = 0.004$ and 0.001). Additionally, the amount of body fat in study subjects was quantified with computed tomography (CT) at baseline and at 8 weeks, and a significant decrease in the amount of subcutaneous fat was observed in the treatment group versus the control group. This finding is highly encouraging because adult animals were used in this study, more closely approximating the use of bariatric embolization in human adults; growing swine were used in the preceding two studies.

Paxton et al[28] also performed a histopathologic evaluation of the explanted stomachs of treated and control subjects to determine the sequelae of bariatric embolization on a cellular level. Although there was a trend toward increased fibrosis in the gastric fundus of treated animals, this result did not reach statistical significance. However, analysis of the ghrelin-secreting cell density showed a significantly lower cell density in treated animals than in controls ($p = 0.03$). This finding established that the ischemia induced by particle embolization of the stomach is sufficient to destroy ghrelin-secreting cells without causing profound architectural destruction of the gastric wall.

28.6.2 Embolics Used in Bariatric Embolization

The depth of embolic penetration into the arterial bed is likely to affect the degree of ischemia, which may affect the degree of therapeutic response. However, studies in benign and malignant tumors have not demonstrated a clear correlation between the degree of ischemia and particle size, although it is widely believed that smaller particles will induce more profound

ischemia based on deeper penetration into arterioles.[29] Additionally, particle shape and compressibility may also affect the depth of penetration and degree of ischemia.[30] Further confounding this complex interplay is the fact that although increased ischemia may increase damage to or destruction of the ghrelin-secreting cells, increased ischemia may also increase damage to and destruction of the gastric mucosa and wall.

Diana et al[26] embolized the left and right gastroepiploic arteries with 500- to 700-μm microspheres in one group and with 100- to 300-μm microspheres plus coils in another group. The first group demonstrated no significant changes at 3 weeks, whereas the second group demonstrated a significant reduction in serum ghrelin levels. In the study by Paxton et al,[1] 40-μm microspheres were used to successfully induce serum ghrelin reduction, suggesting that smaller particles may be more efficacious. However, in the canine model, Bawudun et al[27] used 500- to 700-μm PVA particles and observed significant decreases in serum ghrelin levels. Furthermore, Diana et al[31] later performed laparoscopic clipping of solely the left gastroepiploic artery with distal embolics and observed significant decreases in serum ghrelin levels. Thus, it appears that there is no obvious correlation between particle size/depth of penetration and decreases in serum ghrelin levels.

28.6.3 Durability of Response to Bariatric Embolization

To date, the longest time interval tested for ghrelin suppression has been 8 weeks.[1] In this study, serum ghrelin depression was sustained, although there appeared to be nonsignificant trend toward baseline over time. All other preclinical studies were performed over 3 to 4 weeks. Given the body's natural inclination toward homeostasis, it is a theoretical possibility that ghrelin-secreting cells may eventually upregulate elsewhere in the body, thus returning serum ghrelin levels to baseline over time. Paxton et al[28] investigated this phenomenon by examining the duodenums of animals undergoing bariatric embolization, as the duodenum is the second-richest source of ghrelin-secreting cells in the body. The population of ghrelin-secreting cells in the duodenum was found to be equivalent in treated and control animals at the 8-week end point, suggesting a lack of ghrelin upregulation. However, it is certainly possible that upregulation may occur more slowly or elsewhere in the body. Further preclinical studies are warranted to examine the durability of bariatric embolization over time, as this information is needed to ascertain the potential role of this procedure in humans.

28.6.4 Ischemic Risks of Bariatric Embolization

Mucosal ulcerations, presumably the result of ischemic injury, have been the only adverse event associated with particle embolization of the gastric fundus, with an incidence ranging from 40 to 50%.[26,28] To date, no cases of transmural necrosis or perforation have been reported. Paxton et al[28] reported endoscopic evidence of mucosal ulcers that were in various stages of healing at 8-week histopathologic analysis.[28] These results demonstrate that the ulcers were not indolent or worsening over time, which is in contradistinction to radioembolization-related ulcers.[32] Although all animals undergoing bariatric embolization did show evidence of gastritis, 83% of control animals undergoing a sham procedure also had evidence of gastritis. It is known that the stress of captivity in a new environment and the use of general anesthesia are sufficient to induce gastritis and ulcers in swine; 79% of swine raised on farms have an ulcer or preulcer changes.[33] Thus, the incidence of ulcers in swine models of bariatric embolization may not be translatable to humans, given this high baseline rate of ulceration. Interestingly, Bawudun et al[27] reported no ulcers with bariatric embolization in a canine model; 500- to 700-μm PVA particles were used in this study. Gastric peristalsis was also assessed at 8 weeks with a barium study of the stomach, and no abnormalities were observed. Histopathologic analysis demonstrated no differences between treated animals and controls in the parietal cell structures.

In additional studies, Paxton et al[34] sought to determine whether gastroprotective agents could mitigate the risk of ulceration by administering sucralfate and a proton-pump inhibitor to animals before and after bariatric embolization.[34] Additionally, the researchers sought to determine whether embolization of fewer arteries would affect the extent and severity of ulceration. In these experiments, the use of gastroprotective agents and the number of arteries embolized were not associated with a change in the extent or severity of ulceration. Gastric ulceration may therefore be an innate risk of bariatric embolization, although particle size may affect this risk. Furthermore, ulcers are not uncommon after bariatric surgeries involving anastomosis with the stomach.[35]

28.6.5 Effect of Arterial Distribution

In preclinical studies, embolization of any or all arteries to the gastric fundus resulted in significant decreases in serum ghrelin levels. Paxton et al[1] embolized all four arteries to the fundus, whereas Diana et al[26] embolized only the gastroepiploic arteries and Bawudun et al[27] embolized only the left gastric artery. Bawudun et al[27] further analyzed decreases in serum ghrelin levels based on the angiographic distribution of the amount of stomach supplied by the left gastric artery and found that greater degrees of stomach embolized were correlated with greater decreases in serum ghrelin levels. Similarly, Paxton et al[34] demonstrated that embolizing fewer arteries was associated with diminished decreases in serum ghrelin levels. Interestingly, embolization of only one artery instead of two or four was associated with significant increases in serum ghrelin levels, although there was no association with weight. Thus, there appears to be a complex and dynamic relationship between the amount of stomach embolized and resultant changes in serum ghrelin levels.

In humans, multiple arteries supply the gastric fundus, including the left gastric artery, short gastric arteries, and left gastroepiploic artery. All of these arteries interconnect with each other and with the arteries that supply the body and antrum of the stomach, including the right gastric artery, right gastroepiploic artery, and gastroduodenal artery. Thus, depending on flow dynamics, infusions of particles or any substance into any one of these arteries could lead to a variable amount of fundal embolization and would almost certainly lead to some degree of embolization of the gastric body and antrum. Because of these extensive interconnections, nontarget embolization of the spleen, pancreas, liver, and duodenum is a risk.

28.7 Human Trials of Bariatric Embolization

Gunn et al[36] retrospectively analyzed the cases of 19 patients who underwent transcatheter embolization of the left gastric artery for the treatment of upper gastrointestinal hemorrhage and compared patient weights with the weights of 28 patients who underwent embolization of any nonleft gastric artery for the treatment of upper gastrointestinal hemorrhage. Analysis of patient weights over 3 months demonstrated a mean 7.3% decrease in body weight for patients undergoing left gastric artery embolization compared to a mean 2% decrease in body weight for those undergoing embolization of a different upper gastrointestinal artery ($p = 0.006$). Embolic agents included particulate agents, coils, or a combination.

Kipshidze et al[37] reported the results of a first-in-man prospective study of left gastric artery embolization using 300- to 500-μm microspheres in five patients with an average BMI of 42.2 and average weight of 128.1 kg. At 6 months, the mean weight had decreased by 16% from baseline and was 17% lower than baseline at final 20- to 24-month follow-up ($p = 0.0008$ and 0.027, respectively). Mean ghrelin levels decreased by 18% from baseline at 6 months, and at final 12 month measurements, the mean ghrelin levels were 22% lower than baseline. Although BMI and weight demonstrated continued decreases at 1, 3, and 6 months after the procedure, serum ghrelin levels demonstrated a maximal decrease at 3 months ($p = 0.0042$ and 0055, respectively). Three patients reported transient abdominal pain. Endoscopy performed in all patients at 1 week after the procedure demonstrated no significant abnormalities.

28.8 Future Directions

In conclusion, bariatric embolization has shown significant promise in preclinical and early clinical studies as a potential endovascular treatment for obesity. However, the number and power of these studies are still somewhat marginal, so additional preclinical studies are needed to further elucidate the mechanisms of this procedure. Given the complex physiology and mechanisms affecting appetite, weight gain, and weight loss, human trials are crucial before this procedure is used clinically. To this end, multiple human trials have been initiated in multiple countries. Although primary efforts in these clinical trials are aimed at demonstrating the safety of this procedure, proving efficacy in terms of ghrelin levels, hunger, and weight loss is also an important goal. The duration of any effects will also be a crucial factor in determining the future use of this promising therapy. Once safety and basic efficacy are demonstrated, randomized clinical trials comparing bariatric embolization to sham treatments or various other treatments for obesity will be required to establish the role of this procedure in the management of obesity. If proven effective and safe, this endovascular method for the treatment of obesity has great promise in helping to treat one of the biggest epidemic health issues worldwide.

References

[1] Paxton BE, Kim CY, Alley CL, et al. Bariatric embolization for suppression of the hunger hormone ghrelin in a porcine model. Radiology. 2013; 266(2): 471–479

[2] World Health Organization. Obesity and overweight fact sheet N311. Updated January 2015. Available at: http://www.who.int/mediacentre/factsheets/fs311/en/

[3] Caballero B. The global epidemic of obesity: an overview. Epidemiol Rev. 2007; 29:1–5

[4] National Task Force on the Prevention and Treatment of Obesity. Overweight, obesity, and health risk. Arch Intern Med. 2000; 160(7):898–904

[5] Fontaine KR, Redden DT, Wang C, Westfall AO, Allison DB. Years of life lost due to obesity. JAMA. 2003; 289(2):187–193

[6] Olshansky SJ, Passaro DJ, Hershow RC, et al. A potential decline in life expectancy in the United States in the 21st century. N Engl J Med. 2005; 352 (11):1138–1145

[7] Strader AD, Woods SC. Gastrointestinal hormones and food intake. Gastroenterology. 2005; 128(1):175–191

[8] Kojima M, Hosoda H, Date Y, Nakazato M, Matsuo H, Kangawa K. Ghrelin is a growth-hormone-releasing acylated peptide from stomach. Nature. 1999; 402(6762):656–660

[9] Garin MC, Burns CM, Kaul S, Cappola AR. Clinical review: the human experience with ghrelin administration. J Clin Endocrinol Metab. 2013; 98 (5):1826–1837

[10] Horvath TL, Castañeda T, Tang-Christensen M, Pagotto U, Tschöp MH. Ghrelin as a potential anti-obesity target. Curr Pharm Des. 2003; 9(17):1383–1395

[11] Zorrilla EP, Iwasaki S, Moss JA, et al. Vaccination against weight gain. Proc Natl Acad Sci U S A. 2006; 103(35):13226–13231

[12] Rodgers RJ, Tschöp MH, Wilding JP. Anti-obesity drugs: past, present and future. Dis Model Mech. 2012; 5(5):621–626

[13] Allas S, Abribat T. Clinical perspectives for ghrelin-derived therapeutic products. Endocr Dev. 2013; 25:157–166

[14] Kim HH, Jeon TY, Park DY, et al. Differential expression of ghrelin mRNA according to anatomical portions of human stomach. Hepatogastroenterology. 2012; 59(119):2217–2221

[15] Goitein D, Lederfein D, Tzioni R, Berkenstadt H, Venturero M, Rubin M. Mapping of ghrelin gene expression and cell distribution in the stomach of morbidly obese patients–a possible guide for efficient sleeve gastrectomy construction. Obes Surg. 2012; 22(4):617–622

[16] Aronne LJ, Wadden T, Isoldi KK, Woodworth KA. When prevention fails: obesity treatment strategies. Am J Med. 2009; 122(4) Suppl 1:S24–S32

[17] Cummings DE, Weigle DS, Frayo RS, et al. Plasma ghrelin levels after diet-induced weight loss or gastric bypass surgery. N Engl J Med. 2002; 346(21): 1623–1630

[18] Schindler K, Prager G, Ballaban T, et al. Impact of laparoscopic adjustable gastric banding on plasma ghrelin, eating behaviour and body weight. Eur J Clin Invest. 2004; 34(8):549–554

[19] Beckman LM, Beckman TR, Earthman CP. Changes in gastrointestinal hormones and leptin after Roux-en-Y gastric bypass procedure: a review. J Am Diet Assoc. 2010; 110(4):571–584

[20] Peterli R, Steinert RE, Woelnerhanssen B, et al. Metabolic and hormonal changes after laparoscopic Roux-en-Y gastric bypass and sleeve gastrectomy: a randomized, prospective trial. Obes Surg. 2012; 22(5):740–748

[21] Ramón JM, Salvans S, Crous X, et al. Effect of Roux-en-Y gastric bypass vs sleeve gastrectomy on glucose and gut hormones: a prospective randomised trial. J Gastrointest Surg. 2012; 16(6):1116–1122

[22] Bohdjalian A, Langer FB, Shakeri-Leidenmühler S, et al. Sleeve gastrectomy as sole and definitive bariatric procedure: 5-year results for weight loss and ghrelin. Obes Surg. 2010; 20(5):535–540

[23] Arepally A, Barnett BP, Montgomery E, Patel TH. Catheter-directed gastric artery chemical embolization for modulation of systemic ghrelin levels in a porcine model: initial experience. Radiology. 2007; 244(1):138–143

[24] Arepally A, Barnett BP, Patel TH, et al. Catheter-directed gastric artery chemical embolization suppresses systemic ghrelin levels in porcine model. Radiology. 2008; 249(1):127–133

[25] Monroe P, Morrow CF, Jr, Millen JE, Fairman RP, Glauser FL. Acute respiratory failure after sodium morrhuate esophageal sclerotherapy. Gastroenterology. 1983; 85(3):693–699

[26] Diana M, Pop R, Beaujeux R, et al. Embolization of arterial gastric supply in obesity (EMBARGO): an endovascular approach in the management of morbid obesity. proof of the concept in the porcine model. Obes Surg. 2015; 25(3):550–558

[27] Bawudun D, Xing Y, Liu WY, et al. Ghrelin suppression and fat loss after left gastric artery embolization in canine model. Cardiovasc Intervent Radiol. 2012; 35(6):1460–1466

[28] Paxton BE, Alley CL, Crow JH, et al. Histopathologic and immunohisto-chemical sequelae of bariatric embolization in a porcine model. J Vasc Interv Radiol. 2014; 25(3):455–461

[29] Kishimoto K, Osuga K, Maeda N, et al. Embolic effects of transcatheter mesenteric arterial embolization with microspheres on the small bowel in a dog model. J Vasc Interv Radiol. 2014; 25(11):1767–1773

[30] Rasuli P, Hammond I, Al-Mutairi B, et al. Spherical versus conventional polyvinyl alcohol particles for uterine artery embolization. J Vasc Interv Radiol. 2008; 19(1):42–46

[31] Diana M, Halvax P, Pop R, et al. Gastric supply manipulation to modulate ghrelin production and enhance vascularization to the cardia: proof of the concept in a porcine model. Surg Innov. 2015; 22(1):5–14

[32] Yim SY, Kim JD, Jung JY, et al. Gastrectomy for the treatment of refractory gastric ulceration after radioembolization with 90Y microspheres. Clin Mol Hepatol. 2014; 20(3):300–305

[33] Swaby H, Gregory NG. A note on the frequency of gastric ulcers detected during post-mortem examination at a pig abattoir. Meat Sci. 2012; 90(1): 269–271

[34] Paxton BE, Arepally A, Alley CL, Kim CY. Bariatric embolization: pilot study on the impact of gastroprotective agents and arterial distribution on ulceration risk and efficacy in a porcine model. J Vasc Interv Radiol. 2016; 27(12):1923–1928

[35] Coblijn UK, Lagarde SM, de Castro SM, Kuiken SD, van Wagensveld BA. Symptomatic marginal ulcer disease after Roux-en-Y gastric bypass: incidence, risk factors and management. Obes Surg. 2015; 25(5): 805–811

[36] Gunn AJ, Oklu R. A preliminary observation of weight loss following left gastric artery embolization in humans. J Obes. 2014; 2014:185349

[37] Kipshidze N, Archvadze A, Bertog S, Leon MB, Sievert H. Endovascular bariatrics: first in humans study of gastric artery embolization for weight loss. JACC Cardiovasc Interv. 2015; 8(12):1641–1644

29 Intra-Abdominal Fluid Collections

Stephen R. Lee, Ashraf Thabet, and Peter R. Mueller

29.1 Introduction

In this chapter, the percutaneous management of intra-abdominal fluid collections will be discussed. The rationale, technique, and issues related to postprocedure care of intra-abdominal abscesses will be reviewed. Special clinical scenarios, deep pelvic collections and peripancreatic collections, will be considered. Finally, an overview of the pathophysiology enterocutaneous fistulas (ECFs), traditional management strategies, and new interventional techniques for treating ECFs will be provided.

29.2 Indications/Contraindications

Drainage of intra-abdominal fluid collections can serve three main purposes: treatment of infection, characterization of fluid, and relief of symptoms. Most commonly, interventional radiologists are asked to drain fluid collections in the setting of sepsis to provide source control. At other times, a fluid collection is incidentally discovered on imaging and sampling may be required to determine its source. This commonly occurs in the postoperative setting; in such cases, the fluid collection may represent a hematoma, urinoma, lymphocele, or abscess. Less commonly, a fluid collection may be a source of discomfort for a patient. Examples include symptomatic hepatic cysts, lymphoceles, or pancreatic pseudocysts.

Contraindications to drainage of intra-abdominal fluid collections are generally relative. The risk of not intervening must be weighed against the risk of any potential procedural complications (e.g., the risk of not achieving source control by draining an abscess in a patient with sepsis vs. the risk of bleeding complications in the setting of mild coagulopathy or recent antiplatelet medication use). Relative contraindications include uncorrectable coagulopathy, hemodynamic instability, and absence of a safe window for catheter placement.

29.3 Preprocedural Preparation and Planning

Because these procedures are typically performed with moderate conscious sedation, patients are typically instructed to take nothing by mouth for 8 hours before the procedure (or otherwise per institutional guidelines). In our own practice, a combination of an opioid (e.g., fentanyl) and a benzodiazepine (e.g., midazolam) is administered intravenously with cardiorespiratory monitoring.

The Society of Interventional Radiology (SIR) consensus guidelines provide recommendations regarding management of anticoagulant medications as well as goal laboratory values in the setting of thrombocytopenia or coagulopathy.[1] Abscess drainage is categorized as a procedure with "moderate risk of bleeding," so an international normalized ratio (INR) of less than 1.5 and a platelet count of greater than 50,000/uL is recommended.

In the setting of a possibly infected fluid collection, antimicrobial therapy is most effective if it is initiated up to 3 hours

before percutaneous drainage.[2] Most intra-abdominal abscesses are polymicrobial, so broad-spectrum antibiotics to cover gram-negative rods and anaerobes are recommended.[3]

Computed tomography (CT) or ultrasound is typically used for catheter drainage of intra-abdominal fluid collections. In general, CT offers better visualization of the targeted fluid collection, especially in larger patients or for collections that are deeper in the abdomen or pelvis. For complex, loculated fluid collections, CT also offers the advantage of ensuring complete drainage after initial catheter placement and can assist the interventionalist in identifying additional fluid collections that may need to be addressed. Unlike ultrasound imaging, CT images are not degraded by air within the targeted fluid collection or in the bowel.

Ultrasound does offer some distinct advantages in certain circumstances. In the setting of hemodynamic instability, ultrasound can be employed at the patient's bedside, obviating the need to transport a critically ill patient to the interventional suite and risking decompensation during the process. Draining a collection with the use of ultrasound is also typically more expedient than draining a collection with the use of CT, as catheter position is confirmed with real-time ultrasound imaging. In the pediatric population, use of ultrasound is generally strongly considered because ultrasound visualization of the targeted collection may be sufficient, obviating the need to expose the patient to ionizing radiation. Another advantage of ultrasound is that it may be performed in a traditional interventional fluoroscopy suite. This is particularly useful for complex fluid collections. Access to the collection can be achieved with ultrasound guidance; then, under fluoroscopic guidance, contrast can be injected to define the extent and configuration of the collection. Using the Seldinger technique, a wire and directional catheter can be used to navigate through the collection to ensure appropriate catheter position (▶ Fig. 29.1).

29.4 Catheter Placement Technique

There are two techniques by which a catheter can be placed into a fluid collection: tandem trocar and modified Seldinger techniques. In the tandem trocar technique, a 20- or 21-gauge needle is placed into the targeted collection under CT guidance. A small aspirate may be obtained to determine the nature of the collection. If catheter drainage is desired, the needle can then be used as a guide for catheter placement. The skin is anesthetized with local anesthesia, a skin nick is made, and the tract is bluntly dissected with Kelly forceps. The catheter is then assembled with the metal stiffener and inner trocar in place. The catheter is inserted parallel to the guiding needle to a depth determined on the planning CT. The catheter is fed off of the metal stiffener and trocar assembly, and the retention string is pulled to lock the pigtail. After the catheter position is confirmed with CT, the catheter is secured to the skin with a suture.

In the modified Seldinger technique, access may be obtained using a micropuncture technique or a larger 18-gauge needle.

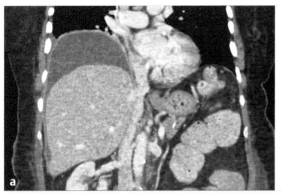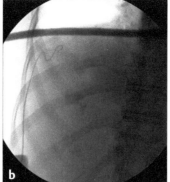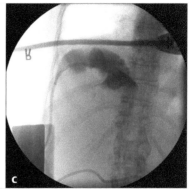

Fig. 29.1 (a) Contrast-enhanced CT scan shows a large subphrenic collection. (b) Ultrasound and fluoroscopic guidance was selected because of the absence of a safe CT window, which would have resulted in transpulmonic placement. After access from a subcostal approach was achieved with a 19-gauge thin-wall needle using ultrasound, a 0.035-inch wire was directed superiorly under fluoroscopic guidance. (c) A multisidehole catheter was placed using a modified Seldinger technique. Use of fluoroscopy allows for precise catheter placement. Note the radiopaque marker on the catheter demarcating the most proximal sidehole, which is appropriately positioned within the collection.

After confirmation of needle position with CT, a wire is passed into the collection. Wire position is confirmed with CT, and serial dilation from 8-Fr up to the catheter size is then performed in 2-Fr increments. The catheter is then placed over the wire with the internal metallic or plastic stiffener, and position is confirmed with CT. The catheter is advanced, and the retention string is pulled to lock the pigtail.

The decision regarding whether to use the tandem trocar technique or the modified Seldinger is typically based on operator preference and experience. No randomized clinical trials have compared the two techniques. However, in our experience, each technique offers distinct advantages. The tandem trocar technique is quicker and does not require wire placement and sequential tract dilation. Because there is decreased instrumentation and manipulation within the collection, there is less risk for causing sepsis. Furthermore, even when best technique is followed, each exchange of the dilator over the wire increases the chance for wire dislodgement out of the collection, particularly for small collections. The modified Seldinger technique allows for very precise catheter placement and is preferable to the trocar technique when only a small window of access is present. Also, because the wire is typically left in place before catheter deployment, the catheter can be repositioned or advanced with relative ease. A variety of catheters may be deployed with the modified Seldinger technique, including multisidehole or biliary drainage catheters, which do not typically come packaged with a sharp trocar.

29.5 Postprocedural Care

Catheter occlusion due to viscous drainage is one of the most common complications after placement of a drainage catheter. To prevent this complication, a three-way stopcock may be connected between the catheter and the drainage bag. The risk of catheter occlusion may be minimized by routinely flushing the catheter with enough volume to fill the dead space of the catheter and connecting tubing. In our practice, 5 mL of normal saline is instilled toward the catheter and 5 mL toward the drainage bag every 8 hours.

Criteria that can be used to assess the appropriateness of catheter removal include: (1) decrease in output to less than 10 mL/d, (2) absence of a residual collection on imaging (i.e., CT, ultrasound, or abscessogram), and (3) absence of significant fistula between the abscess cavity and adjacent structures that could promote redevelopment of abscess (e.g., pancreatic or biliary ducts, bowel, or bladder).

Although a decrease in catheter output may mean that the abscess cavity has collapsed, it may also suggest catheter obstruction or highly viscous collection contents. If imaging shows a residual collection and the catheter flushes with ease, this suggests that the cause of decreased output is a highly viscous collection. In this setting, tissue plasminogen activator (tPA) can be administered via the catheter into the collection. A dose of 4-mL tPA diluted in 25-mL sterile saline is administered into the catheter; the total volume instilled is smaller than the cavity volume. The catheter is clamped for 30 minutes and unclamped thereafter. This can be performed twice daily for 2 to 3 days. This protocol has been shown to be effective in reducing the need for additional catheter placement or surgical drainage. In one series of 46 abscesses refractory to initial drainage, complete evacuation of 41 abscesses (89%) was achieved after tPA was administered.[4] Notably, there were no bleeding complications directly attributable to tPA administration.

29.6 Special Considerations

29.6.1 Peripancreatic Collections

Surgical management of necrotizing pancreatitis has evolved over the past few years.[5] Minimally invasive surgical necrosectomy is now being performed in some centers with promising results. Mortality rates have been shown to be lower with the minimally invasive approach when compared to open necrosectomy (19 vs. 38%, respectively).[6] These techniques rely on a drainage catheter placed via a percutaneous retroperitoneal approach for access. During surgery, the drain is followed into the peripancreatic collection. The collection is opened, and a laparoscopic camera is inserted. The necrotic cavity is vigorously debrided with continuous lavage via two drains.[7]

When placing drainage catheters for potential video-assisted retroperitoneal debridement of a peripancreatic collection, interventionalists should be mindful of a few points. The

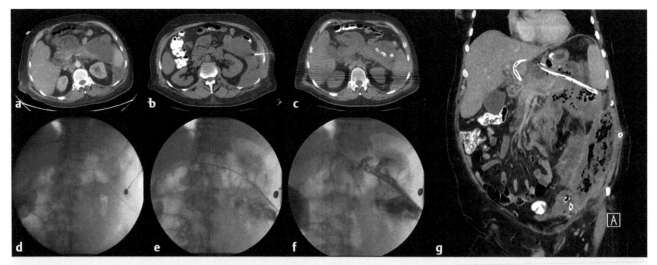

Fig. 29.2 **(a)** CT scan shows a large peripancreatic fluid collection from necrotizing pancreatitis. **(b)** Access to the fluid collection was achieved under CT guidance with a 19-gauge thin-wall needle. **(c)** A 16-French catheter was placed into the collection. Note that the more medial component of the collection is not drained by the catheter. **(d)** The patient was brought to the fluoroscopy suite the next day for catheter repositioning. **(e)** Under fluoroscopic guidance, a wire and Kumpe catheter were navigated to the more medial component of the collection. **(f)** Final injection of the catheter shows that the catheter is well-centered within the collection. **(g)** Diagnostic CT scan performed after catheter repositioning shows position of the catheter. This precise placement would have been difficult to achieve with the use of CT guidance only.

standard surgical approach for video-assisted retroperitoneal debridement is to dissect into the left retroperitoneum from a subcostal entry site along the percutaneous catheter into the region of peripancreatic necrosis. Therefore, attempts are made to place the catheter via a left retroperitoneal approach, anterior to the left kidney and posterior to the descending colon. The material drained from pancreatic necrosis is highly viscous and debris-filled. Accordingly, the potential for catheter clogging is high if the catheter selected is too small. At our institution, catheters up to 24-Fr are routinely placed. Inadvertent traversal of adjacent organs and large blood vessels by these large catheters can be avoided by noting the position of the organs and vessels on the preprocedural scan. In our practice, these catheters are typically placed using the modified Seldinger technique (▶ Fig. 29.2).

29.6.2 Deep Pelvic Collections

Deep pelvic collections can pose a challenge for even the most seasoned interventionalist. A safe percutaneous window is frequently obscured by the bowel or bladder in such cases. Review of imaging before the patient's arrival to the interventional suite may alert the interventionalist to the need to decompress the bladder by having the patient void or by placing a urinary catheter. In general, an anterior approach is preferable if there is a safe window to the collection, as supine positioning is typically more tolerable during the procedure. Additionally, in our experience, there is less risk of dislodgement for catheters placed via an anterior approach compared to those placed via a posterior approach. If a safe anterior approach cannot be achieved, a transgluteal approach may be a good option (▶ Fig. 29.3). Inadvertent injury to the sciatic nerve and gluteal arteries can be avoided by ensuring that the course of the catheter remains close to the lateral margin of the sacrum. Transrectal and transvaginal approaches under ultrasound guidance are also options for drainage of deep pelvic collections

if a percutaneous approach is not feasible. However, one of the drawbacks to these techniques is that catheter dislodgement after placement is common because of difficulty in adequately securing the catheter.

29.7 Enterocutaneous Fistulas

29.7.1 Pathophysiology/Classification

ECFs can be classified based on their anatomy, etiology, or physiology. Anatomically, an ECF is defined by the portion of the gastrointestinal (GI) tract from which it originates. ECFs most commonly arise, in descending order, from the small bowel, colon, stomach, and duodenum. ECFs can also be classified according to their volume of daily output. ECFs with an output of < 200 mL/d are classified as low output, those with an output of 200 to 500 mL/d are classified as moderate output, and those with an output of > 500 mL/d are classified as high output.

The etiologies of ECFs are variable but can be recalled with the mnemonic "FRIEND" (▶ Table 29.1). Approximately 80% of ECFs are associated with a previous surgery, most commonly surgeries related to malignancy, inflammatory bowel disease, and adhesions. Approximately 20% of ECFs are spontaneous, with no specific inciting event. The most common causes of spontaneous fistulas are malignancy and inflammatory bowel disease. Although most ECFs occur postoperatively, interventionalists are likely to encounter spontaneous fistulas more frequently, as these patients are typically poor surgical candidates in whom conservative management is more likely to fail.

Classification of ECFs based on their anatomy, etiology, and physiology is important, as all of these factors may provide some prognostic value with regard to spontaneous closure and overall mortality (▶ Table 29.2).[8] In one of the earliest series of patients with ECFs, Edmunds et al[9] noted an overall mortality rate of 54% in patients with high-output small bowel ECFs compared to 16% in patients with low-output colonic fistulas. The

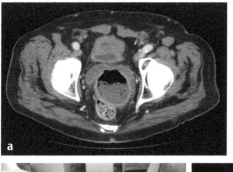
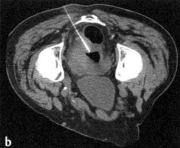
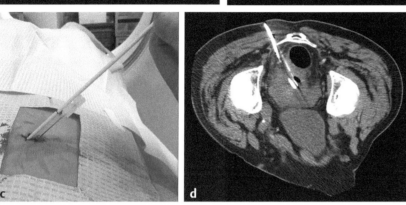

Fig. 29.3 (a) Diagnostic CT scan shows a large diverticular abscess in the deep pelvis. (b) A transgluteal approach was selected as there was not a safe anterior window because of intervening bowel and bladder. A 20-gauge needle was placed into the collection under CT guidance. (c) Tandem trocar technique was employed. Note the parallel orientation between the 20-gauge guiding needle and the catheter. (d) Catheter in appropriate position. Note its proximity to the lateral margin of the sacrum to avoid injury to vascular and nerve structures.

higher mortality rate of high-output fistulas was confirmed in a more recent series by Lévy et al,[10] who reported a mortality of 50 versus 26% in high- and low-output fistulas, respectively. In a series spanning 30 years and 404 patients, Soeters et al[11] also noted higher complication rates, specifically uncontrolled infection and malnutrition, with high-output small bowel fistulas. These fistulas were also less amenable to medical or surgical treatments. Although the mortality associated with high-output fistulas has decreased significantly over the past few decades,[12] the mortality differences discovered in earlier series elucidate key differences among the natural histories of different types of fistulas and help clinicians to create informed treatment strategies.

Fistulas occur in 17 to 43% of patients with Crohn's disease (CD),[13] and ECFs associated with CD have unique features.[14] Patients with CD frequently have more than one site of active disease that needs to be addressed. The optimal medical management strategy for CD has also evolved over the past 20 years with the introduction of biological medical therapy and immunomodulation. Infliximab, a monoclonal antibody against tumor necrosis factor, has been shown to be effective in reducing the number of fistulas and ensuring a sustained response with an overall reduction in fistulizing disease.[15,16] This highlights the importance of a multidisciplinary approach when treating patients with ECFs related to CD, as optimal medical management is recommended before any invasive intervention.

However, in spite of best medical therapy, many patients will require interventional or surgical management for fistulizing CD. In a series of 26 patients, Poritz et al[17] found that although either a partial or complete response to infliximab was seen in 61% of patients, 73% either required surgery or had abscesses remaining after medical therapy. Surgical techniques must also be adapted in patients with CD (although this is beyond the scope of this chapter). For instance, in a subgroup analysis of their series of 203 patients who underwent surgical

Table 29.1 Mnemonic for enterocutaneous fistula etiologies

F	Foreign body
R	Radiation
I	Inflammation
E	Epithelialization
N	Neoplasia
D	Distal obstruction

Table 29.2 Predictive factors for spontaneous closure and/or mortality

Factor	Favorable	Unfavorable
Organ of origin	Esophageal Duodenal stump Pancreatic, biliary Jejunal Colonic	Gastric Lateral duodenal Ligament of Treitz Ileal
Etiology	Postoperative (anastomotic leakage) Appendicitis, diverticulitis	Malignancy Inflammatory bowel disease
Output	Low (< 200–500 mL/d)	High (> 500 mL/d)
Fistula characteristics	Tract > 2 cm Defect < 1 cm	Tract < 1 cm Defect > 1 cm
Nutritional status	Well-nourished Transferrin > 200 mg/dL	Malnourished Transferrin < 200 mg/dL
Sepsis	Absent	Present
State of bowel	Intestinal continuity Absence of obstruction	Bowel discontinuity Distal obstruction Large abscess Previous radiation

Source: Data from Evenson and Fischer.[8]

Table 29.3 Mnemonic for enterocutaneous fistula management principles

S	Sepsis control
N	Nutritional support
A	Anatomy definition
P	Plan

Source: Data from Rahman and Stavas.[20]

management of ECF, Lynch et al[18] reported a higher recurrence rate in patients with CD who underwent oversewing than those who underwent resection (75 vs. 15%, respectively).

29.7.2 Principles of Management

In 1964, Chapman et al[19] reported on their experience in the management of ECF, and the principles of management they presented more than 50 years ago remain the foundation of ECF management today (and can be remembered with the mnemonic shown in ▸ Table 29.3).[20] These principles state that patients should be stabilized and volume repleted upon presentation; electrolyte derangements, specifically hypokalemia, are quite common. Control of the ECF effluent may be achieved via stoma devices or negative pressure wound dressings (vacuum-assisted devices). Local skin care may also be aggressively managed.

Upon volume repletion and correction of electrolyte abnormalities, the search should begin for sources of intra-abdominal infection, typically with cross-sectional imaging or, less frequently, with exploratory laparotomy in the setting of peritonitis and concern for uncontained infection. Empiric antibiotic treatment should be initiated early in the setting of sepsis. In the absence of sepsis, however, antibiotics are best used judiciously. Broad-spectrum antibiotics can be tailored to the targeted pathogens when feasible. In the absence of signs of infection, indiscriminate use of antibiotics may result in the selection of resistant bacteria.

Although the anatomy of the fistula can frequently be delineated with CT, fistulography with fluoroscopy may be required to provide more functional anatomic detail. Communication between the referring surgeon and the radiologist performing the fistulogram is important to ensure that the appropriate images are obtained for surgical planning and that an adequate and thorough evaluation has been performed.

Nutritional support of the patient is paramount throughout all phases of care. As Chapman et al[19] showed, mortality rates were significantly lower in patients receiving 3,000 kcal/d compared to those with suboptimal caloric intake. Early studies showed that using total parenteral nutrition (TPN) not only ensures that caloric requirements are met, but also decreases the volume of effluent, which facilitates local skin care and decreases skin complications.[21,22] More recently, the reliance on TPN has become controversial. Some advocate the use of TPN only as an adjunct to distal enteral feeding, whereas others advocate bowel rest and rely on TPN solely for nutritional support.[23,24]

Definitive management strategies for ECF have traditionally been surgical. These operations are classically herculean undertakings, requiring hours of meticulous dissection, adhesiolysis, and mobilization of the GI tract. Resection of the affected portion of bowel, reestablishment of GI continuity, and reconstruction of the abdominal wall are the goals of the operation. Success rates between 58 and 89% for fistula resection have been reported in the surgical literature.[18,25] Mortality rates have ranged from 3.5 and 7% in modern surgical series.[18,25]

Percutaneous management strategies, which will be discussed in detail below, are relatively new to the field of ECF treatment and can provide an additional approach when traditional methods fail or when patients are poor surgical candidates. The recent emergence of bioadhesives and extracellular matrix materials has allowed percutaneous approaches to evolve beyond catheter drainage. Although endoscopic approaches using similar closure materials have been described, identification of the internal fistula origin remains a challenge and major limitation of this technique.

29.7.3 Interventional Techniques

Preprocedural Imaging

As with any interventional procedure, careful and methodical planning is requisite for success. This is especially true in cases of ECF closure; many factors that can impede closure must be addressed during preprocedural evaluation. ECF location and anatomy and associated complicating factors (i.e., distal obstruction, abscesses, strictures) are best fully investigated before the start of any intervention.

Fistulography

Fluoroscopic imaging remains the workhorse and modality of choice for ECF evaluation today. The following observations must be made: (1) location of the fistula, (2) size of the fistula (i.e., tract length, width, course, and relationships), (3) continuity of the bowel (i.e., end vs. side fistula), (4) presence of distal obstruction, (5) associated findings in the adjacent bowel (i.e., stricture, inflammation), and (6) presence of associated abscess with or without communication to the fistula (▸ Fig. 29.4).[21]

Technique Fistulography

A scout plain film of the abdomen is obtained to document evidence of previous surgical intervention and to provide anatomic landmarks of the fistula before the injection of contrast. Water-soluble contrast is recommended for the initial assessment of the fistula. Although barium, with its higher radiographic density, provides greater mucosal detail and better contrast, it incites significant peritoneal inflammation if extravasation into the peritoneal cavity occurs. Therefore, water-soluble contrast can be used primarily and, once the absence of peritoneal communication is ensured, barium may be used if imaging with water-soluble contrast provides inadequate anatomic detail. However, administered barium may severely limit the utility of subsequent CT scans.

The skin area surrounding the fistula is prepared and draped in a sterile fashion. Lidocaine gel may be administered for local anesthesia. A straight- or angle-tipped 5-Fr angiographic catheter is gently inserted into the fistula orifice. Depending on the size of the fistula, a variety of other catheters may be used. For fistulas with larger orifices, urinary catheters may be a better

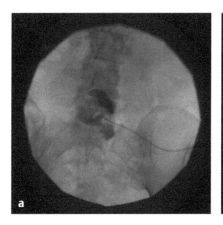
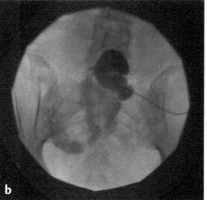

Fig. 29.4 (a) Fistulogram performed to evaluate for possible plug procedure. (b) The fistulous tract between the skin and loop of small bowel was noted to be too short for plug placement (<2 cm).

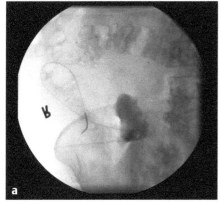
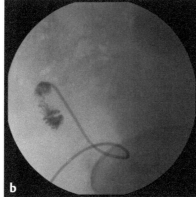

Fig. 29.5 (a) Fistulogram performed to evaluate for possible plug procedure. A Kumpe catheter is navigated from the skin fistula site into the small bowel. The distance between the skin entry site and the bowel lumen was approximately 5 cm, appropriate for plug placement. Note the extravasation of contrast near the skin entry site. (b) A catheter was placed to maintain access to the fistula.

choice, as the larger catheter diameter and the ability to inflate the retention balloon minimizes the risk of pericatheter leakage during administration of contrast. If resistance is met upon advancement of a standard straight- or angle-tipped diagnostic angiography catheter into the fistula, a 5- or 8-Fr pediatric feeding catheter may be used. These catheters, with their round leading edge, are designed to be atraumatic during blind advancement, making them well suited for blind cannulation of ECFs.

Gentle injection of contrast can prevent unnecessary trauma to the commonly friable adjacent soft tissues and may prevent the creation of false passages. There is at least one report of pancreatic pseudocyst rupture during fistulogram due to over-aggressive injection of contrast (▶ Fig. 29.5).[26]

Once the course of the fistula is identified, images from multiple projections are obtained. Although excess manipulation in the fistula increases the chance for creation of false passages, the catheter must be manipulated, advanced, and repositioned as needed to ensure that additional tracts and/or fluid collections are not present. Magnification views, when used judiciously, may increase the diagnostic quality of the examination by increasing the sensitivity for detection of additional tracts or collections.

Percutaneous Approaches

Catheter Drainage

In spite of optimal medical management, a certain proportion of ECFs will fail to spontaneously close. Spontaneous closure rates reported in modern series are widely variable and range from 15 to 46%.[27] Until the early 1980s, radiology's role in the management of ECFs was limited to diagnosis and preoperative planning. The first description of the use of interventional radiology to manage ECFs was published in 1982 by McLean et al.[28] In their series of 12 patients with postoperative ECFs, a closure rate of 100% was achieved with the use of T-tubes to control the bowel effluent and adjacent catheters to sump any additional fluid adjacent to the bowel wall. Although subsequent studies failed to achieve the same degree of success, the concept these authors introduced remains the foundation on which modern interventional radiology management techniques are built.[29,30,31] Namely, by reducing and controlling the path of the bowel effluent and evacuating any adjacent collections, the surrounding soft tissues are given an opportunity to heal, and spontaneous fistula closure is promoted. It is important to note that up to 44% of ECFs are associated with an abscess, which must also be addressed.[32]

Technique of Catheter Drainage

Relevant imaging results are reviewed, with particular attention paid to any fluid collections that may need to be addressed. Associated fluid collections that do not directly communicate with the fistula are drained using standard techniques under CT or ultrasound guidance (see preceding section on intra-abdominal fluid collections).

After any adjacent fluid collections are addressed with percutaneous drainage, a catheter may be placed directly into the fistula to control bowel effluent and/or to drain any collections in communication with the fistula. The skin is prepared and draped in the usual sterile fashion. Lidocaine may be administered subcutaneously or as a topical gel for local anesthesia. Moderate conscious sedation is generally not required.

The fistula can be cannulated using a standard 5-Fr straight or directional angiographic catheter. If initial access with a standard 5-Fr catheter is difficult, a 5- or 8-Fr pediatric feeding catheter may be advanced in an atraumatic fashion until the catheter has reached a stable position. From there, a directional catheter may be exchanged over a wire. If a 5-Fr pediatric feeding catheter is used for initial cannulation, the exchange wire needs to be a 0.018-inch wire, as a 0.035-inch wire is too large to fit into the inner lumen. A variety of wires and catheters can be used to navigate to the deepest part of the abscess–fistula complex. In general, softer wires (e.g., 3J, Bentson) are favored over stiffer wires (e.g., Amplatz) to minimize the amount of trauma to the surrounding tissues. Intermittent injection of contrast can be performed during catheter navigation to ensure that the catheter is still within the abscess–fistula complex. Once final catheter position has been achieved, the 5-Fr catheter is exchanged over the wire for a drainage catheter.

Selection of the type of drainage catheter depends on the length and size of the abscess–fistula complex. To reduce the risk of catheter clogging, catheter diameters larger than 10-Fr are recommended. For smaller cavities, standard pigtail catheters with sideholes along the curved portion only may be placed. For more complex or longer tracts, multisidehole catheters may be employed, as these catheters have sideholes along a longer portion of the catheter than standard pigtail catheters. When using a multisidehole catheter, it is important to ensure that the sideholes do not extend beyond the desired area of drainage, as this may be a source of pericatheter leakage. If the selected multisidehole catheter has too many sideholes, a standard pigtail catheter may be modified by cutting additional holes along its side, taking care not to ligate the retention string.

One of the challenges of catheter placement within an abscess–fistula complex is ensuring catheter retention after placement. Although skin sutures may be placed, the skin surrounding the fistula is often friable and prone to breakdown. Creative strategies often have to be employed with the assistance of a stoma or wound care specialist. If a stoma device is used, the catheter can be secured to the stoma rather than to the patient's skin.

Tract Closure

Techniques to actively close ECF tracts emerged in the 1990s with the development of fibrin sealant. This represented a shift in the interventional radiologic treatment of ECFs. Previously, catheter management relied on the body's ability to spontaneously close an ECF after promoting enteral diversion and healing. One of the earliest reports of the successful use of fibrin sealant was published by Brady et al,[33] who described the use of Tisseel to close a duodenal fistula caused by a duodenal stump leak. Since then, a variety of techniques to actively close ECF tracts have been reported.

Materials used in ECF tract closure fall broadly into two categories: bioadhesives and extracellular matrix materials. Fibrin glues are the most common type of bioadhesives used in ECF

tract closure. Fibrin glues are packaged as separate solutions of fibrinogen and thrombin that coagulate immediately when mixed together. The coagulum not only functions as a mechanical plug, but also promotes growth of granulation tissue, resulting in a connective tissue scar. Two commonly used fibrin glues are Tisseel and Evicel. BioGlue is another type of bioadhesive that consists of a separate 45% bovine serum albumin and 10% glutaraldehyde solution. Exposure of the two components results in immediate polymerization and creates a strong scaffold. The use of a combination of n-butyl-2-cyanoacrylate (NBCA) glue and Lipiodol in a ratio of 1:5 has also been reported.[34]

Extracellular matrix materials are a newer type of device used in ECF tract closure. Extracellular matrix materials provide a biologic scaffold and promote tissue growth. The Cook Biodesign fistula plug was designed to treat anal, enterocutaneous, and rectovaginal fistulas. The plug is derived from decellularized porcine intestinal submucosa, which provides a scaffold for tissue growth. The plug is deployed fluoroscopically via an 18- or 21-Fr sheath and has a radiopaque internal retention flange that seals against the intraluminal bowel wall. The plug is retained by an external disc that is positioned against the patient's skin.

Technique with Bioadhesives

After cannulation of the ECF tract with a 4- or 5-Fr catheter, normal saline is flushed through the catheter to remove residual contrast and debris from the tract. The catheter is then positioned at the enteric opening of the fistula, just outside of the bowel lumen. Depending on the type of bioadhesive selected, the catheter may need to be primed with a solution per the manufacturer's instructions (e.g., 5% dextrose if NBCA is used). The bioadhesive is then slowly injected under fluoroscopic guidance while the catheter is withdrawn to the skin surface (▶ Fig. 29.6).

Technique with Extracellular Matrix Materials

After cannulation of the ECF tract with a 4- or 5-Fr catheter, the tract is dilated in the standard fashion to accept the selected 18- or 22-Fr delivery sheath. The tract is denuded with a bronchoscopic brush to incite local hyperemia. The tract is then thoroughly flushed with 1% hydrogen peroxide. The plug is advanced through the delivery sheath until the retention flange is deployed within the bowel lumen. The plug is hydrated with normal saline, and the sheath is removed. Gentle traction is maintained on the plug to ensure adequate intraluminal seal of the retention flange. The external portion is then secured to the skin with a Molnar disc (▶ Fig. 29.7).

Postprocedural Care

Patients and referring providers should be counseled regarding the expected postprocedural course. Early leakage may occur; this is not considered a sign of procedural failure. In our practice, patients are instructed to take nothing by mouth for the first 24 hours and are allowed to ingest clear liquids after 48 hours. A high-fiber diet is recommended thereafter to assist in reducing the volume of liquid effluent from the ECF. TPN can be considered for patients who are unable to meet their nutritional goals. An abdominal binder is placed, and patients are instructed to refrain from strenuous activity for 6 weeks. In our

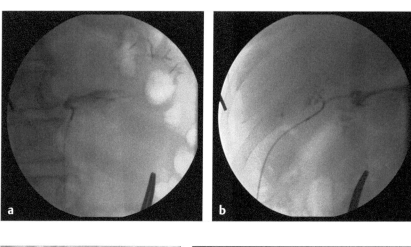

Fig. 29.6 (a) Fistulogram performed in preparation of bioadhesive tract closure. A Kumpe catheter was navigated through the gastrocutaneous fistula. Injection of contrast shows rugal folds, confirming intraluminal position of the catheter tip. (b) The catheter was positioned just outside the gastric lumen. The bioadhesive (Tisseel) was injected as the catheter was withdrawn to the skin surface.

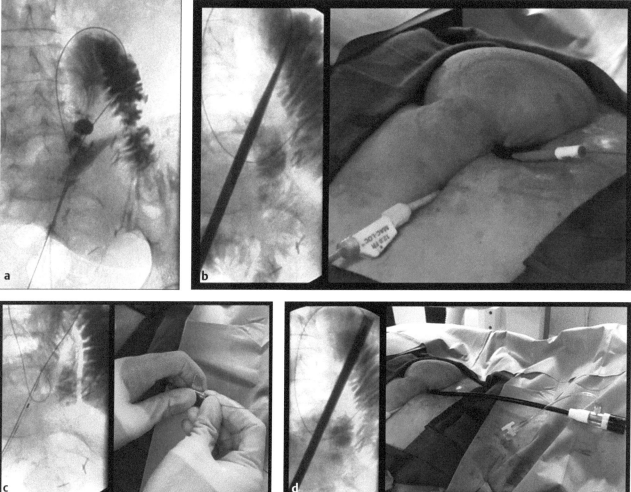

Fig. 29.7 (a) Initial fistulogram in preparation for plug deployment. (b) The tract is dilated to accept the 22-French delivery sheath. (c) An endoscopic biopsy brush is inserted to denude the tract to promote fistula closure. (d) The 22-French delivery sheath is positioned. (*continued*)

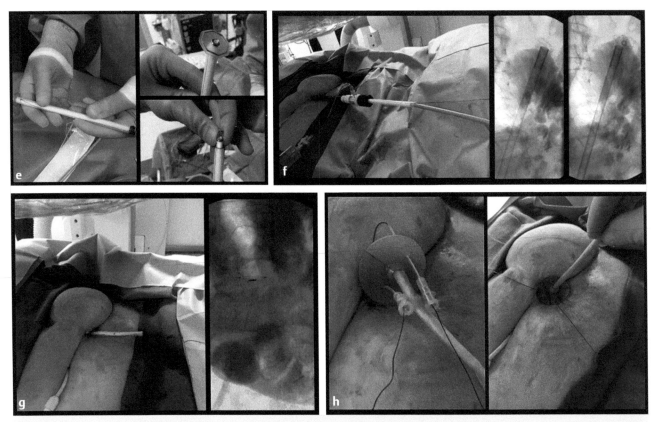

Fig. 29.7 (*continued*) **(e)** Back-table preparation of the fistula plug. The pliable octagonal flange is loaded into the delivery system. This flange will appose the inner wall of bowel lumen. **(f)** The plug is loaded into the delivery sheath. The flange is advanced into the bowel lumen. **(g)** The delivery sheath system is removed and the plug is left in place. The plug is positioned to ensure good apposition of the flange against the inner bowel wall. **(h)** The Molnar disc is apposed to the skin surface.

practice, patients are seen in the clinic for follow-up 2 to 4 weeks after the procedure. The Molnar disc and internal flange will typically spontaneously fall away 2 to 4 weeks after placement.

References

[1] Patel IJ, Davidson JC, Nikolic B, et al. Standards of Practice Committee, with Cardiovascular and Interventional Radiological Society of Europe (CIRSE) Endorsement, Standards of Practice Committee of the Society of Interventional Radiology. Addendum of newer anticoagulants to the SIR consensus guideline. J Vasc Interv Radiol. 2013; 24(5):641–645

[2] McDermott VG, Schuster MG, Smith TP. Antibiotic prophylaxis in vascular and interventional radiology. AJR Am J Roentgenol. 1997; 169(1):31–38

[3] Venkatesan AM, Kundu S, Sacks D, et al. Society of Interventional Radiology Standards of Practice Committee. Practice guidelines for adult antibiotic prophylaxis during vascular and interventional radiology procedures. Written by the Standards of Practice Committee for the Society of Interventional Radiology and Endorsed by the Cardiovascular Interventional Radiological Society of Europe and Canadian Interventional Radiology Association [corrected]. J Vasc Interv Radiol. 2010; 21(11):1611–1630, quiz 1631

[4] Beland MD, Gervais DA, Levis DA, Hahn PF, Arellano RS, Mueller PR. Complex abdominal and pelvic abscesses: efficacy of adjunctive tissue-type plasminogen activator for drainage. Radiology. 2008; 247(2):567–573

[5] da Costa DW, Boerma D, van Santvoort HC, et al. Staged multidisciplinary step-up management for necrotizing pancreatitis. Br J Surg. 2014; 101(1):e65–e79

[6] Raraty MGT, Halloran CM, Dodd S, et al. Minimal access retroperitoneal pancreatic necrosectomy: improvement in morbidity and mortality with a less invasive approach. Ann Surg. 2010; 251(5):787–793

[7] Horvath KD, Kao LS, Wherry KL, Pellegrini CA, Sinanan MN. A technique for laparoscopic-assisted percutaneous drainage of infected pancreatic necrosis and pancreatic abscess. Surg Endosc. 2001; 15(10):1221–1225

[8] Evenson AR, Fischer JE. Current management of enterocutaneous fistula. J Gastrointest Surg. 2006; 10(3):455–464

[9] Edmunds LH, Jr, Williams GM, Welch CE. External fistulas arising from the gastro-intestinal tract. Ann Surg. 1960; 152:445–471

[10] Lévy E, Frileux P, Cugnenc PH, Honiger J, Ollivier JM, Parc R. High-output external fistulae of the small bowel: management with continuous enteral nutrition. Br J Surg. 1989; 76(7):676–679

[11] Soeters PB, Ebeid AM, Fischer JE. Review of 404 patients with gastrointestinal fistulas. Impact of parenteral nutrition. Ann Surg. 1979; 190(2):189–202

[12] Schecter WP. Management of enterocutaneous fistulas. Surg Clin North Am. 2011; 91(3):481–491

[13] Schwartz DA, Pemberton JH, Sandborn WJ. Diagnosis and treatment of perianal fistulas in Crohn disease. Ann Intern Med. 2001; 135(10):906–918

[14] Orangio GR. Enterocutaneous fistula: medical and surgical management including patients with Crohn's disease. Clin Colon Rectal Surg. 2010; 23(3):169–175

[15] Present DH, Rutgeerts P, Targan S, et al. Infliximab for the treatment of fistulas in patients with Crohn's disease. N Engl J Med. 1999; 340(18):1398–1405

[16] Sands BE, Anderson FH, Bernstein CN, et al. Infliximab maintenance therapy for fistulizing Crohn's disease. N Engl J Med. 2004; 350(9):876–885

[17] Poritz LS, Rowe WA, Koltun WA. Remicade does not abolish the need for surgery in fistulizing Crohn's disease. Dis Colon Rectum. 2002; 45(6):771–775

[18] Lynch AC, Delaney CP, Senagore AJ, Connor JT, Remzi FH, Fazio VW. Clinical outcome and factors predictive of recurrence after enterocutaneous fistula surgery. Ann Surg. 2004; 240(5):825–831

[19] Chapman R, Foran R, Dunphy JE. Management of intestinal fistulas. Am J Surg. 1964; 108:157–164

[20] Rahman FN, Stavas JM. Interventional radiologic management and treatment of enterocutaneous fistulae. J Vasc Interv Radiol. 2015; 26(1):7–19, quiz 20

[21] Aguirre A, Fischer JE, Welch CE. The role of surgery and hyperalimentation in therapy of gastrointestinal-cutaneous fistulae. Ann Surg. 1974; 180(4):393–401

[22] Reber HA, Roberts C, Way LW, Dunphy JE. Management of external gastrointestinal fistulas. Ann Surg. 1978; 188(4):460–467

[23] Visschers RG, Olde Damink SW, Winkens B, Soeters PB, van Gemert WG. Treatment strategies in 135 consecutive patients with enterocutaneous fistulas. World J Surg. 2008; 32(3):445–453

[24] Martinez JL, Luque-de-Leon E, Mier J, Blanco-Benavides R, Robledo F. Systematic management of postoperative enterocutaneous fistulas: factors related to outcomes. World J Surg. 2008; 32(3):436–443, discussion 444

[25] Draus JM, Jr, Huss SA, Harty NJ, Cheadle WG, Larson GM. Enterocutaneous fistula: are treatments improving? Surgery. 2006; 140(4):570–576, discussion 576–578

[26] Alexander ES, Weinberg S, Clark RA, Belkin RD. Fistulas and sinus tracts: radiographic evaluation, management, and outcome. Gastrointest Radiol. 1982; 7(2):135–140

[27] Schein M. What's new in postoperative enterocutaneous fistulas? World J Surg. 2008; 32(3):336–338

[28] McLean GK, Mackie JA, Freiman DB, Ring EJ. Enterocutaneous fistulae: interventional radiologic management. AJR Am J Roentgenol. 1982; 138(4):615–619

[29] Papanicolaou N, Mueller PR, Ferrucci JT, Jr, et al. Abscess-fistula association: radiologic recognition and percutaneous management. AJR Am J Roentgenol. 1984; 143(4):811–815

[30] LaBerge JM, Kerlan RK, Jr, Gordon RL, Ring EJ. Nonoperative treatment of enteric fistulas: results in 53 patients. J Vasc Interv Radiol. 1992; 3(2):353–357

[31] D'Harcour JB, Boverie JH, Dondelinger RF. Percutaneous management of enterocutaneous fistulas. AJR Am J Roentgenol. 1996; 167(1):33–38

[32] Kerlan RK, Jr, Jeffrey RB, Jr, Pogany AC, Ring EJ. Abdominal abscess with low-output fistula: successful percutaneous drainage. Radiology. 1985; 155(1):73–75

[33] Brady AP, Malone DE, Tam P, McGrath FP. Closure of a duodenal fistula with fibrin sealant. J Vasc Interv Radiol. 1993; 4(4):525–527, discussion 527–529

[34] Cambj Sapunar L, Sekovski B, Matić D, Tripković A, Grandić L, Družijanić N. Percutaneous embolization of persistent low-output enterocutaneous fistulas. Eur Radiol. 2012; 22(9):1991–1997

30 Pediatric Gastrointestinal Interventions

Shellie C. Josephs, Lisa Kang, and Kristi Bogan Oatis

30.1 Introduction

Gastrointestinal (GI) interventions in children are very similar to those performed in adults; however, in children they are performed only on a smaller scale, both in number of patients treated and in the size of the target of intervention. Diseases affecting the liver in children range from benign steatosis to portal hypertension and cirrhosis. Some focal lesions, such as infantile hepatic hemangioma (IHH) and hepatoblastoma, are unique to the pediatric population. Pediatric patients are more likely to undergo liver transplant to cure their underlying condition, and biliary and vascular complications after the transplant frequently require interventional skills for less invasive management. Interventional radiologists may additionally encounter vascular tumors and congenital shunts in this population. This chapter discusses manifestations of GI disease specific to children and presents evidence regarding interventional radiology treatment options.

30.2 General Considerations for Pediatric Interventional Procedures

Pediatric patients have an increased sensitivity to ionizing radiation compared to adults; physician awareness of this fact can promote optimal radiation safety practices. Image Gently, Step Lightly is a campaign designed to promote minimization of radiation dose in pediatric interventions, in accordance with the principle of "as low as reasonably achievable" (ALARA).[1] ▶ Table 30.1 lists measures recommended by the Image Gently, Step Lightly campaign that can be employed to reduce radiation exposure.

Table 30.1 Image gently/step lightly

Document X-ray exposure, review prior exposure

Use lowest dose protocol for patient size

US for procedure guidance

Pulsed fluoroscopy

Optimize patient positioning prior to fluoroscopy
- Position appropriately under image intensifier
- Avoid tissue overlap

Collimate, excluding eyes, gonads, and breasts

Decrease dose digitally
- Use digital zoom rather than magnification
- Use last image hold function rather than exposure

Minimize extended runs (i.e., into venous) when not needed

Acknowledge the fluoroscopy time
- Use a fluoroscopic timer during the exam
- Record and review exposure post-procedure

Data from www.imagegently.org/Procedures/Interventional-Radiology/StepsforSafetyPedIR. Accessed January 28, 2016.[1]

30.2.1 Anesthesia and Sedation

Most of the GI procedures discussed in this chapter are performed under general anesthesia to reduce patient and respiratory motion, as well as patient anxiety and pain. Anesthesiologists trained specifically in the care of children are critical to this effort, as medication dosing is weight based and a small volume of blood loss can have significant physiologic effects.

30.2.2 Fluids and Contrast

In neonates and young infants, care must be taken to minimize the volume of intravascular fluid administered, as small amounts can have a significant effect on overall fluid balance.[2] Iodinated contrast must be accounted for; careful coordination and communication between the radiologist and anesthesiologist are critical in this matter. Senthilnathan et al[3] reviewed the cases of more than 2,300 pediatric patients who underwent cardiac catheterization and concluded that adverse events, including contrast-induced nephropathy, were exceedingly rare in patients who receive iodinated contrast doses of 6 mL/kg or less. Hyponatremia and increased serum osmolality have been documented in pediatric patients undergoing cardiac catheterization who received higher doses of nonionic contrast (mean, 6.1 mL/kg).[4] The Joint Quality Improvement Guidelines by the Society of Interventional Radiology (SIR) and Society of Pediatric Radiology Interventional Committee state that contrast volume should not exceed 4 to 5 mL/kg in infants and 6 to 8 mL/kg in older children.[5] Dilution of contrast material with up to an equal volume of saline does not cause significant image degradation in small children.

30.2.3 Patient Safety

Padding of pressure spots and patient positioning are important for examinations performed under anesthesia. Hypothermia is a serious risk in the interventional suite; neonates and infants are especially susceptible. Minimizing thermal loss by limiting skin exposure, especially when the patient is wet, and providing continuous external warming are important measures for decreasing this risk.[2] Chlorhexidine gluconate/isopropyl alcohol preparations can safely be used to clean the skin with little to no absorption. Povidone iodine can be transcutaneously absorbed, especially in young infants, and is therefore not commonly used.[6]

30.2.4 Arterial Access

Obtaining arterial access in pediatric patients can be challenging, especially in neonates. Children's arteries are significantly smaller and more likely to exhibit vasospasm or arterial dissection than arteries in adults. Occlusion is also more common and may be caused by the larger ratio of catheter diameter to vessel lumen size and by the application of excessive pressure when obtaining hemostasis. In general, ultrasound (US) guidance and single-wall puncture technique are recommended. The smallest diameter catheter with which the task can be accomplished (typically 3–4 Fr) should be used. Sheaths are rarely used unless embolization is being performed. In the absence of a contraindication, systemic heparin is usually administered; doses range from 50 to 100 IU/kg depending on the estimated duration of the procedure.[5] Puncture site complications are more common in patients younger than 1 year, with an incidence of up to 7 to 10%.[7]

30.3 Liver Biopsy

Over the past decade, many tertiary-care institutions have shifted toward the practice of having a dedicated pediatric interventional radiologist perform liver biopsies.[8,9] Imaging guidance for this procedure has been shown to be safe and cost effective[10,11] and has facilitated the use of outpatient biopsies so that hospital admission is no longer routinely required. Preprocedural measures used for pediatric patients, including laboratory evaluation of coagulation parameters and withholding of anticoagulant/antiplatelet medications, are the same as those used for adults, with guidelines for percutaneous image-guided biopsy published by the SIR.[12] Contraindications to both percutaneous and transjugular biopsy are also similar to those in the adult population. However, there are some pediatric-specific special considerations for percutaneous and transjugular biopsies.

30.3.1 Percutaneous Liver Biopsy

For percutaneous biopsy in small patients, the left hepatic lobe is often accessed via the subxiphoid approach. However, the left liver lobe in very small infants may be too small to accommodate the biopsy needle throw; the right lobe, from a subcostal approach, can provide the increased length and width needed for adequate sampling in these cases. Note that on sonographic images, the available liver for biopsy can appear deceptively large. The use of electronic caliper measurement is recommended in very small children when planning the needle trajectory. The intercostal approach is associated with greater postprocedural pain and is therefore reserved for cases in which other approaches are not feasible.[13]

An 18-gauge cutting core biopsy needle with an approximate 20-mm throw is typically used for pediatric patients. Introducer needles are seldom used for random liver biopsies or for biopsies of easily accessible focal lesions. However, an introducer is used for the rare lesions that require computed tomography (CT) guidance, to speed up the procedure and decrease radiation dose by reducing the number of scans needed for needle positioning. Diagnostic quality samples are obtained in a high percentage of percutaneous liver biopsies, with most studies reporting rates of 98.5 to 100%.[8,9,10,13,14] Nondiagnostic results are more common if the specimen length is short (1.4 vs. 1.7 cm) as reported by Short et al in a study of over 200 liver pediatric liver biopsies.[15]

30.3.2 Transjugular Liver Biopsy

Transjugular liver biopsy has been performed in infants weighing as little as 4 kg.[16] The smallest available biopsy set has a shorter guiding cannula but still uses a 7-Fr sheath, requiring a

minimum vein diameter of approximately 3 to 3.5 mm.[2] In the largest series of pediatric transjugular liver biopsies reported to date, Habdank et al[17] performed 74 biopsies in 64 patients over a period of 8 years. Adequate samples were obtained in 98.6% of the procedures. The authors used simultaneous transabdominal sonography to visualize the needle path and suggested that this method could be used to decrease the risk of puncturing the liver capsule or gallbladder, especially in small children and patients with reduced liver transplants. Diagnostic quality specimens for transjugular liver biopsy were, overall, slightly lower than with percutaneous biopsy, with a rate of > 95% reported.[17,18]

30.3.3 Complications of Liver Biopsy

Several recent pediatric-specific studies of percutaneous liver biopsies performed by interventionalists reported complications that were categorized as major or minor according to SIR guidelines for adult image-guided percutaneous biopsy.[19] Hemorrhage was the most common major complication. Major bleeding complication rates after percutaneous biopsy in children range from 0 to 4.6%.[8,9,10,13,14,20] Studies suggest a higher incidence of hemorrhage in infants, with major hemorrhage occurring in 4.6 to 8.7% of patients,[8,10,15] including one fatal hemorrhage in a 2.6-kg infant.[15] Lower weight, lower preprocedural hematocrit, and suspected metabolic disease have been associated with increased risk of hemorrhagic complications.[15] Interestingly, Matos et al[13] observed no increase in bleeding complications when using 16-gauge biopsy needles in a series of 513 pediatric patients. Aside from hemorrhage, other reported major complications include pneumothorax, sepsis, hemobilia, and abdominal wall pseudoaneurysm.[8,9]

Although bleeding is also the most common complication of transjugular liver biopsy, the risk appears to be lower than with the percutaneous technique. In the series reported by Habdank et al,[17] the bleeding complication rate was reduced from 11 to 5% after the addition of transabdominal US to evaluate the needle path. The reported rate of capsular perforation is 3.5%; clinically significant bleeding has been reported in only 0.35% of cases.[18]

30.4 Interventions for Portal Hypertension

Extrahepatic portal vein occlusion (EHPVO) is the cause of portal hypertension in 70% of pediatric patients and is the most common cause of upper GI bleeding in children (▶ Fig. 30.1).[21] Thrombosis is idiopathic in up to 50% of patients with EHPVO; the remaining cases are attributed to umbilical vein catheterization, intra-abdominal infections, hypercoagulable states, dehydration, and other chronic liver disease. Cirrhosis can be a late finding in EHPVO but is more often associated with chronic cholestasis. ▶ Table 30.2 lists the potential causes of portal hypertension in this patient population.[22]

Doppler US is a useful initial examination in the evaluation of EHPVO. This modality can be used to evaluate the extent of EHPVO, assess the general size of intrahepatic portal veins, and determine patency of the splenic and left renal veins in case a splenorenal shunt is needed.

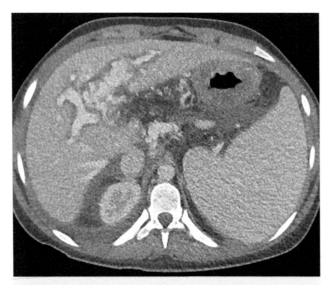

Fig. 30.1 CT with contrast demonstrating EHPVO with patent intrahepatic portal veins, splenomegaly and ascites.

30.4.1 Meso-Rex Bypass

The treatment of patients with EHPVO is directed toward reducing episodes of GI bleeding resulting from varices. The preferred operative intervention in children with portal hypertension related to EHPVO is meso-Rex bypass (MRB). This surgical shunt, which extends from the superior mesenteric vein to the left portal system at the Rex recess (RexR), decompresses the splanchnic circulation in a more normal physiologic route. This treatment option should be considered before complications of portal hypertension and bleeding develop.[23] A Rex vein of at least 2 mm in size is needed for adequate bypass.[24]

When MRB is planned, sonographic visualization of the left portal vein can be limited because of small size and low flow. Cross-sectional imaging with magnetic resonance (MR) or CT imaging is often needed for additional information (▶ Fig. 30.2a–c).

Wedged hepatic venous portography via the left hepatic vein may also be useful in evaluating the left portal vein at the RexR when this entity is not observed on other imaging studies. In

Table 30.2 Etiologies of portal hypertension

Presinusoidal	Umbilical vein instrumentation
	Omphalitis
	Congenital malformations
	Blunt trauma
	Intra-abdominal infections
Presinusoidal, intrahepatic	Congenital
	Schistosomiasis
Sinusoidal	Cirrhosis
Post	Cirrhosis
	Budd-Chiari syndrome
	Suprahepatic IVC webs
	Venooclusive disease
	Cardiac disease

Data from Kleinman et al.[22]

one small series, Lawson et al[25] reported a sensitivity of 80% and a specificity of 100% in visualizing a vein suitable for creation of a MRB using wedged hepatic venous portography. Another small series by Chaves et al[24] demonstrated a sensitivity of 92% for identification of the left portal vein via wedged portography compared to 86 and 95% for CT angiography and MR venogram, respectively. In both series, a 4-Fr catheter was wedged into a left hepatic vein, with portography performed in the frontal, cranial oblique, and caudal oblique projections using iodinated contrast.

Shunt Revision

As with any other type of operative bypass procedure, serial follow-up examinations are needed after MRB, usually with Doppler US. Reversal of flow in the proximal intrahepatic left portal vein is a normal postoperative finding. Flow is hepatopetal through the shunt into the liver and hepatofugal in the proximal left portal vein as it crosses to the right portal vein (▶ Fig. 30.2d). Depending on the conduit used, the lumen frequently becomes smaller in caliber before the anastomosis to the left portal vein, which may cause an increase in velocity at this site. This does not represent pathologic shunt stenosis when there is a gradual increase in size of the intrahepatic portal veins and a decrease in splenic size on serial Doppler US examinations.[26] Interventions to improve or reestablish flow through a stenotic or occluded bypass have been reported, with the largest series performed by Lautz et al.[27] Nine of 15 patients (60%) were treated successfully, with 3 technical failures requiring surgical revision. Stents were placed in five of the nine patients. Stenosis was more common at the hepatic end of the shunt, likely because of the angulation and turbulent flow at this site.

In accessing the shunt via a transhepatic approach, sonographic and fluoroscopic guidance is used, similar to how this guidance is used in biliary drainage procedures, with direct puncture followed by slow retraction of the needle and contrast injection until the portal vein branches are identified. This guidance is necessary because a patent right portal vein branch target may not be readily apparent due to decreased intrahepatic portal flow. Procedural success is defined as normalization of the hemodynamic gradient. Stents are used much more conservatively in children because of issues of future growth and stent durability. The choice between a balloon-expandable stent and a self-expanding stent is often determined based on the angulation at the site of stenosis.

30.4.2 Recanalization of Chronic Portal Vein Occlusion

Scattered case reports of stent recanalization of chronic portal vein occlusion in children have been published. The first reported case by Cwikiel et al[28] described successful transhepatic access into a patent right portal vein. Transplenic access to the portal vein, with or without partial splenic artery embolization, has also been described.[29,30] Although there are increasing reports of transjugular intrahepatic portosystemic shunt (TIPS) placement in the adult population, the use of this technique in children is less common, likely because of the increased technical difficulties resulting from the small size of the vessels. If a

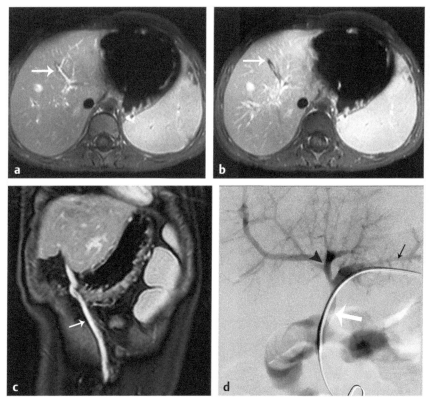

Fig. 30.2 (a) Axial contrast enhanced MR THRIVE image with arrow marking location of access of left portal vein in Rex recess along falciform ligament. (b) Axial contrast enhanced MR THRIVE image with arrow marking location of Rex recess along falciform ligament. (c) Coronal contrast enhanced MR THRIVE image with arrow marking recanalized paraumbilical vein that can be used as conduit for MRB. (d) Portogram with patent MRB. White arrow denotes MRB with hepatopetal flow from superior mesenteric vein to left portal vein, arrowhead at the anastomosis. Small black arrow is the segment 2 portal vein branch. Black arrowhead is the native bifurcation of the right and left portal veins. (The image is provided courtesy of Dr. Stanley Kim.)

child is not a candidate for an MRB and has had multiple episodes of refractory bleeding, an experienced interventionalist (with multidisciplinary consensus) may consider recanalization. Multidisciplinary discussion should include consideration of the stent location to preserve the ability to perform liver transplant in the future.

30.4.3 Transjugular Intrahepatic Portosystemic Shunts

TIPS procedures in children were first performed in 1997, with a series of 12 procedures in 9 children.[31] The original technical success rate of 78% reflects the difficulty of performing this procedure in small children. Small hepatic and portal vein size, short parenchymal tract length, and significant periportal fibrosis make this procedure technically challenging (▶ Fig. 30.3). Technical success rates of up to 100% have more recently been reported, although repeat interventions are common.[32] Bare metal stents are frequently used because of a lack of available lengths of endografts. Two recent case series described the use of the VIATORR endoprostheses in patients ranging in age from 18 months to 19 years.[33,34] Eight- and 10-mm diameter endoprostheses were used based on preprocedural and intraprocedural measurements of the portal and hepatic vein sizes, with initial tract dilation to 5 to 8 mm. Portosystemic gradients over 12 mm Hg determined whether further dilation was required. Technical success rates were 92 to 100%, with one failure in a patient with chronic portal vein thrombosis. Three of 23 patients developed shunt dysfunction requiring angioplasty and/or additional stent placement. In another case report, a VIATORR stent was successfully placed in a 7-month-old, 6.4-kg child despite the patient's small size. The patient died of

progression of intestinal failure–associated liver disease 2 weeks after TIPS placement without further GI bleeding.[35]

Continued longitudinal growth of the child and organ growth of the liver can lead to shunt inadequacy. Regular sonographic surveillance of the TIPS is necessary, as shunt revision, including the addition of overlapping stents, is frequently required. Although placement of a VIATORR stent in a very small child may be feasible, clinicians should carefully consider the length of the uncovered segment remaining in the portal vein to ensure that this will not preclude future transplant, which is the ultimate treatment for all pediatric patients with complications of portal hypertension.

30.4.4 Partial Splenic Embolization

In children with EHPVO and portal hypertension, variceal hemorrhage is more difficult to treat when it occurs concomitantly with thrombocytopenia. The effect of TIPS placement on the spleen, including spleen-related effects on platelet function, is variable. Vo et al[33] reported an overall decrease in the mean splenic length after TIPS placement with a modest improvement in platelet count in a small series of eight patients. Di Giorgio et al[34] reported no significant change in spleen length or platelet count after TIPS placement.

Partial splenic embolization (PSE) should be considered as a means to both improve circulating platelet cell volume and, theoretically, decrease splanchnic venous flow (▶ Fig. 30.4).[36] Early reports of PSE included very high complication rates with occurrences of abscess formation, prolonged pain, and death. However, in a review of the available literature, Koconis et al[36] noted a change in the rate of reported complications over 30 years of experience with the procedure. Later reports showed

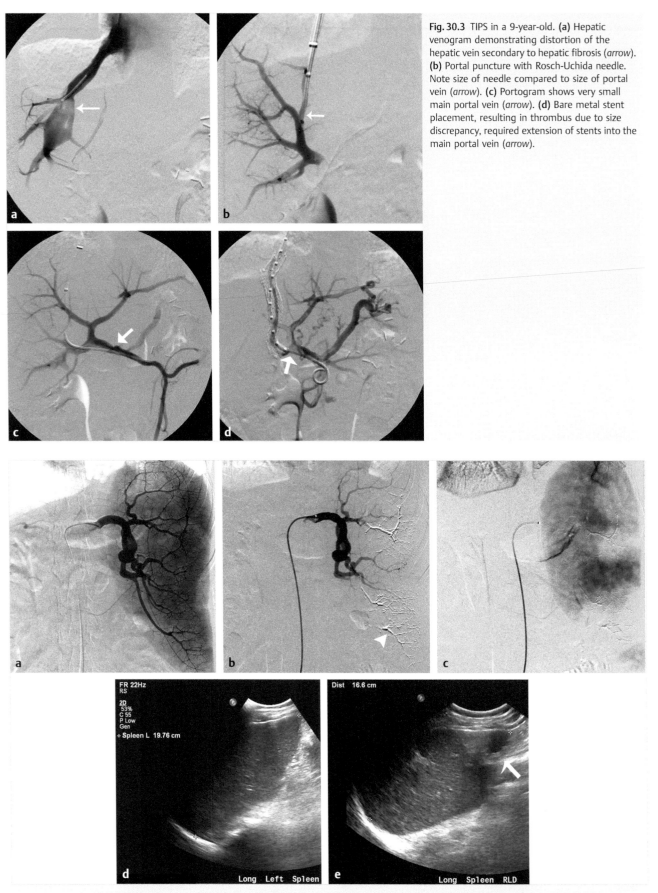

Fig. 30.3 TIPS in a 9-year-old. **(a)** Hepatic venogram demonstrating distortion of the hepatic vein secondary to hepatic fibrosis (*arrow*). **(b)** Portal puncture with Rosch-Uchida needle. Note size of needle compared to size of portal vein (*arrow*). **(c)** Portogram shows very small main portal vein (*arrow*). **(d)** Bare metal stent placement, resulting in thrombus due to size discrepancy, required extension of stents into the main portal vein (*arrow*).

Fig. 30.4 Partial splenic embolization in a 15-year-old with EHPVO, portal hypertension, and cirrhosis. **(a)** Preembolization arteriogram mapping with marked splenomegaly. **(b)** Arteriogram after selective embolization of middle and lower pole branches with *n*-butyl cyanoacrylate (*arrowhead*). **(c)** Delayed parenchymal phase showing devascularized portions of the spleen. **(d)** Pretreatment sonogram showing marked splenomegaly. Platelet count 43,000. **(e)** Postembolization follow-up sonogram showing substantial decrease in splenic size with atrophied lower pole (*arrow*). Platelet count peaked at 2 weeks at 341,000.

that the volume of the spleen infarcted was critical to success. Embolization of too much splenic parenchyma led to more complications; embolization of too little (less than 50%) yielded a high rate of recurrent hypersplenism.[37] The goal of 60 to 70% infarcted splenic volume has been associated with the highest improvement in hematologic parameters of leukocyte count, red blood cell count, and, most importantly, platelet count. Clinical durability of this procedure at 7 and 14 years has been documented in patients with cystic fibrosis–related liver disease and hypersplenism,[38,39] and long-term efficacy at 5 years has been reported in 70% of children, including patients with cirrhosis from biliary atresia, EHPVO, and idiopathic causes.[40]

There is no overall consensus regarding the best agent for embolization. Very small particles are not necessary, as penetration of the embolic agent to the splenic capsule is not required for infarction to occur and may in fact contribute to increased pain. Still, particles no larger than 600 to 800 µm are recommended.[41] Additionally, sparing of the upper pole of the spleen may reduce the amount of diaphragmatic inflammation and associated atelectasis.[41]

30.4.5 Balloon-Occluded Retrograde Transvenous Obliteration

There are few case reports describing the use of balloon-occluded retrograde transvenous obliteration (BRTO) in children for bleeding related to gastric varices, likely because of the prevalence of EHPVO. The use of BRTO in patients with EHPVO should be considered very carefully, as these engorged veins may be the primary drainage source of the splanchnic circulation, and disruption of these pathways may lead to mesenteric ischemia. With cavernous transformation, careful evaluation of the flow to the liver and assessment of the risks are needed before this intervention is performed.[30,42]

Sodium tetradecyl sulfate (STS) 3% is the most commonly used sclerosant in the United States because of its availability.[43] Adverse effects of STS 3% in doses exceeding 0.5 mL/kg have been reported in children who underwent treatment of vascular malformations. Complications included hemoglobinuria, oliguria,[44] and renal failure.[45] Mason et al[46] also documented alterations in coagulation factors, with decreased fibrinogen and platelets, when larger volumes were used.

30.5 Liver Transplant Interventions

There is a higher reported rate of posttransplant complications in the pediatric population. Causes of complications are widely varied but are believed to center around technical difficulties due to donor–recipient size differences, smaller caliber recipient vessels, and a small operative field.[47,48,49,50,51] Patient and organ growth is also cited as factor complicating pediatric liver transplants.[48,49] For both the early detection and management of complications, detailed familiarity with the type of liver graft transplanted is needed. For radiologic detection of early complications, a Doppler US examination has become the primary tool to establish a baseline and screen for complications. US has been shown to detect arterial complications before any

elevation in liver enzymes or bilirubin occurs.[52] Contrast-enhanced MR and MR cholangiopancreatography (MRCP) imaging can be used when US imaging is equivocal or technically inadequate.[53]

30.5.1 Hepatic Arterial Complications

Historically, the most common posttransplant complication affecting pediatric liver transplants was hepatic artery thrombosis (HAT), occurring in up to 40% of cases. With the use of newer microsurgical techniques and more routine use of antiplatelet agents, the incidence of HAT has fallen to less than 5%.[47,53,54,55] Early HAT is defined as HAT occurring within the first month after transplant, with peak incidence in the first 2 weeks.[56] Doppler US findings of HAT can be subtle. Arterial collateral formation is robust in children. Detection of collateral flow within the liver parenchyma can be falsely reassuring; in such cases, confirmatory imaging with CT angiography (CTA) or angiography is useful (▶ Fig. 30.5a,b). Unfortunately, collateral flow is insufficient to prevent biliary necrosis and graft failure in many cases.[53,54] If HAT is detected early, revascularization can improve 20-year graft survival from 24 to 77%.[57] The immediate choice of surgical or interventional treatment with thrombolysis varies among institutions. Early thrombolysis has been successfully performed in infants as young as 6 months and as early as 4 days after transplant and may be used in conjunction with angioplasty and possibly stenting.[52,58] Dosing of thrombolytics is not well documented, and there are no formal studies assessing the use of tissue plasminogen activator in pediatric patients. A median dose of 0.3 mg/kg/h for arterial thrombolysis has been reported in the literature; however, major bleeding occurred in 11% of patients and minor bleeding occurred in 43% of patients.[59] Lower dose protocols of 0.03 to 0.1 mg/kg/h have been shown to be effective in venous thrombolysis in children.[59]

Hepatic artery stenosis at the surgical anastomosis plagues the pediatric population and has become more common than HAT. Doppler US detection of this complication is challenging in a small child, but low resistive indices (<0.5), delayed acceleration times (>80 ms), and tardus parvus waveforms within the intrahepatic arteries (▶ Fig. 30.5c–f) should prompt close monitoring or further workup.[53,60] Increased systolic velocities at the anastomotic site within the first 72 hours can be normal, and serial monitoring with Doppler US can help differentiate elevated velocities from postoperative edema.[60]

Treatment with angioplasty and reserved stent placement in pediatric patients is similar to treatment in the adult population, with refractory cases requiring surgical revision.[47,60] Preprocedural initiation of aspirin therapy is recommended. The greatest difference between the adult and pediatric populations is the small size of the pediatric artery. Short length (1–1.5 cm) coronary angioplasty balloons with diameters ranging from 2 to 5 mm are usually required in pediatric patients. Arterial spasm is very common and should be pretreated with either nitroglycerine[61] or a calcium channel blocker, usually intra-arterial verapamil. The largest reported series of stent placements in pediatric patients included seven children aged 5 to 16 years treated with a combination of stent types, including two covered stents for angioplasty-induced rupture. Five patients survived, and stent patency was documented in four of these patients on follow-up at 9 to 40 months.

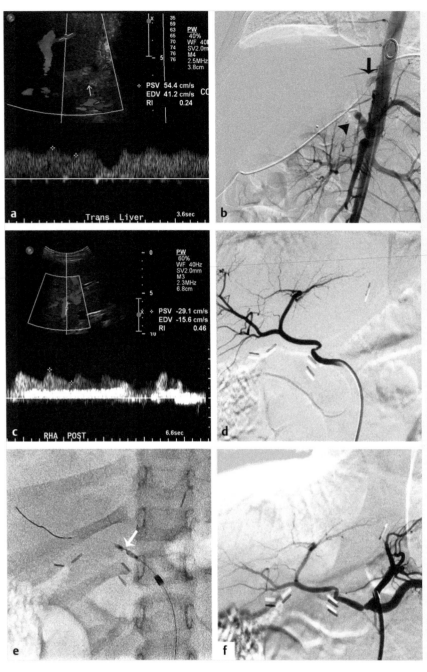

Fig. 30.5 Hepatic arterial thrombosis of liver transplant in a 2-year-old with thrombophilia. **(a)** Doppler ultrasound demonstrating collateral artery supply at the periphery of the left lobe of the liver with high diastolic flow and low resistive index. No arterial flow identified centrally, near the hilum of the liver. **(b)** Diagnostic arteriogram confirming complete occlusion of the main hepatic artery (*arrowhead*) and supraceliac conduit (*arrow*) in a 2-year-old with diagnosis of thrombophilia. **(c)** Doppler US with low resistive indices and tardus parvus waveform 18 months posttransplant in a 5-year-old. **(d)** Hepatic arteriogram demonstrating stenosis at anastomosis with pressure gradient of > 40 mm Hg. **(e)** Angioplasty with a 2.5-mm-diameter, 10-mm-long coronary balloon. Note very tight waist on balloon (*arrow*). **(f)** Postangioplasty arteriogram with no residual stenosis.

30.5.2 Portal Venous Complications

Portal vein stenosis occurs in up to 8% and thrombosis in 5.5% of pediatric patients undergoing liver transplant.[48,53,60] Complications are more common with reduced-size grafts.[53] Doppler US in these patients may show hypoechoic thrombus or slow flow (< 30 cm/s) with low resistive indices (< 0.65).[60,62] A continuous downward trend of these measurements from postoperative baseline scans should also raise the question of stenosis. Portal vein stenosis appears as elevated velocities, with a poststenotic to prestenotic segment ratio of greater than 3.[53,62,63] Clinically, patients may be asymptomatic or may exhibit decreased platelet count or splenomegaly.[64] Treatment of portal vein thrombosis and stenosis can be performed from a transhepatic or transsplenic approach.[48,62] A transjugular approach may

be suitable if coagulopathy or ascites is present. Thrombolysis has also been used for acute thrombosis. Treatment of portal vein stenosis usually involves angioplasty and, rarely, stenting. Refractory lesions require surgery.[51,62,63,65]

30.5.3 Biliary Complications

Biliary complications are the most common reason for intervention after transplant, with an incidence ranging from 10 to 45%.[66,67] Postoperative bile leaks or bilomas are easily detected with US and can be treated by percutaneous biloma drainage and biliary drainage and diversion.[68] Biliary strictures can be subtle or even occult on US, resulting in delay of diagnosis and increased morbidity.[53,69,70] MRCP can be performed as second-line imaging when a stricture is suspected, although often no

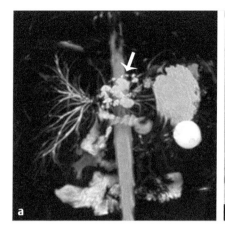 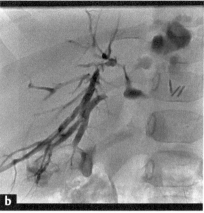

Fig. 30.6 Biliary ischemia secondary to hepatic artery thrombosis in a 1-year-old liver transplant recipient. **(a)** MRCP showing classic beaded appearance of left hepatic lobe biliary radicles (*arrow*) from alternating stenotic and dilated segments characteristic of biliary necrosis from loss of crucial hepatic arterial supply. **(b)** PTC showing the same beaded appearance of the left lobe biliary ducts with multifocal strictures of the right bile ducts and central hilar stricture.

biliary dilation is evident despite the presence of a high-grade stenosis (▶ Fig. 30.6). Percutaneous cholangiography (PTC) and drain placement are performed when biliary stenosis is clinically suspected despite nonconfirmatory imaging.[53,70,71] MRCP provides a useful map of the often altered posttransplant biliary anatomy before intervention.[66,70] PTC is challenging in children with nondilated ducts (often measuring less than 2 mm in size); US guidance is a necessity. Once the stricture is crossed, cholangioplasty can be performed with balloons ranging from 4 to 7 mm in diameter. Biliary drainage catheters are often too long for these patients. Instead, standard pigtail drainage catheters measuring 6 to 12 Fr with intraprocedural modifications of added side holes are needed. Ensuring the side holes are within the ductal system is imperative to prevent bile leak or bleeding. Some advocate repeating balloon dilation every 4 weeks with progressively increasing balloon sizes; an average number of four sessions is usually required in these cases.[58] Cholangiogram with complete passage of contrast from the biliary tree within 3 minutes is indicative of relief of the stenosis.

30.5.4 Hepatic Venous Complications

Hepatic venous outflow-related complications are more common in children, as these complications are more likely to occur in patients with split and reduced grafts.[49,72] The overall incidence remains low, with rates of up to 6% reported. Most narrowings affecting the hepatic outflow are thought to be due to twisting or torque of the veins as the patient grows.[48,49,50,72] Stenoses due to this twisting at the anastomosis have become less common because of improvements in surgical techniques specifically designed to lessen organ movement and prevent torsion.[49,50] US, contrast-enhanced CT, and/or MR venogram should be used to investigate other potential causes of vessel narrowing such as mass effect from adjacent fluid collections, lymphadenopathy, or recurrent tumor before intervention is attempted (▶ Fig. 30.7). Balloon venoplasty remains the gold standard for treating stenotic and thrombotic causes of venous outflow issues. Repeat venoplasty may be required, with a 50% reintervention rate reported in a small study by Cheng et al.[73] In this study, stents were used for restenosis. Pulmonary edema occurred in three patients who received stents; this was thought to be related to acute elevation of central venous pressure. Stent placement in the pediatric patient is associated with an increased risk of stent migration if the child outgrows the

stent.[48,49] Some advocate using self-expandable stents and upsizing the stent as much as possible to prevent growth-related migration.[48,49]

30.6 Vascular Lesions of the Liver

Hepatic vascular lesions can be divided into two categories based on pathology: congenital malformations and vasoproliferative neoplasms.[74] Congenital nontumorous vascular malformations lack the cellular proliferating parenchymal component seen in neoplastic lesions. Shunting of blood can occur in both types of lesions and can be (1) arterial to systemic or portal or (2) portal to systemic. Shunting may lead to a wide variety of secondary issues including the development of focal nodular hyperplasia, irreversible pulmonary arterial hypertension, and even metastatic hepatocellular carcinoma (HCC) and congestive heart failure (CHF) in the most severe cases.[75,76,77] Early recognition and treatment are key to preventing irreversible complications. Flow pattern on Doppler US, including evaluation of the direction of flow in the hepatic arteries, main portal vein, and hepatic veins, can be used to further characterize the lesion. An absence of intrahepatic portal vein flow may also be seen.[78] Imaging with dynamic contrast-enhanced MR/MR angiography imaging is complementary and can lead to a specific diagnosis in most cases.

30.6.1 Congenital Hepatic Low-Flow Vascular Lesions

Venous Malformations

Low-flow vascular malformations of the liver are nonproliferative, nonneoplastic lesions that grow proportionally with the child. The term "cavernous hemangioma" is a misnomer for what is truly a low-flow venous malformation. Most lesions can be easily diagnosed on MR imaging by their characteristic dynamic contrast-enhancement pattern: discontinuous, nodular peripheral enhancement with gradual centripetal filling. Although these lesions do not spontaneously involute, they rarely require treatment. Treatments are usually for symptoms related to mass effect. If the lesion is relatively small, direct puncture sclerotherapy is an option for treatment. For large lesions, there are rare reports of the effective use of transarterial embolization for treatment.[79]

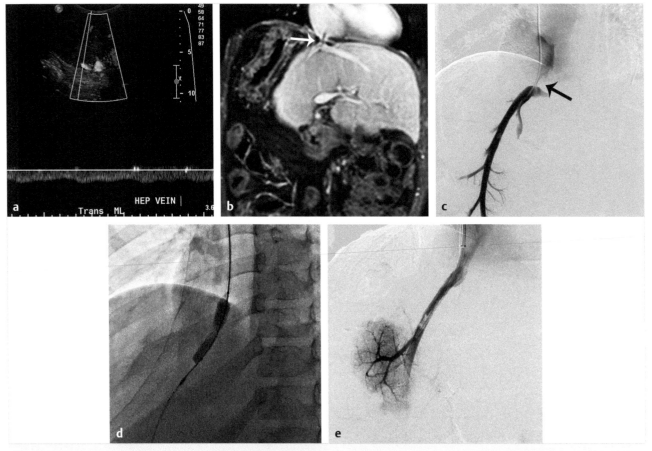

Fig. 30.7 (a) Posttransplant hepatic venous Doppler showing monophasic wave form characteristic of hepatic vein stenosis. Normal hepatic venous waveforms should be either tri- or biphasic. (b) Coronal MRV showing hepatic vein stenosis with turbulent flow jet (*arrow*). (c) Transjugular hepatic venogram demonstrating high-grade stenosis in the main hepatic vein (*arrow*). (d) Percutaneous venoplasty balloon dilatation across the stenosis. (e) Postvenoplasty confirmation of reestablishment of flow.

Congenital Portosystemic Shunts

Diagnosis of congenital portosystemic shunts (PSS) can be somewhat complicated, as these shunts can present at any age depending on the type and severity.[75,76,77] Symptomatic patients demonstrate cholestasis, hyperammonemia, or hypergalactosemia and present with jaundice, encephalopathy, hepatopulmonary syndrome, pulmonary hypertension, or liver tumors. Many classification schemes for congenital PSS have been proposed based on anatomy[80,81,82] or clinical severity.[75] For this discussion, we separate the lesions into two categories, intrahepatic and extrahepatic.

Intrahepatic Portosystemic Shunts

Although the location and number of intrahepatic PSS are highly variable among patients, the most common presentation is a single connection from the right portal vein to the inferior vena cava (IVC). Persistence of the ductus venosus, a vein connecting the left portal vein to the left hepatic vein near the IVC, can be considered a congenital intrahepatic PSS (▶ Fig. 30.8a–c). Complete closure of the ductus usually occurs in the first 17 days of life.[83] Some delay in closure may be seen with congenital heart disease. Spontaneous closure of intrahepatic shunts may occur within the first 2 years of life; thus, early treatment

is not necessary unless there are significant symptoms. Concomitant hypoplasia of the intrahepatic portal veins is not uncommon and is likely the consequence of diverted flow. Shunt closure is usually successful at "growing" these intrahepatic portal vein branches.

Extrahepatic Portosystemic Shunts

Extrahepatic PSS, or portacaval shunts, include the classic "Abernethy malformation," initially described in 1793 by Dr John Abernethy. This malformation features a portacaval shunt occurring at the level of the renal veins with azygous continuation of the IVC above the diaphragm.[80] Current terminology separates these malformations into two types. Type 1 consists of an end-to-side termination of the portal vein to the IVC with absent intrahepatic portal veins; type 2 is a side-to-side communication of the portal vein to the IVC with hypoplastic portal veins. Appropriate diagnosis often involves some combination of US, MR, and/or CTA. MR and CT are also very helpful in identifying hepatic lesions that may be associated with PSS such as hepatic adenomas and focal nodular hyperplasia (▶ Fig. 30.8d–i). Venography with temporary balloon occlusion of the shunt and intraprocedural portography with pressure measurements are the gold standard for determining the presence of intrahepatic portal vein branches and subsequent treatment options.[76,84] When severely atretic

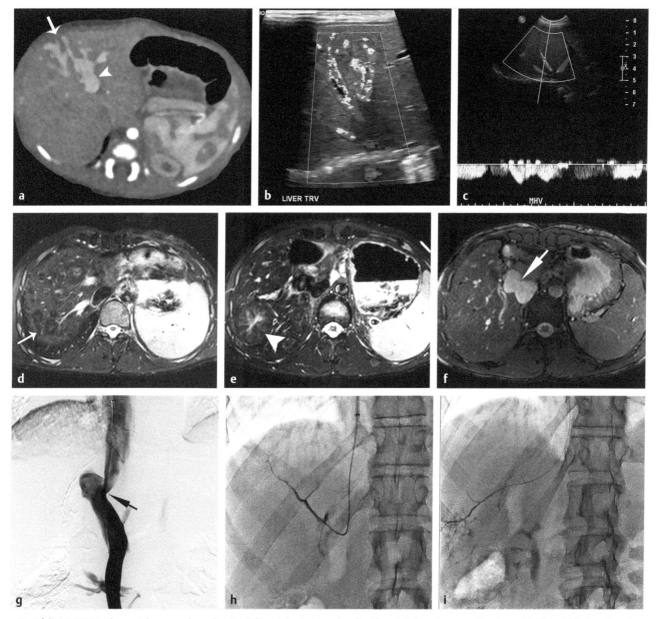

Fig. 30.8 (a) CECT in the portal venous phase showing left portal vein (*arrowhead*) with an intrahepatic connection (*arrow*) to the middle hepatic vein (*arrow*) in this intrahepatic type PSS in a 1-week-old with cholestasis and jaundice. (b) Color Doppler in the same patient showing the intrahepatic connection between the left portal vein (*red*) and the middle hepatic vein (*blue*) with aliasing from turbulent flow due to portal to systemic shunting. (c) Follow-up color Doppler 5 months later showing spontaneous resolution of the shunt connection and return of normal color flow patterns, without the need for percutaneous intervention. (d) Axial STIR MRI with multifocal hepatic lesions, likely regenerating nodules (*white arrow*) in a 19-year-old. (e) Axial STIR MRI with characteristic focal nodular hyperplasia in same patient (*arrowhead*). (f) Axial white blood sequence demonstrating large connection between main portal vein and IVC denoted by *arrow*. (g) Catheter enters from SVC to superior mesenteric vein. *Black arrow* at portacaval connection. (h,i) Selective catheter placement in atretic right portal vein branches.

portal branches are present, assessment of the portal system may require up to 15 minutes of shunt balloon occlusion to allow appreciation of small intrahepatic branches.[76,84,85]

Treatment of Congenital Portosystemic Shunts

Treatment methods for intrahepatic and extrahepatic PSS are based on two primary considerations: the presence and size of the intrahepatic portal veins and the pressure in the portal veins with balloon occlusion. Although these lesions are rare,

there are increasing reports of percutaneous closure, either as a primary one-step treatment or in a staged approach with gradual reduction of the shunt. Staging may be performed with surgical ligature placement or via interventional means with reducing stents or shunt occlusion plus simultaneous TIPS placement.[86] In the largest series to date among children with PSS, 10 of 22 patients underwent surgical closure; half performed as staged procedures after one patient treated with direct surgical shunt ligation developed portal vein thrombosis acutely.[77] This patient had portal pressures of 35 mm Hg on

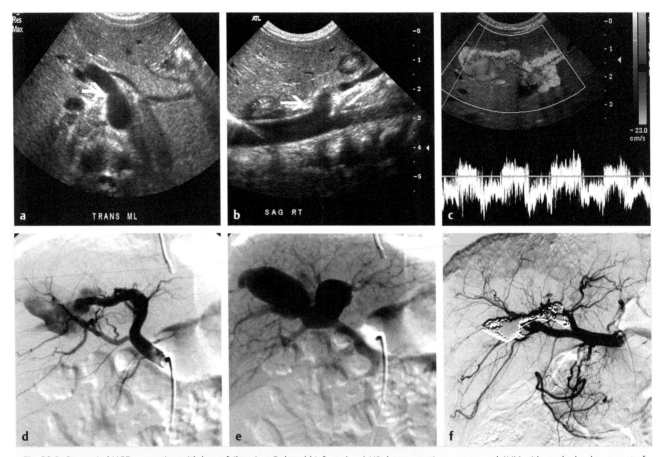

Fig. 30.9 Congenital IAPF presenting with heart failure in a 5-day-old infant. **(a–c)** US demonstrating a presumed AVM with marked enlargement of celiac trunk (*arrow*), equal in size as aorta on axial image and tapering of aorta beyond celiac on sagittal view. Color Doppler with hypervascular mass and significant spectral broadening. **(d,e)** Arteriogram demonstrating arterial to portal fistula with venous phase filling of the portal vein. **(f)** Five years postembolization. IAPF no longer fills, however, clinical evidence of portal hypertension with splenomegaly and varices. Selective hepatic artery injections (not shown) demonstrate areas of peripheral hepatofugal flow into small portal vein branches thought to be the cause of portal hypertension.

preoperative balloon occlusion portography and therefore staged procedures were recommended on patients with portal vein pressure above 32 mm Hg and absent or severely hypoplastic portal veins. Hepatic regenerative nodules and adenomas were shown to regress after closure, but there was persistence of pulmonary hypertension in many of the patients. Liver transplant may be used for patients with truly absent portal veins, especially if there are complications related to PSS closure.[76,84]

30.6.2 Congenital High-Flow Fistulas and Malformations

Congenital Intrahepatic Arterioportal Fistula

Congenital intrahepatic arterioportal fistulas (IAPF), a cause of portal hypertension, can be classified as simple or complex. In simple IAPF, there is a single communication between the hepatic arterial and portal venous systems. Complex lesions involve more than one artery or portal vein branch and have the appearance of an arteriovenous malformation (AVM).[23] GI bleeding, often related to portal hypertension and varices, is the most common presentation, seen in two-thirds of patients.

Other presenting manifestations include hypoglycemia, encephalopathy, failure to thrive, and chronic diarrhea.[87] High-output heart failure is uncommon except in the presence of a persistent ductus venosus (▶ Fig. 30.9a–c).

IAPF may benefit from coil or glue embolization, especially in patients with the simple type of fistula (▶ Fig. 30.9d,e). Embolization of complex lesions is more difficult and may cause ischemia if there are corresponding abnormalities or occlusions of portal venous branches. Cirrhosis may be a late development due to longstanding portal hypertension.[23] In published reports, persistent portal hypertension with hepatofugal portal flow after embolization occurred in less than 10% of patients (▶ Fig. 30.9f).[87]

Hepatic Arteriovenous Malformations

Hepatic AVMs usually present in the neonatal period with high-output heart failure, hepatomegaly, or anemia. Infantile hepatic AVMs are in some instances associated with hereditary hemorrhagic telangiectasia; this disorder should therefore be considered, especially in patients with a positive family history.[88] Treatment with coil or glue embolization may be appropriate for some patients with hepatic AVMs, although liver transplant may be required in patients with diffuse involvement.

30.6.3 Infantile Hepatic Hemangioma

IHH is the most common benign liver tumor that occurs during infancy. A variety of names have been used for IHH in the past (e.g., hepatic hemangioendothelioma, hepatic hemangioma, capillary hemangioma, and cavernous hemangioma). This has led to confusion with other hepatic lesions including borderline malignant epithelioid hemangioendothelioma and benign hepatic hemangiomas, both of which are distinct lesions that occur in adults.[89] Confusion persists today, as there are significant differences in the clinical presentation and outcomes of various IHHs.

At histology, IHHs are subcategorized based on endothelial staining for GLUT1, an erythrocyte-type glucose transporter protein.[90] GLUT1-positive lesions are referred to as hepatic infantile hemangioma (HIH). Imaging of HIHs demonstrates multiple small nodules without arteriovenous shunting or calcification (► Fig. 30.10a,b). GLUT1-positive lesions are typically asymptomatic and follow a benign course with eventual involution. GLUT1-negative lesions are generally referred to as hepatic vascular malformation with capillary proliferation (HVMCP), although this is not a universally accepted term. These lesions are generally symptomatic and do not undergo spontaneous involution. They are analogous to the rapidly involuting congenital hemangioma (RICH) lesion found elsewhere in infants. HVMCPs are more likely to fail to respond to corticosteroids or medical management without embolization or surgery. Clinical manifestations of HVMCP include abdominal distention and mass effect, cardiomegaly with or without CHF, Kasabach–Merritt syndrome (thrombocytopenia and consumptive coagulopathy), and anemia. Imaging of HVMCP typically demonstrates a single large mass with central necrosis, calcification, and arterial enlargement (► Fig. 30.10c,d).

An additional diffuse lesion type has been described for which GLUT1 immunostaining characteristics are not yet established. In this third category, lesions tend to be larger and associated with more significant clinical abnormalities including mass effect, compartment syndrome, and severe hypothyroidism but without clear CHF (► Fig. 30.10e–g). The clinical course and potential for spontaneous regression of these lesions are not yet defined. However, these lesions are thought to demonstrate a poor response to medical therapy; in some cases, these patients may therefore benefit from early transplant.[89,91] Lesions with significant high flow often demonstrate enlarged hepatic arteries and veins, tapering of the abdominal aorta below the celiac axis, and areas of hepatic arteriovenous and arterioportal shunting. Typically, dynamic centripetal enhancement pattern on MR imaging is diagnostic[92]; biopsy is generally avoided because of the bleeding risk.

Medical management of these high-flow hepatic lesions in symptomatic infants includes treatment with propranolol plus corticosteroids and/or vincristine. It is important to address hypothyroidism as a component of medical management, as significant hypothyroidism can aggravate heart failure. Kassarijian et al[92] found that only the presence of CHF predicted the need for therapy and that the presence of a shunt predicted the inability of medical therapy to control symptoms. The presence of Kasabach–Merritt syndrome is an indicator for more aggressive treatment; usually with the addition of vincristine to the medical regimen.[93] It is important to note that the effects of medical treatment require time, often up to 6 weeks. In some cases, embolization can be used for temporary stabilization while awaiting the effects of medical treatment.

Overall survival is approximately 90% in all cases.[92] However, in patients with significant shunt lesions and CHF, mortality may be higher. In the series presented by Kassarjian et al,[92] of the 55 patients diagnosed with IHH, 28 presented with CHF (51%) and 13 (24%) underwent embolization. The overall mortality rate was 11%, including one patient who underwent embolization. The technical aspects of embolization are based on the degree of arteriovenous shunting in individual patients, with microcoils and particulate agents commonly used.

30.6.4 Acquired Tumors of the Liver

Hepatoblastoma

Hepatoblastoma is the most common malignant hepatic tumor in children and usually occurs in late infancy, with most lesions discovered by the time the patient is aged 18 months. This tumor rarely occurs in newborns, which helps distinguish it from IHH. Elevated alpha fetoprotein (AFP) levels are present in more than 90% of patients with hepatoblastoma. In contrast, elevated AFP levels are uncommon in IHH and, when present, the elevation is mild.[89] Surgical resection is the primary treatment for hepatoblastoma, and neoadjuvant chemotherapy is often used to increase the resectability of lesions. Transplant is used in patients with unresectable lesions. Transarterial chemoembolization (TACE) has been described as a preoperative technique to allow resection; however, because of the infrequent use of TACE in patients with hepatoblastoma, most reports are grouped with those of TACE for the treatment of pediatric HCC.

Hepatocellular Carcinoma

HCC is rare in children, with a median age at diagnosis of 12 years. Most HCCs in children arise de novo. However, liver diseases including chronic viral hepatitis and inherited metabolic diseases are risk factors.[94] In children, metastases are frequently present at the time of diagnosis and commonly involve regional lymph nodes (38%) and distant metastasis to the lungs and bones (33%) (► Fig. 30.11). With metastatic disease, the overall 5-year survival is reduced to < 30%.[95] The fibrolamellar variant of HCC demonstrates similar poor survival in patients treated with chemotherapy and surgery.[96] Surgery is the mainstay for the treatment of HCC, with the goal of complete excision. However, this is often not possible because of tumor size and metastatic disease. As in adults, juvenile HCC is well known to be chemoresistant. Although TACE has become well established for the treatment of HCC in adults, little is known about the efficacy of TACE in juvenile HCC because of the rarity of the lesion and the protocol-driven treatment algorithms prevalent in pediatric cancers.

Interventional Treatment Options

Chemoinfusion

Arcement et al[97] assessed the use of intra-arterial chemoinfusion, with or without concomitant embolization with Gelfoam, in 14 children with unresectable liver tumors (7 with hepatoblastoma

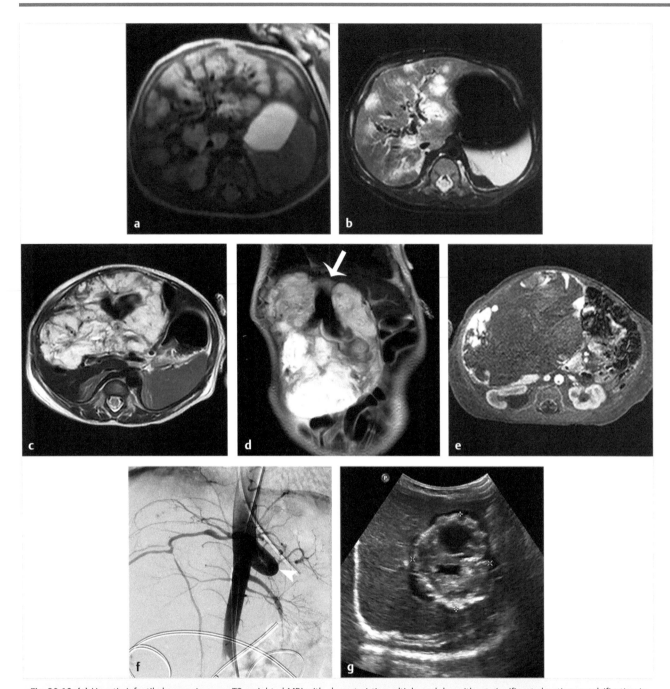

Fig. 30.10 (a) Hepatic infantile hemangioma on T2-weighted MRI with characteristic multiple nodules without significant shunting or calcification in asymptomatic infant. (b) Same infant at 6 months after treatment with propranolol. Note significant decrease in size of lesions. Enlarged arteries are present but without shunting. (c) T2-weighted MRI of newborn with large abdominal mass and high output heart failure. (d) Coronal postcontrast MRI with peripheral enhancement of mass and massive enlargement of middle hepatic vein (*arrow*) indicating shunting. (e) Axial postcontrast MRI of a newborn without CHF but significant Kasabach–Merritt and intracranial hemorrhage. Large liver mass that demonstrated classic peripheral enhancement. (f) Angiography and coil embolization performed to help improve platelet count. Note absence of significant shunting and enlarged celiac (*arrowhead*). (g) US performed 3 months after embolization and continued medical therapy demonstrate decreased size of mass and decreased vascularity (not shown).

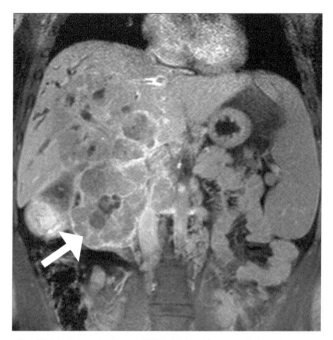

Fig. 30.11 Contrast-enhanced MRI with large hepatocellular carcinoma with extrahepatic nodal disease (*arrow*) and biliary obstruction at presentation.

and 7 with HCC). Intra-arterial cisplatin (dose, 90–150 mg/m^2) and Adriamycin (dose, 30 mg/m^2) were delivered by an infusion pump over 30 minutes. Embolization with Gelfoam pledgets was performed before infusion in tumors with rapid blood flow. The protocol was changed during the course of the study, and the final eight patients were treated with embolization before or after infusion with a goal of minimal residual blood flow in the targeted hepatic artery branch. In the first treatment group, including patients who did not consistently undergo embolization, none of the patients experienced a significant decrease in tumor size, and a decrease in AFP level was observed in only one patient. In the subgroup of eight patients who underwent Gelfoam embolization, AFP levels decreased; however, the tumors did not significantly decrease in size. By the end of the study, three of these eight patients had received transplants and remained alive, one was alive and awaiting transplant, and four had died.

Transarterial Chemoembolization

A small study assessed the toxicity of TACE in six children with unresectable or recurrent hepatoblastoma, three with HCC, and two with undifferentiated hepatic sarcoma (mean age, 4.2 years).[98] All but one patient with HCC had received prior systemic chemotherapy. A transient elevation in transaminase and bilirubin levels was seen in all patients. Fever occurred in 68% of patients, and 63% of patients experienced nausea and vomiting despite aggressive pretreatment with antiemetics. These symptoms resolved within 2 to 3 days. Transient coagulopathy occurred in 63% of patients, and pain occurred in 47%. One patient with a large HCC who received the entire treatment volume developed tumor lysis syndrome and disseminated intravascular coagulopathy immediately after the procedure and myelosuppression and mucositis as a later complication. This

patient received significantly higher systemic dosing of the chemotherapeutic agents than would have been prescribed if a size-based dosing regimen had been used. Severe myelosuppression resulting in sepsis and death was observed by Czauderna et al[99] in an infant with hepatoblastoma treated with TACE. Fatal and nonfatal lipiodol embolization to the lungs was reported in another series.[100]

Tumor response to TACE was variable in the study by Malogolowkin et al.[98] None of the patients with sarcoma responded, and all others exhibited only a partial response. Five of 11 patients underwent resection after TACE; however, only 3 patients survived with no evidence of disease.

Drug-Eluting Beads

There are currently no series reporting the use of drug-eluting beads in children. The clinical benefits of this technique and the importance of procedural standardization have been demonstrated in adults. Dosing has not been established in children, but weight-based dosing would likely be appropriate.

Radioembolization

Radioembolization in children with hepatoblastoma and HCC is under investigation. Hawkins et al[101] assessed the technical feasibility of radioembolization with ^{90}Y resin microspheres in two patients, ages 12 and 17 years, with unresectable HCC. Dosing was calculated using a body surface area formula, and the dose was then reduced by 25% because of the use of prior sorafenib therapy in both patients.[102,103] One patient had only mild procedural complications consisting of transient transaminitis and fatigue. However, the other patient developed intratumoral bleeding, severe pain, transient liver dysfunction, pancreatitis, and severe thrombocytopenia and required prolonged hospitalization. This patient died of cancer progression and progressive liver failure 4 months after radioembolization; the other patient had stable liver disease but experienced progression of extrahepatic disease.

Ablative Therapies

There are limited pediatric-specific case series on the use of ablative therapies such as radiofrequency ablation (RFA) and cryoablation for the treatment of recurrent or metastatic liver tumors.[104,105] Gómez et al[105] reviewed the existing literature on the subject of regional ablative therapies in children and found data on 28 patients, including 5 with hepatic lesions—2 primary hepatoblastomas, 2 metastases (Wilms' tumor and adrenocortical carcinoma), and 1 hepatic adenoma. Ablation was performed under US guidance with a mean lesion diameter of 19 mm. Technical and clinical success was achieved in all cases. Hoffer et al[106] published the only prospective evaluation of the toxicity of RFA in children. The authors reported on 16 patients who underwent a total of 37 RFA sessions. RFA was used in this series primarily to treat pulmonary metastatic disease; the series also included one patient with fibrolamellar HCC who had a total of seven hepatic lesions treated. The patient with HCC experienced a grade 4 toxicity (elevation of transaminases) and grade 2 toxicities (myoglobinuria and hemoglobinuria), although no additional treatment was required. Localized grounding pad site skin burns occurred in 3 of the 16 patients.

Additional skin burns occurred in the extremities of several patients. These burn complications highlight the importance of careful monitoring and attention to technique in pediatric patients, in whom thinner skin may increase the risk of burns.

Combination Therapies

Combination therapy with TACE plus regional ablation is being used with increasing frequency in adults but has been reported only rarely in the pediatric population. One early study involved 12 children with unresectable hepatoblastoma treated with TACE and high-intensity focused US (HIFU). TACE was performed with a suspension of carboplatin (dose, 100 mg/m^2) or Adriamycin (dose, 10–15 mg/m^2) and 3 to 8 mL of lipiodol. Approximately 2 to 3 weeks after TACE, HIFU was performed with real-time sonographic guidance. Survival rates at 1 and 2 years were 91.7 and 83.3%, respectively. Transient, mild postprocedural transaminitis occurred and rib malformations were noted in two patients after HIFU.[107]

30.7 Enteric Access in Children

In pediatric patients, preprocedural planning for gastrostomy or gastrojejunostomy tube placement includes an upper GI examination, including an esophagram. This examination is needed to define the anatomy, assess the size of the esophagus, and exclude malrotation.[2] Given the limited window to access the stomach in smaller pediatric patients, great care must be taken in delineating the structures outlining this window. Sonography is used to delineate the margins of the liver, spleen, and rectus muscle. Gastrostomy positioning lateral to the rectus muscle is preferred; midline placement is another option. The last resort is puncture through the rectus muscles, as this increases the risk of injury to the superior epigastric artery and subsequent bleeding. Water-soluble contrast is placed per the rectum to demarcate the colon, especially the transverse colon. This is particularly useful in infants, as large and small bowel loops are difficult to distinguish in these patients. If gaseous distention of the colon precludes a safe window, a 27-gauge needle may be used to decompress the colon.[108] Additionally, sonography may be used again to delineate the liver after gaseous distention of the stomach, as the stomach may push the liver margin superiorly. If the patient has had repair of the abdominal wall such as closure of an omphalocele defect, any graft, mesh, or other surgical material used for closure should be avoided. The needle puncture for the gastrostomy should not be too close to the pylorus, and attention should be paid to ensure that the retention mechanism, whether a disc or balloon, does not result in gastric outlet obstruction.

Both retrograde-type ("push") and anterograde-type ("pull") gastrostomy tubes have been placed in pediatric patients. Techniques for retrograde and anterograde placement of gastrostomy tubes in children are similar to those used for adults. A 16-Fr tube is safe to place with the pull technique in small children and infants and is sufficient in size to allow a coaxial jejunal feeding tube if needed.[2] The anterograde approach is not a viable option for patients with significant esophageal abnormalities such as narrowing or severe mucositis or significant facial deformities, as these would preclude dragging the anterograde tube through the mouth and into the stomach.

However, this approach is preferred when possible as it does not require serial dilation and decreases the risk of leakage of gastric contents into the peritoneum.[2]

There is a lack of data comparing interventional radiology gastrostomy (IRG), percutaneous endoscopic gastrostomy (PEG), and surgical gastrostomy in children.[109] A retrospective review comparing IRG to surgical PEG placement demonstrated similar major complication rates (1% for PEG, 3% for IRG).[110] Major complications included gastrocolic fistula, which occurred in 2 of 195 patients who underwent IRG, highlighting the importance of demarcating the colonic anatomy. Another study that included children as young as 12 years of age found that IRG had a higher success rate than PEG and lower morbidity than PEG or surgically placed gastrostomy.[111]

Gastrojejunostomy tubes have been placed in lieu of the combination of gastrostomy plus fundoplication. Reports comparing these two techniques are inconclusive, as there remains a paucity of data in the pediatric population. Studies have suggested that there are fewer major complications with percutaneous gastrojejunostomy tube placement but more minor complications.[112] A disadvantage of gastrojejunostomy tube feeding through the jejunal limb is that feeding is usually continuous, whereas feeds through a gastrostomy are often much shorter bolus feeds.

30.8 Conclusion

The application of interventional techniques to GI disease in the pediatric population is still in its infancy. As techniques such as locoregional therapy in liver cancers and vascular stent placement for transplant hepatic artery stenosis are shown to improve outcomes in adults, they will be more readily accepted and modified for diseases in children. Uncommon conditions and a small number of patients make establishing treatment algorithms for many GI diseases in pediatric patients very difficult without collaboration among centers. Longevity is expected for children, even in the face of multiple chronic illnesses, so careful consideration of every procedural detail is important to reduce radiation exposure and prevent harm.

References

[1] Image Gently. Step Lightly Checklist. Available online at: www.imagegently. org/Portals/6/Procedures/ImGen_StpLight_Chcklst.pdf. Accessed June 1, 2016

[2] Aria D, Vatsky S, Towbin R, Schaefer CM, Kaye R. Interventional radiology in the neonate and young infant. Semin Ultrasound CT MR. 2014; 35(6):588–607

[3] Senthilnathan S, Gauvreau K, Marshall AC, Lock JE, Bergersen L. Contrast administration in pediatric cardiac catheterization: dose and adverse events. Catheter Cardiovasc Interv. 2009; 73(6):814–820

[4] Dennhardt N, Schoof S, Osthaus WA, Witt L, Bertram H, Sümpelmann R. Alterations of acid-base balance, electrolyte concentrations, and osmolality caused by nonionic hyperosmolar contrast medium during pediatric cardiac catheterization. Paediatr Anaesth. 2011; 21(11):1119–1123

[5] Heran MK, Marshalleck F, Temple M, et al. Society of Interventional Radiology Standards of Practice Committee and Society of Pediatric Radiology Interventional Radiology Committee. Joint quality improvement guidelines for pediatric arterial access and arteriography: from the Societies of Interventional Radiology and Pediatric Radiology. J Vasc Interv Radiol. 2010; 21(1):32–43

[6] Tuong B, Shnitzer Z, Pehora C, et al. The experience of conducting Mortality and Morbidity reviews in a pediatric interventional radiology service: a retrospective study. J Vasc Interv Radiol. 2009; 20(1):77–86

[7] Vitiello R, McCrindle BW, Nykanen D, Freedom RM, Benson LN. Complications associated with pediatric cardiac catheterization. J Am Coll Cardiol. 1998; 32(5):1433–1440

[8] Govender P, Jonas MM, Alomari AI, et al. Sonography-guided percutaneous liver biopsies in children. AJR Am J Roentgenol. 2013; 201(3):645–650

[9] Potter C, Hogan MJ, Henry-Kendjorsky K, Balint J, Barnard JA. Safety of pediatric percutaneous liver biopsy performed by interventional radiologists. J Pediatr Gastroenterol Nutr. 2011; 53(2):202–206

[10] Amaral JG, Schwartz J, Chait P, et al. Sonographically guided percutaneous liver biopsy in infants: a retrospective review. AJR Am J Roentgenol. 2006; 187(6):W644–9

[11] Nobili V, Comparcola D, Sartorelli MR, et al. Blind and ultrasound-guided percutaneous liver biopsy in children. Pediatr Radiol. 2003; 33(11):772–775

[12] Malloy PC, Grassi CJ, Kundu S, et al. Standards of Practice Committee with Cardiovascular and Interventional Radiological Society of Europe (CIRSE) Endorsement. Consensus guidelines for periprocedural management of coagulation status and hemostasis risk in percutaneous image-guided interventions. J Vasc Interv Radiol. 2009; 20(7) Suppl:S240–S249

[13] Matos H, Noruegas MJ, Gonçalves I, Sanches C. Effectiveness and safety of ultrasound-guided percutaneous liver biopsy in children. Pediatr Radiol. 2012; 42(11):1322–1325

[14] Pietrobattista A, Fruwirth R, Natali G, Monti L, Devito R, Nobili V. Is juvenile liver biopsy unsafe? Putting an end to a common misapprehension. Pediatr Radiol. 2009; 39(9):959–961

[15] Short SS, Papillon S, Hunter CJ, et al. Percutaneous liver biopsy: pathologic diagnosis and complications in children. J Pediatr Gastroenterol Nutr. 2013; 57(5):644–648

[16] Bergey EA, Sane SS, Kaye RD, Redd DC, Towbin RB. Pediatric transvenous liver biopsy. J Vasc Interv Radiol. 1998; 9(5):829–832

[17] Habdank K, Restrepo R, Ng V, et al. Combined sonographic and fluoroscopic guidance during transjugular hepatic biopsies performed in children: a retrospective study of 74 biopsies. AJR Am J Roentgenol. 2003; 180(5):1393–1398

[18] Kaye R, Sane SS, Towbin RB. Pediatric intervention: an update–part II. J Vasc Interv Radiol. 2000; 11(7):807–822

[19] Cardella JF, Bakal CW, Bertino RE, et al. Society of Interventional Radiology Standards of Practice Committee. Quality improvement guidelines for image-guided percutaneous biopsy in adults. J Vasc Interv Radiol. 2003; 14(9)(,)(Pt 2):S227–S230

[20] Scheimann AO, Barrios JM, Al-Tawil YS, Gray KM, Gilger MA. Percutaneous liver biopsy in children: impact of ultrasonography and spring-loaded biopsy needles. J Pediatr Gastroenterol Nutr. 2000; 31(5):536–539

[21] Sarin SK, Sollano JD, Chawla YK, et al. Members of the APASL Working Party on Portal Hypertension. Consensus on extra-hepatic portal vein obstruction. Liver Int. 2006; 26(5):512–519

[22] Kleinman R, Goulet OJ, Mieli-Vergani G, et al. Walker's Pediatric Gastrointestinal Disease. 5th ed. Hamilton, Ontario: BC Decker Inc; 2008

[23] de Ville de Goyet J, D'Ambrosio G, Grimaldi C. Surgical management of portal hypertension in children. Semin Pediatr Surg. 2012; 21(3):219–232

[24] Chaves IJ, Rigsby CK, Schoeneman SE, Kim ST, Superina RA, Ben-Ami T. Pre- and postoperative imaging and interventions for the meso-Rex bypass in children and young adults. Pediatr Radiol. 2012; 42(2):220–232, quiz 271–272

[25] Lawson AJ, Rischbieter P, Numanoglu A, Wieselthaler N, Beningfield SJ. Imaging the Rex vein preoperatively using wedged hepatic venous portography. Pediatr Radiol. 2011; 41(10):1246–1249

[26] Cárdenas AM, Epelman M, Darge K, Rand EB, Anupindi SA. Pre- and postoperative imaging of the Rex shunt in children: what radiologists should know. AJR Am J Roentgenol. 2012; 198(5):1032–1037

[27] Lautz TB, Kim ST, Donaldson JS, Superina RA. Outcomes of percutaneous interventions for managing stenosis after meso-Rex bypass for extrahepatic portal vein obstruction. J Vasc Interv Radiol. 2012; 23(3):377–383

[28] Cwikiel W, Solvig J, Schroder H. Stent recanalization of chronic portal vein occlusion in a child. Cardiovasc Intervent Radiol. 2000; 23(4):309–311

[29] Cwikiel W, Keussen I, Larsson L, Solvig J, Kullendorff CM. Interventional treatment of children with portal hypertension secondary to portal vein occlusion. Eur J Pediatr Surg. 2003; 13(5):312–318

[30] Saad WE, Anderson CL, Patel RS, et al. Management of gastric varices in the pediatric population with balloon-occluded retrograde transvenous obliteration (BRTO) utilizing sodium tetradecyl sulfate foam sclerosis with or without partial splenic artery embolization. Cardiovasc Intervent Radiol. 2015; 38(1):236–241

[31] Heyman MB, LaBerge JM, Somberg KA, et al. Transjugular intrahepatic portosystemic shunts (TIPS) in children. J Pediatr. 1997; 131(6):914–919

[32] Huppert PE, Goffette P, Astfalk W, et al. Transjugular intrahepatic portosystemic shunts in children with biliary atresia. Cardiovasc Intervent Radiol. 2002; 25(6):484–493

[33] Vo NJ, Shivaram G, Andrews RT, Vaidya S, Healey PJ, Horslen SP. Midterm follow-up of transjugular intrahepatic portosystemic shunts using polytetrafluoroethylene endografts in children. J Vasc Interv Radiol. 2012; 23(7):919–924

[34] Di Giorgio A, Agazzi R, Alberti D, Colledan M, D'Antiga L. Feasibility and efficacy of transjugular intrahepatic portosystemic shunt (TIPS) in children. J Pediatr Gastroenterol Nutr. 2012; 54(5):594–600

[35] Wells LB, Mangat K, Gupte GL. Role of transjugular intrahepatic portosystemic shunt in children with advanced intestinal failure associated liver disease and portal hypertension. J Pediatr Gastroenterol Nutr. 2015; 60(4):e38–e39

[36] Koconis KG, Singh H, Soares G. Partial splenic embolization in the treatment of patients with portal hypertension: a review of the English language literature. J Vasc Interv Radiol. 2007; 18(4):463–481

[37] Sangro B, Bilbao I, Herrero I, et al. Partial splenic embolization for the treatment of hypersplenism in cirrhosis. Hepatology. 1993; 18(2):309–314

[38] Shah R, Mahour GH, Ford EG, Stanley P. Partial splenic embolization. An effective alternative to splenectomy for hypersplenism. Am Surg. 1990; 56(12):774–777

[39] Aslanidou E, Fotoulaki M, Tsitouridis I, Nousia-Arvanitakis S. Partial Splenic Embolization: successful treatment of hypersplenism, secondary to biliary cirrhosis and portal hypertension in cystic fibrosis. J Cyst Fibros. 2007; 6(3):212–214

[40] Nio M, Hayashi Y, Sano N, Ishii T, Sasaki H, Ohi R. Long-term efficacy of partial splenic embolization in children. J Pediatr Surg. 2003; 38(12):1760–1762

[41] Alwmark A, Bengmark S, Gullstrand P, Joelsson B, Lunderquist A, Owman T. Evaluation of splenic embolization in patients with portal hypertension and hypersplenism. Ann Surg. 1982; 196(5):518–524

[42] Al-Osaimi AM, Sabri SS, Caldwell SH. Balloon-occluded retrograde transvenous obliteration (BRTO): preprocedural evaluation and imaging. Semin Intervent Radiol. 2011; 28(3):288–295

[43] Saad WE. Balloon-occluded retrograde transvenous obliteration of gastric varices: concept, basic techniques, and outcomes. Semin Intervent Radiol. 2012; 29(2):118–128

[44] Barranco-Pons R, Burrows PE, Landrigan-Ossar M, Trenor CC, III, Alomari AI. Gross hemoglobinuria and oliguria are common transient complications of sclerotherapy for venous malformations: review of 475 procedures. AJR Am J Roentgenol. 2012; 199(3):691–694

[45] Kok K, McCafferty I, Monaghan A, Nishikawa H. Percutaneous sclerotherapy of vascular malformations in children using sodium tetradecyl sulphate: the Birmingham experience. J Plast Reconstr Aesthet Surg. 2012; 65(11):1451–1460

[46] Mason KP, Neufeld EJ, Karian VE, Zurakowski D, Koka BV, Burrows PE. Coagulation abnormalities in pediatric and adult patients after sclerotherapy or embolization of vascular anomalies. AJR Am J Roentgenol. 2001; 177(6):1359–1363

[47] Sanada Y, Wakiya T, Hishikawa S, et al. Risk factors and treatments for hepatic arterial complications in pediatric living donor liver transplantation. J Hepatobiliary Pancreat Sci. 2014; 21(7):463–472

[48] Uller W, Knoppke B, Schreyer AG, et al. Interventional radiological treatment of perihepatic vascular stenosis or occlusion in pediatric patients after liver transplantation. Cardiovasc Intervent Radiol. 2013; 36(6):1562–1571

[49] Sommovilla J, Doyle MM, Vachharajani N, et al. Hepatic venous outflow obstruction in pediatric liver transplantation: technical considerations in prevention, diagnosis, and management. Pediatr Transplant. 2014; 18(5):497–502

[50] Rodriguez-Davalos MI, Arvelakis A, Umman V, et al. Segmental grafts in adult and pediatric liver transplantation: improving outcomes by minimizing vascular complications. JAMA Surg. 2014; 149(1):63–70

[51] de Ville de Goyet J, Lo Zupone C, Grimaldi C, et al. Meso-Rex bypass as an alternative technique for portal vein reconstruction at or after liver transplantation in children: review and perspectives. Pediatr Transplant. 2013; 17(1):19–26

[52] Sevmis S, Karakayali H, Tutar NU, et al. Management of early hepatic arterial thrombosis after pediatric living-donor liver transplantation. Transplant Proc. 2011; 43(2):605–608

[53] Berrocal T, Parrón M, Alvarez-Luque A, Prieto C, Santamaría ML. Pediatric liver transplantation: a pictorial essay of early and late complications. Radiographics. 2006; 26(4):1187–1209

[54] Bekker J, Ploem S, de Jong KP. Early hepatic artery thrombosis after liver transplantation: a systematic review of the incidence, outcome and risk factors. Am J Transplant. 2009; 9(4):746–757

[55] Heffron TG, Welch D, Pillen T, et al. Low incidence of hepatic artery thrombosis after pediatric liver transplantation without the use of intraoperative microscope or parenteral anticoagulation. Pediatr Transplant. 2005; 9(4):486–490

[56] Kivelä JM, Kosola S, Kalajoki-Helmiö T, et al. Late hepatic artery thrombosis after pediatric liver transplantation: a cross-sectional study of 34 patients. Liver Transpl. 2014; 20(5):591–600

[57] Ackermann O, Branchereau S, Franchi-Abella S, et al. The long-term outcome of hepatic artery thrombosis after liver transplantation in children: role of urgent revascularization. Am J Transplant. 2012; 12(6):1496–1503

[58] Miraglia R, Maruzzelli L, Caruso S, et al. Minimally invasive endovascular and biliary treatments of children with acute hepatic artery thrombosis following liver transplantation. Pediatr Radiol. 2014; 44(1):94–102

[59] Manco-Johnson M, Grabowski EF, Hellgreen M, et al. Recommendations for tPA thrombolysis in children. On behalf of the Scientific Subcommittee on Perinatal and Pediatric Thrombosis of the Scientific and Standardization Committee of the ISTH. Thromb Haemost. 2002; 88(1):157–158 Accessed June 1, 2016

[60] Jamieson LH, Arys B, Low G, Bhargava R, Kumbla S, Jaremko JL. Doppler ultrasound velocities and resistive indexes immediately after pediatric liver transplantation: normal ranges and predictors of failure. AJR Am J Roentgenol. 2014; 203(1):W110–6

[61] Maruzzelli L, Miraglia R, Caruso S, et al. Percutaneous endovascular treatment of hepatic artery stenosis in adult and pediatric patients after liver transplantation. Cardiovasc Intervent Radiol. 2010; 33(6):1111–1119

[62] Cheng YF, Ou HY, Yu CY, et al. Section 8. Management of portal venous complications in pediatric living donor liver transplantation. Transplantation. 2014; 97 Suppl 8:S32–S34

[63] Cho YP, Kim KM, Ha TY, et al. Management of late-onset portal vein complications in pediatric living-donor liver transplantation. Pediatr Transplant. 2014; 18(1):64–71

[64] Karakayali H, Sevmis S, Boyvat F, et al. Diagnosis and treatment of late-onset portal vein stenosis after pediatric living-donor liver transplantation. Transplant Proc. 2011; 43(2):601–604

[65] de Ville de Goyet J, Gibbs P, Clapuyt P, Reding R, Sokal EM, Otte JB. Original extrahilar approach for hepatic portal revascularization and relief of extrahepatic portal hypertension related to later portal vein thrombosis after pediatric liver transplantation. Long term results. Transplantation. 1996; 62(1):71–75

[66] Feier FH, Chapchap P, Pugliese R, et al. Diagnosis and management of biliary complications in pediatric living donor liver transplant recipients. Liver Transpl. 2014; 20(8):882–892

[67] Laurence JM, Sapisochin G, DeAngelis M, et al. Biliary complications in pediatric liver transplantation: Incidence and management over a decade. Liver Transpl. 2015; 21(8):1082–1090

[68] Westra SJ, Zaninović AC, Hall TR, Busuttil RW, Kangarloo H, Boechat MI. Imaging in pediatric liver transplantation. Radiographics. 1993; 13(5):1081–1099

[69] Teplisky D, Urueña Tincani E, Halac E, et al. Ultrasonography, laboratory, and cholangiography correlation of biliary complications in pediatric liver transplantation. Pediatr Transplant. 2015; 19(2):170–174

[70] Atchie B, Kalva S, Josephs S. Pediatric biliary interventions. Tech Vasc Interv Radiol. 2015; 18(4):276–284

[71] Lorenz JM, Funaki B, Leef JA, Rosenblum JD, Van Ha T. Percutaneous transhepatic cholangiography and biliary drainage in pediatric liver transplant patients. AJR Am J Roentgenol. 2001; 176(3):761–765

[72] Lorenz JM, Van Ha T, Funaki B, et al. Percutaneous treatment of venous outflow obstruction in pediatric liver transplants. J Vasc Interv Radiol. 2006; 17(11)(,)(Pt 1):1753–1761

[73] Cheng YF, Chen CL, Huang TL, et al. Angioplasty treatment of hepatic vein stenosis in pediatric liver transplants: long-term results. Transpl Int. 2005; 18(5):556–561

[74] Lowe LH, Marchant TC, Rivard DC, Scherbel AJ. Vascular malformations: classification and terminology the radiologist needs to know. Semin Roentgenol. 2012; 47(2):106–117

[75] Witters P, Maleux G, George C, et al. Congenital veno-venous malformations of the liver: widely variable clinical presentations. J Gastroenterol Hepatol. 2008; 23(8)(,)(Pt 2):e390–e394

[76] Bernard O, Franchi-Abella S, Branchereau S, Pariente D, Gauthier F, Jacquemin E. Congenital portosystemic shunts in children: recognition, evaluation, and management. Semin Liver Dis. 2012; 32(4):273–287

[77] Franchi-Abella S, Branchereau S, Lambert V, et al. Complications of congenital portosystemic shunts in children: therapeutic options and outcomes. J Pediatr Gastroenterol Nutr. 2010; 51(3):322–330

[78] Gallego C, Miralles M, Marín C, Muyor P, González G, García-Hidalgo E. Congenital hepatic shunts. Radiographics. 2004; 24(3):755–772

[79] Firouznia K, Ghanaati H, Alavian SM, et al. Management of liver hemangioma using trans-catheter arterial embolization. Hepat Mon. 2014; 14(12):e25788

[80] Abernethy J. Account of two instances of uncommon formation in the viscera of the human body. Philos Trans R Soc. 1793; 83:59–66

[81] Morgan G, Superina R. Congenital absence of the portal vein: two cases and a proposed classification system for portasystemic vascular anomalies. J Pediatr Surg. 1994; 29(9):1239–1241

[82] Park JH, Cha SH, Han JK, Han MC. Intrahepatic portosystemic venous shunt. AJR Am J Roentgenol. 1990; 155(3):527–528

[83] Stringer MD. The clinical anatomy of congenital portosystemic venous shunts. Clin Anat. 2008; 21(2):147–157

[84] Kanazawa H, Nosaka S, Miyazaki O, et al. The classification based on intrahepatic portal system for congenital portosystemic shunts. J Pediatr Surg. 2015; 50(4):688–695

[85] Barsky MF, Rankin RN, Wall WJ, Ghent CN, Garcia B. Patent ductus venosus: problems in assessment and management. Can J Surg. 1989; 32(4):271–275

[86] Stewart JK, Kuo WT, Hovsepian DM, Hofmann LV, Bonham CA, Sze DY. Portal venous remodeling after endovascular reduction of pediatric autogenous portosystemic shunts. J Vasc Interv Radiol. 2011; 22(8):1199–1205

[87] Norton SP, Jacobson K, Moroz SP, et al. The congenital intrahepatic arterioportal fistula syndrome: elucidation and proposed classification. J Pediatr Gastroenterol Nutr. 2006; 43(2):248–255

[88] Al-Saleh S, John PR, Letarte M, Faughnan ME, Belik J, Ratjen F. Symptomatic liver involvement in neonatal hereditary hemorrhagic telangiectasia. Pediatrics. 2011; 127(6):e1615–e1620

[89] Chung EM, Cube R, Lewis RB, Conran RM. From the archives of the AFIP: Pediatric liver masses: radiologic-pathologic correlation part 1. Benign tumors. Radiographics. 2010; 30(3):801–826

[90] Mo JQ, Dimashkieh HH, Bove KE. GLUT1 endothelial reactivity distinguishes hepatic infantile hemangioma from congenital hepatic vascular malformation with associated capillary proliferation. Hum Pathol. 2004; 35 (2):200–209

[91] Christison-Lagay ER, Burrows PE, Alomari A, et al. Hepatic hemangiomas: subtype classification and development of a clinical practice algorithm and registry. J Pediatr Surg. 2007; 42(1):62–67, discussion 67–68

[92] Kassarjian A, Zurakowski D, Dubois J, Paltiel HJ, Fishman SJ, Burrows PE. Infantile hepatic hemangiomas: clinical and imaging findings and their correlation with therapy. AJR Am J Roentgenol. 2004; 182(3):785–795

[93] Moore J, Lee M, Garzon M, et al. Effective therapy of a vascular tumor of infancy with vincristine. J Pediatr Surg. 2001; 36(8):1273–1276

[94] Emre S, McKenna GJ. Liver tumors in children. Pediatr Transplant. 2004; 8 (6):632–638

[95] Lau CS, Mahendraraj K, Chamberlain RS. Hepatocellular carcinoma in the pediatric population: a population based clinical outcomes study involving 257 patients from the Surveillance, Epidemiology, and End Result (SEER) database (1973–2011). HPB Surg. 2015; 2015:670728

[96] Katzenstein HM, Krailo MD, Malogolowkin MH, et al. Fibrolamellar hepatocellular carcinoma in children and adolescents. Cancer. 2003; 97(8): 2006–2012

[97] Arcement CM, Towbin RB, Meza MP, et al. Intrahepatic chemoembolization in unresectable pediatric liver malignancies. Pediatr Radiol. 2000; 30(11): 779–785

[98] Malogolowkin MH, Stanley P, Steele DA, Ortega JA. Feasibility and toxicity of chemoembolization for children with liver tumors. J Clin Oncol. 2000; 18(6): 1279–1284

[99] Czauderna P, Zbrzezniak G, Narozanski W, Korzon M, Wyszomirska M, Stoba C. Preliminary experience with arterial chemoembolization for hepatoblastoma and hepatocellular carcinoma in children. Pediatr Blood Cancer. 2006; 46(7):825–828

[100] Yamaura K, Higashi M, Akiyoshi K, Itonaga Y, Inoue H, Takahashi S. Pulmonary lipiodol embolism during transcatheter arterial chemoembolization for hepatobla-stoma under general anaesthesia. Eur J Anaesthesiol. 2000; 17(11): 704–708

[101] Hawkins CM, Kukreja K, Geller JI, Schatzman C, Ristagno R. Radioembolisation for treatment of pediatric hepatocellular carcinoma. Pediatr Radiol. 2013; 43(7):876–881

[102] Ye J, Shu Q, Li M, Jiang TA. Percutaneous radiofrequency ablation for treatment of hepatoblastoma recurrence. Pediatr Radiol. 2008; 38(9):1021–1023

[103] Kennedy AS, McNeillie P, Dezarn WA, et al. Treatment parameters and outcome in 680 treatments of internal radiation with resin 90Y-microspheres for unresectable hepatic tumors. Int J Radiat Oncol Biol Phys. 2009; 74(5):1494–1500

[104] van Laarhoven S, van Baren R, Tamminga RY, de Jong KP. Radiofrequency ablation in the treatment of liver tumors in children. J Pediatr Surg. 2012; 47(3):e7–e12

[105] Gómez FM, Patel PA, Stuart S, Roebuck DJ. Systematic review of ablation techniques for the treatment of malignant or aggressive benign lesions in children. Pediatr Radiol. 2014; 44(10):1281–1289

[106] Hoffer FA, Daw NC, Xiong X, et al. A phase 1/pilot study of radiofrequency ablation for the treatment of recurrent pediatric solid tumors. Cancer. 2009; 115(6):1328–1337

[107] Wang S, Yang C, Zhang J, et al. First experience of high-intensity focused ultrasound combined with transcatheter arterial embolization as local control for hepatoblastoma. Hepatology. 2014; 59(1):170–177

[108] Wiebe S, Cohen J, Connolly B, Chait P. Percutaneous decompression of the bowel with a small-caliber needle: a method to facilitate percutaneous abdominal access. AJR Am J Roentgenol. 2005; 184(1):227–229

[109] Baker L, Beres AL, Baird R. A systematic review and meta-analysis of gastrostomy insertion techniques in children. J Pediatr Surg. 2015; 50(5): 718–725

[110] Nah SA, Narayanaswamy B, Eaton S, et al. Gastrostomy insertion in children: percutaneous endoscopic or percutaneous image-guided? J Pediatr Surg. 2010; 45(6):1153–1158

[111] Wollman B, D'Agostino HB, Walus-Wigle JR, Easter DW, Beale A. Radiologic, endoscopic, and surgical gastrostomy: an institutional evaluation and meta-analysis of the literature. Radiology. 1995; 197(3):699–704

[112] Livingston MH, Shawyer AC, Rosenbaum PL, Jones SA, Walton JM. Fundoplication and gastrostomy versus percutaneous gastrojejunostomy for gastroesophageal reflux in children with neurologic impairment: A systematic review and meta-analysis. J Pediatr Surg. 2015; 50(5):707–714

Index

Note: Page numbers set **bold** or *italic* indicate headings or figures, respectively.